OXFORD MEDICAL PUBLICATIONS

Oxford American Handbook of Nephrology and Hypertension

Published and forthcoming Oxford American Handbooks

Oxford American Handbook of Anesthesiology
Oxford American Handbook of Clinical Dentistry
Oxford American Handbook of Clinical Medicine
Oxford American Handbook of Surgery
Oxford American Handbook of Critical Care
Oxford American Handbook of Emergency Medicine
Oxford American Handbook of Nephrology and Hypertension
Oxford American Handbook of Obstetrics and Gynecology
Oxford American Handbook of Otolaryngology
Oxford American Handbook of Pediatrics
Oxford American Handbook of Psychiatry
Oxford American Handbook of Pulmonary Medicine

Oxford American Handbook of Nephrology and Hypertension

Paul J. Scheel, Jr., MD
Associate Professor and Director
Division of Nephrology
Johns Hopkins Hospital
Baltimore, Maryland

Michael J. Choi, MD
Associate Professor
Division of Nephrology
Johns Hopkins Hospital
Baltimore, Maryland

with

Simon Steddon
Neil Ashman
Alistair Chesser
John Cunningham

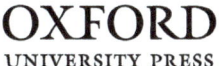

OXFORD
UNIVERSITY PRESS

Oxford University Press is a department of the University of Oxford.
It furthers the University's objective of excellence in research, scholarship,
and education by publishing worldwide.

Oxford New York
Auckland Cape Town Dar es Salaam Hong Kong Karachi
Kuala Lumpur Madrid Melbourne Mexico City Nairobi
New Delhi Shanghai Taipei Toronto

With offices in
Argentina Austria Brazil Chile Czech Republic France Greece
Guatemala Hungary Italy Japan Poland Portugal Singapore
South Korea Switzerland Thailand Turkey Ukraine Vietnam

Oxford is a registered trade mark of Oxford University Press
in the UK and certain other countries.

Published in the United States of America by
Oxford University Press
198 Madison Avenue, New York, NY 10016

© Oxford University Press 2008

First issued as an Oxford University Press paperback, 2014.

All rights reserved. No part of this publication may be reproduced, stored
in a retrieval system, or transmitted, in any form or by any means, without
the prior permission in writing of Oxford University Press, or as expressly
permitted by law, by license, or under terms agreed with the appropriate
reproduction rights organization. Inquiries concerning reproduction outside
the scope of the above should be sent to the Rights Department,
Oxford University Press, at the address above.

You must not circulate this work in any other form
and you must impose this same condition on any acquirer.

Library of Congress Cataloging-in-Publication Data
Scheel, Paul J.
Oxford American handbook of nephrology and hypertension/Paul J.
Scheel Jr., Michael J. Choi.
p. ; cm.—(Oxford American handbooks)
Adapted from: Oxford handbook of nephrology and hyper-tension/
edited by Simon Steddon . . . [et al.]. 2006.
Includes index.
ISBN 978-0-19-938464-8
1. Kidneys—Handbooks, manuals, etc. 2. Nephrology—Handbooks,
manuals, etc. 3. Hypertension—Handbooks, manuals, etc.
I. Choi, Michael J. II. Oxford handbook of nephrology and hypertension.
III. Title. IV. Title: Handbook of nephrology and hy-pertension.
V. Title: Nephrology and hypertension. VI. Series.
[DNLM: 1. Kidney Diseases—Handbooks. WJ 39 S314o 2008]
RC903.S33 2008
616.6'1—dc22   2007044661

Oxford University Press makes no representation, express or implied, that the drug dosages in this book are correct. Readers must therefore always check the product information and clinical procedures with the most up-to-date published product information and data sheets provided by the manufacturers and the most recent codes of conduct and safety regulations. The authors and the publishers do not accept responsibility or legal liability for any errors in the text or for the misuse or misapplication of material in this work.

Preface

Nephrology as a subspecialty of internal medicine has historically been a discipline that has challenged even the brightest of internal medicine residents. Routed deep in the science of physiology, nephrology has evolved and expanded over the past thirty years to include areas of dialysis, hypertension, transplantation, glomerulonephritis, nephrolithiasis, toxicology, and numerous metabolic syndromes. This evolution has made mastering such a complex and diverse group of diseases even more intimidating.

This handbook is designed to provide the basics of nephrology to every clinician, whether a student or a seasoned physician, with practical and easily accessible information that will enhance both learning and patient care.

In this edition, we have updated the sections on chronic kidney disease, glomerulonephritis, hypertension, and medical aspects of renal transplantation to reflect the latest in science and practice guidelines. We hope that the material contained in this handbook will enhance readers' learning, make them better clinicians, and stimulate them to explore the rapidly expanding discipline of nephrology.

Paul J. Scheel, Jr., M.D.
Michael J. Choi, M.D.

Contents

Preface *vi*
Detailed contents *ix*
Symbols and abbreviations *xxi*

1	Clinical assessment of the renal patient	1
2	Acute renal failure (Acute kidney injury)	69
3	Chronic kidney disease	151
4	Renal replacement therapy	207
5	Hypertension	287
6	Diseases of the kidney	359
7	The kidney in systemic disease	437
8	Urinary tract obstruction	495
9	Fluids and electrolytes	519
10	Pregnancy and the kidney	567
11	Drugs and the kidney	591
12	Appendices	611

Index *649*

Detailed contents

1 Clinical assessment of the renal patient 1
History *2*
Physical examination *8*
The urine *12*
Proteinuria *18*
Red blood cells *20*
Cells, organisms, and casts *22*
Crystals *24*
Determining renal function *26*
Creatinine *28*
Diagnostic imaging *36*
  Ultrasound (US) *38*
  Intravenous urography (IVU) *40*
  Computerized tomography (CT) *42*
  Nuclear medicine *43*
  Angiography and urology *45*
Clinical syndromes *48*
  Proteinuria *48*
  Hematuria *52*
  Chronic kidney disease *58*
  The uremic syndrome *59*
  Other clinical syndromes *60*
  Pulmonary renal syndromes *61*
  Changes in urine volume *63*
  Pain *64*
  Tubular syndromes *65*
  Bladder outflow obstruction *67*

2 Acute renal failure (Acute kidney injury) 69

Definition and epidemiology *70*

Causes and classification *74*

Prevention *76*

Clinical approach to ARF *78*

Acute renal failure or chronic kidney disease? *80*

Assessing ARF *82*

Rapidly progressive glomerulonephritis and myeloma screen *86*

Assessing ARF: imaging and histology *90*

Prerenal ARF *92*

Causes of prerenal ARF *94*

Volume replacement in prerenal ARF *96*

Intrinsic renal ARF *98*

Acute tubular necrosis (ATN) *100*

Pathophysiology of ischemic ATN *102*

Management of ARF 1: a checklist *104*

Management of ARF 2: hyperkalemia *106*

Management of ARF 3: reducing total body K^+ *110*

Management of ARF 4: pulmonary edema *112*

Management of ARF 5: electrolytes and acidosis *114*

Management of ARF 6: other strategies *116*

Management of ARF 7: nutrition *118*

Management myths *122*

Renal replacement therapy in ARF *126*

Prescribing acute hemodialysis *128*

Peritoneal dialysis in ARF *132*

The hepatorenal syndrome (HRS) *134*

Management of HRS *136*

Rhabdomyolysis *138*

Management of rhabdomyolysis *140*

Contrast-induced nephropathy (CIN) *142*
Tumor lysis syndrome (TLS) *144*
ARF in sepsis *146*
Managing septic shock and ARF *148*

3 Chronic kidney disease — 151

What is chronic kidney disease (CKD)? *152*
Pathogenesis of CKD *154*
Diagnosing CKD *156*
Progression of CKD *158*
Preventing progression: blood pressure *159*
Preventing progression: other measures *160*
Managing CKD *162*
Complications of advanced CKD *164*
Uremia *166*
Anemia of CKD *168*
Erythropoietin *170*
Prescribing erythropoietin *172*
Iron stores and iron therapy in CKD *174*
Renal bone disease 1 *176*
Renal bone disease 2: physiology *178*
Renal bone disease 3: clinical features *180*
Renal bone disease 4: treatment *182*
Hyperphosphatemia *184*
Vitamin D analogues *186*
Calcimimetics *188*
Parathyroidectomy *190*
Calciphylaxis *192*
Cardiovascular disease in CKD *194*
Pretransplant workup *196*
Diet and nutrition in CKD *198*

Malnutrition in CKD *200*
Endocrine problems in CKD *202*
Palliative treatment of advanced CKD *204*

---

4 Renal replacement therapy 207

A brief history of renal replacement therapy (RRT) *208*
Introduction *210*
Hemodialysis (HD) *212*
Dialysers and membranes *216*
HD prescription *218*
Variables in the dialysis prescription *220*
Vascular access *222*
Complications of vascular access *224*
Acute HD complications *226*
Peritoneal dialysis (PD) *228*
Types of PD *230*
PD fluids *232*
Prescribing PD *234*
Peritonitis *236*
Other complications *240*
PD adequacy *242*
Ultrafiltration failure *244*
The well PD patient *246*
Basic transplantation *248*
Compatibility *250*
Pretransplant assessment *252*
Living donor transplantation *254*
Pretransplant management *256*
The transplant operation *258*
Post-transplant management *260*

Principles of recipient management *262*
Immunosuppression *264*
Surgical complications *266*
Graft dysfunction *268*
Acute rejection *270*
Chronic allograft nephropathy (CAN) *272*
Post-transplant infections *274*
Cytomegalovirus (CMV) *276*
BK virus nephropathy *278*
Post-transplant malignancy *280*
Expanding the donor pool *282*
Kidney–pancreas transplantation *284*

5 Hypertension 287

Hypertension facts and figures *288*
What is hypertension? *290*
Pathogenesis *292*
BP measurement *298*
Clinical assessment *300*
Classification of hypertension *302*
Treatment thresholds *304*
Lifestyle measures *306*
Secondary hypertension *308*
Primary hyperaldosteronism *310*
Specific causes of hyperaldosteronism *312*
Other "hyperaldosteronism" syndromes *314*
Other causes of secondary hypertension *316*
Drug management of hypertension *318*
Drug treatment of hypertension *320*
Clinical trials in hypertension *324*
The ASCOT study *330*

Diuretics *332*
β-blockers *336*
α-blockers *338*
Calcium channel blockers (CCBs) *340*
ACE inhibitors (ACEIs) *342*
Angiotensin II receptor blockers (ARBs) *344*
Other antihypertensives *346*
Resistant hypertension *348*
Hypertensive urgencies and emergencies *350*
Assessing urgencies and emergencies *352*
Management of urgencies and emergencies *354*
Orthostatic hypotension *356*

6 Diseases of the kidney 359

Approaching glomerular disease *360*
Histology of glomerular disease *362*
Focal and diffuse glomerulonephritis *364*
Approaching focal and diffuse glomerulonephritis *366*
General principles of management of focal and diffuse glomerulonephritis *367*
Immunosuppressive management of glomerulonephritis *368*
IgA nephropathy *372*
Management of IgA nephropathy *374*
Postinfectious glomerulonephritis *376*
Membranoproliferative glomerulonephritis (MPGN) *378*
Hereditary nephropathies *380*
Other forms of glomerulonephritis *382*
The nephrotic syndrome *384*
Minimal change nephropathy *388*

Membranous nephropathy (MN) *390*
Focal and segmental glomerulosclerosis (FSGS) *394*
Treatment of FSGS *396*
Thrombotic microangiopathy (TMA) *398*
Thrombotic thrombocytopenic purpura (TTP) *400*
Hemolytic-uremic syndrome (HUS) *401*
Management of HUS, TTP, and TMA *402*
Tubulointerstitial diseases *404*
Chronic tubulointerstitial diseases *406*
Analgesic nephropathy *408*
Renovascular disease *410*
Management of ARAS *412*
Other renovascular diseases *414*
Adult polycystic kidney disease (APKD) *416*
Complications of APKD *418*
Other cystic kidney diseases *420*
Urinary tract infections (UTIs) *422*
Reflux nephropathy *428*
Nephrolithiasis *430*
Investigating recurrent stone-formers *432*
Acute renal colic *435*

7 The kidney in systemic disease 437

Diabetic nephropathy (DN) *438*
Management of diabetic nephropathy *442*
Management of ESRD in diabetes *444*
The kidney in multiple myeloma *446*
Managing myeloma kidney *448*
Renal amyloidosis *450*
Other non-amyloid dysproteinemias *453*
Sickle cell nephropathy *454*

Vasculitis and renal disease 456
ANCA-positive vasculitis 458
Treatment of ANCA-positive vasculitis 460
Churg–Strauss syndrome 462
Classical polyarteritis nodosa 464
Goodpasture's or anti-GBM disease 466
Lupus nephritis 468
Management of lupus nephritis 470
Anti-phospholipid syndrome 472
Scleroderma renal crisis 474
Rheumatoid arthritis (RA) 476
Sarcoidosis 478
HIV and renal disease 480
Hepatitis B–related renal disease 482
Hepatitis C–related renal disease 484
The kidney in infective endocarditis 486
Renal tuberculosis 488
Schistosomiasis 490
Malaria 492

8 Urinary tract obstruction 495

Approaching obstruction 496
Imaging urinary tract obstruction 498
Acute obstruction 500
Chronic obstruction 502
UPJ and UVJ obstruction 504
Retroperitoneal fibrosis (RPF) 506
Investigation of a renal mass 508
Renal cell carcinoma (RCC) 510
Urothelial tumors 512
Benign prostatic hypertrophy (BPH) 514

Prostate cancer *516*
Management of prostate cancer *518*

9 Fluids and electrolytes 519
Sodium: salt and water balance *520*
Hyponatremia *522*
Management of hyponatremia *526*
Hypernatremia *528*
Edema and its treatment *531*
Diuretics *532*
Potassium *534*
Hypokalemia *536*
Bartter's, Gitelman's, and Liddle's syndromes *538*
Calcium, magnesium, and phosphorus *540*
Hypocalcemia *542*
Hypercalcemia *544*
Hypomagnesemia *546*
Hypermagnesemia *548*
Hypophosphatemia *549*
Hyperphosphatemia *550*
Acid–base *552*
Metabolic acidosis *554*
Renal tubular acidosis (RTA) *556*
Lactic acidosis *559*
Metabolic alkalosis *560*
Mixed acidosis and alkalosis *564*
Tubular rarities *566*

10 Pregnancy and the kidney 567
Renal physiology in pregnancy *568*
UTI in pregnancy *570*

Acute renal failure in pregnancy 572
Hypertension in pregnancy 574
Gestational hypertension 575
Preeclampsia and eclampsia 576
Managing preeclampsia and eclampsia 578
Chronic hypertension in pregnancy 580
Preexisting renal disease 582
Disorders of the renal tract in pregnancy 585
Pregnancy while on dialysis 586
Renal transplantation and pregnancy 588

11 Drugs and the kidney — 591
Prescribing in renal impairment 592
The septic ESRD patient: drug issues 594
Cardiac drugs in renal failure 596
NSAIDs and the kidney 598
Analgesia in renal failure 600
Opioids in renal failure 602
Poisoning and dialysis 604
Lithium and salicylate poisoning 606
Ethylene glycol poisoning 608

12 Appendices — 611
The glomerulus 612
Regulation of GFR 614
Tubular function 616
The proximal convoluted tubule 618
The loop of Henle 620
Solute transport in the loop 622
The distal convoluted tubule 624
The collecting duct 626

Insertion of hemodialysis catheters *628*

Renal biopsy *634*

Preparing chronic kidney disease patients for surgery *638*

Plasma exchange *640*

Clinical practice guidelines *644*

Useful Web sites *648*

Index *649*

Symbols and abbreviations

⚠	warning
▶	important
▶	don't dawdle
♂	male
♀	female
∴	therefore
~	approximately
?	question/ask about
↑	increased
↓	decreased
→	leading to
1°	primary
2°	secondary
📖	page reference
α	alpha
β	beta
💣	controversial topic
AAA	ACE-inhibitor after anthracycline (study)
AAA	abdominal aortic aneurysm
ABG	arterial blood gas
ABPM	ambulatory blood pressure monitoring
ACEI	angiotensin converting enzyme inhibitor
ACR	albumin/creatine ratio
ACS	acute coronary syndrome
ACT	activated clotting time
ACTH	adrenocorticotropic hormone
ADMA	asymmetric dimethyl arginine
ADQI	Acute Dialysis Quality Initiative
AG	anion gap
AGE	advanced glycosylated end-products
AII	angiotensin II
AIN	acute interstitial nephritis
AKI	acute kidney injury
ANA	anti-nuclear antibodies
ANCA	anti-neutrophil cytoplasmic antibodies

ANP	atrial natriuretic peptide
APD	automated peritoneal dialysis
APKD	adult polycystic kidney disease
APS	anti-phospholipid syndrome
ARAS	atherosclerotic renal artery syndrome
ARB	angiotensin-receptor blocker
ARDS	acute respiratory distress syndrome
ARF	acute renal failure
ASO	anti-streptolysin O
ATG	anti-thymocyte globulin
ATN	acute tubular necrosis
AVF	arteriovenous fistula
AVM	arteriovenous malformation
AVP	arginine vasopressin
BCG	Bacillus Calmette–Guérin
bid	twice daily
BMD	bone mineral density
BMI	body mass index
BMR	basal metabolic rate
BOO	bladder outflow obstruction
BP	blood pressure
BPH	benign prostatic hypertrophy
CAH	congenital adrenal hyperplasia
CAN	chronic allograft nephropathy
CAPD	continuous ambulatory peritoneal dialysis
CBC	complete blood count
CCB	calcium channel blocker
CCF	chronic cardiac failure
CCPB	calcium-containing phosphate binder
CCPD	continuous cycling peritoneal dialysis
CD	collecting duct
CDC	complement-dependent cross-match
cfu	colony forming units
CHF	congestive heart failure
CHR	corticotropin-releasing hormone
CKD	chronic kidney disease
CLL	chronic lymphocyte leukemia
CMV	cytomegalovirus
CNI	calcineurin inhibitor
CO	cardiac output
COX	cyclo-oxygenase

CPAP	continuous positive airway pressure
CrCl	creatinine clearance
CRF	chronic renal failure
CRP	C-reactive protein
CT	computerized tomography
CTA	CT angiography
CTL	cytotoxic T lymphocyte
CV	cardiovascular
CVA	costovertebral angle
CVP	central venous pressure
CVVH	continuous venovenous hemofiltration
CVVHD	continuous venovenous hemodialysis
CVVHDF	continuous venovenous hemodiafiltration
DASH	Dietary Approach to Hypertension (trial)
DBP	diastolic blood pressure
DCT	distal convoluted tubule
DDD	dense deposit disease
DI	diabetes insipidus
DIC	disseminated intravascular coagulopathy
DM	diabetes mellitus
DSA	donor-specific antigen
DT	distal tubule
DTPA	diethylenetriamine penta-acetic acid
EABV	effective arterial blood volume
EBCT	electron-beam computerized tomography
EBV	Epstein–Barr virus
ECF	extracellular fluid
EDD	extended-duration dialysis
EMU	early-morning urine
ENaC	epithelial sodium channel
EPO	erythropoietin
ESP	erythropoiesis-stimulating protein
ESR	erythrocyte sedimentation rate
ESRD	end-stage renal disease
FDP	fibrinogen degradation products
FFP	fresh frozen plasma
FGN	fibrillary glomerulonephritis
FHR	fetal heart rate
FMD	fibromuscular dysplasia
FSGS	focal and segmental glomerulosclerosis
GBM	glomerular basement membrane

GDP	glucose degradation products
GFR	glomerular filtration rate
GH	growth hormone
GN	glomerulonephritis
GRA	glucocorticoid remediable aldosteronism
Hb	hemoglobin
Hct	hematocrit
HCV	hepatitis C virus
HD	hemodialysis
HIT	heparin-induced thombocytopenia
HIVAN	HIV-associated nephropathy
HLA	human leukocyte antigen
HMW	high molecular-weight
hpf	high-powered field
HRS	hepatic-renal syndrome
HRT	hormone replacement therapy
HSP	Henoch-Schönlein purpura
HSV	herpes simplex virus
HUS	hemolytic-uremic syndrome
ICAM	intercellular adhesion molecule
Ig	immunoglobulin
IgAN	immunoglobulin A nephropathy
IHD	ischemic heart disease
IM	intramuscular
ISH	isolated systolic hypertension
IV	intravenous(ly)
IVDSA	intravenous digital subtraction angiography
IVI	intravenous injection
IVP	intravenous pyelogram
IVU	intravenous urography
JVP	jugular venous pressure
KDIGO	Kidney Disease Improving Global Outcomes
KDOQI	Kidney Disease Outcomes Quality Initiative
KUB	kidney, ureter, bladder
LCDD	light-chain deposition disease
LDH	lactate dehydrogenase
LFT	liver function test
LMW	low molecular-weight
LUTS	lower urinary tract symptoms
LV	left ventricular
LVH	left ventricular hypertrophy

MAG3	mercaptoacetylglycine
MAP	mean arterial pressure
MARS	molecular adsorbed recirculating system
Mb	myoglobin
MCGN	mesangiocapillary glomerulonephritis
MCN	minimal change nephropathy
M,C&S	microscopy, culture and sensitivity
MDRD	Modification of Diet in Renal Disease (study, measure)
MI	myocardial infarction
MM	multiple myeloma
MMF	mycophenolate mofetil
MPA	microscopic polyangiitis; mycophenolic acid
MRA	magnetic resonance angiography
MRI	magnetic resonance imaging
MRSA	methicillin-resistant *Staphylococcus aureus*
MSA	membrane stabilizing activity
MSH	melanocyte-stimulating hormone
MW	molecular weight
NG	nasogastric
NHL	non-Hodgkin's lymphoma
NIPD	nighttime intermittent peritoneal dialysis
npo	nothing by mouth
NO	nitric oxide
NOS	nitric oxide synthase
nPCR	normalized protein catabolic rate
NSAID	nonsteroidal anti-flammatory drug
OC	oral contraceptive
od	once daily
OSA	obstructive sleep apnea
osm	osmolality
PAC	plasma aldosterone concentration
PAF	platelet activating factor
PAN	polyacrylonitrile; polyarteritis nodosa
PAWP	pulmonary capillary wedge pressure
PC	pelvicalyceal
PCA	patient-controlled analgesia
PCR	protein/creatinine ratio; polymerase chain reaction
PCT	proximal convoluted tubule
PD	peritoneal dialysis
PEEP	positive end-expiratory pressure
PET	peritoneal equilibrium tests

Plt	platelets
pmp	per million population
PN	papillary necrosis
po	by mouth
POTS	postural tachycardia syndrome
PP	pulse pressure
PR	per rectum
PRA	panel-reactive antibody; plasma renin activity
PRCA	pure red cell aplasia
PSA	prostate specific antigen
PTC	proximal tubular cells
PTFE	polytetrafluoroethylene
PTH	parathyroid hormone
PTLD	post-transplant lymphoproliferative disease
PTRA	percutaneous transluminal renal angioplasty
PUJ	pelviuretic junction
PVD	peripheral vascular disease
PVR	postvoid residual urine volume
qid	four times daily
QOL	quality of life
RA	rheumatoid arthritis
RAS	renin–angiotensin system; renal artery stenosis
RBC	red blood cells
RBF	renal blood flow
RCC	renal cell carcinoma
RF	rheumatoid factor
RIFLE	risk, injury, failure, loss, and end-stage disease
RN	reflux nephropathy
RPGN	rapidly progressive glomerulonephritis
RRT	renal replacement therapy
RTA	renal tubular acidosis
RVD	renovascular disease
SAA	serum amyloid A
SAH	subarrachnoid hemorrhage
SBP	systolic blood pressure
SC	subcutaneous(ly)
SCC	squamous cell carcinoma
SEP	sclerosing encapsulating peritonitis
SGA	subjective global assessment
SHPT	secondary hyperparathyroidism
SIADH	syndrome of inappropriate antidiuretic hormone secretion

SIRS	systemic inflammatory response syndrome
SLE	systemic lupus erythematosus
SLED	sustained low-efficiency dialysis
SNS	sympathetic nervous system
SPEP	serum protein electrophoresis
SS	systemic sclerosis
SVC	superior vena cava
SVR	systemic vascular resistance
T1DM	type I diabetes mellitus
T2DM	type II diabetes mellitus
TB	tuberculosis
TBW	total body water
TCC	transitional cell carcinoma
TEAP	transurethral ethanol ablation of the prostate
TIA	transient ischemic attack
tid	three times daily
TGF	tubuloglomerular feedback
TIN	tubulointerstitial nephritis
TIPS	transjugular intrahepatic portosystemic shunts
TMA	thrombotic microangiopathy
TMP	transmembrane pressure
TNF	tumor necrosis factor
TNM	tumor node metastates
TOD	target organ damage
TOR	target of rapamycin
TPN	total parenteral nutrition
TRUS	transrectal ultrasound
TTP	thrombotic thrombocytopenic purpura
TUNA	transurethral needle ablation
TURBT	transurethral resection of bladder tumor
TURP	transurethral resection of the prostate
UA	urinalysis
U&E	urea and electrolytes
UF	ultrafiltration
UO	urine output
UPJ	ureteropelvic
Ur	urea
URR	urea reduction ratio
US	ultrasound scan
USRDS	U.S. Renal Data Service
UTI	urinary tract infection

UVJ	ureterovesicular junction
VCUG	voiding crysturethrography
VF	ventricular fibrillation
VHL	von Hippel–Lindau
VUJ	vesicoureteric junction
VUR	vesicoureteral reflux
vWF	von Willebrand factor
WBC	white blood cells
WG	Wegener's granulomatosis

Chapter 1

Clinical assessment of the renal patient

History 2
Physical examination 8
The urine 12
Proteinuria 18
Red blood cells 20
Cells, organisms, and casts 22
Crystals 24
Determining renal function 26
Creatinine 28
Diagnostic imaging 36
  Ultrasound (US) 38
  Intravenous urography (IVU) 40
  Computerized tomography (CT) 42
  Nuclear medicine 43
  Angiography and urology 45
Clinical syndromes 48
  Proteinuria 48
  Hematuria 52
  Chronic kidney disease 58
  The uremic syndrome 59
  Other clinical syndromes 60
  Pulmonary renal syndromes 61
  Changes in urine volume 63
  Pain 64
  Tubular syndromes 65
  Bladder outflow obstruction 67

CHAPTER 1 Clinical assessment of the renal patients

History

In nephrology, as in all branches of medicine, a competent clinical assessment is crucial. This should endeavor to incorporate symptoms and signs.
- arising locally from the kidneys and urinary tract;
- resulting from impaired salt and water handling;
- caused by failing renal excretory and metabolic function;
- relating to a systemic disease causing or contributing to renal dysfunction.

Three further factors need to be considered:
- Asymptomatic patients often require assessment following the discovery of an abnormal blood pressure (BP), urinalysis, or creatinine (Cr) level.
- Symptoms, signs, and investigation findings are organized into clinically useful clinical syndromes (see Box 1.1).
- Biochemistry, radiology, or histopathology is almost always required for accurate diagnosis (although a thorough clinical assessment will lessen overreliance on expensive and invasive tests).

Past medical history
- Urinary problems in childhood (e.g., infections, nocturnal enuresis)
- Previously documented renal or urinary disease of any kind. Ask specifically about infections, stone disease, and, in ♂, prostatic disease.
- Hypertension. When was it diagnosed? Who is responsible for follow-up? Treatment? Level of control?
- Relevant systemic disease (e.g., diabetes mellitus, connective tissue disorder, gout, vascular disease).
- Insurance or employment medical histories can provide invaluable historical benchmarks. Can the patient recall a BP check or providing a urine specimen? Have they had blood tests in the past?

Box 1.1 Renal clinical syndromes
- Asymptomatic urinary abnormalities
  - Proteinuria (p. 48)
  - Microscopic hematuria (p. 20)
- Macroscopic hematuria (p. 20)
- Nephritic syndrome (p. 60)
  - Rapidly progressive glomerulonephritis (RPGN)
- Pulmonary renal syndromes (p. 60)
- Nephrotic syndrome (p. 50)
- Renal tubular syndromes (p. 65)
- Hypertension (Chapter 5)
- Acute renal failure (ARF) (Chapter 2)
- Chronic renal failure (CRF)/chronic kidney disease (CKD) (Chapter 3)

Local symptoms of urinary tract disease

- Pain
  - Loin pain
  - Ureteric colic
  - Suprapubic pain
- Hematuria
- Change in urine appearance
- Changes in urine volume
  - Polyuria
  - Oliguria and anuria
- Lower urinary tract symptoms
  - Obstructive (voiding) symptoms:
    —Acute retention of urine
    —Impaired size or force of the urinary stream
    —Hesitancy or abdominal straining
    —Intermittent or interrupted flow
    —Sensation of incomplete emptying
  - Storage (filling) symptoms:
    —Nocturia
    —Daytime frequency
    —Urgency
    —Urge incontinence
    —Dysuria
- Urethral discharge

Review of systems

This may provide clues to an underlying systemic condition such as connective tissue disorder or vasculitis.
- Skin rashes
- Painful, stiff, or swollen joints
- Myalgia
- Raynaud's phenomenon
- Dry, red, or painful eyes
- Thromboembolic episodes
- Fevers
- Night sweats
- Sinusitis, rhinitis, epistaxis
- Hemoptysis
- Mouth ulcers
- Photosensitivity
- Sicca symptoms
- Hair loss

Drug and treatment history

This often tells its own story. Ask about compliance.
- Antihypertensive therapy—past and present. Side effects
- Analgesics—ask specifically about common nonsteroidal anti-inflammatory drugs (NSAIDS) (by their over-the-counter names if necessary). Then ask again.
- Any recent courses of therapy that may not be mentioned as part of regular treatment, e.g., recent antibiotics (interstitial nephritis).
- Oral contraceptive.
- Steroids, immunosuppressives—type and duration.
- Nonprescription, recreational (cocaine, intravenous drug use [IVDU], and herbal (🕮 p. 74) medicines.
- Exposure to important nephrotoxic drugs (see Table 1.1).

Sexual, menstrual, and obstetric history

- Decreased libido and impotence are extremely common in both ♂ and ♀ with CKD.
- Irregular menses and subfertility are frequently encountered in ♀. Amenorrhea is common in end-stage renal disease (ESRD).
- Previous pregnancies and any complications (urinary tract infection [UTI], proteinuria, ↑BP, preeclampsia). Were there any miscarriages or terminations? Were infants healthy and born at term?
- In CKD, maternal and fetal outcomes are closely related to severity (🕮 p. 582).
- Cytotoxic drugs used in the treatment of glomerular disease, can → premature menopause. This may influence treatment in a ♀ of child-bearing age.

Dietary history

This involves changes in appetite and weight. Ask about dietary habits (vegan, ethnic diet, alcohol). Dietetics is an important part of the management of several renal disorders (↑BP, ARF, CKD, the nephrotic syndrome, stone disease, dialysis) (see Table 1.1).

Ethnicity and renal disease

- IgA nephropathy: Caucasians and certain Asian populations (China, Japan, and Singapore).
- Diabetic nephropathy: African Americans, Mexican Americans, Pima Indians (a Native American tribe in Southern Arizona, beloved of epidemiologists and geneticists). This is an increasing problem in the immigrant Asian population in the UK.
- Systemic lupus erythematosus (SLE): Asians and African Americans.
- Hypertension: African Americans.

Table 1.1 Important nephrotoxins

"Prerenal" renal insufficiency
Diuretics
Any hypertensive agent (in particular, ACE inhibitors and ARBs aggravate other prerenal states)

Hemodynamically mediated
NSAIDs and COX-2 inhibitors
ACE inhibitors and ARBS
Cyclosporin
Tacrolimus
Vasoconstrictors

Glomerulopathy
NSAIDs
Penicillamine
Gold
Hydralazine
Interferon α
Anti-thyroid drugs
Carbon tetrachloride and other organic solvents (e.g., glue sniffing)

Thrombotic microangiopathy
Chemotherapeutic agents:
- Mitomicin C
- Cisplatin
- Bleomycin

Immunosuppressive agents:
- Cyclosporin
- Tacrolimus
- Clopidogrel
- Quinine
- Oral contraceptive

Tubular crystal formation
Acyclovir
Ethylene glycol (antifreeze)
Sulfonamide antibiotics
Methotrexate
Indinavir

Acute tubular necrosis
Aminoglycosides
Antifungals:
- Amphotericin
- Ifosfamide
- Foscarnet

Antivirals:
- Adefovir
- Cidofovir
- Tenofovir

Cisplatin
Heavy metals (arsenic, mercury, and cadmium)
Herbal remedies
Interleukin-2
Intravenous immunoglobulin
Acetaminophen
Paraquat
Pentamidine
X-ray contrast agents

Interstitial nephritis (these and many, many others)
Antibiotics:
- Penicillins
- Cephalosporins
- Quinolones
- Rifampicin
- Sulphonamides

Allopurinol
Cimetidine (rarely ranitidine)
NSAIDS and COX-2 inhibitors
Diuretics
5-aminosalicylates (sulfasalazine and mesalazine)
Analgesics
Omeprazole

Chronic interstitial disease
Lead
Lithium
Analgesics
Chinese herbs

Social history
- Smoking: general cardiovascular (CV) risk, renovascular disease, urothelial malignancy (2- to 5-fold risk), pulmonary hemorrhage in Goodpasture's disease, progression of CKD.
- Occupational history: risk factors for urothelial malignancy (📖 p. 512).
- Hepatitis and HIV risk factors.
- Physical activity.
- Renal diseases are often chronic disorders incurring appreciable social morbidity. Social circumstance will exert an important influence on choice of, and ability to cope with, a particular dialysis modality. Livelihood may also be affected—one of the goals of renal replacement therapy (RRT) should be to keep an individual in employment.

Family history
- Essential hypertension: more common if one or both parents affected.
- Diabetes mellitus (I and II): more common if close relative affected.

Inherited kidney diseases
- Cystic kidney diseases:
  - Adult and juvenile polycystic kidney disease
- Alport syndrome and variants
- Metabolic diseases with renal involvement:
  - Nonglomerular—cystinosis, primary hyperoxaluria, urate nephropathy
  - Glomerular—Fabry disease
- Nonmetabolic diseases:
  - Glomerular—congenital nephrotic syndrome, nail-patella syndrome
  - Nonglomerular—nephronophthisis
- Cystic disease:
  - Tuberous sclerosis (renal angiomyolipoma)
  - Von Hippel–Lindau disease (renal cell carcinoma)
- Primary glomerulonephritides:
  - IgA nephropathy (occasionally)
  - Other focal and segmented glomerulosclerosis (FSGS) (rarely)
- Tubular disorders:
  - Cystinuria
  - Various inherited tubular defects
- Disorders with a "genetic influence":
  - Vesicoureteric reflux
  - Hemolytic-uremic syndrome

Approach to the patient on renal replacement therapy

When faced with a dialysis or transplant patient, a few direct questions will help you get familiar with their treatment (and reassure the patient). These will also facilitate discussion with the patient's dialysis unit.

The patient on hemodialysis
- Where does the hemodialysis treatment take place?
- How many times per week do they dialyse and how many hours is each treatment?
- What is the patient's current access for dialysis (e.g., an AVF)?
- What is their usual fluid gain between treatments?
- Do they receive activated vitamin D with dialysis? What dosage?
- Do they have any documented allergies to dialysis membranes?

The patient on peritoneal dialysis
- How many exchanges do they perform in a day?
- How many liters is each exchange?
- Are they on continuous ambulatory peritoneal dialysis (CAPD) or automated peritoneal dialysis (APD)?
- Do they need assistance to perform an exchange?
- Do they measure their own blood pressure at home? What have the readings been recently?
- Is the exit site of their dialysis catheter clean and dry?
- Are the dialysis bags clear or cloudy on drainage?
- When was their last episode of peritonitis?

All dialysis patients
- What is the patient's dry (aka target) weight?
- How much urine do they pass, if any?
- What is their daily fluid allowance?
- Do they adhere to a renal diet?
- Do they know the cause of their ESRD?
- How long have they been on dialysis?
- Do they take regular injections of erythropoietin? Who gives these injections? What is the dose?
- Have they ever received parenteral iron? Have they ever had an allergic reaction to parenteral iron?
- Have they always been on the same modality of dialysis?
- Have they previously received a transplant?
- How are they coping with dialysis?

The transplant patient
- When and where was the transplant performed?
- What immunosuppression is the patient taking?
- Do they have any side effects to the immunosuppressive medication?
- Do they know if they had any rejection episodes?
- Who is responsible for their follow-up?
- Do they know their baseline Cr?
- Was the transplant from a living or cadaveric donor?
- Have they had any serious infections since the transplant?
- Do they use sun block and attend a skin clinic?
- Do they know the cause of their ESRD?
- What mode of dialysis were they on prior to transplantation?

Physical examination

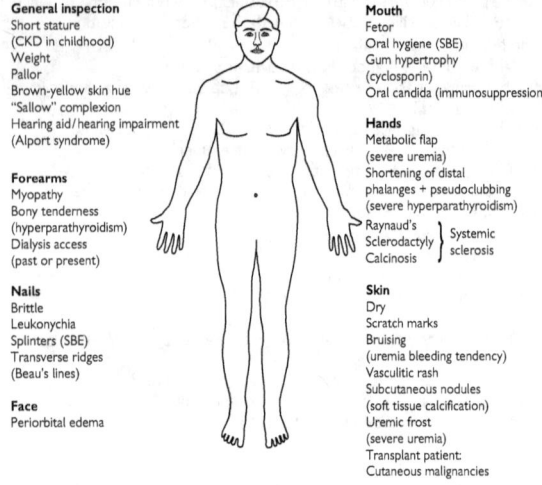

General inspection
Short stature
(CKD in childhood)
Weight
Pallor
Brown-yellow skin hue
"Sallow" complexion
Hearing aid/hearing impairment
(Alport syndrome)

Forearms
Myopathy
Bony tenderness
(hyperparathyroidism)
Dialysis access
(past or present)

Nails
Brittle
Leukonychia
Splinters (SBE)
Transverse ridges
(Beau's lines)

Face
Periorbital edema

Mouth
Fetor
Oral hygiene (SBE)
Gum hypertrophy
(cyclosporin)
Oral candida (immunosuppression)

Hands
Metabolic flap
(severe uremia)
Shortening of distal
phalanges + pseudoclubbing
(severe hyperparathyroidism)
Raynaud's ⎫
Sclerodactyly ⎬ Systemic sclerosis
Calcinosis ⎭

Skin
Dry
Scratch marks
Bruising
(uremia bleeding tendency)
Vasculitic rash
Subcutaneous nodules
(soft tissue calcification)
Uremic frost
(severe uremia)
Transplant patient:
Cutaneous malignancies

Fig. 1.1A Elements of physical examination.

Examination by system

Neurological
Conscious level
Mental state
Myoclonic jerks
Seizures
Tetany
(hypocalcemia)
Peripheral neuropathy

Cardiorespiratory
Respiratory pattern
(? Acidosis)
Blood pressure
JVP
Edema
Carotid bruits
Apex beat
Heart sounds
Pericardial rub
Pleural effusion
Pulmonary edema

Musculoskeletal
Bony deformity
Joint inflammation
Osteoarthritis (? NSAIDs)

Ophthalmic
Dry, red, or painful eyes
(iritis, episcleritis)
Corneal calcification

Retina
Hypertension
Diabetes mellitus
Vasculitis
Cholesterol emboli

Abdomen
Scars
? Tenckhoff catheter
Ascites
Palpation:
Loin tenderness
Palpable kidney(s)
Palpable bladder
Transplant kidney
(right or left iliac fossa)
Abdominal bruit
Rectal (prostate) } Obstruction
Pelvic exam

Legs
Peripheral pulses
Edema
Femoral bruits
Restless legs

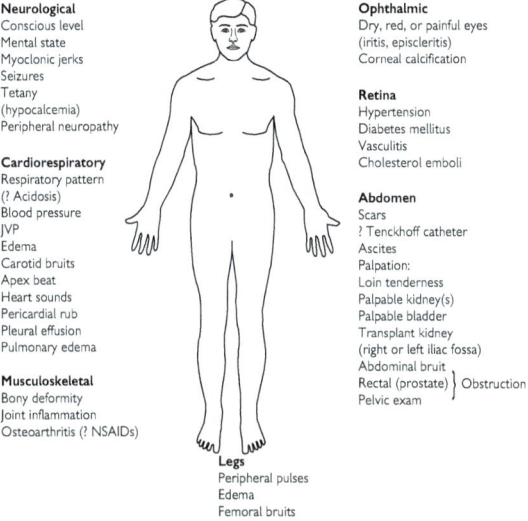

Fig. 1.1B Physical examination by system.

Examination: the circulation

▶ The ability to assess the volume status of a patient is critical to the practice of renal medicine. In the vast majority of cases it can be achieved at the bedside without invasive monitoring.

Hypovolemia

Salt and water or blood loss leads to ↓ effective circulating volume and may lead to shock. Signs include the following:
- ↓BP (and ↓ pulse pressure)
- Postural ↓BP (fall in SBP >10 mmHg)
- Sinus tachycardia and postural ↑ heart rate (HR) (↑ in HR >10 beats/min)
- ↓ jugular venous pressure (JVP). Neck veins are flat even if supine.
- Cool peripheries and peripheral venoconstriction (⚠ septic patients may be vasodilated and warm)
- Poor urine output.

Less reliable signs include the following:
- ↓ capillary refill
- Poor skin turgor (forehead and anterior triangle of the neck)
- Dry mouth and mucous membranes
- Sunken eyes.

Hypervolemia

↑ Extracellular fluid (ECF) volume may be found with ↑ intravascular volume, ↑ interstitial space volume, or both. ⚠ It is possible to be simultaneously salt and water overloaded and intravascularly depleted (e.g., with cirrhosis or in nephrotic patient receiving diuretics).

Increased circulating volume
- ↑BP
- Elevation of JVP.

Increased interstitial fluid
- Peripheral or generalized edema
- Pulmonary edema (tachypnea, tachycardia, a third heart sound ± basal crackles)
- Pleural effusion(s)
- Ascites.

The urine

Examination of the urine should be considered a routine extension of the physical examination in all patients.

Appearance
- Depending on concentration, normal urine is clear or given a light yellow hue by urochrome and uroerythrin pigments.
- Cloudy urine may result from high concentrations of leukocytes, epithelial cells, or bacteria. Precipitation of phosphates can also produce turbidity in urine refrigerated for storage.
- Blood causes a pink to black discoloration depending on the number of red blood cells (RBCs) and length of time present.
- Jaundice (conjugated hyperbilirubinemia) may cause dark yellow or brown urine.
- Hemoglobinuria from intravascular hemolysis (p. 141) and myoglobinuria from muscle breakdown (p. 138) are both causes of dark urine that tests positive for blood on dipstick examination. If the sample is centrifuged, the supernatant will remain colored and continue to test positive. No red cells are seen on microscopy. Specific assays for hemoglobin and myoglobin are available.
- Normal urine tends to darken on standing (urobilinogen oxidizes to colored urobilin). See Box 1.2.
- Chyluria is a rare cause of turbid urine. It has a milky appearance (particularly after fatty meals) and settles into layers on standing. It results from a fistulous connection between the lymphatic and urinary systems (usually a malignancy, though lymphatic obstruction by *Filaria bancrofti* is more important worldwide).
- Beets can produce red urine due to enhanced intestinal absorption of the pigment betalaine in genetically susceptible individuals. It rarely causes diagnostic confusion.

Odor
Offensive urine usually denotes infection (bacterial ammonium production). Sweet urine suggests ketones. Certain rare metabolic diseases confer characteristic smells—one can only hope to encounter maple-syrup urine disease before isovaleric acidemia ("sweaty feet urine").

Box 1.2 Urine discoloration

Causes of a colored urine
- Beet ingestion (red)
- Blood (pink/red to brown/black)
- Chloroquine (brown)
- Chyluria (milky white)
- Hemoglobin (pink/red to brown/black)
- Hyperbilirubinemia (yellow/brown)
- Methylene blue (er ... blue)
- Myoglobin (pink/red to brown/black)
- Nitrofurantoin (brown)
- Onchronosis (black)
- Phenytoin (red)
- Propofol (green)
- Rifampicin (orange)
- Senna (orange)

Urine that darkens on standing
- Alkaptonuria (homogentisic acid)
- Imipenem-cilastin
- Melanoma (melanogen)
- Methyl dopa
- Metronidazole
- Porphyria (porphobilinogen)

Chemical analysis

Osmolality and specific gravity

Specific gravity refers to the weight of a solution with respect to an equal weight of distilled water (normal range, 1.003–1.035 in urine). It can be estimated with a dipstick, but for accurate measurement an osmometer (urinometer) is required.

Osmolality refers to the solute concentration of a solution. It cannot be measured with a dipstick. In the absence of significant glycosuria, the concentrations of Na^+, Cl^-, and urea are the most important determinants in urine. The ability to vary urine osmolality (range, 50–1350 mOsmol/kg) plays a central role in the regulation of plasma osmolality (maintained across a narrow range: 280–305 mOsm/kg).

Generally speaking, the two measurements correlate. An exception is when relatively large particles such as glucose, proteins, and radiocontrast media are present in the urine. These produce an ↑ in specific gravity with little change in osmolality.

Uses

These two measurements are used for investigation of polyuria and hypo- or hypernatremic states (p. 63). Recurrent stone formers can monitor their own urine-specific gravity to maintain a dilute urine.

Isosthenuria

CKD leads to a progressive ↓ in the range of urinary osmolality that the kidneys can generate. In advanced renal insufficiency, the osmolality becomes relatively fixed at ~300 mOsmol/kg (~1.010 specific gravity), close to that of glomerular filtrate. In this situation, the urine cannot be adequately concentrated or diluted in response to Na^+ and water depletion and overload, respectively.

Urinary pH

Urinary pH ranges from 4.5 to 8.0 (usually 5.0–6.0), depending on systemic acid–base status. Most people (except vegans) pass an acid urine most of the time. Isolated urinary pH measurements provide very little useful information. Their main clinical use is the investigation of systemic metabolic acidosis. In this situation, a fall in urinary pH (to around 5) is expected as acid is excreted. Failure of this response may indicate renal tubular acidosis (p. 556). Most urine dipsticks have an indicator strip for estimation of pH, but if a tubular disorder is suspected, a pH meter should be used.

In certain situations the therapeutic manipulation of urinary pH might be useful (see Box 1.3).

Box 1.3 Therapeutic urinary alkalinization

(● See Chapter 2)
- Urinary stone disease (cystine and urate stones)
- Poisoning
  - Salicylates
  - Barbiturates
  - Methotrexate
- Rhabdomyolysis
- ARF secondary to myeloma

Further dipstick tests

Leukocyte esterase and nitrites
These are increasingly used as indicators of infection. Detection of neutrophil esterase activity identifies pyuria, while the nitrite test exploits the ability of some urinary pathogens (though not all—notably certain gram-positive organisms such as *Streptococcus faecalis*, *Staphylococcus albus*, *Neisseria gonorrheae*, as well as many *Pseudomonas* sp p. and mycobacteria) to reduce nitrate → nitrite. Positivity requires an adequate dietary nitrate intake and an adequate bladder dwell time (preferably >4 hours).

When combined, these methods possess good specificity (i.e., take seriously if positive), though only modest sensitivity (i.e., treat a negative result with caution if infection is likely clinically). They can serve as a useful screening test in at-risk populations, but are not a substitute for microscopy and culture.

Bilirubin and urobilinogen
Conjugated (∴ water-soluble) bilirubin → biliary excretion → small bowel → converted to urobilinogen → distal reabsorption → partially excreted in the urine. So (1) unconjugated (water-insoluble) bilirubin does not pass into the urine (∴ dipstick positive bilirubin indicates hepatic or cholestatic disease), and (2) absence of dipstick urobilinogen in a jaundiced patient suggests biliary obstruction.

Glucose
Glycosuria results when tubular reabsorptive capacity for glucose is exceeded (plasma level >180 mg/dl). A glucose test is a valuable screening tool, but it is less useful for diagnosis and monitoring of diabetes mellitus (DM).

"Renal" glycosuria occurs when proximal tubular injury leads to a failure to reabsorb filtered glucose (📖 p. 66).

Causes of a positive dipstick for ketones

Dipsticks semi-quantitatively detect acetoacetate (but not β-hydroxybutyrate). A positive test can be seen in the following:
- Diabetic ketoacidosis (and occasionally severe intercurrent illness in T2DM)
- Prolonged fasting and starvation diets (e.g., Atkins' diet)
- Alcoholic ketoacidosis
- Severe volume depletion
- Isopropyl alcohol poisoning (hand rubs, solvents, and deicers)

Urinary test strips

A variety of test strips for urinalysis are available. Some have a specific purpose—e.g., Clinistix® (glucose), Hemastix® (blood), and Albustix® (albumin). Others cast a wider net with various combinations of the following:
- Specific gravity
- pH
- Leucocytes
- Nitrites
- Glucose
- Urobilinogen
- Bilirubin
- Ketones
- Albumin or protein*
- Blood

* Dipsticks able to detect microalbuminuria are also available.

Proteinuria

Urinary protein excretion should not exceed 150 mg/day, of which <20 mg is albumin (the remainder consists mainly of non-serum-derived tubular mucoprotein such as Tamm–Horsfall/uromodulin). ↑ excretion of albumin is a sensitive marker of renal, particularly glomerular, disease (📖 p. 48).

> *Proteinuria* (total protein) and *albuminuria* (albumin) are not strictly interchangeable terms. When screening for renal disease, specific tests for albumin are preferable.

Protein excretion can be measured in untimed ("spot") or timed (usually 24-hour) samples.

Dipsticks
These are convenient, highly specific, but less sensitive. They contain pH-sensitive indicators that change color when bound to negatively charged proteins. They predominantly detect albumin (some are albumin specific; e.g., Albustix®) and may not identify large amounts of other proteins, e.g., Bence–Jones. Dipstick tests have completely superseded sulphosalicylic acid turbidity testing.

A positive result occurs with protein excretion ≥300 mg/L. Lower amounts of proteinuria, particularly in the context of diabetes, are termed *microalbuminuria* (📖 p. 48) (usually defined as 30–300 mg/day). This is usually measured by ELISA or radioimmunoassay, although sensitive dipsticks are available.

Dipsticks are semi-quantitative. As a *rough* guide:

Trace	~15–30 mg/dL
+	~30–100 mg/dL
++	~100–300 mg/dL
+++	~300–1,000 mg/dL
++++	>1,000 mg/dL

⚠ Changes in urinary concentration affect the result. If volumes are high and the urine dilute, large amounts of protein can go undetected (specific gravity may be a clue). Concentrated morning samples are ∴ preferable.

▶ If a patient has a positive dipstick test of ≥1+, repeat test after 1–2 weeks. If persistent, verify with one of the quantitative methods below.

Timed collections
For many clinicians a 24-hour urine collection remains the gold standard, but there are important drawbacks:
- Inaccurate collection
- The processing is time consuming.

Timed collections are gradually being supplanted by protein/creatinine ratio (PCR) or albumin/creatinine ratio (ACR). See Box 1.4.

24-hour collection: what to tell the patient

- Use a non-acidified, clearly labeled, container.
- Pick a convenient day with minimum commitments.
- Discard first urine void on that day.
- Start collection—all subsequent urine into the container (including overnight)
- First void the following day goes into the collection
- Since Cr excretion, or creatinine clearance (CrCl) (p. 29), should be similar in two successive samples from the same patient, their measurement in "back to back" 24-hour collections may enhance reliability (i.e., disregard the result if CrCl differs greatly between the two).

Box 1.4 The albumin/creatinine ratio (ACR)

Untimed ("spot") urine samples can (and many say should[1]) be used to detect and monitor proteinuria. The ACR corrects for variations in urinary concentration (caused by changes in hydration) and correlates well with measurements obtained from timed collections.

A first-morning urine specimen is preferable. Urinary excretion of creatinine generally remains constant.

- Interpretation
- In the United States and in labs where urinary Cr is measured in mg/dL rather than mmol/L, ACR is expressed as mg/g (normal: <30 mg/g, microalbuminuria: 30–300 mg/g, overt proteinuria: >300 mg/g).
- ACR will underestimate proteinuria when Cr excretion is high (muscular build) and overestimate proteinuria when Cr excretion is low (in elderly, cachectic). However, the ACR remains useful for serial monitoring in individual patients.
- The total protein/creatinine ratio (PCR) is an adequate alternative to ACR in most circumstances. ACR is more sensitive if screening for early disease in high-risk groups (especially diabetes). A PCR 500 mg/g of creatinine indicates significant proteinuria.
- Dipsticks that estimate the PCR (e.g., Multistix Pro®) await further validation.

1 Kidney Disease Outcomes Quality Initiative (K/DOQI) Clinical practice guidelines.

Red blood cells

Hematuria is defined (arbitrarily) as the presence of 2 RBCs per high-powered field (hpf) in spun urine. The amount determines whether it is visible to the naked eye (macroscopic hematuria) or requires a dipstick or microscopy for detection (microscopic hematuria). Causes and investigation are considered later (📖 p. 21).

Dipstick

Hemoglobin (Hb) induces a color change (usually green) in a dye linked to organic peroxide. Dipsticks detect as little as 2 RBCs per field and are at least as sensitive as microscopic examination (though with an appreciable false negative rate). If dipstick is positive, it is still desirable to perform confirmatory microscopy.

Dipsticks detect Hb and remain positive even after RBC lysis. They also detect hemoglobinuria from intravascular hemolysis and myoglobin from muscle breakdown, though red cells will be absent on microscopy in both situations.

Urine sediment

Microscopic examination of the urine sediment is still the gold standard.

Urinary RBCs may have variable morphology. Those that have passed through the glomerular basement membrane and suffered osmotic stress in the tubules may have an abnormal appearance; they are best appreciated under phase-contrast microscopy.

In expert hands, the presence of these "dysmorphic" red cells can help distinguish glomerular from lower urinary tract bleeding (Fig. 1.2). ⚠ The presence of dysmorphic cells does not rule out a lower-tract lesion.

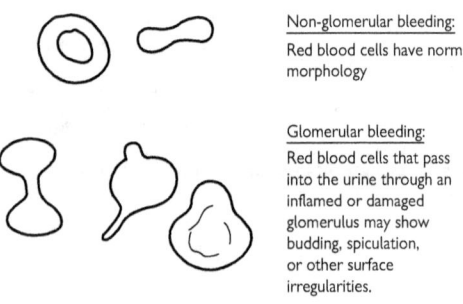

Non-glomerular bleeding:
Red blood cells have normal morphology

Glomerular bleeding:
Red blood cells that pass into the urine through an inflamed or damaged glomerulus may show budding, spiculation, or other surface irregularities.

Fig. 1.2 Characteristics of red blood cells in glomerular and nonglomerular hematuria.

Examination of the urine sediment

- Tell the patient to discard the first few milliliters of urine and then collect ~20 mL into a universal container.
- Process and analyze the sample within a few hours (red cell lysis).
- Centrifuge a 10 mL aliquot at $400 \times g$ for 10 minutes.
- Remove 9.5 mL of supernatant with a pipette.
- Resuspend the pellet in the remaining 0.5 mL of urine (gently!).
- Transfer a drop of resuspended urine to a slide.
- Cover the sample (unstained) with a coverslip.
- Examine with a microscope at 160x and 400x.
- Cellular elements are quantitated as number per high-power field.
- Look also for casts and other elements.
- Use polarized light to identify crystals.
- Clean the microscope and discard all the urine!

In an urgent situation, e.g., for rapid diagnosis of a UTI, an unspun sample may be examined. It may be necessary to acidify the urine to prevent precipitation of (view-obscuring) phosphate crystals.

Should we screen for hematuria with urinary dipsticks?

The benefit of screening the general population for hematuria is yet to be established.

Argument for
Dipstick examination is easy, acceptable to patients, and inexpensive. It may assist in the early diagnosis of both urological malignancies (where early intervention may be life saving) and intrinsic renal disease (where intervention may delay or prevent progression to ESRD).

Argument against
The basic criteria for general population screening are not fulfilled. Dipstick examination is not a sufficiently specific test and the predictive values for urothelial malignancy and renal disease are quite poor. In both cases the benefits of early detection have not been established.

At present the relevant advisory bodies do not advocate population screening.

Cells, organisms, and casts

Leukocytes

Neutrophils
Leukocytes are a prominent feature of urinary infection, but may be present in inflammatory renal conditions (glomerulonephritis [GN], tubulointerstitial nephritis [TIN]). *Sterile pyuria* refers to the situation when leukocytes are seen consistently on microscopy but subsequent culture is sterile.

Causes of sterile pyuria
- Partially treated UTI or fastidious organism (e.g., *Chlamydia*)
- Calculi
- Prostatitis
- Bladder tumor
- Papillary necrosis
- TIN
- Tuberculosis (TB) (send 3x EMUs, 📖 p. 488)
- Appendicitis

Lymphocytes
These are a feature of chronic tubulointerstitial disease. *Eosinophils* are tested by Hansel's or Wright's stain. They are associated with TIN (📖 p. 404), but are also possible in several other conditions, including RPGN, prostatitis, and atheroemboli. *Renal tubular cells* are large, oval cells. Present in normal urine, but ↑ in tubular damage (acute tubular necrosis [ATN] or TIN). *Squamous epithelial cells* are large cells with small nuclei and an urethral origin (or skin/vaginal contaminant). *Transitional epithelial (urothelial) cells* suggest cystitis. Special stains, immunocytochemistry, and flow cytometry all aid in detection of malignant cells.

Microorganisms
- **Bacteriuria:** Normal urine is sterile. Concomitant presence of leukocytes suggests true infection, rather than contamination. Gram staining enables initial identification and cell count, while culture and sensitivities are pending.
- **Fungi:** Candida is the most frequent. Typical appearance is a small, pale green cell, often with visible budding. It may result from genital contamination. Risk factors for colonization are indwelling plastic (ureteric stents, bladder catheter), DM, antibiotic therapy, and immunosuppression.
- **Trichomonas:** Oval and flagellate (motile if alive). Usually a genital contaminant is involved.
- **Schistosoma haematobium:** Ova detection is an important technique in endemic areas.

Urine culture

Microscopy, culture, and sensitivity (M,C&S) differentiate contamination from true infection and guides treatment. A pure growth of >10^5 colony-forming units (cfu)/mL is the conventional diagnostic criterion for urinary tract infection (📖 p. 422).

Casts

Casts are plugs of Tamm–Horsfall mucoprotein within the renal tubules, conferring a characteristic cylindrical shape. They are classified according to appearance and the cellular elements embedded in them. Though produced in normal kidneys, they can be valuable clues to the presence of renal disease.

Noncellular casts
- *Hyaline casts:* Mucoprotein alone and virtually transparent. A nonspecific finding, these occur in concentrated urine.
- *Granular casts:* Granular material (aggregates of protein or cellular remnants) is embedded in the cast. They are often pathological, but nonspecific.
- *Broad or waxy casts:* Hyaline material with a waxy appearance under the microscope. They form in dilated, poorly functioning tubules of advanced CKD.

Cellular casts
- *Red cell casts*
  ▶ These are virtually diagnostic of GN.
- *White cell casts* are characteristic of acute pyelonephritis—they may help to distinguish upper from lower tract infection. They also occur in TIN.
- *Epithelial cell casts* are sloughed epithelial cells embedded in mucoprotein. They are a nonspecific feature of ATN and are also found in GN.
- *Fatty casts:* contain either lipid-filled tubular epithelial cells or free lipid globules. They are distinguished from other casts by their "Maltese cross" appearance under polarized light. They occur in the lipid-laden urine of the nephrotic syndrome. Lipids may also appear as droplets or crystals. When clumped these are referred to as oval fat bodies.
- *Other casts:* Under the right conditions any constituent of the urine (microorganisms, crystals, bilirubin or myoglobin) may become entrapped in a mucoprotein cast.

Crystals

Crystals are detected by examining the urine under polarized light. Most crystals are irrelevant.

Uric acid
Crystals of this type are usually lozenges with a yellow-brown hue. They precipitate at acid pH. A few may be normal (e.g., high meat intake), but ↑quantities may indicate hyperuricosuria. They may be present in acute urate nephropathy (tumor lysis syndrome 📖 p. 144).

Calcium oxalate
These crystals may be monohydrated (ovoid) or bihydrated (pyramidal—like the back of an envelope) (Fig. 1.3). They prefer an acidic pH, but not always. A few may be normal (spinach and chocolate), but may denote hypercalciuria or hyperoxaluria (see 📖 p. 566). They are a diagnostic clue in ethylene glycol poisoning (📖 p. 608).

Calcium phosphate
Heterogeneous in appearance (needles, prisms, stars), these crystals have alkaline pH. They might be a risk factor for calcium stone formation.

Magnesium ammonium phosphate (triple phosphate)
These crystals are birefringent prisms ("coffin-lids") with alkaline pH. If present, check for a proteus UTI.

Amorphous phosphates
Unattractive clumps in (alkaline) urine cooled for storage. No clinical significance.

Cystine
Cystine crystals are hexagonal. Cystine is not a constituent of normal urine, so it is always significant. It prefers an acid urine and is a marker of cystinuria (📖 p. 566).

Cholesterol
Cholesterol crystals take the shape of thin plates with sharp edges. They occur with heavy proteinuria.

Drug-induced crystalluria

Many drugs can precipitate in the renal tubule. In severe cases this may → ARF.
- Antibiotics: sulfadiazine, amoxicillin
- Antiviral agents: acyclovir and indinavir
- Methotrexate
- Primidone (a barbiturate)
- Triamterene
- Vitamin C (calcium oxalate deposition)

Uric acid

Calcium oxalate
Bihydrated   Monohydrated

Calcium phosphate

Magnesium ammonium phosphate

Cystine

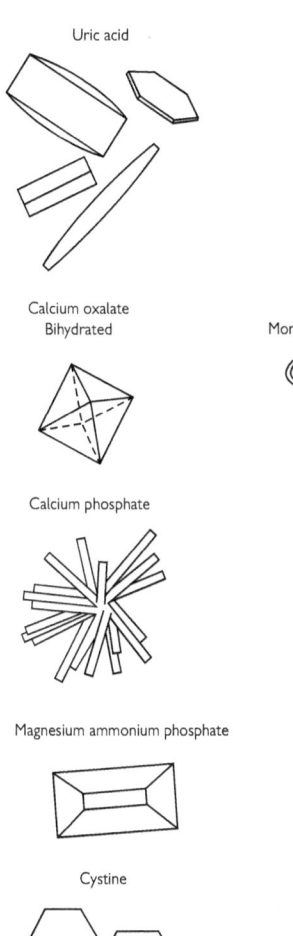

Fig. 1.3 Urinary crystals.

Determining renal function

Several aspects of renal function can be measured (see Box 1.5). The most important one is the *glomerular filtration rate* (GFR), which refers to the ultrafiltrate of plasma that crosses the glomerular barrier into the urinary space. The GFR is measured per unit time (usually expressed mL/min) and represents the sum of filtration rates in all functioning nephrons (∴ a surrogate for the amount of functioning renal tissue).

The GFR is useful for the following:
- Providing a consistent measure of kidney function
- Monitoring progression of CKD (and response to treatment)
- Forecasting the need for RRT
- Determining appropriate drug dosing in renal impairment.

It provides no information on the cause of renal insufficiency.

Measurement of GFR
- GFR is measured indirectly by evaluating clearance from plasma of a (renal excreted) marker substance.
- Clearance is the volume of plasma from which this substance is removed per unit time.
- Suitable markers require certain characteristics, shown below, and may be endogenous (e.g., Cr) or exogenous (e.g., inulin).

Characteristics of an ideal clearance marker
- Safe, economical, and easy to measure
- Freely filtered at the glomerulus
- Not protein bound (able to distribute in the extracellular space)
- Present at a stable plasma concentration
- No extrarenal elimination
- Not reabsorbed, secreted, or metabolized by the kidney

- *Inulin*, a fructose polysaccharide for which we have the Jerusalem artichoke to thank, remains the gold standard. Cost and technical considerations (it requires a continuous infusion) prohibit its routine use.

In clinical practice, GFR is estimated by one of the following means:
- Serum Cr (and to a lesser extent urea)
- Formulas based on the serum creatinine (estimated, or eGFR)
- Creatinine clearance (CrCl) from a 24-hour urine collection
- Isotopic clearance (EDTA-GFR or DTPA-GFR)

Box 1.5 Aspects of renal function

- Glomerular filtration rate (GFR)
- Tubular function (including Na^+ and K^+ handling and urinary concentrating or diluting capacity)
- Acid–base balance
- Endocrine function
  - Renin–angiotensin system
  - Erythropoietin production
  - Vitamin D metabolism

Not measured in clinical practice

- Autocrine
  - Production of endothelins, prostaglandins, natriuretic peptides, nitric oxide
- Protein and polypeptide metabolism (e.g., insulin catabolism)

Creatinine

Serum creatinine

This test is convenient and inexpensive and the most commonly used indirect measure of GFR.
- Generated from nonenzymatic metabolism of creatine in skeletal muscle. Production is proportional to muscle mass (20 g muscle → ~1 mg Cr). There is little short-term variation in an individual.
- ~25% is derived from dietary meat intake.
- $U_{cr} \times V$ is relatively constant in the formula for CrCl.

    So   CrCl = (Urine Cr × V)/Plasma Cr

    Becomes   CrCl = constant/Plasma Cr

Hence, serum Cr varies inversely with GFR: ↓GFR → ↑Cr (until a new steady state is reached).
- ↓ muscle mass (elderly, cachectic) → ↓Cr production → overestimates GFR.
- Cr meets many, but not all, of the criteria for a clearance marker. Shortcomings are the following:
  - It is secreted by the proximal tubule (~10%–20% when GFR is normal), so the amount excreted in the urine exceeds the amount filtered. As GFR falls, there is a progressive ↑ in tubular secretion until saturation occurs at Cr ~132–176 μmol/L. Beyond this, Cr rises as expected (see Fig. 1.4).
  - It undergoes extrarenal elimination by secretion and degradation in the gastrointestinal tract (GI) tract. This becomes more important as GFR falls.
- When ↓GFR is rapid, it takes time for a steady state to be reached and Cr to ↑; i.e., Cr may initially be normal after a catastrophic renal insult.
- Cr is traditionally measured by the Jaffé alkaline pictrate colorimetric assay. Interference by non-creatinine chromogens created a tradition of overestimating Cr. Enzymatic methods on modern autoanalyzers are generally more accurate.
- Certain substances interfere with Cr, either through competitive inhibition of tubular secretion (cimetidine, trimethoprim, amiloride, spironolactone, triamterene) or assay interference (in the Jaffé reaction: ketoacids, vitamin C, glucose, and cephalosporins).

Creatinine clearance

CrCl is calculated as:
 CrCl × plasma creatinine (P_{Cr}) = urine creatinine (U_{Cr}) × volume (V)
 ∴ CrCl = (U_{Cr} × V)/P_{Cr}.

Example
- Serum Cr = 1.5 mg/dL
- Urine Cr = 55 mg/dL
- Urine volume = 2.0 L
- CrCl = (U_{Cr} × V)/P_{Cr}
- CrCl = (55 × 2.0)÷1.5 = 73.3 L/day

Conventionally CrCl is shown in mL/min ∴ ×1000/1440
- (73.3 × 1000)/1440 = 50.9 mL/min

Normal range: ♀: 95 ± 20 mL/min; ♂: 120 ± 25 mL/min

Limitations
- Tubular secretion of Cr means that GFR is overestimated.
- It requires accurate urine collection.
- It is heir to all the pitfalls inherent in Cr measurement.
- Even if collections are accurate, there is marked serial variation (15%–20%).

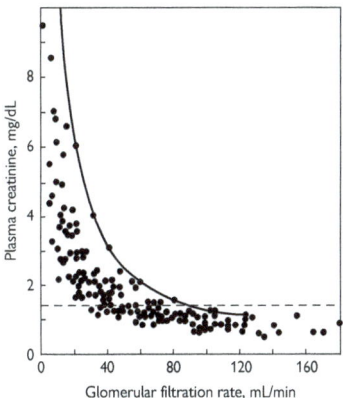

Fig. 1.4 Relationship between Cr concentration and GFR (measured as inulin clearance) in 171 patients with glomerular disease. The hypothetical relationship between GFR and Cr is shown in the continuous line, assuming that only filtration of Cr takes place. The broken horizontal line represents the upper limit of normal serum Cr (1.4 mg/dL or 115 µmol/L). It can be seen that because of Cr secretion, serum Cr consistently overestimates GFR. Reproduced from Shemesh O, Golbertz H, Kriss JP, et al. (1985). Limitations of creatinine as a filtration marker in glomerulopathic patients. *Kidney Int* **28**: 830–8.

eGFR: formulas based on creatinine (see also p. 153)

Recent guidelines emphasize the need to diagnose and monitor kidney function with equations based on serum Cr, which attempt to correct for the confounding effects of body weight, age, gender, race, and muscle mass. Such equations are still nonetheless based on Cr and do not take into account tubular secretion, extrarenal elimination, or differences in production between individuals of the same age and gender, or the same individual over time.

Cockcroft–Gault (CG)

$$\text{eGFR (mL/min)} = \frac{\{140 - \text{age (yr)}\} \times \text{weight (kg)}}{\text{Cr (mg/dl)} \times 72}$$

Multiply × 0.85 in ♀ to correct for reduced creatinine production.

MDRD

Developed from data in the Modification of Diet in Renal Disease (MDRD) study, this formula remains unvalidated in children (age <18 years), the elderly (age >70 years), during pregnancy, in ethnic groups other than Caucasians and African Americans, and in those without CKD.

eGFR, in mL/min per 1.73 m^2

$$= (170 \times (\text{PCR [mg/dL]}) \exp[-0.999]) \times (\text{Age} \exp[-0.176])$$
$$\times ((S_{\text{Urea}}\text{[mg/dL]})\exp[-0.170]) \times ((\text{Albumin [g/dL]})\exp[+0.318])$$

- Multiply × 0.762 if the patient is female.
- Multiply × 1.180 if the patient is black.

Simplified version:

$$\textbf{eGFR} = 186.3 \times ((\text{serum creatinine}) \exp[-1.154])$$
$$\times (\text{Age} \exp[-0.203]) \times (0.742 \text{ if female})$$
$$\times (1.21 \text{ if African American})$$

The CG tends to overestimate and the MDRD to underestimate GFR. Up to 25% of patients will be misclassified if either is used to categorize patients according to the KDOQI CKD classification (p. 58).

The formulas are available as Web-based and downloadable calculators from the following Web sites:
- www.nephron.com
- www.hdcn.com
- www.renal.org
- www.nkdep.nih.gov/healthprofessionals/tools/

Reciprocal of plasma creatinine

There is an inverse relationship between GFR and Cr:

   CrCl = constant/Cr

Plotting the reciprocal of Cr (1/Cr) against time will often, though not always, produce a straight line, the slope of the curve representing change in GFR with time. A logarithmic plot of Cr can be used in a similar way.

This may be useful in two settings:
- Extrapolation of the line can help predict when CKD is likely to reach ESRD and ∴ assist timely planning of RRT.
- A change in the slope of the curve can be used to monitor treatment: a ↓ in the slope indicates slowed progression; an ↑ may indicate a second insult (acute on chronic renal failure).

Other methods of GFR measurement

Isotopic GFR
Several radiopharmaceuticals (^{51}Cr-EDTA, ^{99m}Tc-DTPA, ^{125}I-Iothalamate) compare favorably to inulin for GFR measurement.

Method
A single IV injection is followed by venous sampling at regular intervals (intervals ↑ as expected GFR ↓). Post-injection, plasma isotope activity ↓ rapidly as it distributes throughout the ECF. A slower exponential decline (renal elimination) then follows, allowing GFR to be determined. Protocols based on urine collection are also described.

With DTPA, renal elimination is often measured with a gamma camera positioned directly over the kidneys. While not as precise as venous sampling, it allows assessment of each kidney's contribution to total GFR ("split function") (📖 p. 43).

Note: isotopic techniques are expensive.

Cystatin C
Cysteine protease inhibitor is produced by all nucleated cells. It is easy to measure, has a stable production rate, is freely filtered at the glomerulus, and is not influenced by age, gender, muscle mass, diet, or inflammation. This measure correlates well with GFR, with ↑ concentration in advance of Cr as GFR falls. This test is not yet available in routine clinical practice.

β_2-microglobulin
Early ↑ in plasma levels occurs as GFR ↓. Susceptible to nonrenal elevation (lymphoid malignancy, inflammatory states), this test is expensive.

MRI
Gadolinium, a paramagnetic contrast agent, undergoes renal elimination and is well tolerated in renal insufficiency. MRI could potentially provide both structural and functional information.

Renal function in the elderly

Functioning renal mass declines with age, with progressive glomerulosclerosis from age ~30. This is accompanied by sclerosis of the renal vasculature and altered renal hemodynamics.

The Baltimore longitudinal study (1958–1981) used serial measurements of CrCl to show a ↓GFR of 0.75 mL/min/year. Recent studies have used inulin clearances to show that, although GFR is lower in older age groups, it generally stays in the normal range. Associated comorbidity (↑BP, vascular disease, CCF, etc.) may have more of an impact than age itself.

Clinical relevance
- In the absence of disease, a major age-related ↓ in GFR is uncommon.
- ↓ Muscle mass in the elderly → ↓Cr ∴ ↑Cr usually represents a significant ↓GFR.

Urea (Ur)

- Synthesized in the liver as a means of ammonia excretion
- Rate of production not constant (unlike Cr)
- Inverse relationship with GFR
- Influenced by a number of factors independent of GFR

↑Ur	↓Ur
High dietary protein intake	Low protein diet
GI bleeding	Liver disease
Catabolic states	Pregnancy
• Hemorrhage	
• Trauma	
• Corticosteroids	
Tetracyclines	

- Freely filtered at the glomerulus but reabsorbed in the tubules
  - Ur movement is linked to water (under vasopressin influence) in the distal nephron
  - ↓ renal perfusion → ↑Ur reabsorption → disproportionate ↑Ur compared to Cr
  - Can be used to differentiate "prerenal" renal dysfunction (p. 92)

Diagnostic imaging

To select the most appropriate investigation (and maintain healthy relations with the radiology department), the requesting clinician should understand the indications and limitations of imaging in renal disease.

Plain X-ray
- "KUB" (kidneys–ureter–bladder). This is essentially a supine abdominal X-ray centered on the umbilicus.
- Its main role is identification and surveillance of calcification (Table 1.2). Lateral and oblique films may differentiate calcification *in line with* as opposed to *in* the renal tract.
- The medial edges of both psoas muscles are usually visible. Disappearance suggests a perinephric mass or retroperitoneal collection.
- Tomography keeps one particular image plane in focus, blurring out images in front and behind. Moving the plane can produce serial "cuts" used to detect small calculi and establish the exact location of calcification. It is superseded by CT.

Where are the kidneys on a plain abdominal X-ray?
- Differences in attenuation between renal tissue and perinephric fat mean that the kidneys are (just) visible.
- The kidneys are usually adjacent to the upper border of the T11 through to the lower border of L3.
- Normal renal size is 11–15 cm (in adults). Kidneys appear bigger on an abdominal X-ray than on ultrasound.
- The right kidney is usually shorter than the left (upper limit of variation in length between right and left is 1.5 cm).

Table 1.2 Causes of renal tract calcification

Urinary calculi (most are radio-opaque to some degree; exceptions are pure uric acid and xanthine stones)

Localized calcification
- Tuberculosis
- Tumors

Nephrocalcinosis
- Medullary
  - Disturbed calcium metabolism:
    —Hyperparathyroidism
    —Sarcoidosis
    —Vitamin D excess
    —Idiopathic hypercalciuria
    —Oxalosis*
  - Tubular diseases:
    —Distal renal tubular acidosis
    —Bartter's syndrome
  - Other:
    —Medullary sponge kidney
    —Papillary necrosis
  - Cortical:
    —Trauma
    —Cortical necrosis
    —Oxalosis*

* Causes both medullary and cortical calcification.

Ultrasound (US)

This is the front-line investigation in most forms of renal disease. Its pros are that it is noninvasive and relatively quick to do, and requires little patient preparation. Its disadvantages are that it is operator dependent, provides poor pelviureteric detail and no functional information, and may miss small stones and masses.

Main uses
- Document 1 or 2 kidneys
- Diagnosis of obstruction (pelvicalyceal [PC] dilatation)
- Measurement of renal size in CKD (see Table 1.3)
- Evaluation of renal masses (cystic vs. solid)
- Screening for polycystic disease
- Identify nephrocalcinosis and calculi
- Evaluate bladder emptying
- Estimate prostate size (may require a rectal probe)
- Guide percutaneous procedures (e.g., renal biopsy, nephrostomy)
- Doppler US can be used to evaluate arterial and venous blood flow. It is widely used for transplant assessment, but its role as a screening tool in renovascular diseases remains uncertain (p. 410).

Normal appearances
- Renal length 9–12 cm
- Smooth outline
- Cortex >1.5 cm
- Echotexture: medulla is darker than cortex. ↓ corticomedullary differentiation in ↑ age and parenchymal disease (e.g., acute GN)
- Pelvicalyceal (PC) system is poorly visualized
- Bladder is examined when full. Normal bladder wall is thin and hard to delineate.

Table 1.3 Causes of abnormal renal size on imaging

Large kidneys
- Unilateral:
  - Tumor
  - Cyst
  - Unilateral hydronephrosis
  - Compensatory hypertrophy
- Bilateral:
  - Polycystic kidney disease (and other cystic diseases)
  - Infiltration (e.g., lymphoma, HIV, AIN, sarcoid)

Small kidneys
- Unilateral:
  - Congenital hypoplasia
  - Renal artery stenosis
- Bilateral:
  - Small smooth kidneys
    - Chronic glomerulonephritis
    - Chronic interstitial nephritis
    - Virtually any chronic renal disorder, except diabetic nephropathy
  - Small irregular kidneys
    - Reflux nephropathy
    - Congenital dysplastic syndromes
    - TB
    - Renal infarction

Intravenous urography (IVU)

This technique provides a good overview of the urinary tract, particularly the PC system and ureters (Fig. 1.5). It is good for detecting calculi.

The procedure
- Ensure good bowel prep, with patient npo for 4 hours pre-procedure. If GFR is normal, a fluid restriction of ~500 mL/prior 24 hours assists contrast concentration (⚠ dangerous if ↓GFR ∴ often avoided).
- Includes (film sequence altered according to clinical situation):
  - Plain control film (?opacities pre-contrast)
  - Post-contrast: bilateral nephrograms (delayed: poor perfusion, obstruction, ATN, venous thrombosis) renal outline (?ischemic scars, reflux, TB)
  - Further exposures at 5 and 10 minutes (PC filling defects: clot, tumor, sloughed papilla, stone; PC deformity: reflux)
- Mild abdominal compression delays contrast excretion and may improve PC system views.
- Post-voiding film is used to assess bladder outflow.
- Delayed films (2, 6, 12, and 24 hours) may establish a level of obstruction.

Modifications
- *IVU with furosemide:* furosemide exaggerates and distinguishes PUJ obstruction from normal anatomical variants ("baggy" pelvis).
- *High-dose IVU:* used if ↓GFR limits contrast excretion. Superseded by US and CT.

Contrast media

- Organic radio-opaque iodides excreted by glomerular filtration
- Nonionic, iso-osmolar agents are better tolerated than their ionic, hyperosmolar (~1500 mOsm/kg) predecessors.
- Minor contrast reactions (urticaria, itching, nausea, vomiting, sneezing, metallic taste) are common (5%–10%), especially if there is a history of allergy. These are usually self-limiting, but antihistamines may help. They are not necessarily associated with reaction on re-challenge.
- Severe reactions include ↓BP, shock, pulmonary edema, bronchospasm, and anaphylaxis. ▶ Access to resus equipment is mandatory. Mortality is estimated at 1 in 30,000 to 1 in 75,000; it is lower with nonionic media.
- Corticosteroids (e.g., prednisolone 30 mg bid for 24 hours pre- + post-procedure) are often used if there is a history of atopy or asthma (⚠ do not guarantee non-reaction).
- Nephrotoxicity is dose dependent and ↑ if there is dehydration, DM, preexisting ↓GFR, ↑ age, or poor CV function (📖 p. 142).

DIAGNOSTIC IMAGING 41

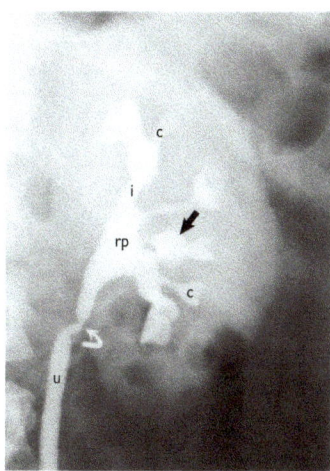

Fig. 1.5 Intravenous urography: magnified view of the left kidney. Calyx (c), infundibulum (i), renal pelvis (rp), proximal ureter (u). Calyx which projects posteriorly is seen en face (arrow). Normal fold of the ureter is at the ureteropelvic junction (curved arrow). Reproduced with permission from Davison AMA, Cameron JS, Grunfeld J-P, et al. (eds) (2005). *Oxford Textbook of Clinical Nephrology*, 3rd ed. Oxford: Oxford University Press.

⚠ Metformin

Ingestion in the 48 hours prior to an IVU → risk of lactic acidosis post-procedure. ▶ Stop ≥24 hours beforehand in all elective cases and recheck Cr at 48 hours before restarting.

Computerized tomography (CT)

More widespread availability, better image resolution, and progressively shorter scanning times have increased the routine use of CT in the investigation of the urinary tract.

Indications
- Characterization of a renal or perirenal mass
  - Differentiation of simple cysts from tumors (📖 p. 508)
- Tumor staging
- Delineate renal or perirenal collections and abscesses
- Renal and ureteric calculi (CT–KUB) (📖 p. 430)
- Trauma
  - Defines extent of renal and associated intra-abdominal injuries
- Retroperitoneal disease
  - Abdominal aorta, adrenal glands, retroperitoneal masses, fluid collections, lymphadenopathy
  - Investigation of choice in retroperitoneal fibrosis (📖 p. 506)
- Obstruction
  - Presence, level, and etiology (📖 p. 498)
- Parenchymal infection
  - Pyelonephritis may not show on US or IVU
  - Exclude associated pyonephrosis
- ✸ Renovascular disease (📖 p. 410).

CT angiography (CTA)
Software reconstructs 3D images of the intra-abdominal vasculature.

Electron beam CT (EBCT)
A tool for monitoring vascular, particularly coronary, calcification (📖 p. 187), EBCT is not widely available.

MRI

Indications
- Evaluation of a renal mass and tumor staging
  - Selected cases; e.g., venous invasion
- MR urography (the MR equivalent of an IUP—growing in popularity)
- Renal insufficiency
  - Gadolinium is not nephrotoxic and is safe when there has been a previous adverse allergic reaction to iodinated contrast.[1]
- ✸ Renovascular disease (📖 p. 410)
  - MR angiography (MRA)

---

[1] Very recently, MRI contrast agents have been implicated in the development of nephrogenic systemic fibrosis, a rare, painful, and often disabling, skin lesion that can progress to involve internal organs.

Nuclear medicine

Nuclear techniques provide functional as well as structural information (see Fig. 1.6) and can complement other imaging modalities. There are three types:
- GFR estimation (e.g., ^{51}Cr-EDTA) (📖 p. 32)
- Dynamic (e.g., ^{99m}Tc-DTPA, ^{99m}Tc-MAG 3): serial scans track renal uptake, transit, and excretion of isotope. A time-activity curve is generated.
- Static (e.g., ^{99m}Tc-DMSA): isotope is taken up and retained within functioning tissue. This demonstrates nonfunctioning ("scarred") renal tissue.

Radiopharmaceuticals
- **^{99m}Tc-DTPA.** Filtered at the glomerulus and neither reabsorbed or secreted by the tubules. A good marker of GFR, but limited utility in renal failure (Cr >200).
- **^{99m}Tc-MAG 3.** Principally excreted by tubular secretion, so useful if there is ↓GFR. Less background uptake than DTPA, but more expensive.
- **^{99m}Tc-DMSA.** Filtered at the glomerulus then reabsorbed and retained in the proximal tubules. Subsequent excretion is slow. Used for parenchymal imaging.

Applications
- Split function (DTPA, MAG3, DMSA)
- Congenital abnormalities (DMSA)
  - e.g., horseshoe kidney, ectopic pelvic kidneys
- Chronic pyelonephritis and vesicoureteric reflux (DMSA) (📖 p. 428)
  - Focal scarring (more than one cause)
  - DTPA-cystogram: reflux follow-up and sibling screening
- Renal transplantation
  - Perfusion and obstruction (📖 p. 240)
- Acute renal failure (📖 p. 68)
- Dilated vs. obstructed renal pelvis
  - A dilated pelvis may not indicate true obstruction.
  - Diuretic renography (DTPA or MAG3) may differentiate the two.
- Arterial occlusion (DTPA, MAG3)
  - Failure of perfusion
- Captopril renography in renovascular disease (📖 p. 90)
  - In renal artery stenosis, perfusion and GFR are maintained by AII-mediated efferent arteriolar constriction. ACEI blocks this and alters uptake and excretion of DTPA or MAG3
  - Positive scan
    —Asymmetry of size and function
    —Delayed time to peak activity
    —Cortical isotope retention
  - Sensitivity ↓ if there is bilateral disease, ↓GFR, or preexisting ACEI therapy (stop 4–5 days prior).

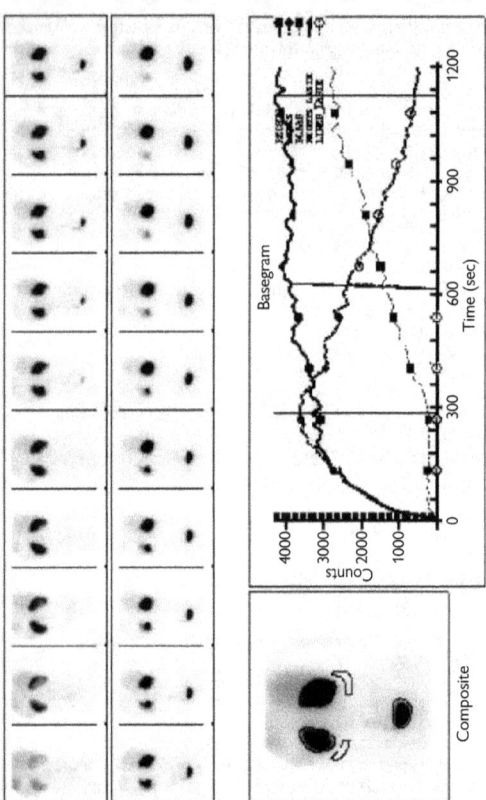

Fig. 1.6 Diuretic renogram showing "true" obstruction of the right kidney. The collecting system does not empty and the curve remains flat (note: ↓GFR causes slow filling of the renal pelvis and ↓ response to frusemide). Reproduced with permission from Davison AMA, Cameron JS, Grunfeld J-P, et al. (eds) (2005). *Oxford Textbook of Clinical Nephrology*, 3rd ed. Oxford: Oxford University Press.

Angiography and uroradiology

Angiography
This remains the gold-standard investigation in renovascular disease.

Technique

A retrograde catheter is passed under fluoroscopic guidance via a femoral puncture. A flush aortogram reveals the number and location of renal arteries, before selective catheterization. Intravenous digital subtraction angiography (IVDSA) is generally inadequate. Contrast nephrotoxicity (📖 p. 142) is a concern, but CO_2 or gadolinium are alternatives to iodinated media.

Indications
- Renovascular disease
  - Invasive ∴ not an ideal screening test (📖 p. 410)
- Acute renal ischemia
  - Acute emboli or thrombosis, traumatic occlusion, dissection
  - Therapeutic intervention (e.g., thrombolysis) may be possible.
- Unexplained hematuria
  - Vascular lesions (e.g., arteriovenous malformation [AVM], angioma). May allow embolization
- Classical polyarteritis nodosa (PAN) (📖 p. 482)
  - Intrarenal microaneurysms
- Renal transplantation
  - Evaluation of donor anatomy prior to live kidney donation (📖 p. 254)
- Bleeding postrenal biopsy
  - Identify bleeding source (± embolization)

Uroradiology

Urethrography and cystography

Contrast → urethra ± bladder. Indications are trauma, urethral stricture, bladder diverticulae or fistulas. CT cystography is increasingly used.

Voiding cysturethrography (VCUG)

A contrast-filled bladder and urethra are visualized during voiding. VCUG is the gold standard for diagnosis of vesicoureteral reflux [VUR] (📖 p. 428). It demonstrates reflux and dilatation/distortion of the ureters and PC system. Pressure-flow videocystometrography involves measurement of bladder pressures and urine flow rate in addition to imaging.

Retrograde ureteropyelography

The ureteric orifices are cystoscopically cannulated and contrast injected under fluoroscopic screening. The ureter, pelviuretic junction [PUJ], and PC system can be visualized. This technique may precede insertion of a retrograde ureteric stent.

Antegrade ureteropyelography (percutaneous nephrostomy)
A needle is placed percutaneously into the renal pelvis under fluoroscopic or US guidance. Contrast media is injected to evaluate PC, ureteric, and bladder anatomy. Urine → culture and cytology. Pressure studies can be undertaken in suspected UPJ obstruction (Whitaker test). (p. 500).

Indications include relief of urinary obstruction (p. 504), dilation of ureteric strictures, antegrade stent placement, and removal of calculi.

Ileal loopography
The loop is filled with contrast following the introduction of a Foley catheter. Upper-tract dilatation is common after ileal diversion and free reflux of contrast into the ureters is almost universal—if not, obstruction at the ureteric insertion (most common site) should be suspected.

Cysturethroscopy, ureteroscopy, and ureterorenoscopy

Cysturethroscopy or cystoscopy involves visual inspection of the inside of the urethra and bladder using either a flexible or rigid cystoscope. It is undertaken by urologists rather than radiologists. Indications include:
- Micro- and macroscopic hematuria
- Recurrent UTIs
- Unexplained lower tract symptoms
- Surveillance of bladder tumors

Flexible ureteroscopy involves passing a small, flexible fiber-optic transurethral endoscope through the bladder and as far up as the renal pelvis. Ureteroscopy provides for direct visualization of the ureter and renal pelvis and is used for obtaining biopsies and removal of stones.

Clinical syndromes

Proteinuria (p. 18)
Protein excretion <150 mg/day is normal; ~30 mg of this is albumin, the rest is low molecular-weight (LMW) protein, including β_2-microglobulin, enzymes, and peptide hormones. A small proportion is secreted by the renal tubules, including Tamm–Horsfall mucoprotein (uromodulin).

Why is abnormal proteinuria important?
1. It is a marker of intrinsic renal disease, particularly glomerular injury.
2. It is a risk factor for the progression of renal insufficiency.
3. It is an independent risk factor for CV morbidity and mortality.

What is the relevance of a positive dipstick for protein?
- Dipsticks predominantly detect albumin (p. 18). They test positive if protein excretion is >300 mg/day.
- Dipstick proteinuria has a prevalence of around 5% in healthy individuals (usually *trace* to 1 + range).
- Further evaluation is mandatory to distinguish benign from pathological proteinuria.

What is pathological proteinuria?
Persistent protein excretion >150 mg/day implies renal or systemic disease (see Table 1.4). The amount and composition depend on the nature of renal injury. Urinary electrophoresis can distinguish the source:
- *Glomerular.* Failure of the glomerular barrier allows passage of intermediate and high molecular-weight protein, the most important cause of proteinuria in clinical practice. The predominant protein is albumin.
- *Tubular.* LMW proteins, such as Ig light chains and β_2-microglobulin, normally pass through the glomerulus and are reabsorbed by proximal tubular cells. Damage to the proximal tubule disrupts this cycle and results in tubular proteinuria. Not detectable on dipstick examination.
- *Overflow.* Overproduction of LMW plasma proteins exceeds the capacity of a normal proximal tubule to reabsorb them. Causes are (1) Ig light chains in myeloma; (2) lysozyme in monomyelocytic leukemia. Dipstick examination will be negative—specific assays are required.
- *Secretory proteinuria.* Protein is added to the urine lower in the urinary tract (e.g., bladder tumor, prostatitis). Blood (>50 mL/24 h) will also cause proteinuria (not albuminuria).

What is microalbuminuria?
- Albuminuria above the normal range (>30 mg), but below the threshold of traditional dipsticks (<300 mg)
- A misleading term, implying that the albumin is of lower molecular weight–the *micro-* prefix simply signifies the low amount
- A sensitive indicator of (1) early renal disease and (2) CV risk in DM, ↑BP, and several other conditions
- Detected by radioimmunoassay on a 24-hour urine collection, ultra-sensitive dipstick, or spot microalbumin/creatinine ratio, p. 19.

When is proteinuria "benign"?

Transient
- Fever
- Exercise
- Extreme cold
- Seizures
- Congestive heart failure (CHF)
- Severe acute illnesses

Persistent

Postural (orthostatic) proteinuria is persistent.
- Normal subjects demonstrate a small ↑ in protein excretion on standing. Postural proteinuria is an exaggeration of this.
- Relatively common in young adults (~3%–5%). Rare over age 30.
- Usually <1 g/24 h.
- Diagnose with a "split" urine collection: 16 hours daytime and 8 hours overnight collection (simpler: negative dipstick on waking, positive at night).
- Renal function remains normal, even after prolonged follow-up.
- This condition remits with time (remains in ~50% cases at 10 years and <25% at 20 years).

Possible mechanisms include (1) trivial glomerular lesion; (2) ↑ circulating AII and noradrenaline when upright → ↑ glomerular permeability; and (3) renal vein entrapment between the aorta and superior mesenteric artery → local hemodynamic disturbance ("nutcracker" syndrome; ?also a cause of microscopic hematuria).

Table 1.4 Levels of proteinuria

Daily protein excretion	Cause
0.15–2.0 g/24 h	Mild glomerulopathies
	Orthostatic proteinuria
	Tubular proteinuria
	Overflow proteinuria
2.0–4.0 g/24 h	Probably glomerular
> 4.0 g/24 h	Virtually always glomerular

NB Proteinuria >3 g/24 h does not necessarily result in the nephrotic *syndrome* but is often referred to as nephrotic *range*. Proteinuria with accompanying microscopic hematuria strongly suggests glomerular disease.

Clinical consequences
Mild proteinuria does not produce clinical sequelae (Fig. 1.7). When it is more severe (>3–5 g/day) a distinct clinical entity—the nephrotic syndrome—may result. Heavy proteinuria may cause a frothy urine (↓ surface tension).

The nephrotic syndrome (📖 p. 50)
Urine albumin loss → ↓ serum albumin → edema (through a variety of mechanisms). The concomitant loss of other serum proteins → hyperlipidemia, thrombotic tendency, and ↑ susceptibility to infection.

Selectivity
Selectivity refers to the size discrimination at the glomerulus.
- Highly selective proteinuria
  - Only albumin and proteins of similar molecular weight
- Nonselective proteinuria
  - Larger proteins, including Igs.

Selectivity is calculated by comparison of IgG and albumin (or transferrin) clearance. It requires a sample of plasma and "spot" urine specimen.

$$\text{Selectivity index } \frac{\text{urine IgG} \times \text{serum Alb}}{\text{serum IgG} \times \text{urine Alb}} \times 100$$

≤ 10% highly selective
11%–20% moderately selective (limited discriminatory value)
≥ 21% poorly selective

- It may have a limited prognostic value—nonselective proteinuria denotes more severe injury to the glomerular apparatus.
- In children the selectivity index identifies the highly selective proteinuria of minimal change disease, circumventing the need for biopsy.

Microalbuminuria and cardiovascular risk

- Microalbuminuria is a marker of CV risk.
- It applies to the general population, not just DM or ↑BP.
- The mechanisms underpinning this association are poorly understood. Microalbuminuria, endothelial dysfunction, and chronic inflammation are interrelated processes that develop and progress together.
- Microalbuminuria can be correlated to the risk of stroke, myocardial infarction (MI), left ventricular (LV) dysfunction, peripheral vascular disease (PVD), and death.
- BP reduction is the key to microalbuminuria reduction—renin–angiotensin system (RAS) blockade with angiotensin converting enzyme inhibitors (ACEIs) or angiotensin-receptor blockers (ARBs) (or both) appears to be the treatment of choice.
- There is no present consensus on microalbuminuria screening in nondiabetics, although screening of hypertensive patients (and other high-risk groups) is increasingly advocated.

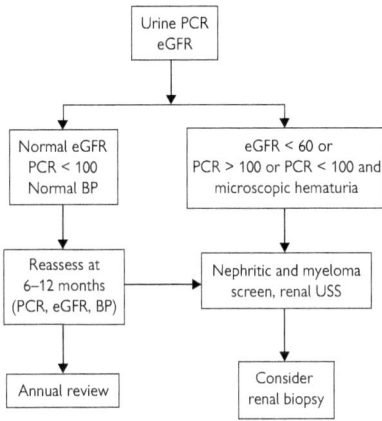

Fig. 1.7 Suggested management of asymptomatic proteinuria. Nephritic and myeloma screen: anti-nuclear antibodies (ANA), anti-neutrophil cytoplasmic antibodies (ANCA), anti-GBM (globular basement membrane) antibodies, complement components, hepatitis B and C serology, protein electrophoresis, immunoglobins, and urinary Bence–Jones proteins (p. 86).

Hematuria

This can result from bleeding at any site in the urinary tract. Causes range from benign to serious (Table 1.5).

Classification
Macroscopic vs. microscopic
- *Macroscopic*: Blood is visible to the naked eye. Gross hematuria startles the patient and ∴ presents early—the patient may not recognize blood and report discoloration (pink, smoky, cola, or tea-like). ▶ Macroscopic hematuria always requires investigation (presenting complaint in 85% of bladder and 40% of renal tumors). Heavy bleeding with clot formation almost never occurs in glomerular disease.
- *Microscopic*: Blood is only visible under high-powered microscopy. It is often found on dipstick examination in an asymptomatic patient.

Glomerular vs. nonglomerular
This classification provides a framework for considering pathology. Both forms can present with macro- or microscopic bleeding (particularly non-glomerular hematuria). Locally agreed nephrological and urological referral and investigation pathways are desirable.

"Transient" hematuria
- Exercise ("joggers' nephritis")
- Menstruation
- Sexual activity
- Viral illnesses
- Trauma

Table 1.5 Important causes of hematuria by age and source

Origin	Age <40 years	Age ≥40 years
Glomerular	IgA nephropathy	IgA nephropathy
	Thin basement membrane disease	Alport syndrome
	Alport syndrome	Mild focal GN of other causes
	Mild focal GN of other causes (e.g., lupus nephritis)	
	Other GN (variably present in membranous and diabetic nephropathies)	
Nonglomerular		
Upper urinary tract	Renal stones	Renal stones
	Pyelonephritis	Renal-cell carcinoma
	Polycystic kidney disease	Polycystic kidney disease
	Medullary sponge kidney	Pyelonephritis
	Hypercalciuria/hyperuricosuria ± stones	Transitional-cell tumor
	Renal trauma	Papillary necrosis
	Papillary necrosis	Renal infarction
	Ureteral stricture and hydronephrosis	Ureteral stricture and hydronephrosis
	Sickle cell trait or disease in black patients	Renal TB
	Renal infarction or arteriovenous malformation	Renal vein thrombosis
	Renal TB (?HIV)	
	Renal vein thrombosis	
Lower urinary tract	Cystitis, prostatitis, and urethritis	Cystitis, prostatitis, and urethritis
	Benign bladder, ureteral polyps, and tumors	Bladder cancer
	Bladder cancer	Prostate cancer
	Prostate cancer	Benign ureteral/bladder tumors
	Urethral stricture	
	Schistosoma hematobium	
Uncertain	Exercise hematuria	Exercise hematuria
	Unexplained hematuria	Over-anticoagulation (usually warfarin)
	Over-anticoagulation (usually warfarin)	
	Factitious hematuria	

History
- How much bleeding is there? Is the urine discolored or frankly bloody?
- Is there recent trauma? It may be relatively trivial, e.g., contact sports.
- Are there previous episodes?
- Is there a history of stone disease?
- Are there relevant medications? Anticoagulants should not cause hematuria if the INR is in the required range.
- Is there recent instrumentation of the urinary tract?
- Are there any associated urinary symptoms? Urinary infection?
- Is there pain? Sudden onset of colicky flank pain suggests a stone. Suprapubic pain may indicate infection or clot colic. ▶ Painless macroscopic hematuria indicates a tumor until proven otherwise.
- What part of the stream is involved?
  - Initial hematuria suggests an anterior urethral lesion.
  - Terminal hematuria usually arises from the posterior urethra, bladder, bladder neck, or trigone.
  - Continuous hematuria usually originates at or above the level of the bladder.
  - Cyclical hematuria in ♀ suggests endometriosis of the urinary tract.
- Are there risk factors for urothelial malignancy (p. 512)?
- Recent skin or throat infection indicates post-streptococcal GN.
- Episodic macroscopic hematuria with throat infections is a classical presentation of IgA nephropathy; p. 372.
- Has the patient traveled recently? Schistosomiasis is the most common cause of hematuria worldwide (don't swim in lake Malawi!).
- Are there systemic symptoms (e.g., arthralgia, rashes) to suggest an underlying inflammatory disorder?
- Is there a family history of deafness (Alport syndrome).

Physical examination (signs usually scarce)
- Is the patient hemodynamically stable?
- Anemia
- Bruising or bleeding (bleeding diathesis)
- Skin or throat infections
- Rashes, swollen joints
- Cardiorespiratory
  - Endocarditis
  - ↑BP and edema (glomerular disease)
- Abdomen
  - Flank tenderness (stone disease, pyelonephritis)
  - Masses
  - Bruit (AVM)
  - Testicles and prostate
  - ±VE (?misinterpreted vaginal bleeding).

Investigation of macroscopic hematuria
- Urinalysis
  - A negative dipstick in a patient with documented macroscopic hematuria should not stop further investigation.
  - In heavy bleeding the dipstick often tests positive for protein: interpret with caution.
- Urine M,C+S. Verify dipstick. Is there evidence of infection? Ova of *Schistosoma haematobium* (if relevant)?
- Urine cytology. Are there malignant cells? Casts and dysmorphic cells?
- CBC, urea and electrolytes (U&E), clotting, group and screen (G&S) (± cross-match when severe), prostate-specific antigen (PSA) assay, Hb electrophoresis in black patients.
- Imaging. CT is the investigation of choice. If this is unavailable, do an US + IVU.
- Cystoscopy (in all patients) ± ureterography, 📖 p. 46
- ± Angiography. This may demonstrate a vascular lesion.

Microscopic hematuria

Definition
Arbitrary. >2 red cells/hpf (📖 p. 20) (~10^7 red cells/24 h). It is usually a positive dipstick, not a cell count, that triggers investigation (dipsticks detect 2–5 cells/hpf).

Epidemiology
Reported prevalence varies widely (0.19%–16.1%), reflecting differences in the definition used and population screened (particularly age). Microscopic hematuria is common in both adults and children.

Predictive value
The proportion of individuals who have (or develop) significant disease depends on the group studied and the thoroughness of investigation. The overall risk of malignancy (2%–10%) is less than that for macroscopic hematuria (5%–22%), but ↑ with age.

Table 1.6

↑ Chance of malignant lesion	↑ Chance of glomerular lesion
• Age>40	• Proteinuria
• History of gross hematuria	• Dysmorphic red cells and red cell casts (📖 p. 20)
• Analgesic abuse	• Renal impairment
• Smoking	• ↑BP
• Alcohol abuse	
• Occupational exposures (📖 p. 407)	
• Pelvic irradiation	
• Previous cyclophosphamide treatment	

Evaluation
- See Figure 1.8.
- Casts and dysmorphic cells (📖 p. 20).
- Imaging: CT is the investigation of choice. If this is unavailable, a combination of US (used alone it may miss small stones and renal tumors <3 cm diameter) and IVU (used alone it may miss tumors not involving the PC system) is used.
- Nephrology workup: measure BP, CBC, UA, and eGFR; quantify proteinuria; consider nephritic screen (📖 p. 86) ± renal biopsy (📖 p. 635).
- "High risk": See left-hand column in Table 1.6.

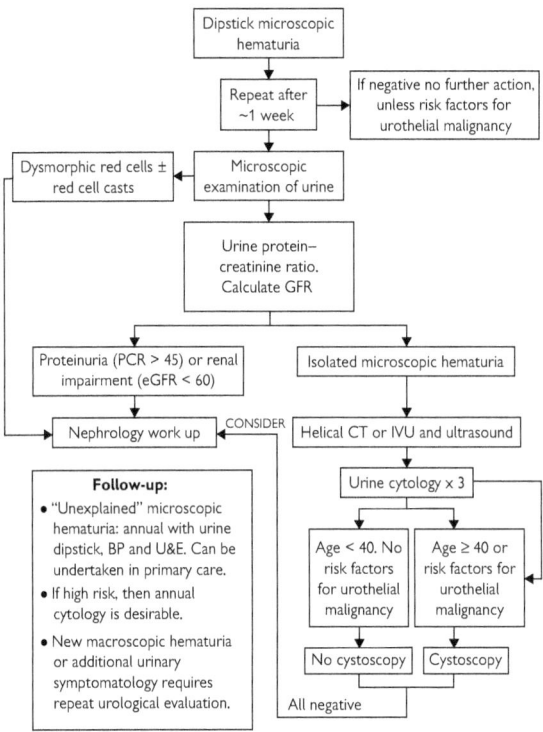

Fig. 1.8 Suggested management of microscopic hematuria.

Chronic kidney disease (see Chapter 3)

This is the end result of any process causing renal parenchymal damage. It implies irreversible reduction in the number of functioning nephrons and is characterized by progressive inability of the kidneys to fulfill their homeostatic responsibility (see Table 1.7). ⚠ Make sure reversible factors have been excluded.

Definition
CKD was previously termed chronic renal failure, with an arbitrary definition. Its definition was recently clarified by the K/DOQI (📖 p. 152).

Nomenclature
Uremia (or uremic syndrome) is the constellation of symptoms and signs produced as GFR declines (originally chosen to imply retention of urine in the blood). This is a multisystem disorder with a complex pathophysiological basis (📖 p. 166). Correlation of Ur and Cr with symptomatology is poor, so the diagnosis is part clinical, part biochemical.

Azotemia is used to imply retention of nitrogenous compounds. It usually refers to early CKD, sparing *uremia* for symptomatic patients. The term also attempts to play down the role of Ur itself.

End-stage renal disease (ESRD) is generally defined as a GFR ≤10 mL/min. The initiation of renal replacement therapy (RRT) is required for the patient's continued well-being (note: RRT does not have to wait until the patient is symptomatically uremic 📖 p. 167).

Table 1.7 Introduction to CKD

Stage	Description	GFR mL/min 1.73 m^2
1	Asymptomatic urinary abnormalities	>90
2	Mild	60–89
3	Moderate	30–59
4	Severe	15–29
5	Approaching ESRD	<15 or on dialysis

The uremic syndrome

Water, electrolyte, and acid–base balance
- Breathlessness secondary to volume overload and Kussmaul breathing secondary to acidosis
- Postural hypotension caused by volume depletion
- Effects of ↑ or ↓ potassium

Hematological system
- Symptomatic anemia and bleeding tendency

Cardiorespiratory
- Cardiac failure associated with fluid overload, ↑BP, anemia, and impaired LV function
- Accelerated atherosclerosis (angina, stroke, PVD) and vascular calcification
- Pleuropericarditis
- Cardiac arrhythmias secondary to ↑ electrolyte disturbances

Musculoskeletal
- Weakness, bone pain, and deformity secondary to osteodystrophy
- Gout

Nervous system
- Hypertensive stroke and encephalopathy
- Anxiety, depression, and other psychological disturbances
- Impaired cognitive function
- Peripheral and autonomic neuropathy
- Involuntary movements (including restless legs)
- Decreased conscious level and seizures (late)

Gastrointestinal
- Nausea, anorexia, and malnutrition
- GI bleeding (↑ peptic ulceration and angiodysplasia)
- Fetor, constipation, and diarrhea

Skin
- Dry skin, nail changes, and pruritus
- Bullous eruptions
- Pallor, pigmentation, and uremic frost (late)

Eyes
- Conjunctival calcium deposits and retinal vascular disease

Immunity
- Impaired cellular and humoral immunity (↑ infection and malignancy)

Endocrine
- Aberrant vitamin D and parathyroid hormone (PTH) metabolism
- Impaired IGF-1 production (growth retardation in children)
- Hyperprolactinemia (gynecomastia in ♂)
- Multiple other subclinical abnormalities

Sexual function
- Sexual dysfunction
- Decreased fertility

Other clinical syndromes

The nephritic syndrome (📖 p. 366)

Acute postinfectious GN, particularly following pharyngitis or cellulitis with group A β-hemolytic streptococci, provides a historical prototype but is now uncommon in developed countries. It may be associated with a variety of other conditions (📖 p. 376).

Clinical features
- Hematuria (usually microscopic)
- Proteinuria
- ↑BP
- Oliguria
- Circulatory overload and edema
- ↓GFR

Rapidly progressive glomerulonephritis (RPGN)
This represents the dramatic end of the nephritic spectrum with a rapid ↓GFR and (usually) oligoanuria. It is caused by an aggressive glomerular lesion with extensive crescent formation (📖 p. 366). Other renal diseases can produce an identical clinical picture (e.g., thrombotic microangiopathy).

▶ Seek expert help. Recovery of renal function is rare without early treatment.

Hypertension (📖 Chapter 5)

Hypertension in renal disease
- Underlying renal disease is found in a minority of patients with ↑BP, although the possibility should always be considered.
- ↑BP may be a feature of any renal disease, although it is particularly common in glomerular and vascular diseases.
- Hypertension has an important bearing on the progression of renal disease (📖 p. 157).

Renal disease in hypertension
- The normal kidney plays an important role in the pathogenesis of essential hypertension (📖 p. 291).
- The kidney is an important site of end-organ damage caused by ↑BP.
- The kidney has been described as both "villain" and "victim" in ↑BP.

Acute renal failure (ARF) (📖 Chapter 2).

Pulmonary renal syndromes

The combined presentation of acute GN and pulmonary hemorrhage is one of the most dramatic in clinical medicine.

Causes

ANCA-positive vasculitis (p. 458) occurs in ~60% cases. Anti-GBM disease, also known as Goodpasture's disease (p. 466), occurs in ~20%. SLE (p. 468), Henoch–Schönlein purpura (p. 373), and rheumatoid vasculitis (p. 476) are other causes.

History

The first report of a condition simultaneously affecting the lungs and kidney was presented in 1919 by Ernest Goodpasture, following post-mortem studies during the 1918–19 influenza pandemic. Four decades later the eponymous term Goodpasture's syndrome was adopted to describe comparable clinicopathological presentations. Subsequent realization that pulmonary renal syndromes are not a single clinical entity brought about further refinements to nomenclature—Goodpasture's *disease* is now reserved for lung hemorrhage and crescentic GN in the context of anti-GBM disease (p. 466). With hindsight, it is likely that Goodpasture's original patient had a systemic vasculitis and not the disease that now bears his name.

Clinical features

- Acute nephritic syndrome (rapidly progressive renal failure with an active urinary sediment)
- Features of an underlying systemic condition may be present (e.g., cutaneous vasculitis, sinusitis, arthritis)
- Pulmonary hemorrhage:
  - Cough
  - Dyspnea
  - Hemoptysis (extensive bleeding)
  - Anemia (and iron deficiency)
  - Hypoxemia and respiratory failure
  - Chest X-ray: diffuse or patchy alveolar shadowing (indistinguishable from pulmonary edema or acute respiratory distress syndrome [ARDS])
  - CT: confirms air space filling
  - Lung function: ↑ diffusion capacity for carbon monoxide (KCO)
  - Bronchoscopy: bloody bronchoalveolar lavage.

Other "pulmonary renal" syndromes
Pulmonary hemorrhage is rare, but respiratory dysfunction and/or chest X-ray abnormalities are common in ARF.
- Pulmonary edema
- Infection
  - ARF may accompany pneumonia and vice versa
  - A vasculitis patient receiving immunosuppressive therapy will be at risk of opportunistic infections including fungi, viruses, and TB
  - Hantavirus
- Pulmonary emboli
- Acid–base disturbances
- Acute respiratory distress syndrome (ARDS)

Changes in urine volume
- Polyuria: >3 L/24 h
- Oliguria: <400 mL/24 h
- Anuria: <100 mL /24 h

Polyuria
This is characterized by excretion of a urine volume in excess of normal; >3 L/day is an arbitrary cutoff. H_2O excretion is tightly controlled, so daily volumes vary widely in an individual.

It is usually frequency of micturition (especially overnight) secondary to the larger volume, rather than the volume itself, that causes the patient to present (although most patients with frequency do not have polyuria). Obtain a 24-hour urine collection for volume before undertaking further investigation.

Polyuria is seen in three clinically important situations:
1. Excessive fluid intake
2. Increased tubular solute load, e.g., hyperglycemia
3. Failure of the renal tubules to concentrate the urine (diabetes insipidus 📖 p. 530).

Oliguria
This entails passage of a urine volume inadequate for excretion of the end products of metabolism, <400 mL/24 h (~20 mL/h). The causes of oliguria (and anuria) are analogous to those of ARF.

Anuria
Anuria is passage of <100 mL/24 h, or the absence of urine flow.

▶ Address the following questions urgently if anuria is present:
1. Is the urinary tract obstructed?
2. Are the kidneys perfused?

Pain

Loin pain
Renal pain is usually experienced in the loin near the costovertebral angle. Anterior radiation may cause confusion with intraperitoneal pain. It may also radiate to the genitalia. Pain is usually associated with distension of the renal capsule and described as a constant, dull ache.

The differential is nerve root irritation (commonly T10–T12).

⚠ An aggressive and destructive renal disease may be painless.

Ureteric colic
This pain consists of sudden-onset, extremely severe (pale, distressed, unable to settle) colic. It is caused by a combination of ureteral stretching, local inflammation, and hyperperistalsis (spasm of ureteral smooth muscle). Pain may not completely fade between exacerbations.

Causes
Passage of a stone (common), blood clot, or sloughed papillae. Ureteral pathology that develops slowly or produces only partial obstruction may be painless (small stone → excruciating colic; large, nonobstructing, staghorn calculus → no pain).

The pattern of referred pain can sometimes help determine the level of ureteric obstruction.
- Upper ureter → loin
- Mid-ureter → ipsilateral iliac fossa. May → testicle in ♂, labium in ♀, and upper thigh in both.
- Lower ureter → bladder irritability (frequency, dysuria, urgency), and suprapubic discomfort. May → urethra and tip of penis.

The bladder
Suprapubic pain
- Usually overdistension of the bladder (acute retention) or local inflammation (cystitis)
- Cystitis: signs of bladder irritability (below) and sharp, stabbing pain towards the end of voiding
- Slowly progressive distension (e.g., neurogenic bladder) may cause no pain.
- Constant suprapubic pain, unrelated to retention, may not originate in the bladder. In ♀ consider gynecological causes.

Bladder irritability
- Dysuria, frequency, and urgency are among the most common symptoms encountered in clinical practice.
- Urinary infection, causing inflammation of the urethra, trigone, and bladder, is (by far) the most frequent cause (p. 424).
- ⚠ About one-third of patients with bladder cancer present with bladder irritability.

Tubular syndromes

A degree of tubular dysfunction may occur with any renal injury (though the clinical picture is usually dominated by ↓GFR). Several distinct clinical syndromes result from tubular defects in the context of a normal GFR.

Generalized tubular dysfunction (Fanconi syndrome)

Multiple tubular defects produce a distinct clinical phenotype referred to as the Fanconi syndrome. Components may be present to a variable degree.

- *Phosphaturia and bone disease.* Impaired PO_4 reabsorption → phosphaturia → hypophosphatemia. This, along with impaired 1α hydroxylation (activation) of 25-hydroxyvitamin D_3 in proximal tubular cells, produces skeletal abnormalities including rickets (children), osteomalacia (adults), and osteoporosis.
- *Aminoaciduria.* Amino acids are usually filtered at the glomerulus before reabsorption by multiple transport carriers in the proximal tubule. Fanconi syndrome → all amino acids appearing in the urine in excess. There are no clinically significant sequelae and supplementation is unnecessary.
- *Glycosuria.* The amount varies, but serum glucose is usually normal. Clinical sequelae are rare, although hypoglycemia occurs in some forms (e.g., Fanconi–Bickel syndrome or glycogenosis).
- *Renal tubular acidosis (RTA).* Defective bicarbonate reabsorption in the proximal tubule results in systemic acidosis (a form of type II RTA, 📖 p. 556).
- Na^+ *loss.* If severe → postural ↓BP, ↓Na^+, and metabolic alkalosis. Salt supplementation is occasionally necessary.
- *Hypokalemia.* ↑delivery of Na^+ to the distal tubule → Na^+ reabsorption at the expense of K^+. Acidosis and RAS activation by volume depletion also → K^+ loss. Clinical sequelae are common (muscle weakness, constipation, polyuria, cardiac arrhythmias) and supplementation is often required.
- *Proteinuria.* LMW proteinuria is common ($β_2$-microglobulin, lysozyme, and other tubular proteins), although excretion rates are usually low to moderate.
- *Polyuria.* Polyuria, polydipsia, and dehydration can be prominent. It is caused by ↓K^+ and impaired concentrating ability in the distal tubule.
- *Hypercalciuria.* Rarely → nephrolithiasis/calcinosis (?protective effect of polyuria), although these may be precipitated by treatment with vitamin D metabolites (further ↑ urinary Ca^{2+}). Serum Ca^{2+} is usually normal.

Isolated tubular defects

Renal glycosuria
- ↓ Proximal tubular glucose reabsorption → glycosuria (despite normal blood glucose).
- Clearance studies allow differentiation into different patterns implicating several defective tubular transport mechanisms.
- The amount can be quite significant (normally 1–30 g/24 h), but generally this is a benign condition with no clinical sequelae.
- ⚠ It always needs to be distinguished from DM.
- Genetic mechanisms are involved, but inheritance is unpredictable.

Aminoaciduria
- Causes:
  - Inborn error of metabolism → ↑ plasma levels and "overflow."
  - Renal aminoaciduria → defective tubular transport mechanisms. Amino acid transport is complex, involving transporters specific to single or chemically related groups of amino acids.
- The most important isolated aminoaciduria is cystinuria, a cause of recurrent cystine stone formation. It is autosomal recessive (📖 p. 430).

Phosphaturia
- Defective phosphate transport → phosphaturia, hypophosphatemia, and disorders of the skeleton.
- Several varieties are described, including X-linked hypophosphatemic rickets (vitamin D resistant rickets).

Bladder outflow obstruction

The main causes are shown in Box 1.6. The likelihood of each is influenced by age and gender. Presentation is with
- Acute retention of urine
- Lower urinary tract symptoms (LUTS)

LUTS are divided into two groups (see Table 1.8). Symptoms correlate poorly with underlying urinary pathology, so it is best to remain as descriptive as possible.

"Prostatism" is no longer favored to describe outflow symptoms (age-matched ♀ report similar symptoms).

Examination
Palpate for bladder enlargement, rectal examination, pelvic examination in ♀, examine the legs neurologically, and test anal tone/sensation.

Investigations
- Urine C&S, urinalysis (UA), and PSA assay (in males >40 years)
- *Imaging.* Bladder US to measure residual volume post-micturition (correlation to outflow obstruction is poor)
- *Uroflowmetry.* The full bladder is emptied into a flowmeter to generate a flow curve (rate vs. time). Normal max flow is >20mL/s. Further urodynamic assessment will distinguish nonobstructive causes of low flow (e.g., detrusor failure).
- *Pressure-flow studies (cystometrography).* These are more sensitive and specific but invasive. Bladder and rectal catheters record filling and voiding bladder pressures (normograms relate pressure to flow).
- *Videocystometrography.* This involves fluoroscopic screening of the ureters, bladder, and urethra. It is useful in the investigation of neurological bladder dysfunction.
- *Retrograde urethrography.* ?Urethral stricture.

Table 1.8 Lower urinary tract symptoms

Obstructive (voiding) symptoms	Storage (filling) symptoms*
• Impaired size or force of stream	• Nocturia
• Hesitancy or straining	• Daytime frequency
• Intermittent or interrupted flow	• Urgency
• Sensation of incomplete emptying	• Urge incontinence
	• Dysuria

* Also called irritative.

CHAPTER 1 Clinical assessment of the renal patients

Box 1.6 Causes of bladder outflow obstruction
- Congenital
  - Urethral valves and strictures
- Structural
  - Benign prostatic hyperplasia
  - Carcinoma of the prostate
  - Bladder neck stenosis
  - Urethral stricture
- Functional
  - Bladder neck dyssynergia
  - Neurological disease—spinal cord lesions, multiple sclerosis (MS), diabetes
  - Drugs—anticholinergics, antidepressants

Prostatic enlargement (p. 517)
- Prostate size correlates poorly with degree of obstruction on urodynamic assessment.
- Impaired flow is a function of two separate components:
  - Dynamic: ↑ sympathetic tone of prostatic smooth muscle
  - Static: mass effect of enlargement

Chapter 2

Acute renal failure (Acute kidney injury)

Definition and epidemiology 70
Causes and classification 74
Prevention 76
Clinical approach to ARF 78
Acute renal failure or chronic kidney disease? 80
Assessing ARF 82
Rapidly progressive glomerulonephritis and myeloma screen 86
Assessing ARF: imaging and histology 90
Prerenal ARF 92
Causes of prerenal ARF 94
Volume replacement in prerenal ARF 96
Intrinsic renal ARF 98
Acute tubular necrosis (ATN) 100
Pathophysiology of ischemic ATN 102
Management of ARF 1: a checklist 104
Management of ARF 2: hyperkalemia 106
Management of ARF 3: reducing total body K^+ 110
Management of ARF 4: pulmonary edema 112
Management of ARF 5: electrolytes and acidosis 114
Management of ARF 6: other strategies 116
Management of ARF 7: nutrition 118
Management myths 122
Renal replacement therapy in ARF 126
Prescribing acute hemodialysis 128
Peritoneal dialysis in ARF 132
The hepatorenal syndrome (HRS) 134
Management of HRS 136
Rhabdomyolysis 138
Management of rhabdomyolysis 140
Contrast-induced nephropathy (CIN) 142
Tumor lysis syndrome (TLS) 144
ARF in sepsis 146
Managing septic shock and ARF 148

Definition and epidemiology

Acute renal failure (ARF) is the syndrome arising from a rapid fall in GFR (over hours to days). It is characterized by retention of both nitrogenous (including BUN and Cr) and non-nitrogenous waste products of metabolism, as well as disordered electrolyte, acid–base, and fluid homeostasis.

Definition
- Despite its relative insensitivity to acute changes in GFR, most definitions have been based on serum Cr, either as an absolute value or as a change from baseline. Other definitions incorporate urine output (UO) or need for dialysis support.
- Until recently, there has been no consensus on a clinical definition of ARF, making it difficult to compare and interpret studies of prevention, incidence, and treatment. A survey of 598 participants at a critical-care nephrology conference in 2004 revealed 199 different criteria to define ARF, and 90 for initiating RRT.[1]

The RIFLE classification
- In 2004, a multilayered definition of ARF was proposed by the Acute Dialysis Quality Initiative (ADQI). In this model, ARF is stratified into five stages based on severity and duration of injury: **R**isk, **I**njury, **F**ailure, **L**oss, and **E**nd-stage disease (RIFLE), as shown in Table 2.1.
- More recently, as a modification of the RIFLE criteria, the concept of acute kidney injury (AKI) has emerged and is likely to be widely adopted as the standard over the next few years.

Acute kidney injury classification
- AKI is defined as functional or structural abnormalities, or markers of kidney damage (including abnormalities in blood, urine, tissue tests or imaging studies), present for <3 months.
- Diagnostic criteria include an abrupt (within 48 hours) reduction in kidney function as classified in Table 2.2. This assumes adequate fluid resuscitation and that obstruction has been excluded.

---

1 Ricci Z, Ronco C, D'Amico G, et al. (2006). Practice patterns in the management of acute renal failure in the critically ill patient: an international survey. *Nephrol Dial Transplant* **21**: 690–6.

Table 2.1 Risk, Injury, Failure, Loss and End-stage disease (RIFLE) classification of ARF[1]

	GFR criteria	Urine output criteria
Risk	Cr increased 1.5x or GFR decrease >25%	<0.5 mL/kg/h for 6 h
Injury	Cr increased 2.0x or GFR decrease >50%	<0.5 mL/kg/h for 12 h
Failure	Cr increased 3.0x or Cr >4 mg/dl when there was an acute rise of 0.5 mg/dL or GFR decrease >75%	<0.3 mL/kg/h for 24 h or anuria for 12 h
Loss	Persistent ARF; complete loss of kidney function for >4 weeks	
End-stage renal disease	ESRD for >3 months	

Acute renal failure is divided into three severity categories: risk, injury, and failure, and two clinical outcome categories: loss and end-stage renal disease (ESRD). Criteria can be fulfilled through changes in Cr, urine output (UO), or both (the measure leading to the more severe ranking is used). Note: the F component of RIFLE is present even if the ↑ in Cr is <3x, as long as the new Cr is >4.0 mg/dL (355 μmol/L) with an acute ↑ of at least 44 μmol/L (0.5 mg/dL). The designation $RIFLE_{FC}$ is used to denote acute on chronic disease. Similarly, when $RIFLE_F$ is achieved by UO criteria, a designation of $RIFLE_{FO}$ is used to denote oliguria.

1 2nd International Consensus Conference of the Acute Dialysis Quality Initiative (ADQI) Group; Bellomo R, Ronco C, Kellum J A, et al. (2004). *Critical Care* **8**(4):R204–12.

Table 2.2 Acute kidney injury (AKI) classification

Stage	CR criteria	Urine output criteria
1	↑Cr of ≥25 μmol/L (≥0.3 mg/dL) or ↑ to ≥150%–200% baseline	<0.5 mL/kg/h for >6 h
2	↑Cr to >200%–300% baseline	<0.5 mL/kg/h for >12 h
3	↑Cr to >300% baseline or Cr ≥350 μmol/L (≥4.0 mg/dL) with an acute rise of at least 45 μmol/L (0.5 mg/dL). Or on RRT	<0.3 mL/kg/h for 12 h or anuria for 12 h

Only one criterion (i.e., Cr or UO) needs to be met. If both are present, then select the one that places the individual in the higher stage.

Incidence

This depends on the population studied and definition used.

Hospital
- 7% of hospitalized patients
- 20%–25% of patients with sepsis and ~50% with septic shock
- By AKI criteria, ~65% of ICU admissions (mortality 43%–88%).

Community
- Community-based studies in the UK (Cr >3.4 mg/dl) estimate 486–620 per million population (pmp). Incidence is age and comorbidity related (17 pmp in age <50 years and 949 pmp in age 80–89 years).
- Dialysis-dependent ARF: ~200 pmp annually.

Prognosis
Mortality

Overall mortality in dialysis-requiring ARF remains >50% (reflecting a high incidence in the elderly and those with multiorgan failure). This rate is despite improvements in many aspects of clinical care (particularly nutrition and dialysis support). Using the new AKI classification[2]:

Rise in Cr	Odds ratio for hospital mortality
≥0.3 mg/dL (27 µmol/L)	4.1
≥0.5 mg/dL (45 µmol/L)	6.5
≥1.0 mg/dL (90 µmol/L)	9.7
≥2.0 mg/dL (180 µmol/L)	16.4

2 Chertow GM, Burdick E, Honour M, et al. (2005). Acute kidney injury, mortality, length of stay, and costs in hospitalized patients. *J Am Soc Nephrol*, **16**:3365–70.

Recovery of renal function depends on the underlying diagnosis. ARF is irreversible in ~5% (~16% in the elderly).

Causes and classification

ARF is caused by, or complicates, a wide range of disorders and may be the result of multiple precipitants (Fig. 2.1). Three clinical syndromes can be used to direct diagnosis and therapy.

1. Prerenal ARF
- Decreased renal blood flow (RBF) decreases GFR.
- Decreased RBF may be secondary to decreased effective arterial blood volume (decreased cardiac output, systemic vasodilatation in sepsis, splanchnic vasodilatation in cirrhosis).
- Glomerular hemodynamic changes may occur with medications (preglomerular vasoconstriction with NSAIDs, cyclosporine/tacrolimus, intravenous contrast, Amphotericin B, severe hypercalcemia; efferent vasodilatation with ACEI/ARB).
- Prerenal ARF is reversed by restoration of RBF.
- Kidneys remain structurally normal.

2. Intrinsic renal ARF
- The renal parenchyma itself is damaged through injury to the renal vasculature, glomerulus, tubules, or interstitium.
- The most common cause (by far) is acute tubular necrosis (ATN), which is the end product of an ischemic or nephrotoxic injury (p. 100).
- The diagnosis of ATN implies the following:
  - Glomerular, vascular, and other interstitial diseases are not responsible for intrinsic ARF. Be cautious; these disorders often require specific treatment and a delay in their diagnosis can have severe consequences for long-term kidney function. They may coexist with ATN. Seek expert help (e.g., anti-GBM disease) if you are uncertain.
  - Recovery of renal function should occur if supportive measures are adequate (so make sure that they *are* adequate).
  - There may have been a potentially reversible phase that has passed during which ATN could possibly have been avoided.

3. Postrenal ARF (p. 495)
- The kidneys may produce urine, but there is obstruction to its flow.
- Increased back pressure leads to decreased tubular function.
- Obstruction may occur at any level in the urinary tract.
- ARF results when both kidneys are obstructed or when there is obstruction of a solitary functioning kidney.
- Obstruction eventually causes structural (and permanent) damage.

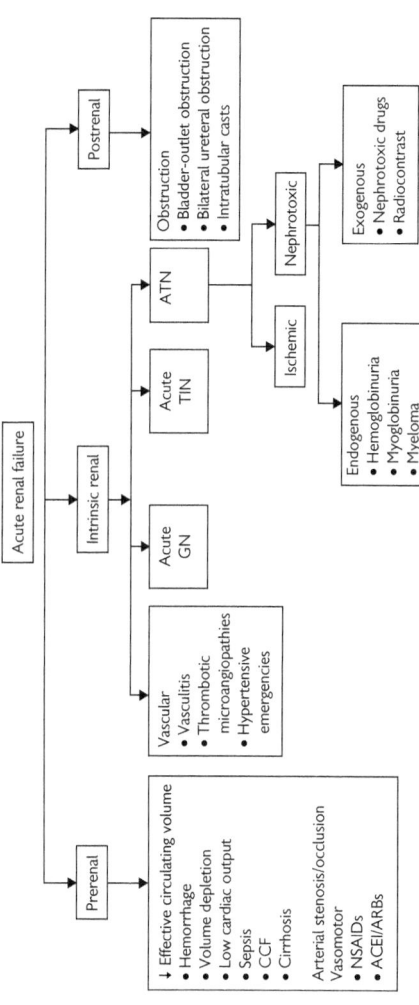

Fig. 2.1 Classification and major causes of acute renal failure. ACEI, angiotensin converting enzyme inhibitor; ARB, angiotensin-receptor blocker; ATN, acute tubular necrosis; CCF, chronic cardiac failure; GN, glomerulonephritis; TIN, tubulointerstitial nephritis.

Prevention

▶ Many cases of ARF should never occur in the first place.

Who is at risk?
- The elderly
- Those with preexisting renal disease
  - Increased Cr, decreased eGFR, or proteinuria (dipstick positive)
- Those undergoing surgery (especially if with another risk factor)
  - Trauma and burns surgery (hypovolemia, sepsis, myoglobinuria)
  - Cardiac surgery (poor LV function, intraoperative hemodynamic instability, cardiopulmonary bypass, aprotinin use)
  - Vascular surgery (suprarenal aortic cross-clamping disturbs renal perfusion and may cause atheromatous emboli to kidneys). Risk of emergency abdominal aortic aneurysm (AAA) repairs > elective (25% vs. <5% ARF).
  - Hepatic and biliary surgery (over 70% of lives transplants are complicated by ARF). Biliary surgery with severe jaundice is also high risk.
- Those with diabetes mellitus (DM) (especially if there is established diabetic nephropathy with elevated Cr)
- Those with volume depletion (NPO, bowel obstruction, vomiting, burns)
- Those with LV dysfunction and other CV disease
- Other causes of decreased effective arterial blood volume (cirrhosis)
- Those on drugs causing renal vasomotor changes (NSAID, ACEI, ARB)
- Those with jaundice (hyperbilirubinemia)
- Those with multiple myeloma (It may be that these patients are often dehydrated with a degree of renal insufficiency to start with.)

Common nephrotoxins
- NSAIDs, COX-2 inhibitors
- Diuretics, ACEI, ARB in volume-depleted patients or those with renovascular disease
- Antibiotics: aminoglycosides, vancomycin, pentamadine
- Antiviral or highly active antiretroviral therapy: ritonovir, foscarnet, cidofovir, tenofovir
- Amphotericin B (Lipid preparation is ONLY 50% less nephrotoxic than a non-lipid, and may still cause ARF.)
- Immunosuppressants (e.g., cyclosporin, tacrolimus) and chemotherapeutic agents (e.g., cisplatin, mitomycin C, ifosfamide)
- IV contrast (see 📖 p. 142).

Using nephrotoxic drugs
Use with caution:
- Definite indication
- No therapeutic alternative
- Precautions to minimize toxicity undertaken
- Renal function closely monitored
- Regular drug levels where possible (e.g., gentamicin).

Reducing risk perioperatively

Three principles
1. Avoid volume depletion (use 0.9% NaCl [NS] as replacement).
2. Avoid nephrotoxins (contrast agent, NSAIDs, aminoglycosides).
3. Review clinical status and renal function in those at risk.

- Optimize volume status preoperatively
  - No patient should ever go to surgery volume depleted.
  - Review daily weights, chart input/output, CVP, check postural BP if able.
  - Calculate losses, especially in patients NPO.
  - Use correct IV fluid replacement (NS, not 5% dextrose).
- Optimize blood sugar control in diabetics (sliding scale).
- Optimize nutrition (with parenteral nutrition if indicated).
- Catheterize those with prostatic disease.
- Avoid surgery if possible immediately after a contrast procedure.
- Stop antihypertensive agents (especially diuretics, ACEI/ARB) for 24–48 hours.
- Find out how the procedure and patient progressed in surgery. Check intraoperative records for blood loss, fluid, BP, and drugs administered.
- Review the patient early postoperatively.

Clinical approach to ARF

ARF occurs in the context of a wide range of underlying conditions with multiple possible causes, and the patient is often extremely ill.

Recognize the problem

Patients may be asymptomatic during the early stages of ARF, despite nearly nonfunctional kidneys. They may be very symptomatic by the time the diagnosis is apparent. This is why it is so important to be familiar with at-risk patients in high-risk situations (see p. 76).

Presenting features of ARF
Usually
- Increased BUN and serum Cr
- Decreased UO (UO <400 mL/day (oliguria) is frequent [~50%] but not invariable).

Frequently
- Volume depletion *OR*
- Volume overload: pulmonary edema
- Hyperkalemia (arrhythmias or cardiac arrest)
- Nonspecifically sick patient

Rarely
Uremic symptoms (see p. 166).

▶ Check renal function and K^+ in all acutely ill patients, especially if the following are present:
- Decreasing or low UO, or anuria
- Persistent nausea and vomiting, or prolonged NPO
- Drowsiness or impaired conscious level
- Signs of systemic sepsis
- Hypertension or hypotension, particularly if severe
- Pulmonary or peripheral edema
- Puzzling ECG abnormalities (peaked T-wave changes and conduction delays)
- Metabolic acidosis.

▶▶ Make the patient safe

Evaluate if the patient is critically ill as per protocol: airway, breathing, circulation (ABC). The standard priorities of resuscitation override thoughts as to the underlying cause. Two specific questions must be addressed urgently:

▶ How high is the K^+?
▶ What is the volume status?

Hyperkalemia (see p. 106) and pulmonary edema (see p. 112) may kill your patient quickly.

Look for a reversible cause of ARF

Consider the following questions first; relatively straightforward interventions can have a big impact in such situations.
- Is the patient septic?
- Is the patient making urine—if so, how much? What does it look like?
- Is it prerenal (see p. 74)?
  - Are there predisposing factors in the history?
  - Carefully assess the patient's volume and hemodynamic status (obtain lying and standing BP, if able).
  - Is invasive monitoring going to be needed? (usually not required)
- Is it postrenal (see p. 74)?
  - Are there predisposing factors in the history?
  - Is there a *palpable bladder* or symptoms of prostatism?
  - Arrange an urgent ultrasound
  - Determine if Foley catheter placement is required.
- What are the medications (see p 76.)?
  - Stop all nephrotoxins if possible. Check levels of suspected culprits (gentamicin).
- Has any contrast been administered, and if so, what volume?
- Have you looked at the urine (see p. 82)?

If there is increased serum Cr or decreased eGFR, is it ARF or acute or chronic kidney disease?

See next section, 📖 p. 80.

Acute renal failure or chronic kidney disease?

Patients are often found to have elevated serum Cr or decreased eGFR, or oliguria on presentation with unrelated medical or surgical conditions. Differentiating true ARF from stable (long-standing) CKD or even an acute deterioration on preexisting renal impairment is often very important.

Much is made of the ability to distinguish the two after an initial clinical assessment and blood tests. Many of these features, even when present, are at best suggestive and, at worst, misleading. The only two consistently useful discriminators are the following:

1. Previous measurements of renal function
    - Where could this be documented? Has the patient been admitted previously?
    - Search your laboratory pathology system and pull hospital notes.
    - Ask the patient's primary-care physician to send records.

2. Ultrasound
    - Long-standing renal disease leads to loss of renal parenchyma and decreases renal size.
    - Small (<9–10 cm in length), echogenic and often cystic kidneys are characteristic of CKD. Increased echogenicity by itself is not specific for CKD.

⚠ Normal-sized kidneys in patients with CKD should arouse suspicion of ARF. Exceptions are diabetic nephropathy (see p. 438) or amyloidosis.

Laboratory findings suggesting ARF rather than CKD

These are *rarely* as helpful as textbooks imply. Err on the side of caution (assume ARF until proven otherwise).

- Anemia might suggest a chronic decreased synthesis of erythropoietin by scarred kidneys: a *normal* Hb argues against CKD, but anemia occurs in both ARF and CKD
- ↓Ca^{2+} suggests impaired vitamin D synthesis (as found with CKD). However, disturbances of mineral metabolism may occur *rapidly* in ARF. ↑PO_4 may be due to either acute or chronic kidney disease.

▶ In many situations, particularly when renal size is normal, a biopsy may be necessary to determine the nature of the renal lesion and the extent of reversibility (📖 p. 638).

Assessing ARF

Urinalysis

▶ The urinalysis should be performed unless a patient is not making any urine. Always exclude bladder outflow obstruction. Different urinary findings lead to a diagnosis, particularly when suspecting glomerulonephritis. See Fig 2.2.

After collecting a urine sample for dipstick:
- ▶ Send a mid-stream urine sample for microscopy (or do it yourself) and culture.
- Consider spot urine protein: Cr ratio (PCR), urine electrolytes.

Urine biochemical indices

In prerenal ARF, tubular function is intact with avid salt retention, whereas in ATN the reabsorptive and concentrating capacity of the kidney is lost. Urinary biochemical indices (Table 2.3) can ∴ differentiate the two and are most helpful in oliguric patients.
- "Typical" prerenal ARF
  - ↓UNa, ↑UUN, ↑UCr, urine osmolality is high
- "Typical" ATN
  - ↑UNa, urine osmolality is relatively isoosmolal

⚠ In everyday practice, these indices are of limited value.
- They are not sufficiently sensitive or specific.
- Diuretics confound the analysis (→ dilute urine with ↑UNa content).
- Exceptions that by urinary indices appear prerenal, but are not:
  - Hepatorenal syndrome
  - Contrast nephropathy
  - Early obstruction
  - Acute GN and vasculitis
- They will often not influence management.

Table 2.3 Urine indices in ARF

	Prerenal ARF	ATN
Urine-specific gravity	>1.020	~1.010
Urine osmolality (mOsm/kg H_2O)	>500	~300–350
Urine: plasma osmolality	>1.5	<1.1
UNa (mEq/L)	<20	>40
Fractional Na^+ excretion % (FE_{Na+})[1] traditionally considered the best index!	<1	>2
Fractional urea nitrogen excretion % ($FE_{urea\ nitrogen}$)	<35	>50
Plasma urea: creatinine ratio	>10	<15
Urine: plasma urea nitrogen ratio	>8	<3
Urine: plasma creatinine ratio	>40	<20
Renal failure index[2]	<1	>1

[1] (urine Na/plasma Na)/(urine Cr/plasma Cr) × 100.
[2] urine Na/(urine creatinine/plasma creatinine) × 100.

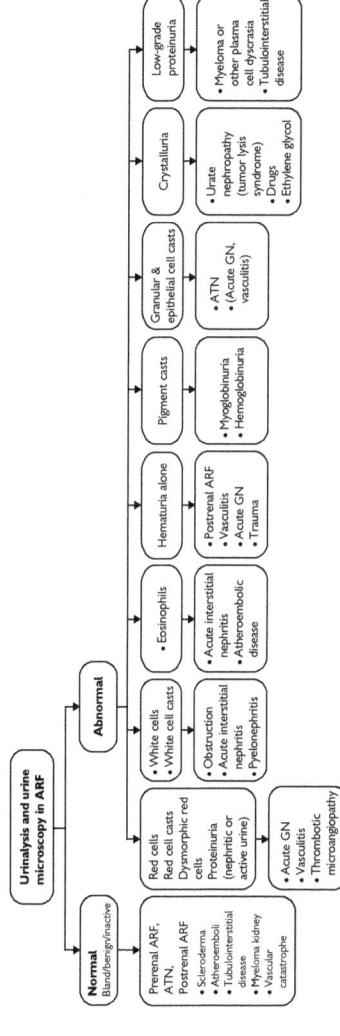

Fig. 2.2 Findings on urinalysis and urine microscopy in ARF.

Blood work
Managing and diagnosing renal impairment requires regular and informed testing. Order investigations sensibly rather than simply requesting everything below.

Hematology
- Complete blood count (CBC) and erythrocyte sedimentation rate (ESR)
  - ↓Hb develop early, typically 8–11 g/dL. ⚠ Hemolysis, GI bleeding
  - ↑ white blood cells (WBC): infection (rarely tissue infarction or vasculitis). Eosinophilia is an uncommon feature of interstitial nephritis, occurring more frequently with penicillins. ↓WBC: severe sepsis (rarely SLE)
  - ↓ platelets (Plt): disseminated intravascular coagulation (DIC) or thrombotic microangiopathy (→ check clotting and ask for a blood smear). ↑Plt: vasculitis
  - Pancytopenia: ?marrow infiltration (?myeloma or other malignancy)
  - ↑ESR with any inflammatory condition, but especially vasculitis
- Clotting
  - ?Liver disease (↑INR) or DIC (↑PT, ↑aPTT, ↑D-dimers)
- Type and screen if anemic
- Blood smear if ↓ plts, or ?microangiopathy
  - Fragmented red cells. If found, send lactate dehydrogenase (LDH), haptoglobin, retic count.

Biochemistry
- Electrolytes, BUN, and creatinine
  - ↑ BUN:Cr ratio may indicate prerenal ARF (but see 📖 p. 92).
  - ↑K^+ ▶▶ Needed urgently
  - Serum Na^+ is usually normal; ↓Na^+ may occur if there is volume overload or with diuretics.
  - ↓Venous HCO_3^- from metabolic acidosis (may not need arterial blood gas [ABG])
- Liver function tests (LFTs)
  - ↓ albumin may imply GN
  - ?↑ bilirubin, ?hepatorenal syndrome (📖 p. 134), ?acetaminophen OD
  - ⚠ ↑transaminases may be of muscle origin → check creatine kinase (CK)
- Ca^{2+} and PO_4
  - ↑Ca^{2+} is a cause of ARF (?myeloma, sarcoidosis, malignancy)
  - ↓Ca^{2+} and ↑PO_4 present in most cases
- ESR/C-reactive protein (CRP) as a marker of any infection or inflammation
- CK if rhabdomyolysis is likely
- Uric acid if tumor lysis or preeclampsia is possible
- Lactate to assess tissue ischemia or underperfusion
- PSA
- Others if glomerular disease is suspected.

Microbiology
- Urine and blood culture if there is any clinical suspicion of sepsis
- Hepatitis serologies

Arterial blood gas
A venous HCO_3^- may be enough to assess the acidosis of ARF, particularly if O_2 saturations are normal. However, have a low threshold for ABG, especially in deteriorating or critically ill patients.

Minimum ARF labs
- Urinalysis
- CBC, electrolytes, BUN, creatinine, Ca^{2+}, phosphate, albumin, LFTs, CK, and ESR/CRP
- Venous HCO_3^- or ABG.

Rapidly progressive glomerulonephritis and myeloma lab tests

▶ Order these quickly if a rapidly progressive glomerulonephritis or myeloma as an intrinsic cause of ARF (but not ATN) is suspected, as timely initiation of therapy is required, but use common sense. These are costly assays that careful clinical assessment can put in perspective.

Anti nuclear antibodies (ANA)

ANA tests are the serological hallmark of some autoimmune diseases. They are further defined by specific assays against target antigens (see Table 2.4).
If a clinical suspicion is strong, the specific assay may be necessary despite a negative ANA. ⚠ False positive ANAs are common.

Anti neutrophil cytoplasmic antibodies (ANCA)

These are a set of autoantibodies directed against components of neutrophil cytoplasm, characteristic of small vessel vasculitis (📖 p. 458 here are two patterns:
- Cytoplasmic ANCA (C-ANCA). Diffuse cytoplasmic staining on immunofluorescence. The antigen is proteinase 3 (ELISA assay for PR3-ANCA) (e.g., positive in Wegener's granulomatosis).
- Perinuclear ANCA (P-ANCA). Perinuclear staining on immunofluorescence. There are several antigens, myeloperoxidase being the most important (ELISA for MPO-ANCA) (e.g., positive in microscopic polyangiitis).
- Screening for ANCA in many labs is performed using immunofluorescence. Positive results are then confirmed with more specific ELISA tests.

Anti glomerular basement membrane antibody (anti-GBM)

This antibody is highly sensitive and specific for anti-GBM disease (📖 p. 466).

Table 2.4 Assays against target antigens in autoimmune diseases

Antigen	Association
Double-stranded DNA	SLE
Sm (Smith)	SLE
Ro/SSA and La/SSB	SLE, Sjogren syndrome
Scl-70	Diffuse systemic sclerosis (SS)
Centromere	CREST syndrome (limited SS)
RNA polymerase	Renal involvement in systemic sclerosis
RNP	Mixed connective tissue disease (overlap)

Anti-streptolysin O titers (ASO)

Post-streptococcal GN is the historical prototype for the acute nephritic syndrome, although incidence is falling (📖 p. 376). It is sensitive for the diagnosis of streptococcal pharyngitis, but less so for skin infections.

Protein electrophoresis (serum and urine)

- Serum: M band in multiple myeloma
- Urine: monoclonal light chains (Bence–Jones proteinuria)
- Free serum light chains may be indicated (📖 p. 446).

Immunoglobulins

Serum IgG, IgA, and IgM levels are of interest.
- Uninvolved immunoglobulins may be reduced in myeloma.
- IgA is raised in ~50% IgA nephropathy but is not diagnostic (📖 p. 372).
- Polyclonal ↑Ig occurs in HIV infection and Sjogrens syndrome.

Rheumatoid factor (RF)

This may be positive in vasculitis associated with RA (📖 p. 476), or in cryoglobulinemia with IgM (📖 p. 485).

Viral serology

This includes hepatitis B surface antigen, anti-hepatitis C antibody, and anti-HIV antibody.
- Hepatitis B is associated with PAN (📖 p. 482).
- Hepatitis C is associated with membranoproliferative GN and cryoglobulinemia (📖 p. 485).
- HIV may present with many renal manifestations.

Hepatitis B status is important for hemodialysis machine disinfection.

Cryoglobulins (📖 p. 485)

Send a sample if there is an unexplained rash, peripheral neuropathy, hypocomplementemia (see Box 2.1), known hepatitis C, known lymphoproliferative disorder, or positive RF (a useful screening test). The sample needs to be transported at 37°C, so either oversee lab handling or take the sample to the lab yourself (in a water bath—your armpit is second best) within minutes. Inform the lab that it is coming.

Antiphospholipid antibodies

These are not routine. They are associated with the primary and secondary anti-phospholipid syndrome (📖 p. 472). Request IgG and IgM anti-cardiolipin antibodies, anti-B2 glycoprotein I, and the lupus anticoagulant.

Box 2.1 Complement

Common investigations are immunoassays for C3 and C4 and a functional assay for the total hemolytic component (CH50). C3 and C4 can be used to screen for abnormalities in the classical and alternative pathways, with diseases associated with high levels of circulating immune complexes associated with hypocomplementemia. CH50 measures red cell lysis and is a good screen for overall complement activity (e.g., a patient with recurrent infections).

Disorder	C3 & C4
SLE	↓C3, ↓C4, ↓CH50
Infective endocarditis	↓C3, ↓C4, ↓CH50
Shunt nephritis	↓C3, ↓C4, ↓CH50
Post-strep GN	↓C3, ↓/↔C4, ↓CH50
Cryoglobulinemia	↔C3, ↓C4, ↓CH50
MPGN type II	↓C3, ↔C4, ↓CH50 ?C3 nephritic factor (p. 377)

Assessing ARF: imaging and histology

▶▶ Get a chest X-ray with shortness of breath or positive lung physical findings (pulmonary edema, infection, pulmonary hemorrhage).

Any clinical indication in its own right (tachypnea, ↓O_2 saturation, hemoptysis, occult infection, or suspected associated primary lung disease) obviously merits a chest X-ray, but much important information about ARF may be gathered:
- Cardiac size—?left ventricular hypertrophy (LVH) is consistent with long-standing ↑BP. ? Pericardial effusion
- Hilar lymphadenopathy, lytic lesions.

▶▶ Get an ultrasound (US) of the renal tract as soon as possible.

Imaging rarely makes a specific diagnosis. It has two principal aims:
- To exclude reversible obstruction (postrenal failure)
- To confirm the presence of two kidneys and quantify renal size. Renal length is used as a surrogate for the time course of renal impairment. Long-standing CKD → parenchymal scarring and loss of volume.
  - >10–12 cm = normal (∴ probable ARF)
  - <9 cm suggests CKD (▶ acquired cysts strongly suggest CKD)

▶ 📖 p. 498 for imaging in suspected acute obstruction.

Isotope studies in ARF

These are not considered first line, but they can occasionally be useful.
- Acute loss of renal perfusion associated with renal artery occlusion or embolism can be diagnosed with nuclear scans.
- Cortical necrosis (after severe hemorrhagic shock, particularly post-partum) is readily demonstrated.
- Early vascular complications in the immediate postrenal transplantation setting can be evaluated.
- In partial obstruction, delayed transit in the ureteric phase can be helpful, 📖 p. 43.
- A furosemide renogram differentiates a dilated collecting system with or without true obstruction.
- ARF vs. CKD—one may detect cortical scars (acute or chronic pyelonephritis).

Renal biopsy in ARF

Consider this after pre- and postrenal factors have been addressed. It is required in a minority of cases. Most intrinsic ARF is caused by ATN—histological confirmation will not alter management and prognosis, for renal recovery is generally good. The aims of biopsy should be to:
- Establish a tissue diagnosis
- Assess prognosis (?is renal function salvageable)
- Guide therapy.

Potential indications
- Unexplained ARF (initial assessment unhelpful/equivocal)
- Suspected glomerular disease (hematuria ± RBC casts, marked proteinuria, nephrotic syndrome)
- Serological or other evidence of systemic disease
  - ANCA, ANA, anti-GBM, complements, monoclonal protein spike, HIV, etc.
- Suspected thrombotic microangiopathy (HUS/TTP) if platelet count allows.
- Presumed ATN persists >2–4 weeks (especially if anuric)
- Preexisting glomerular disease
- Suspected interstitial disease (acute interstitial nephritis [AIN]) or drug allergy.

Intrinsic renal disease presenting as ARF
- Acute primary GN (p. 367)
- Systemic vasculitis affecting the kidney (p. 456)
- Infection-associated GN (p. 376)
- Thrombotic microangiopathies (p. 398)
- ATN
- AIN (p. 404)
- Myeloma cast nephropathy (p. 446)
- Atheroembolic disease (p. 414).

Prerenal ARF

Any cause of *apparent* volume depletion may compromise renal perfusion, as ↓RBF → ↓GFR. The kidneys are structurally intact, but functionally compromised. As a general rule, the metabolically susceptible proximal tubule can withstand relative hypoperfusion (and hypoxia) for a period of days (and often as much as 5 days) before true cellular injury supervenes (ATN).

Causes of hypoperfusion

Hypoperfusion is *not* the same as volume depletion. Renal perfusion is a product of effective arterial blood volume, cardiac output, and peripheral vascular resistance.

⚠ Any cause of a fall in effective arterial blood volume (📖 p. 94) will cause prerenal failure, despite the total body volume status of the patient:
- Hypovolemia
- Cardiogenic shock (or cardiac failure)
- Systemic (sepsis) or splanchnic (cirrhosis) vasodilatation.

Physiological response to hypoperfusion

Systemic response

Systemic hypoperfusion is sensed as an ↓ in arterial fullness by carotid and arterial baroreceptors. Activation of the sympathetic nervous system (SNS) and renin–angiotensin–aldosterone axis (RAA), as well as ↑ vasopressin release then act in concert to maintain BP and preserve blood flow to vital organs. This is accomplished by the following (Fig. 2.3).
- Vasoconstriction in "dispensable" vascular beds (e.g., cutaneous)
- ↑ cardiac output and heart rate
- ↑ thirst and ↓ sweating
- ↑ renal conservation of salt and water.

Renal response (renal autoregulation)

GFR is initially maintained because intraglomerular pressure is preserved despite the fall in systemic BP through renal autoregulation and is dependent on the balance between dilatation of the preglomerular afferent arteriole (prostaglandins and nitric oxide [NO]) and constriction of the efferent post-glomerular arteriole (mainly angiotensin II).

If perfusion continues to fall, prerenal ARF results. As RBF drops, the GFR and urine output fall as well. Below a mean arterial pressure (MAP) of ~80 mmHg, GFR ↓ rapidly. Lesser degrees of hypotension may provoke prerenal ARF in susceptible individuals:
- The elderly
- Those with preexisting afferent arteriolar pathology (e.g., hypertensive nephrosclerosis or diabetic nephropathy)
- Those taking ACEI or ARBs, where constriction of the efferent arteriole is blocked
- NSAIDS/Cox-2 inhibitors, where vasodilatation of the afferent arteriole is prevented.

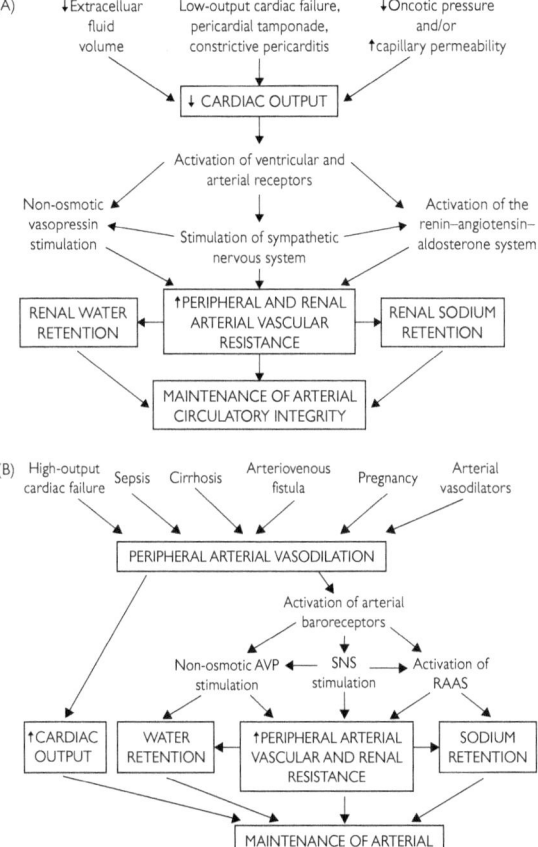

Fig. 2.3 (A) Sequence of events in which reduced cardiac output initiates renal sodium and water retention. (B) Sequence of events in which peripheral arterial vasodilatation initiates renal sodium and water retention. Reproduced with permission from Schrier RW, Chen YC, and Cadnapaphomchai MA (2004). *Neuroscience* **129**: 897–904.

Causes of prerenal ARF

Hypovolemia
This results from any cause of ↓ intravascular volume.
- ECF depletion (usually both Na^+ and H_2O depletion—when losses are predominantly H_2O, ECF volume is usually preserved until late)
  - Inadequate fluid intake: limited access to fluid (children, elderly patients with poor mobility, endurance sports), NPO status, inadequate IV fluids
  - GI losses: diarrhea and vomiting, nasogastric (NG) drainage, GI bleeding
  - Renal losses: diuretic therapy, uncontrolled DM (osmotic diuresis), salt losing nephropathy (rare—📖 p. 502), post-obstructive diuresis, diabetes insipidus
  - Skin losses: excessive sweating, febrile patients, burns
- Hemorrhage
  - Trauma, surgery (and surgical drains), GI bleeding
- "Third-space" compartmental losses
  - Intestinal obstruction, peritonitis, pancreatitis, major fractures

(*Third space* was originally coined to refer to a fluid compartment that is not in equilibrium with the ECF.)

Impaired cardiac output
- Cardiac pump failure → ↓BP → ↓RBF
  - Ischemic heart disease → angina or MI
  - Arrhythmias (including rapid atrial fibrillation)
  - New or established LV dysfunction (including myocarditis and cardiomyopathy of any cause)
  - Pericardial disease: ⚠ tamponade
- In CHF the ECF volume may be normal or ↑ (with edema and ascites), but the kidneys respond as though it were inadequate (↓ "effective arterial blood volume"). See 📖 p. 92 and 📖 p. 520.

Peripheral vasodilatation
- Septic shock causes failure of peripheral circulatory control (📖 p. 95). Systemic vasodilatation → ↓MAP → ↓RBF → ARF
- Interactions between intraglomerular vasodilating and constricting mediators resulting from sepsis also contribute to ↓GFR.

Splanchnic vasodilatation
- Cirrhosis causes splanchnic vasodilatation and renal vasoconstriction.

Intrarenal vasomotor changes
- NSAIDs impede prostaglandin-mediated afferent arteriolar dilatation.
  ▶ Postoperative patients are prescribed NSAIDs.
- Radiocontrast administration (📖 p. 142)
- Renovascular disease (📖 p. 410).
- ACEI and ARB oppose angiotensin II–induced efferent arteriolar constriction. ▶ Volume depleted elderly patient still taking an ACEI.

Is it prerenal ARF?
- Is the patient volume depleted?
- Is cardiac function good?
- Is the patient septic ± vasodilated, or cirrhotic?

Physical examination
Many signs have been described as representing volume depletion. Some are key to the diagnosis.
- Blood pressure: check lying and standing if possible.
- Heart rate
- Peripheral perfusion
  - Warm with bounding pulse → vasodilatation (? sepsis)
  - Cold and shut down with ↓ capillary refill → volume depletion or low cardiac output
- JVP: may be elevated with pump failure. *Not* ↑ with hypovolemia or vasodilatation
- Urine output.

Poor signs
- Dry mucous membranes (most sick patients mouth breathe)
- ↓ Skin turgor (better sign in children)

▶▶ Proceed to try and elicit a cause for the signs.

Classically
1. Volume depletion (hypovolemic or hemorrhagic shock):
   - (Orthostatic) hypotension
   - May be peripherally shut down
   - JVP ↓

2. Poor cardiac output (cardiogenic shock)
   - Hypotension with narrow pulse pressure
   - Peripherally shut down
   - JVP ↑

3. Systemic vasodilatation (septic shock)
   - Hypotension with ↑ pulse pressure
   - Peripherally warm
   - JVP ↓

Volume replacement in prerenal ARF

Prompt fluid resuscitation reverses prerenal ARF due to volume depletion. The key to fluid management is repeated clinical assessment of a patient's volume status.

Which fluid?
Crystalloids
NS is the initial treatment of choice in virtually all patients. Even in critically ill patients with capillary leak, early resuscitation with NS is indicated.

⚠ Ringers lactate solutions contain K^+ ∴ avoid in ARF.

Sodium bicarbonate
$NaHCO_3$ solutions can be useful in volume-depleted patients with severe acidosis (pH < 7–7.1). You can use D5W and 1–3 amps of $NaHCO_3$ or your pharmacy may be able to make IV $NaHCO_3^-$ 150 mEq/L. The underlying cause of acidosis needs to be treated. It is controversial if IV $NaHCO_3^-$ is better than NS for prevention of contrast-induced nephropathy.

Hypotonic crystalloids
Combined 0.45% ("half-normal") saline and 5% dextrose distribute rapidly throughout total body water and are of limited use for the restoration of intravascular volume. Avoid unless the patient has hypernatremia as well.

Colloids—human albumin solutions
"Physiological colloid" is expensive. Although a Cochrane meta-analysis concluded that its use was associated with ↑ mortality in the critically ill, the more recent (and well-designed) SAFE study suggested equivalence with saline in terms of mortality. Some favor it when volume depletion occurs in the context of hypoalbuminemia. It has proven to be of benefit in one situation—ARF in the context of cirrhosis with spontaneous bacterial peritonitis (📖 p. 236).

- Isotonic (4%–5%). Usually comes in 100–500 mL bottles. It is used to restore circulatory volume.
- Concentrated (20%–25%). Usually comes in 50–100 mL bottles. It is used to expand circulatory volume when general salt and water restriction is desirable—i.e., in an edematous, hypoalbuminemic patient who is intravascularly depleted (e.g., nephrotic syndrome, cirrhosis).

How much fluid?

The volume required to restore euvolemia is the amount that improves clinical signs of volume depletion. These might include the following:
- Improving tachycardia
- Better peripheral perfusion
- Improving BP (▶ postural drop). If ↓BP continues despite apparently adequate filling, consider cardiogenic or septic shock.
- Visible JVP
- Improving UO.

⚠ Beware of volume overload: ↑BP, ↑RR, lung crackles, ↓O_2 saturations.

How quickly?

Resuscitation
Infusion of fluids (± blood products) is required to restore BP and tissue perfusion. If in doubt, try a bolus of 250 mL NS IV, and reassess clinical parameters. Repeat as required.

Replacement
If a patient is not in shock, the optimal infusion rate depends on:
- Degree of hypovolemia
- Ongoing losses
- Whether the patient is oligoanuric
- Cardiovascular status.

The following is a *rough* guide to getting things under way:
- Give first liter over ≤2 hours, *then reassess*.
- Give second liter over 4 hours, *then reassess*.
- Give third liter over 6 hours, *then reassess*.

⚠ Slower replacement is needed in the elderly and in those with poor LV function. In the face of ongoing losses (e.g., diarrhea), input should aim to exceed measured and unmeasured (insensible, ~30 mL/h) losses by 100 mL/h. If you think you have overdone it, stop all fluids and reassess the patient.

Maintenance
Once euvolemic status is attained, and assuming there are no other losses, match UO + 30 mL on an hourly basis. Insensible losses will be higher if the patient is febrile.

⚠ Reassess the patient at least twice a day.

When do you need a central venous pressure (CVP) line?
- Not often
- Managing prerenal failure rarely requires a CVP line. Accurate bedside assessment is not difficult. ▶ Putting central lines into hypovolemic patients is not easy and offers a real risk of complication.

However, a CVP line may be useful in ARF in conjunction with
- septic shock and capillary leak;
- cardiogenic shock, or where the CV status is precarious and you feel it would be dangerous or unwise to give significant fluids without a more accurate baseline and continuous monitoring.
- The target for euvolemia is a CVP of 8–12 cm H_2O.

Intrinsic renal ARF

This encompasses all causes of ARF in which the renal parenchyma has been damaged. ▶ ATN accounts for 80% of all intrinsic ARF (Fig. 2.4).

⚠ Exclude or correct prerenal ± postrenal factors prior to diagnosis.

Differential diagnosis of acute intrinsic renal failure

- Vascular
  - ACEI + bilateral renovascular disease (📖 p. 410)
  - Renal artery occlusion due to thrombosis or dissection
  - Cholesterol emboli (📖 p. 414)
  - Renal vein thrombosis (📖 p. 414)
  - Thrombotic microangiopathies
- Acute glomerulonephritis (📖 p. 364)
  - Malignant hypertension (📖 p. 350) or scleroderma renal crisis (📖 p. 474)
- Diseases of the tubulointerstitium
  - Acute interstitial nephritis (📖 p. 404)
  - Cast nephropathy (complicating multiple myeloma) (📖 p. 446)
  - Tumor lysis or acute uric acid nephropathy (📖 p. 144)
- Acute tubular necrosis (📖 p. 100).

Is it intrinsic renal ARF?

▶ Have pre- and postrenal causes been excluded?

Vascular

History
- Cardiovascular
  - Risks: smoking, diabetes, lipids, ↑BP, age
  - Disease: claudication, stroke, ischemic heart disease (IHD)
  - Intervention: invasive radiological procedures or vascular surgery
- Source of embolus: atrial fibrillation, prosthetic valve, cardiomyopathy
- Nephrotic syndrome: renal vein thrombosis (📖 p. 414).

Examination
This includes atrial fibrillation, missing pulses, dilated heart, bruits, aortic aneurysm, ischemic lesions on toes, ↑BP (though very nonspecific), edema (?nephrotic).

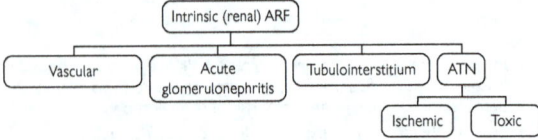

Fig. 2.4 Classification of intrinsic ARF.

Acute glomerulonephritis

History
- No other cause is evident.
- Recent infection: particularly skin or throat (post-streptococcal GN)
- Symptoms suggesting a deep-seated infection: fevers, night sweats
- Known or symptoms of systemic disorder, e.g., SLE, scleroderma, vasculitis
- Symptoms suggesting an underlying connective tissue disorder or vasculitis (p. 456).

Examination
Look for rash, ↑BP, edema, synovitis, arthropathy, uveitis, mouth ulcers, epistaxis or hearing loss, stigmata of endocarditis, evidence of scleroderma or other connective tissue disorder, and abnormal respiratory findings (pulmonary-renal syndrome).

Investigations
- Urinalysis (p. 82)
- Abnormality in RPGN/myeloma screen (p. 86)
- Renal biopsy is often necessary.

Tubulointerstitium

History
- Drugs (p. 5)
- Systemic infection: many are associated, including TB (p. 406)
- Systemic diseases: myeloma, sarcoidosis, Sjogren syndrome, SLE
- Uveitis: tubulointerstitial nephritis and uveitis (TINU) syndrome (p. 405).

Examination
Look for fever or rash, easy bruising multiple myeloma (MM), eosinophilia, eosinophiluria. The patient may have no systemic signs in allergic interstitial nephritis (AIN).

Acute tubular necrosis (ATN)

ATN is by far the most commonly encountered cause of intrinsic ARF. It is widely seen in hospitalized patients, and is predictable in high-risk clinical scenarios (so it is often preventable).

The diagnosis implies that prerenal and postrenal factors have been excluded (or corrected) and that other causes of intrinsic ARF, such as vasculitis or AIN, are deemed unlikely. It suggests that recovery of renal function is likely—but only if the causative insult is removed and adequate supportive measures are put in place. The kidneys are particularly susceptible to nephrotoxic injury because of their rich blood supply and a propensity to concentrate toxic substances within their cortex.

ATN subdivided by cause

Ischemic (including septic)	ANY cause ↓renal perfusion:
	• Hypotension
	• Shock
	  • Hemorrhagic
	  • Cardiogenic
	  • Septic
	• Vascular compromise (including aortic cross-clamping)

Nephrotoxic	• Myoglobin • Hemoglobin • Aminoglycosides • Contrast • Amphotericin B • Cisplatin • Others

Presentation

ATN presents as ARF: ↓GFR → uremia and disordered salt, water, and electrolyte homeostasis.

▶ ATN may be oliguric or nonoliguric.

It is a continuum from prerenal failure, though now with the following:
- Actual structural injury to the renal parenchyma
- Limited (or no) resolution upon restoration of renal perfusion
- Differentiation between prerenal ARF and ATN can be difficult.

Helpful features include (*not* uniformly present):
- Clear evidence of sepsis, hypotension, or nephrotoxin exposure
- Bland urine on dipstick with prerenal (or minor proteinuria)
- Urine biochemistry (*often* not helpful, 📖 p. 82)
  - Uosm ~300–350 mOsm/kg
  - FE_{Na} >2%
  - UNa >40 mEq/L

Histology

▶ A kidney biopsy is rarely required for diagnosis of ATN. ATN is a misnomer—necrotic tubular cells are uncommon. There may be few histological changes even with marked functional renal impairment. Typical features include tubular cell flattening, wide spacing of tubules secondary to interstitial edema, tubular cell vacuolization, loss of proximal tubular cell brush border, tubular cell sloughing into the lumen (→ obstruction), and mitotic figures in regenerating epithelial cells ± leukocyte infiltration. Glomeruli are normal.

Prognosis

ARF secondary to ATN imparts a significant in-hospital mortality of ~19%–37%. The renal prognosis is that:
- 60% can expect a full recovery.
- 30% can expect a recovery short of baseline.
- 5%–10% will eventually require long-term renal replacement therapy.
- Prognosis is worse in ICU patients requiring renal replacement therapy.

Pathophysiology of ischemic ATN

Vessels and endothelium
- Blood flow is not uniform within the kidney—pO_2 falls progressively from the cortex to medulla (10–20 mmHg), despite higher metabolic activity in the latter. ▶ The proximal tubular S3 segment and the medullary thick ascending loop of Henle in outer medullary nephrons are segments most at risk, along with early proximal tubule.
- Any cause of ↓RBF or endothelial injury may ↓ delivered O_2, rendering vulnerable segments of the nephron relatively hypoxic.
- As a result of endothelial cell injury:
  - ↑afferent arteriolar cytosolic Ca^{2+} → ↑ sensitivity to vasoconstrictor and sympathetic stimulation → impaired glomerular autoregulation.
  - Endothelial cell swelling compounds ↓ flow →O_2 delivery.
  - Injured endothelium (or endothelium under the influence of pro-inflammatory mediators (TNF-α, IL-18) → ↑ endothelial adhesion molecules (ICAM-1, VCAM, P-selectin) → ↑leukocyte–endothelial interaction → medullary vascular congestion → medullary hypoxia.
  - Activated leukocytes → local inflammation and local injury.
  - ↓endothelial nitric oxide production + ↑ endothelin and prostaglandin synthesis → enhanced vasoconstriction, further ↓RBF.
- The net result is impeded flow and ↓O_2 delivery to metabolically active and relatively hypoxic tubular segments (see Fig. 2.5): demand exceeds supply.

Tubular cells
- Hypoxic proximal tubular cells (PTC) now become energy depleted.
- Injured PTC generate proinflammatory mediators → recruitment of leukocytes into the interstitium with subsequent inflammation.
- ↓O_2 delivery leads to ↑Ca^{2+} entry into energy-depleted cells.
- ↑Ca^{2+}-dependent cysteine protease activity → actin breakdown → cytoskeletal disruption → loss of cell polarity.
- Loss of polarity → ↓basolateral Na^+/K^+-ATPase pumps and ∴ ↓ proximal Na^+ absorption.
- More Na^+ is delivered to the distal nephron, and sensed at the macula densa. This triggers *tubuloglomerular feedback* (📖 p. 614) → ↓GFR.
- Apical relocation of integrins → loss of cell–cell adhesion → tubular cell desquamation and cast formation → tubular obstruction → ↓GFR.
- Desquamation of PTC exposes the basement membrane and provides a route for misdirected filtrate, further ↑interstitial congestion.
- Necrosis ± apoptosis (*both* are present—ATN is a misnomer)
  - ATP depletion + ↑ reactive O_2 species + intracellular acidosis + ↑cytosolic Ca^{2+} + ↑ phospholipase activity → cell necrosis.
  - Apoptotic stimuli → caspase activation → cell apoptosis.
- Nitric oxide
  - Hypoxia → ↑PTC iNOS expression → NO release → cell death.
  - NO scavenged by O_2 radicals → toxic peroxynitrite generation.
  - (eNOS in the afferent arteriole *protects* against ischemic injury).

Repair

- Post-reperfusion, sublethally injured cells undergo repair and proliferation.
- Nonviable cells die (necrosis and apoptosis) and exfoliate.
- Poorly differentiated epithelial cells appear (?a population of renal stem cells).
- Viable cells enter the cell cycle under regulation of cyclin-dependent kinase inhibitors.
- Growth factors (IGF-1, EGF, HGF, TGF-β → proliferation and differentiation of tubular cells, restoring the epithelium to health.

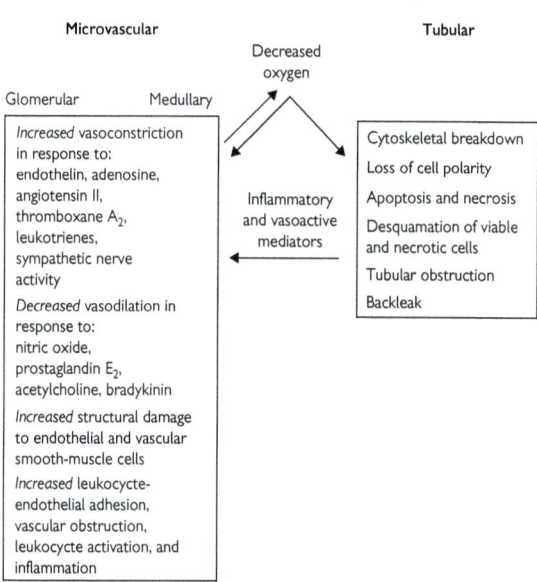

Fig. 2.5 Pathophysiology of ATN Reproduced with permission from Bonventre JV and Weinberg JM (2003). *J Am Soc Nephrol* **14**: 2199–2210.

Management of ARF 1: a checklist

The management of ARF depends on the cause. Nevertheless, as all failing kidneys fail to maintain salt, water, electrolyte, acid–base homeostasis, general principles of management can be described.

Where is information on:
- Resuscitating volume when depleted in prerenal failure? (📖 p. 96)
- Managing hyperkalemia? (📖 p. 164)
- Managing volume overload and pulmonary edema? (📖 p. 112)
- Managing acidosis? (📖 p. 165)
- Maintaining nutrition? (📖 p. 118)
- Instituting dialysis? (📖 p. 126)
- Specific causes of ARF?
  - ATN? (📖 p. 100)
  - Hepatorenal syndrome? (📖 p. 134)
  - Contrast nephrotoxicity? (📖 p. 142)
  - Tumor lysis? (📖 p. 144)
  - Septic shock and ARF? (📖 p. 148)
- Postrenal failure and acute obstruction? (📖 p. 495).

Have you ...
- Checked the result of the serum K^+ and acted appropriately?
- Assessed the patient's volume status and
  - are satisfied clinically and radiologically, the patient is not in pulmonary edema?
  - adequately corrected volume depletion?
- Performed a full history and thorough exam including excluding a palpable bladder?
- Checked a list of *all* the patient's medications? If an inpatient, have you checked regularly dosed and prn medications?
- Stopped nephrotoxins?
- Performed a urinalysis and C+S?
- Arranged renal ultrasound?
- Checked the Hb ± sent a type and screen? (required for renal biopsy)
- Tried to find any old labs (Cr, urinalysis)?
- Checked serum Ca^{2+} and PO_4 and ordered phosphate binder if required?
- Checked acid–base status and intervened appropriately?
- Arranged for the patient to be in ICU or step-down unit if intensive monitoring is required, with strict recording of fluid intake and output?
- Ordered appropriate diet (e.g., K^+/PO_4 restriction)?
- Discussed the patient with your nephrologist?
- Sent labs if ARF is from suspected glomerulonephritis or myeloma?

What you will be asked when you speak to a nephrologist

- What's the history?
- What's the potassium level?
- What is the patient's volume and hemodynamic status?
- Is there anything of note on clinical examination?
- What is the patient's acid–base status?
- What are the patient's medications?
- Is there any illicit drug use?
- What did the urinalysis show?
- Has the patient had a renal ultrasound?
- Does the patient make urine? If so, how much?
- Do you have any record of previous serum creatinines or urinalysis?
- What comorbidities does the patient have?
- Is the patient stable and in the appropriate monitored setting?

Management of ARF 2: hyperkalemia

In excitable tissues, ↑K^+ → depolarization of the membrane resting potential → Na^+ channel inactivation → ↓membrane excitability → neuromuscular depression and cardiac arrhythmias.

What is dangerous ↑K^+?

Chronically hyperkalemic patients may tolerate ↑K^+ of 6.0 mEq/L (but should certainly be treated if >6 mEq/L). Acute ↑K^+ is less well tolerated, particularly if they are among those at risk:
- Elderly
- Patients with associated cardiac disease (especially arrhythmias)
- Oliguric patients (cannot excrete ↑K^+).

Order continuous cardiac monitoring of all patients with ↑K^+ acutely >6.0–6.5 and enhance K^+ removal (📖 p. 110). Treat to urgently lower levels if ↑K^+ ≥6 mEq/L or there are ECG changes.

⚠ Always repeat K^+ to exclude hemolysis or artifact. In the interim, put the patient on a cardiac monitor and start treatment.

The hyperkalemic ECG

ECG manifestations of ↑K^+ are manifold (Fig. 2.6). ⚠ Mild ECG changes can progress to life-threatening disturbances very quickly. All may be exacerbated by coexisting ↓Ca^{2+} and acidosis.

⚠ A normal ECG does *not* rule out cardiac instability.

- Peaking of T waves ("tenting")
- Flattening and disappearance of P waves
- Prolonged PR interval (primary heart block)
- Progressive widening of the QRS complex
- Deepened S waves and merging of S and T waves
- Idioventricular rhythm
- Sine wave pattern
- Ventricular fibrillation (VF) and asystolic cardiac arrest.

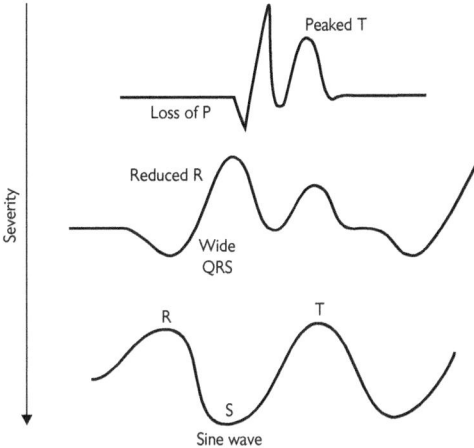

Fig. 2.6 The ECG changes of hyperkalemia.

Treatment of severe hyperkalemia

The following measures will reduce serum K^+ acutely, but NOT affect the elevated total body K^+. Longer-term measures described in the next section are needed in conjunction with emergency treatment.

Calcium
- If $K^+ \geq 6.5$ mEq/L or severe ECG changes (e.g., widened QRS)
- Antagonizes membrane effects of ↑K^+ by a poorly understood mechanism
- 10 mL 10% calcium gluconate (usually 1 ampule—calcium gluconate contains 8.9 mg Ca^{2+}/mL), or 5 mL 10% calcium chloride (usually 1/2 an ampule—$CaCl_2$ 27.5 mg Ca^{2+}/mL)
- Give over 2–5 min. Repeat if there is no ECG improvement after 5 min (up to 40 mL calcium gluconate).
- Acts within minutes but *protective effect lasts <1 hour*
- ⚠ Can induce digitalis toxicity (→ a pragmatic approach: half the initial dose and give more slowly if taking digoxin)

▶ Ca^{2+} is cardioprotective—it does not ↓K^+.

Insulin and glucose
- If $K^+ \geq 6$–6.5 mEq/L or ECG changes
- Insulin in binding its cellular receptor → ↑Na-K-ATPase activity, moving K^+ into cells. Glucose alone will ↓K^+ through endogenous insulin release, but insulin/glucose is more effective.
- 10 units insulin with 50 mL of 50% glucose/dextrose IV over 10 min. Watch carefully for hypoglycemia.
- Expect effect within 10–20 min (peak ~60 min), lasts for 2–4 *hours*. Expect a ↓ of 0.5–1.5 mEq/L.
- Check glucose regularly for 6 hours and infuse 10% dextrose IVI if ↓glucose.
- Can be repeated after 4 *hours*, but should aim for increased K^+ excretion.

Sodium bicarbonate—*usually ineffective as monotherapy*
- If ↑K^+ in the presence of severe acidosis (pH <7.1–7.2).
- ↑Na^+/H^+ exchange → ↑intracellular [Na^+] → ↑Na-K-ATPase activity (i.e., K^+ in for Na^+ out). Additional pH-independent mechanisms.
- Isotonic or ampules (50 mL of 8.4%) IV.
- Unless the patient is severely acidotic, it may have no effect, and if efficacious, it may take hours, not minutes.
- Presents an appreciable Na^+ load (in isotonic solution, 150 mEq/L Na^+ ⚠ Volume overload).
- Rapid correction of acidosis in a patient with ↓Ca^{2+} may induce tetany and seizures as ionized calcium drops rapidly as pH↑.

Reasons not to use β_2-agonists (albuterol)

A dose of 10–20 mg (i.e., big dose) of nebulized albuterol will ↓ serum K^+ by 0.6 to 1 mEq/L by activating Na–K–ATPase, but fails if given as monotherapy in 33%–40% of patients with slower onset of action.

⚠ It may precipitate arrhythmias in those with underlying cardiac disease (2–8 times dose given by nebulizer).

Management of ARF 3: reducing total body K^+

Once (if) the immediate arrhythmic danger is past after shifting K^+ into cells, the aim should be to reduce total body potassium to prevent further hyperkalemic episodes.

1. Urinary K^+ wasting: diuretics
- Only useful in patients expected to make urine, and urine into which K^+ can be excreted. It is particularly useful if the patient is also volume overloaded.
- Acts at renal tubule—K^+ loss is one of several effects.
- Usually furosemide 40–200 mg IV as a bolus, with 10–40 mg/h if patient responds to bolus to a maximum of 800 mg/day. Bumetanide offers a better absorbed oral alternative in CKD, but there is no advantage of IV bumetanide over furosemide.
- Effect depends on onset of diuresis. Patients can lose substantial amounts of K^+ over 24 *hours* with a UO >2 L/day.
- *Much* less effective as GFR deteriorates, as in most patients with hyperkalemia.

2. Gut K^+ removal: cation exchange resins
- Exchanges Na^+ (and small amount of Ca^{2+}) for K^+ in the ileum and colon, so this removes K^+ rather than just redistributing it.
- Sodium polystyrene sulphonate (SPS) (Kayexalate®). Usually give 15–30 g orally (supplied as 60–120 mL of a 20% sorbitol solution) or 50 g suspended in 50 mL of 70% sorbitol + 100 mL water rectally, retained for at least 30–60 min.
- Modest effect seen within 24–48 *hours*. A dose of 60 g on average reduces serum K^+ 1 mEq/L in ARF and 0.6 mEq/L in CKD.
- May cause colonic ulceration and necrosis with ileus (contraindicated in postoperative patients with an ileus or using high doses of opiates).

3. Extracorporeal K^+ removal: dialysis
- If K^+ >6.0–6.5 mEq/L and renal function cannot rapidly be restored
- Lowers K^+ within minutes
- Hemodialysis (HD) using a dialysate K^+ of 0–2 mEql/L is a potent means of removing K^+.
- Continuous renal replacement therapies (p. 126) can lower K^+, though much more slowly.
- Peritoneal dialysis is effective, but rarely indicated acutely (p. 228).
- Does require dialysis access and setup of dialysis or continuous renal replacement machine.

4. Further management

The aim is to prevent further dangerous increases.
- Restrict oral K^+ intake to <60 mEq/day. ▶ Speak to your dietitian (📖 p. 198). K^+ content of enteral and parenteral feeds may need modification.
- No K^+ in IV fluids
- Avoid, if possible, K^+-sparing diuretics, ACEI, ARB, spironolactone, heparin, β-blockers, trimethoprim/sulfamethoxazole, and NSAIDs.
- Refractory ↑K^+ is an indication for dialysis.
- If ↑K^+ persists despite dialysis then do the following:
  - Review dietary intake and compliance.
  - Check for GI or occult bleeding (reabsorbed red cells are rich in K^+) or hemolysis.
  - Exclude concealed tissue or muscle damage (e.g., rhabdomyolysis).
  - Review dialysis access and adequacy (📖 p. 218) and check the dialysate K^+ concentration (📖 p. 217).
  - Recheck the medication chart.

Transfusion

⚠ Caution is needed when transfusing a patient with ARF, particularly if oligoanuric. The volume and K^+ content of red cell transfusions can precipitate pulmonary edema and hyperkalemia, respectively. If the patient requires renal replacement therapy, then transfusions are safest during this time.

Management of ARF 4: pulmonary edema

Oliguric or anuric patients rapidly accumulate sodium and water unless (and even if) they are tightly fluid restricted. Volume overload, often exacerbated iatrogenically, remains a relatively common complication of ARF.

In ARF, the heart is often structurally normal, but sodium and water overload push the heart along the Starling curve. Many patients with ARF may have poor underlying cardiac dysfunction, resulting in high mortality.

Findings

The patient may be cool, clammy, and agitated, with tachycardia, tachypnea, ↑JVP, ↑BP (↓BP in this context is worrying), gallop rhythm, respiratory crackles and wheezes. They may have ascites, pleural effusions and peripheral edema.

Investigations reveal
- Poor O_2 saturation
- Hypoxemia on ABGs
- Chest X-ray showing pulmonary vascular redistribution to alveolar edema.

Management

- Sit the patient up and stop all IV infusions.
- *Oxygen*: Maintain S_aO_2 >95% with nasal canula, non-rebreather face mask, or continuous positive airway pressure (CPAP) if available.
- *Opiates*: Give IV morphine (2–4 mg) as an anxiolytic and venodilator. This can be repeated after 15 min, but opiates accumulate in ARF so resist from giving further doses.
- *Nitrates*: If the systolic BP ≥100 mmHg, start IV nitroglycerin 2–10 mg/h. Start low and titrate every 10 min as tolerated. If systolic BP is <90 mmHg (i.e., ?cardiogenic shock) warn ICU and consider inotropes.
- *Diuretics* (📖 p. 332): Give furosemide IV over 1 *hour* (or partial dose) at a rate not exceeding 4 mg/min to avoid ototoxicity. If this initiates a good diuresis (peak within 30 min), you can follow with a further bolus 6 hours later. If diuresis occurs, but is suboptimal, start a continuous drip and consider adding chlorothiazide IV. If there is no response, refer patient for dialysis.
- *Dialysis*: Oligoanuric patients are likely to need renal replacement therapy (📖 p. 126).
- Consider transfer of patient to ICU.

How to give loop diuretics in ARF

Give 200 mg furosemide IV via infusion pump (rate not exceeding 4 mg/min to avoid ototoxicity).
- If this initiates an adequate diuresis, usually peak after 30 min, give a further 200 mg 6 *hours* later.
- If there is no response, further doses are likely to be futile.
  (▶ Dialysis?)

If there is a reasonable, but transient response, then a continuous infusion 10–40 mg/h over 24 *hours* may promote ongoing diuresis. (Consider adding chlorothiazide 250–500 mg IV).

Consider ventilatory support if there is
- Continuing severe breathlessness
- Falling respiratory rate (tiring patient)
- Hypoxemia and/or rising $PaCO_2$
- Worsening acidosis (pH <7.2).

Continuous positive airways pressure (CPAP)
This provides a constant positive pressure support throughout the respiratory cycle (typically 5–10 cm H_2O), allowing delivery of a higher FiO_2 (80%–100%) and a ↓ in the work of breathing.

⚠ Patients must be conscious, able to protect their airway, and possess sufficient respiratory muscle strength.

Endotracheal intubation and mechanical ventilation
These procedures are carried out in the ICU, probably with positive end-expiratory pressure (PEEP). A preset pressure is added to the end of expiration to prevent airway/alveolar collapse and open up the atelectatic and fluid-filled lung. The tradeoff is a potential ↓ in cardiac output (through ↓ venous return).

Management of ARF 5: electrolytes and acidosis

Hyperphosphatemia

A ↓ in urinary PO_4 excretion → ↑serum PO_4. Particularly marked elevations occur in rhabdomyolysis (□ p. 138), tumor lysis syndrome (□ p. 145), and, rarely, severe hemolysis (tissue injury and cell death → release of intracellular PO_4).

Acute ↑PO_4 is important because it
- Contributes to ↓Ca^{2+} (by a poorly understood mechanism).
- Contributes to secondary hyperparathyroidism.
- Promotes soft tissue/vascular calcification (especially $Ca \times PO_4$ product >55).
- May make the patient pruritic, weak, and anorexic, and severe hyperphosphatemia may contribute to ARF (tumor lysis syndrome).
- May cause arrhythmias.

Treatment (see also □ p. 184)
- Dietary restriction of phosphate (<800 mg/day, □ p. 198)
- Removal wih hemodialysis or continuous renal replacement therapy.
- Oral phosphate binders (reduce intestinal absorption of phosphate)
  - If both ↓Ca^{2+} and ↑PO_4^{2-}, start calcium acetate (667 mg) or calcium carbonate.
  - If patient is hyperphosphatemic and PO_4<6.0 mg/dL, give 1 tablet with each meal.
  - If PO_4>6, give 2–3 tablets with each meal.
- If Ca^{2+}≥9.6, use sevelamer HCl (0.8–2.4 g with meals). Aluminum-based binders may lead to Al toxicity if used >4 weeks—avoid. This agent cannot be crushed (i.e., can't be used with an NG tube).
- Lanthanum chloride is another non-calcium-based phosphate binder that may be used (750–3000 mg/day in divided doses).
- Severe ↑PO_4 may not correct until the patient is on renal replacement therapy or recovers renal function.
- If the patient is being NG or parenterally fed, speak to your dietitian.

Hypocalcemia

Hypocalcemia is common in prolonged or severe ARF. It is caused mainly by ↓1, hydroxylation of 25OH vitamin D synthesis, but also by ↑PO_4. It occurs usually in the corrected range of 6.4–8 mg/dL. Clinical sequelae (e.g., paraesthesia, tetany and seizures) are rare, partly because concomitant acidosis protects by increasing the ratio of ionized to protein bound Ca^{2+}.

⚠ Rapid correction of acidosis with oral or IV HCO_3^- can precipitate symptomatic ↓Ca^{2+}.

Calcium is supplemented orally for concomitant hyperphosphatemia (as above)—the dual phosphate-binding role of calcium salts makes life simple. IV Ca^{2+} (e.g., calcium gluconate) is virtually never required. If Ca^{2+}<8 mg/day/L and the patient is also hypophosphatemic (rare), use calcium carbonate between meals, which will give Ca^{2+} without binding PO_4.

MANAGEMENT OF ARF 5: ELECTROLYTES AND ACIDOSIS

⚠ In rhabdomyolysis (📖 p. 138), Ca^{2+} can precipitate in injured muscle, causing necrosis and ischemic contractures—resist administration of Ca^{2+} unless patient is symptomatic.

Other electrolyte abnormalities found with ARF

Hypokalemia Rare in ARF, but can accompany nonoliguric ATN caused by tubular toxins (e.g., aminoglycosides, amphotericin, cisplatin). It may also develop as GFR recovers, especially if there is polyuria.

Hypomagnesemia ↓Mg^{2+} occasionally occurs with nonoliguric ATN. It is usually asymptomatic, but can → neuromuscular instability, cramps, arrhythmias, resistant ↓K^+, and resistant ↓Ca^{2+}.

Hyponatremia and hypernatremia Problems with water balance may occur in ARF as well. Patients may have hyponatremia due to baseline conditions (CHF, cirrhosis), which may be exacerbated by the kidneys' inability to excrete water. Hypernatremia may also occur with water losses due to diarrhea or diuretics.

Metabolic acidosis

ARF is usually associated with a raised anion gap metabolic acidosis:
- As GFR falls, unmeasured anions (such as HSO_4^- and HPO_4^-) from dietary and metabolic sources accumulate.
- As H^+ is buffered, HCO_3^- is consumed. The injured kidney is unable to reclaim filtered HCO_3^- from the urine (proximal tubule) or generate new HCO_3^- (through production and excretion of NH_4^+) primarily in the collecting duct.

The degree of acidosis is usually modest in uncomplicated ARF (serum HCO_3^- >10, pH >7.2) but more problematic in the critically ill, where it may contribute to circulatory compromise. ⚠ If unexpectedly severe, consider a secondary cause—especially lactic acidosis (sepsis, cardiogenic shock, liver failure), ketoacidosis (diabetes and alcohol), and poisoning (salicylates, methanol, ethylene glycol).

Acidosis per se may be an indication for dialysis, particularly if pH <7.0–7.1, with evidence of cardiovascular compromise.

Management of ARF 6: other strategies

Anemia

▶ Don't always assume anemia is part of the uremic syndrome. Beware of bleeding—especially from the GI tract, or hemolysis.

A Hb of ~8–11 g/dL is a frequent finding in ARF—it does not help distinguish between ARF and CKD. Major contributing factors are impaired erythropoiesis (↓renal EPO production), ↓red cell life span, hemolysis (↑red cell fragility), hemodilution (from fluid overload), and blood loss.

Erythropoietin is rarely effective in ARF, so transfusion may be necessary, particularly if ↓CV reserve means the ↓Hb is poorly tolerated. See 📖 p. 111 for transfusion in oligoanuric patients.

Bleeding

ARF is associated with a bleeding tendency secondary to platelet dysfunction. Uremic toxins disrupt the interaction between platelet GPIIb/IIIa, and adhesion molecules such as von Willebrand factor (vWF) and fibrinogen. ↑Plt nitric oxide synthesis may also inhibit aggregation.

Clinical manifestations are typically mild, with spontaneous bruising, or bleeding at venopuncture sites, though occasionally they are more troublesome.

INR, aPTT, and platelet count are usually normal (if abnormal look for other causes). The bleeding time is prolonged.

Correcting the bleeding tendency of ARF

The two situations that require specific intervention are
- Active bleeding or poorly controlled persistent oozing
- Prior to an invasive procedure (including renal biopsy).

Management
- Stop aspirin, clopidogrel, anticoagulants.
- Correct anemia (transfusion of packed cells). A hematocrit (Hct) ≥25–30% ↓ bleeding time.
- DDAVP (desmopressin): a synthetic analogue of ADH that probably works by ↑ amount of available vWF. It is easy to administer and works. Give 0.3 µg/kg IV in 50 mL of NS over 15–30 min. Effective within 1 hour, it lasts 4–24 hours. It is less effective on repetitive dosing. It can also be given subcutaneously (same dose) and intranasally (3 µg/kg). ⚠ It rarely causes coronary vasospasm—avoid if there is unstable angina.
- Cryoprecipitate: 10 units every 12–24 hours. It is *not* usually required, unless there is catastrophic bleeding.
- Estrogen: 0.6 mg/kg IV for 5 days with peak effect 5–7 days with duration of 1 week or more after therapy is finished.

Dialysis improves bleeding time (although not during actual treatment), presumably through removal of uremic toxins.

▶ Dialysis may require anticoagulation to prevent clotting of the extracorporeal circuit (📖 p. 220).

Infection

▶ Sepsis is an important cause of morbidity and mortality in ARF (76% mortality if ARF + sepsis). It occurs in three contexts:
- ARF is the consequence of a specific infection (e.g., postinfectious GN, endocarditis, malaria, leptospirosis).
- Septicemia → circulatory compromise → prerenal ARF → ATN.
- Localized or systemic infection arises in those with preexisting ATN.

Approach
- Watch carefully for signs of infection such as fever, ↑WCC, ↑CRP.
- Culture (and reculture) blood, urine, sputum, and other secretions.
- Make use of imaging. Repeat chest X-rays frequently. If the source of sepsis remains obscure, consider ± abdominal/chest CT, abdominal US.
- Pay attention to microbiological detail; follow samples, review sensitivities, carefully consider antibiotic options, and speak to your infectious disease specialists about resistance patterns.
- ⚠ Many antibiotics require dose adjustment in ARF and CKD.
- Use strict aseptic technique for central line, dialysis catheter, and bladder catheter insertion. Don't leave bladder catheters in place longer than necessary. Give antibiotic coverage and remove Foley if the urine is a likely source of sepsis.
- Inspect IV cannula sites regularly and look under dressings.
- Consider removing or changing lines as soon as feasible.

▶▶ Treat proven infection aggressively.

Management of ARF 7: nutrition

Both preexisting and hospital-acquired malnutrition → ↑ morbidity and mortality in the critically ill. Preventing malnutrition preserves (respiratory) muscle function, ↑ wound healing, and ↑ resistance to infection.

General rules
- If preexisting nutritional status is normal and a normal diet is likely to be resumed in ≤5 days, support is not initially indicated.
- Avoid feeding within the first 24 hours: there is evidence of harm (feeding during the "insult phase" ↑O_2 requirements and worsens tissue injury).
- If the patient is malnourished, ignore this 5-day rule and start feeding after the first 24 hours.
- If the patient is hypercatabolic (sepsis, trauma, burns), initiate support early.
- Modify nutritional support with changes in GFR and with dialysis.
- Enteral nutrition is always preferable to parenteral, if possible (but these are not mutually exclusive).

Step 1: determine the nutritional status of the patient
- Body weight: Recent unintentional loss >10% body weight is a bad sign.
- Determine body mass index (BMI, as mass in kg/height in m^2). Normal range is 20–25 kg/m^2. ⚠ Beware fluid retention falsely ↑weight.
- Serum albumin (<3 g/dL worrisome), though inflammation may be a confounder. Pre-albumin, transferrin, and cholesterol may also used.
- Subjective global assessment (SGA) combines clinical parameters with albumin, anthropometry, clinical judgment, and others.

Step 2: estimate energy requirements
- Standard formulas (>200 published), e.g., Schofield,[1] revolve around gender-based, weight-adjusted formulas. Ask your dietitian.
- Energy expenditure in "uncomplicated" ARF is actually within the normal range. Energy requirements for those with "complicated" ARF are determined by associated disorders (e.g., sepsis); nevertheless, it is rare for energy requirements to exceed 130% basal unless the patient is hypercatabolic and on dialysis.

▶ Broadly speaking, ♀ should receive 26 kcal/kg/day.

Step 3: estimation of protein (and amino acid) requirements
This depends on associated catabolic stress. Hypercatabolism → ↑UN, which can be used to estimate nitrogen balance. Rules of thumb:
- For "uncomplicated" ARF (nonoliguric, nonhypercatabolic) the daily protein or amino acid requirement is near the recommended allowance of 0.6–1 g/kg/day for normal adults.
- In complicated ARF (hypercatabolic) the requirement is ~1.0–1.3 g/kg/day.
- If dialysis is necessary, add 0.2 g/kg/day up to 1.5 g/kg/day in critically ill patients.
- ≥1.5 g/kg/day may aggravate the situation by stimulating formation of urea nitrogen and other nitrogenous waste products.

1 Schofield WN (1985). *Hum Nutr Clin Nutr* **39**(1): 5–41.

Step 4: decide on route of administration
See Table 2.5.

Step 5: ensure volume and electrolyte content appropriate for ARF
Low volume ± low electrolyte feeds are required if the patient is on intermittent hemodialysis. Standard feed can be used for those on CRRT (📖 p. 126).

CHAPTER 2 **Acute renal failure (Acute kidney injury)**

Table 2.5 Nutrition in treating ARF

Route	What's in it?	Notes	Concerns in ARF	Complications
Oral • Nutrition-dense oral diet • Supplementary sip feeding	Modest protein and energy content	• Many patients can tolerate an oral diet. • Supplementation with nutrition drinks is useful if appetite is poor.	Observe restrictions: • K^+ • PO_4 • Volume	
Enteral	• Enteral feeding formulas specifically for ARF are available, e.g., Nepro® (Ross), Nova source renal® (Novartis). • Ensure correct position of NG tube (aspirate pH or chest X-ray). Allow 4 hours bowel rest in every 24 hours.	Enteral feeding maintains the structural integrity of the gut and protects against translocation of GI bacteria.	• A tailored regimen (i.e., nonstandard feed) may be necessary if the above restrictions apply. • To prevent refeeding syndrome in a malnourished patient, K^+, PO_4, and Mg^{2+} must be checked and corrected prior to starting.	*Mechanical:* dislodged tube. *Gastrointestinal:* abdominal distension, nausea, cramps, and diarrhea *Infectious:* aspiration pneumonia *Metabolic:* hyper/hypoglycemia, electrolyte abnormalities
Parenteral	*Amino acids:* combined essential and nonessential (the latter often become "conditionally" essential in the context of ARF) *Energy:* principally given as glucose, although >5 g/kg/day causes ↑CO_2 production (increasing respiratory demands), ↑lipogenesis (fatty liver), and hyperglycemia. Lipids are used to provide the remainder (usually ≤1g/kg/day to avoid hyperlipidemia). *Vitamins,* trace elements, electrolytes (and sometimes insulin) are added as necessary.	• IV lipids have a low osmolality and can be given into peripheral veins. They do not meet all energy requirements so are mainly a short-term measure. • Full TPN must usually be given centrally (via a dedicated line). • If possible, a small amount of enteral feeds is run concurrently.	• Start feeds slowly. • Continuous renal replacement techniques (e.g., CVVHF) assist the delivery of feeding.	*Catheter insertion:* pneumothorax etc. *Catheter infection* *Metabolic* requires close laboratory monitoring

Management myths

Loop diuretics

Theory: (1) ↑ urinary flow "washes out" cellular debris, casts, and nephrotoxins from tubules; (2) blockade of active transport processes → ↑tubular O_2 consumption and protects against ATN; (3) vasodilator action → ↑RBF.

Evidence: A recent Cochrane meta-analysis showed no improved renal or patient outcome in any ARF setting. The natural history and prognosis of ATN remains unchanged. Some studies have suggested harm, although this may be in unresponsive patients in whom renal replacement therapy is delayed.

▶▶ Give as part of the treatment of pulmonary edema (📖 p. 112).

- If oliguria persists despite correction of prerenal factors, diuretics may ↑UO, simplify fluid balance, and improve pulmonary edema.

Mannitol

This is an osmotic diuretic previously used for the prevention of ATN in high-risk CV surgery. A lack of evidence has led to decreased use. It can paradoxically cause pulmonary edema through volume expansion. Avoid its use.

Dopamine

💊 Despite a lack of evidence for efficacy, dopamine has proved to be a difficult habit to kick. Do not use it for treatment or prophylaxis of ARF.

Theory: Dopamine (DA) is synthesized in the proximal tubule from circulating L-dopa and helps regulate Na^+ excretion and renal vasodilataion through specific DA1 and DA2 receptors. Exogenously administered "low-dose" dopamine should → renal vasodilatation → ↑RBF → ↑ natriuresis and mild ↑GFR. All of these effects are potentially beneficial in ATN (see Table 2.6).

Evidence: Largely anecdotal or from inadequate studies. Some increase in diuresis in CHF patients may because the "renal dose" dopamine is actually acting as an inotrope. Larger trials (e.g., ANZICS) failed to show benefit.

Table 2.6 Dosage and effects of dopamine

μg/kg/min	Effect
0.5–3	Selective DA (mainly DA1) receptor activation → ↑ renal (and mesenteric) blood flow
3–10	Both DA and $β_1$ receptors are activated, the latter → ↑cardiac output (mainly by ↑SV)
10–20	$β_1$ effect predominates. Start to activate α adrenoreceptors
>20	α-adrenergic (vasoconstrictive) effect takes over with ↑SVR

⚠ It may cause **harm**:
- Tachycardia, arrhythmias, myocardial ischemia
- Blunted hypoxemic drive
- Splanchnic vasoconstriction (→ bacterial translocation)
- Digital ischemia
- Impaired pituitary function
- Electrolyte disturbances (even at "renal" dose)
- Dopamine accumulates in renal failure.

Hope for the future? Putative renoprotective agents
- N-acetylcysteine? (see 📖 p. 143 for full discussion)
- Fenoldopam
- Erythropoietin
- NGAL (neutrophil gelatinase-associated lipocalin).

▶ Some of the above may yet become useful agents in managing or preventing ARF—many more have been tried, shown to work in animal models, and been found to have no effect in humans (see Table 2.7).

Table 2.7 Unproven putative renoprotective agents

Pathogenetic mechanism	Interventions of unproven benefit in humans
Renal vasoconstriction	Low-dose dopamine
	Calcium channel blockers
	Atrial natriuretic peptide
	Endothelin receptor antagonists
	Leukotriene receptor antagonists
	PAF antagonists
	iNOS antisense oligonucleotides
Inflammation	Anti-ICAM-1 monoclonal antibody
	Anti-IL-18 monoclonal antibody
	N-acetylcysteine and or other free-radical scavengers
	α-MSH
Tubular obstruction	Diuretics
	RGD peptides
Tubular regeneration	Insulin-like growth factor
	Thyroxine
	Epidermal growth factor
	Hepatocyte growth factor
	Osteopontin
	Protease (e.g., caspase) inhibitors

PAF, platelet activating factor; iNOS, inducible nitric oxide synthase; ICAM-1, intercellular adhesion molecule-1; α-MSH, αα-melanocyte-stimulating hormone; RGD peptides, peptides containing the arginine–glycine–aspartic acid motif (involved in adhesion).

Novel biomarkers and techniques are being tested that may **predict** ARF before it is established, and discriminate between prerenal impairment and ATN. Some of these include the following:
- Blood oxygen level-dependent MRI (a noninvasive method of measuring actual tissue pO_2, useful to gauge medullary ischemia in ATN)
- KIM-1 (kidney injury molecule-1) or IL-18, as urinary markers of injured proximal tubular cells
- NGAL (neutrophil gelatinase-associated lipocalin).

Renal replacement therapy in ARF

Opinion differs on the indications as well as on when to start, when to stop, what method to use, and what "dose" to give. Some generalizations can be made.

Indications

▶ Hyperkalemia
- $K^+ \geq 6.5$ mEq/L or rapidly rising, regardless of ECG changes

▶ Volume overload
- Pulmonary edema with inadequate response to diuretics, particularly if occurring in an oliguanuric patient.
- Intractable acidosis (pH < 7.1), especially if patient is hemodynamically unstable.
- Uremia
  - Uremic pericarditis or encephalopathy
  - Uremic symptoms, especially if BUN >100 mg/dL (⚠ There is no absolute figure that equates with "uremia" and much interpatient variability is seen.)
- Critically ill patients (usually on ICU)
  - Start RRT before accumulation of toxins → circulatory compromise.
  - RRT allows safer administration of volume: feeding, transfusion, other blood products, antimicrobials, other drugs.
  - Diuretic-resistant cardiac failure
- Poison or toxin removal (lithium, ethylene glycol etc.)
- Eponym for indications is AEIOU, which stands for **A**cidosis, **E**lectrolyte abnormalities, **I**ngestion (toxin), **O**verload (volume), **U**remia.

Renal replacement therapy is not without potential problems:
- Complications of vascular access insertion (📖 p. 222)
- Placing a hemodynamic strain on an already sick patient
- Dialysis disequilibrium syndrome with conventional hemodialysis (📖 p. 210)
- ☞ Prolonging ARF duration if there is hypotension during HD treatments.

Modalities (📖 p. 228)

- Generally, intermittent HD may be performed anywhere and continuous renal replacement therapy in ICUs. The latter includes continuous venovenous hemofiltration (CVVH), continuous venovenous hemodialysis (CVVHD), continuous venovenous hemodiafiltration (CVVHDF), and sustained low-efficiency dialysis (SLED) (Fig. 2.7).
- One modality has not been shown to be demonstrably superior over another in mortality or recovery of renal function. Selection may depend on availability.
- However, patients in shock and on vasopressors, those with very large obligate fluid intake requirements, and those with raised intracranial pressure may be better managed with continuous therapies.

📖 p. 212 for explanation of techniques of renal replacement therapy.

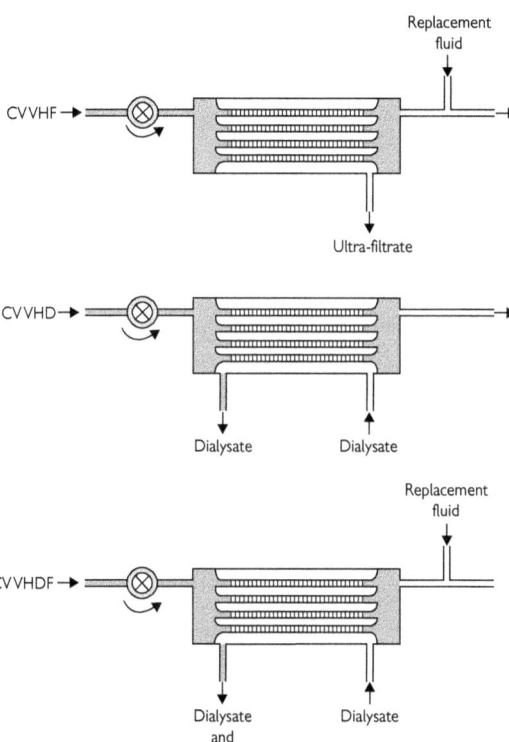

Fig. 2.7 Principles of different continuous renal replacement therapy modalities. Replacement fluids can be given before or after the dialysis membrane (pre-or post-dilution). Reproduced with permission from Levy J, Morgan J, and Brown E (2004). *Oxford Handbook of Dialysis*, 2nd ed. Oxford: Oxford University Press.

Prescribing acute hemodialysis

▶ Experienced dialysis nursing staff may know a great deal (perhaps more than you if you are a novice).

⚠ Rapid overcorrection of uremia may → dialysis disequilibrium. The first dialysis should aim to gently remove uremic wastes.

- Time: first session, 2 hours; second one, 2.5–3 hours; and subsequent ones, 3–4 hours.
- Blood flow: slow at first ~200 mL/min then increase (↑ by 50 mL/min/session for first 3 scssions).
- Frequency: Urea rebound is common, so dialyze daily against symptoms and chemistry for the first 2–3 days. Catabolic patients (e.g., with sepsis) may need to remain on a daily regimen. ? mortality benefit to daily dialysis.
- Dialysis membranes (📖 p. 216): A small dialysis membrane is (≤1.4 m^2) preferable for initiation.
- Fluid removal (ultrafiltration [UF] rate).

▶ Assessment of the patient's volume status is crucial.
  - Hypovolemia: administer saline (1–2 L)—no UF
  - Euvolemia: no UF
  - Overload: Up to 3 L can be removed over 2 hours. If further UF is necessary (patient is still in pulmonary edema), it can be removed by isolated UF (→ dialysate flow turned off leaving fluid removal, not biochemical control, as the primary goal)
  - Avoid hypotension using cool dialysate (35°C), high dialysate Na$^+$, or Na$^+$ modeling (variable Na$^+$ in dialysate) if not contraindicated, with isovolemic connection (prime circuit with NS to minimize preload reduction).

- Anticoagulation-free: Minimize (avoid) heparin if possible, as acutely ill ARF patients are at risk of bleeding: arterial puncture during line insertions, GI bleeding, ↑BP, pericarditis (which may → hemorrhagic tamponade).
- Dialysate
  - Dialysate Na$^+$ of 135–145 mEq/L is typical. If serum Na$^+$<125 mEq/L use a dialysate Na$^+$ ≤15 mEq/L higher to avoid rapid correction.
  - Serum K$^+$ decides dialysate K$^+$. ⚠ Overcorrection → arrhythmias.

Serum K$^+$ (mEq/L)	Dialysate K$^+$ (mEq/L)
>5.5	2.0
4.0–5.5	3.0
<4.0	4.0

K$^+$ free dialysate can be used if ↑↑K$^+$.

- ✒ Adequacy. There is some evidence that daily dialysis → better outcomes. Kt/V (📖 p. 221) is unreliable in ARF, and delivered Kt/V is ~25%< prescribed per treatment. ↑Kt/V may lead to ↑ survival. Aim to keep BUN <70 mg/dL.

Modifications of HD

Modifications of IHD using standard HD equipment may improve tolerability, though overall benefits are unclear.
- Extended-duration dialysis (EDD): 6- to 8-hour treatments with blood and dialysate flows of 200–300 mL/min and 300 mL/min, respectively. This is well tolerated and can achieve good UF volumes (~3 L).
- Sustained low-efficiency dialysis (SLED): 12-hour treatment with blood and dialysate flows of 200 mL/min and 100 mL/min, respectively. This is well tolerated, but circuits are prone to clotting.

Dialysis disequilibrium syndrome

This syndrome is thought to be secondary to cerebral edema: BUN drops rapidly on dialysis, but not as readily across the blood–brain barrier and within cells → water influx into the brain and cerebral edema ± Increased cerebral acidosis (?mechanism) may play a role.
- This is rare if first-dialysis precautions of slow blood flow, small surface area membrane and short treatment are observed.
- Those with higher BUN (>175 mg/dL) are at particular risk.
- Symptoms (during or shortly after dialysis) include nausea, dizziness, headache, visual disturbance, agitation, confusion, ↓GCS, and seizures.
- Exclude hypoglycemia, ↓Na^+, drug toxicity, and intracerebral bleeding, subdural hematoma.
- ✒ Prophylaxis: Some recommend phenytoin 15 mg/kg loading dose, then 200–300 mg/day if BUN >150. Others do not. Treatment: Stop dialysis and supportive treatment (improvement should occur within 24 hours). Give mannitol 12.5 g IV, hypertonic saline, 5–10 mg diazepam IV if patient is seizing.

Prescribing CVVH or CVVHD

See 📖 p. 212 for explanation of technique.
- *Time*: continuous
- *Blood flow*: usually 150–300 mL/min
- *Filter*: high-flux membrane (Polyacrylnitrile (PAN) membranes may precipitate anaphylaxis in patients on ACE inhibitors.)
- *Fluid removal*: Fluid removal is achieved by UF rate exceeding replacement fluid or dialysate rate per hour (e.g., net 100 or 200 mL UF/h).
- *Clearance*: Dialysate or replacement fluid with rates of 15–45 mL/kg/h (usually supplied in 5 L bags) contains:
  - Buffer: HCO_3^- or lactate (liver metabolism to HCO_3^-), but HCO_3^- based solutions are preferable if liver disease, or shock are present.
  - K^+ is generally 0–3 mEq/L and adjusted to serum K.
  - They also contain Na^+ (132–140 mEq/L), Ca^{2+}, Mg^{2+}, and Cl^-.
- *Anticoagulation*: Heparin or citrate is usually preferred if required.
- *Adequacy*: The urea clearance using CVVHD is about 16–34 mL/min, with 1-2 L/h dialysate or replacement rate.
- ✦* ↑ volume of hemofiltration (35–45 mL/kg/h vs. 20 mL/kg/h) may → better outcomes. Adding dialysate to the CVVH dose (CVVHDF-hemodiafiltration) may have better outcomes than the CVVH dose alone.

Peritoneal dialysis in ARF

This is rarely used for ARF in North America, given the availability of CRRT, but it is an important treatment worldwide. Until recently, it was also the most popular technique for the treatment of ARF in children.

Potential advantages
- Technically (relatively) straightforward
- Minimizes hemodynamic instability (making fluid removal easier)
- Gentle correction of biochemical abnormalities. There is no need for vascular access or systemic anticoagulation.
- Dextrose in peritoneal dialysis (PD) fluid boosts caloric intake.

Potential disadvantages
- Bowel perforation during catheter insertion (especially if previous surgery → adhesions)
- ⚠ Infection: peritonitis and catheter exit site
- Relatively slow correction of uremia and ↑K^+
- Unpredictable UF rate (interpatient variability)
- Protein and amino acids are lost in dialysate.
- Catheter problems: migration, poor inflow/outflow, leakage
- Abdominal distension → diaphragmatic splinting → respiratory compromise
- Hyperglycemia (PD fluid uses high-glucose concentrations to generate hypertonicity for fluid removal.)
- Contraindicated by recent abdominal surgery.

Catheter placement
Semi-rigid ("stab PD")
Pros: It is inserted at the bedside under local anesthesia (usually via a Seldinger technique).

Cons: It is non-cuffed, therefore high infection rates can result. It is also uncomfortable and easy to dislodge. There is a higher incidence of bowel perforation. It usually requires removal after 48–72 hours (→ repeated insertions often necessary).

Cuffed catheter (similar to those used in chronic PD)
Pros: The cuff prevents bacterial migration ↓ infection rates. The catheter is softer, so it is more comfortable with less risk of bowel perforation. It is also more compatible with automated cyclers.

Cons: Insertion requires more expertise (though local anesthesia is still possible).

Hemodialysis, hemofiltration, or PD for ARF?
Studies are limited. A recent comparison suggested a worse outcome than for CVVH, though second-rate PD equipment (rigid catheters, home made fluids, acetate buffer, no automated cyclers) was judged against first-rate CVVH technology in highly catabolic patients. PD cannot be considered a first-line treatment for ARF, but may be life saving if HD/CRRT are unavailable.

Prescribing acute PD

- Commercially available dialysate solutions are preferable. Warm to body temperature prior to infusion.
- A correctly positioned catheter should allow inflow and outflow times of <10–15 min. Both proceed under gravity. Ensure complete drainage (remember: more drains out than in if UF has occurred).
- Exchange times of 1 hour are typical.
- With non-cuffed rigid catheters peritonitis risk ↑ dramatically after 72 hours. Cuffed catheters offer uninterrupted treatment.
- Aim for 20–24 exchanges/day (logistically often difficult).
- Record the number of exchanges and bag input:output.
- Dialysate volume: Most patients tolerate 2 L exchanges. Larger volumes (up to 3 L) can → catheter leaks, hernias, and diaphragmatic splinting.
- Dialysis dose is increased by ↑ dialysate volume ± exchange frequency.
- Fluid balance. If the patient is euvolemic, mildly fluid overloaded, or hemodynamically unstable, a 1.5% dextrose concentration is appropriate. Check the subsequent drainage volume to assess UF. Use this figure in combination with repeated clinical assessment to direct the need for higher dextrose concentrations (2.5% or 4.25%).
- Heparin (200–500 U/L) can be added to the dialysate to prevent plugging of the catheter with fibrin clots. It is not absorbed systemically.
- Commercial PD solutions don't contain K^+, so if the patient is hypokalemic, or the serum K^+ is rapidly falling, potassium chloride can be added (usually 2–4 mEq/L) to the dialysate. Monitor closely for hypokalemia.

The hepatorenal syndrome (HRS)

HRS occurs in advanced liver dysfunction, usually cirrhosis, in conjunction with ascites and portal hypertension. HRS has been split into two types based on (1) rapidity of onset, (2) severity of ARF, and (3) prognosis (see Table 2.8).

▶ Not all ARF with cirrhosis is due to the HRS—it is not at the top of the list.

Common causes of combined hepatic and renal dysfunction

- Hypovolemia (GI hemorrhage, diuretics, lactulose-induced diarrhea) → ATN
- Sepsis →ATN
- Nephrotoxins (drugs and ↑bilirubin →ATN)
- Glomerulonephritis (e.g., MPGN with hepatitis C)
- Hepatorenal syndrome.

Pathophysiology

Liver disease is associated with portal hypertension causing marked splanchnic and arterial vasodilatation (→ arterial underfilling and ↓SVR), in part due to excess local NO production (↑ shear stress in portal hypertension), ↑bacterial translocation with endotoxin, and ↑vasoactive gut peptides (glucagons, prostacyclin). As a result, the effective arterial blood volume is sensed to have fallen, leading to intense α-stimulation, secondary hyperaldosteronism, and nonosmotic ADH release (hence salt and water overload). Catecholamine, angiotensin, and endothelin excess result in profound and intense renal vasoconstriction (→ ↓RBF). The kidneys are structurally *normal* and the renal impairment is entirely prerenal in nature—tubular integrity and function are preserved:

- Kidney biopsies are normal.
- Kidneys from HRS patients have been successfully transplanted.

Table 2.8 Classification of HRS

Type I	ARF is the dominant clinical feature
	Rapid ↓GFR (doubling baseline Cr to >2.5 mg/dL or CrCl falling to <20 mL/min in less than 2 weeks)
	Progressive oligoanuria (often profound)
	Median survival 2 weeks
Type II	Ascites (often refractory) is the dominant clinical feature
	Protracted clinical course
	Renal impairment less acute and severe
	Can convert to type I
	Median survival 6 months

HRS: diagnostic criteria

Major criteria
- Acute or chronic liver disease with advanced hepatic failure and portal hypertension
- Renal impairment: serum Cr ≥1.5 mg/dL or CrCl <40 mL/min
- **Absence of** shock, GI fluid losses, excessive diuresis,* or ongoing bacterial infection (▶ spontaneous bacterial peritonitis), recent nephrotoxic drugs (e.g., NSAIDs, aminoglycosides), proteinuria (<500 mg/day) or renal parenchymal disease, or obstruction on US
- No sustained improvement in renal function (serum Cr ↓ to <1.5 mg/dL or ↑ in CrCl >40 mL/min) after 1.5 L of isotonic saline or 20–40 g albumin.

Additional criteria
- Urine volume <500 mL/day
- UNa <10 mEq/L
- Urine osmolality >plasma osmolality
- Urine red blood cells <50/HPF
- Serum Na^+ <130 mmol/L.

* Weight loss <500 mg/day for several days in ascitic patients without (or 1 kg/day in those with) peripheral edema.

From Arroyo V, et al. (1996). *Hepatology* 23: 164–76.

Recognizing deteriorating renal function may not be easy, as cirrhotics often have a ↓muscle mass (low serum Cr may overestimate true GFR). BUN is influenced by GI bleeding and low hepatic production ± variable dietary protein intake and is ∴ unhelpful. The diagnosis depends on the exclusion of other causes of ARF.

Clinical features
- Advanced liver disease: ascites, stigmata of chronic liver disease, portal hypertension (beware of GI bleeding), encephalopathy, jaundice (degree variable), coagulopathy
- Cardiovascular: edema (Na^+ and water retention) and ↓BP (both SVR and effective arterial blood volume are ↓)
- Infection: ↑ susceptibility to sepsis (⚠ pneumonia, line infections, and spontaneous bacterial peritonitis)
- Electrolyte disorders: ↓Na^+ is almost universal (retention of total body Na^+ and even more total body water).
- Nutritional state: usually poor and deteriorating
- Urine output: Oligoanuria is the norm in type I HRS, with urine volumes decreasing as the condition progresses. Anuria is a bad sign.
- Urinalysis is bland, with no proteinuria/hematuria.
- Tubular function is preserved, so the kidneys excrete urine that is low in Na^+ (<10 mmol/L) (indistinguishable from prerenal ARF). It was heavily emphasized in the past, but now considered a minor criterion.
- Normal renal ultrasound as above.

Management of HRS

Identify those at risk on admission to the hospital. Risk factors include:
- Cirrhosis + ascites = 40% 5-year probability of HRS
- Large volume (>5 L) paracentesis without concurrent plasma expansion. (•° Give 5–10 g per 1 L ascites removed.)
- Overdiuresis (possibly—see diagnostic criteria)
- GI bleeding (Variceal bleeding is a well-known precipitant.)
- Sepsis: especially spontaneous bacterial peritonitis (SBP) (~20% develop HRS). Any cirrhotic with ascites should be assumed to have SBP until diagnostic paracentesis proves otherwise.
- Alcoholic hepatitis
- The patient may have no known risk factor other than liver disease.

Preventative measures

These may be effective in specific situations:
- Spontaneous bacterial peritonitis. Administration of IV albumin 1.5 g/kg at diagnosis and 1 g/kg at day 3 in addition to antibiotics (as below) appears to decrease risk.
- Alcoholic hepatitis: pentoxifylline (a TNF inhibitor) 400 mg tid orally.

Managing established HRS

▶ Seek expert help early.
- Volume assessment:
  - IV 20% albumin (salt-poor) for a CVP of 5–10 cmH$_2$O
  - Na$^+$ (80 mEq/24 h) and fluid restriction (<1 L/24 h) if overloaded
- Culture blood, urine, and ascites if you suspect infection; treat with empiric IV antibiotics.
- Consider therapeutic paracentesis if there is tense ascites with ascitic pressure >30 cm H$_2$O (↑intra-abdominal pressure transmitted to kidneys [↑renin release, ↓GFR] and ureters [relative obstruction]).

Specific rescue therapies

- Vasoconstrictors → constriction of the splanchnic bed → improved circulatory (and ∴ renal) function. These are given in combination with albumin 20–40 g daily for 15 days. Aim for MAP >75 mmHg.
  - α-agonists: Midodrine (7.5–12.5 mg po tid) is a selective α$_1$-agonist that may be beneficial in combination with octreotide (100–200 μg SC tid). There are few studies. Aim to ↑MAP by 15 mmHg.
  - Norepinephrine (1–10 μg/min) was successful in one case series.
  - Vasopressin analogues (acting via splanchnic V$_1$ receptors)
  - Terlipressin (0.5–2 mg/4–6 h IV) is the most used agent. Renal response is 42%–92% in various case series. Repeat courses are effective and responders have a better prognosis. It is not available in the United States.
- Transjugular intrahepatic portosystemic shunts (TIPS) may have a role in combination with vasoconstrictors and in selected patients when pharmacotherapy has failed. TIPS are limited by procedure-worsening encephalopathy.

Renal replacement therapy

⚠ RRT does not improve outcome and should be viewed as a bridge to liver transplantation. Perform RRT if liver transplantation is intended or if liver improvement is possible. Continuous RRT is better tolerated than intermittent HD. Standard indications apply (📖 p. 126).

Molecular adsorbent recirculating system (MARS) is an extracorporeal albumin dialysis in which albumin dialysate goes through charcoal and anion-exchanger columns to remove tumor necrosis factor (TNF), IL-6, and NO. Unfortunately, there is no proven benefit and it is usually not available in hospitals.

Liver transplantation

This is the most (only?) effective therapy, but many patients die before transplantation is possible. Organ allocation differs between countries, but in many systems (e.g., MELD) HRS patients are accorded high priority. Most patients have ↑GFR after transplantation, although most do not regain normal renal function (10% incidence of ESRD at 11 years). Patients with pretransplant renal impairment have a ↓long-term survival compared with those with normal GFR.

Rhabdomyolysis

First described as "crush syndrome" during the London blitz of WW II, rhabdomyolysis is a clinical syndrome caused by release of cellular contents after significant striated muscle injury, with CK usually >10,000 in ARF (see Table 2.9).

Injury is caused by either energy-depletion or cell death. Infiltrating leukocytes release oxidant species that cause muscle necrosis. If cell death is widespread, intracellular elements and membrane products are released into the circulation, including creatine kinase (predominantly MM isoenzyme, but also MB), myoglobin, uric acid, electrolytes (especially K^+ and PO_4), and aminotransferase enzymes.

Myoglobin (Mb)

This is the main nephrotoxin in rhabdomyolysis. A 19 kD weak O_2 carrier (similar to Hb but with a single heme moiety), Mb is usually bound to plasma proteins. The ferric form (Fe^{3+}) is freely filtered, and concentrated. Mb causes renal vasoconstriction, intraluminal cast formation, and direct oxidant tubular cell injury. Large quantities of fluid may be retained in inflamed muscle, → profound hypovolemia in addition to toxic renal injury.

▶ Not all rhabdomyolysis → ARF (particularly if you act quickly).

Clinical presentation

Presentation is variable, but the classic triad of myalgias, weakness, and dark urine are rare (~50% have no muscle pain at presentation). Patients may have malaise, fatigue, and nausea. Maintain a high index of suspicion, especially if ↑AST/ALT (initially), ± ↑Cr and ↓UO, with dipstick-positive hematuria and no RBCs on microscopic exam.

⚠ Examine the limbs carefully—don't miss a compartment syndrome. Recurrent rhabdomyolysis after mild exertion → an underlying myopathy.

Investigations

Urine dipstick testing cannot distinguish between myoglobin and hemoglobin. Classically, urine is dipstick positive for blood, but with no red cells on microscopy. About 20% of patients will have a negative urinalysis. Urine microscopy usually shows granular casts.

▶ Urinary Mb is positive (not present in normal urine).
- BUN, Cr, electrolytes (BUN:Cr ratio is often low, perhaps secondary to increased creatinine release from muscle)
- ↑CK (better indicator of amount of muscle damage than likelihood of ARF). ↑ALT, AST
- ↑K^+ (⚠ often ↑↑), ↑↑ PO_4, ↑uric acid, ↑lactate and ↑AG acidosis (organic acids and phosphate)
- ↓↓Ca^{2+}, often with avid calcium sequestration in injured muscle
- Mild DIC is frequent (↓Plt, ↑D-dimers).
- Consider toxicology screen for drugs, viral screen, and thyroid-stimulating hormone (TSH) if cause is not apparent.

Table 2.9 Causes of rhabdomyolysis

Physical causes	Drugs and toxins
Trauma and disasters (crush injury)	Alcohol, heroin, cocaine, amphetamines, and ecstasy
Prolonged immobility	Statins and fibrates
Compartment syndrome	Antimalarials
Muscle vessel occlusion	Zidovudine
Sickle cell disease	Cyclopsorine
Shock and sepsis	Snake and insect venoms
Excessive exertion	Infections
Delirium tremens	Pyomyositis and gas gangrene
Electric shock	Toxic shock, tetanus, legionella, salmonella
Status epilepticus or asthmaticus	Malaria
Neuroleptic malignant syndrome	HIV, influenza, parainfluenza, CMV, EBV, HSV, echovirus, adenovirus, and Coxsackie virus
Malignant hyperthermia	Electrolyte abnormalities
Myopathies	$\downarrow K^+$, $\downarrow Ca^{2+}$, $\downarrow PO_4$, $\downarrow Na^+$, $\uparrow Na^+$
Polymyositis/dermatomyositis	Endocrine disorders (DKA, pheochromocytoma)
McArdle disease and other inherited myopathies	Hypothyroidism
Near drowning/hypothermia	

Management of rhabdomyolysis

Prevention of ARF
In the early phase of the disorder, vigorous resuscitation may protect patients from many of the subsequent complications.
- Aim to resuscitate to euvolemia
  - As much as 12 L may be required per day (and more if there is severe injury).
  - If clinically unsure of volume status, aim for CVP 8–12 cm H_2O.
  - NS. If there is systemic acidosis or immediate injury, consider $NaHCO_3$ (5% dextrose + 2–3 amps of $NaHCO_3$ or $NaHCO_3$ 150 mEq/L if pharmacy is able).
- Maintain a UO ≥150 mL/h, or ≥200–300 mL/h with traumatic injuries.
- Continue therapy until decrease of CK to <5000 occurs.

Urinary alkalinization and mannitol?
※ The role of urinary alkalinization (stabilizes oxidizing form of myoglobin) and forced diuresis (↑ urine flow → ↓tubular precipitation) remains controversial. It has been used in immediate treatment of trauma with the aim of a target UpH >6.5 by using $NaHCO_3$ as above.

▶ The priority is to volume resuscitate the patient. There are no prospective trials, but review of retrospective literature shows no benefit of alkalinization over saline.
- ⚠ Alkalinization → systemic alkalosis and thus symptomatic ↓Ca^{2+}. Alkalinizing urine may lead to increased calcium phosphate deposition in renal tubules worsening ARF.
- Mannitol. Generally avoid this because of general volume depletion. There is limited evidence that it may be helpful in severe rhabdomyolysis (CK> 20,000-30,000). In theory diuretics may ↑flow, thus limiting tubular precipitation. Mannitol, an osmotic diuretic, has been used: as a bolus (e.g., 12.5–25 g as a bolus [= 62.5–125 mL of 20% (200 mg/mL) mannitol solution]) or as an infusion (10 mL/h of 15%–20% mannitol). ⚠ Mannitol ↑osmolar gap and may worsen ARF.

⚠ Once overt renal failure has developed, the only reliable treatment is dialysis. The prognosis is good if the causative insult is removed. Renal function returns to normal in most patients, with slight dysfunction if the patient was dialysis dependent.

Compartment syndrome in rhabdomyolysis
This may occur in two circumstances:
- If the blood supply to a particular limb has been compromised (immobility after seizures, drug overdose, etc.)
- Generalized muscle injury and inflammation (toxic, viral)

Inflammation and edema within a closed muscle compartment → ↑ intracompartment pressure → ↓ O_2 delivery → muscle necrosis.

▶ Always examine the major muscle groups for the characteristic "woody hard" feeling of an evolving or established compartment. Prophylactic fasciotomy in these circumstances may save limb function.

If in doubt, measure the intracompartment pressure. If it is within 20 mm of diastolic pressure, this is worrisome (it is important to remember this in hypotensive patients). If in doubt, recheck every 6 hours.

Hypocalcemia

Usually do not correct ↓Ca^{2+} unless it is symptomatic (tetany, arrhythmias)—there is a risk that the administered calcium will precipitate in injured muscle and a theoretic risk that it may precipitate calcium phosphate in tubules. Rebound hypercalcemia is common during the recovery phase.

⚠ Symptomatic ↓Ca^{2+} may complicate $NaHCO_3$ administration.

Hemoglobinuric ARF

This occurs in the context of massive intravascular hemolysis.
- Transfusion reactions (ABO incompatibility)
- Falciparum malaria (blackwater fever, 📖 p. 492)
- Hemolytic anemias (drug induced, autoimmune)
- Mycoplasma infection
- Snake, insect, and spider venoms.

Free Hb does not enter the urine as freely as Mb, so ARF is relatively rare unless there is massive hemolysis or perhaps underlying glomerular disease.

Investigations
↓Hb, ↓haptoglobin, ↑bilirubin, ↑LDH, ↑K^+, urine is dipstick positive for blood, plasma appears dark

Management
Treat underlying disorder, with volume resuscitation to establish a diuresis.

Contrast-induced nephropathy (CIN)

CIN accounts for ~10% of in-hospital ARF and is associated with significant mortality (x5.5 odds-adjusted risk of death) and may irreversibly ↓GFR (especially in those with preexisting CKD). CIN is associated with ↑length of stay. Overall incidence is ~3.5%, but it rises to >30% if the starting Cr >3 mg/dL.

Why is contrast toxic?
- Direct toxicity: oxidant injury to proximal tubular cells
- Vasoconstrictor: contrast alters afferent/efferent tone and thus perfusion.

▶ Vasoconstriction and ATN result.

Precautions
- Specific measures are listed in Box 2.2.
- Identify those at risk (📖 p. 76).
- Is the procedure necessary? Is there an alternative "non-contrast" technique? Speak to your radiologist.
- Use iso-osmolar, nonionic contrast.
- Minimize contrast volume.
- Optimize volume status pre-study.
- Stop all other nephrotoxins prior to the procedure.
- Where possible, stop diuretics, ACEI, and ARB (❖* Some data suggest ACEI may be protective for 2 days). If they can't be stopped for any reason (e.g., uncontrolled BP or CHF), consider postponement of the procedure.
- Space out multiple procedures whenever possible.
- Inform the renal team of high-risk cases beforehand.

Clinical features
- ↓GFR begins immediately (though Cr may be unchanged initially).
- The earliest (and often only) sign may be oliguria (so ensure that UO is being measured).
- ARF may not be apparent until renal function is rechecked the following day (so make sure it is checked and that you see the result).
- Unlike other causes of ATN, fractional excretion of Na^+ is <1% because of vasoconstricting effects of contrast.

Treatment
Once established, treat patient for ATN as for any other cause. Ensure that the patient remains well hydrated and avoid additional nephrotoxins. Dialysis support may be necessary.

Prognosis
- In most patients, renal dysfunction is mild and transient (though still associated with ↑ mortality).
- Recovery within a week is usual. Those with preexisting advanced CKD are most susceptible to a permanent ↓GFR.

Box 2.2 Strategies to prevent CIN

Hydration
IV fluids correct volume depletion and ↑RBF. Evidence supporting their use is strong.
- NS 1 mL/kg/h for 12 hours before and 12 hours after the procedure (recommended).
- 1.26% $NaHCO_3$ 3 mL/kg/h for 1 hour pre-procedure and 1 mL/kg/h for 6 hours during and post-procedure (may be as good as NS).

Examine the patient first—if overtly volume depleted, then larger volumes are required and the procedure may require postponement. If the patient is already volume overloaded then further fluids are ill advised.

N-acetylcysteine (NAC)
NAC has antioxidant properties, and is *always used in conjunction with IV fluids*. Evidence is controversial, as many randomized trials and meta-analyses have suggested benefits in some and no effect in others. NAC may even ↓Cr independently of GFR, through interference with tubular handling.

▶ It is inexpensive with few side effects.
- 600–1200 mg po bid for day of and day after the procedure.

Others
- Hemofiltration/hemodialysis: prophylactic removal of circulating contrast. Small trials with hemofiltration (CVVH) done pre- and post-procedure show benefit. Hemodialysis shows no benefit, possible harm.
- Theophylline antagonizes adenosine-mediated ↓RBF. There is evidence of benefit, but only in low-risk groups. Further study is required.
- Fenoldopam: specific dopamine$_1$ receptor agonist that ↑RBF. There is no clear current evidence of benefit.

Differential diagnosis

Many patients undergoing invasive vascular studies have diffuse atherosclerotic disease and are at risk of renal atheroemboli. These can occur as a distinctive clinical syndrome (p. 414) but often go unrecognized until the expected recovery of renal function doesn't occur.

Tumor lysis syndrome (TLS)

Tumor lysis usually occurs at initiation of treatment (chemo- or radiation therapy, or even corticosteroids) of lymphoproliferative (and less commonly solid) malignancies, but may occur spontaneously with a large tumor burden. Classically, it is a complication after chemotherapy for high-blast count acute leukemia, lymphoma, myeloma, or germ cell tumors.

It is a result of treatment-induced necrosis of large numbers of purine-rich (actively proliferating) malignant cells, with intracellular and membrane products released abruptly into the circulation. Uric acid and calcium-phosphate precipitation in tubules causes acute renal failure.

Pre- and post-treatment tumor lysis

Uric acid is freely filtered, and in excess precipitates in the tubular lumen to form obstructing crystalline casts (acute uric acid nephropathy). This is more likely in volume-depleted patients with low urinary flow rates (↑ uric acid concentration >15 mg/dL) or if UpH↓. This can occur pretreatment as well as post-treatment. Post-treatment, uric acid elevations may be prevented with allopurinol or rasburicase. Calcium phosphate precipitation occurs in post-treatment tumor lysis as lysed cells release phosphate. (Pretreatment, active malignant cells may utilize phosphate so the serum level may be less elevated.)

Clinical findings

In the context of recent therapy, symptoms and signs are due to electrolyte abnormalities (⚠ ↑K^+ and arrhythmias) and ARF.

Investigations

Within 6–72 hours of therapy:
- ↑K^+: often rapid ↑ to severely elevated levels mEq/L
- ↑PO_4: avidly binds calcium, precipitating hypocalcemia and calcium phosphate deposition in the vasculature and kidney. There is ↓Mg^{2+} for the same reason.
- ↑uric acid: Purine nucleotides are metabolized to hypoxanthine, xanthine, and then uric acid, often rising to >15 mg/dL.
- Electrolytes, BUN, Cr, ↑LDH, Ca^{2+}, PO_4 twice daily, lactate, uric acid
- In TLS, the elevated uric acid level is due to release of purines from ↑ tumor cell turnover. There is an increase in urine uric acid excretion. A spot Uuric acid/UCr >1 implies that the high serum uric acid is from TLS with appropriately high urinary excretion rather than volume depletion where there is
increased tubular reabsorption of uric acid.
- Prevention.

1. Identify at-risk patients (typical or large bulk tumors, first treatment)
2. Prehydration:
    - NS 3–5 L/day for 48 hours pre- and post-therapy for UO >2.5 L/day
3. Prevent uric acid formation. One strategy:
    - If risk is low–moderate: allopurinol 300 mg 12–24 hourly 2 days prior to therapy inhibits xanthine oxidase, preventing the metabolism of hypoxanthine to xanthine (and then urics acid and its salt, urate).
    - If risk of TLS is high (e.g., >50,000 WBC), use preemptive rasburicase.

Treatment of established tumor lysis

- Continue volume expansion with NS and maintain high urine flow.
- Continue allopurinol.
- Rasburicase: a recombinant form of uricase that occurs in most species, but not higher primates. It oxidizes uric acid to soluble allantoin. It rapidly ↓uric acid levels (within 4 hours often to undetectable) and has been shown to prevent dialysis in TLS. Give as 200 µg/kg IVI over 30 min daily for 5 days. ⚠ Avoid if patient is G6PDH deficient.
- ☞ Alkalinize the urine. It is unclear if this is better than saline: $NaHCO_3$ solution aiming for UpH >7.0. Simply maintaining UO at 3–4 L/day may be as good as ↑UpH. It may enhance uric acid solubility, but it is important to watch for metabolic alkalosis, and high UpH may precipitate calcium-phosphate formation in tubules, worsening ARF.
- Institute renal replacement therapy. Consider daily intermittent hemodialysis in oliguric or hyperkalemic patients. This may require long treatment times to remove uric acid or phosphate. Alternatively start continuous therapies at high dialysate or replacement flow rates (2–4 L/hr) to clear elevated serum uric acid and phosphate.

ARF in sepsis

What is the sepsis syndrome?
Sepsis accounts for 2% of all hospital admissions but 10% of admissions to the ICU. ARF is a frequent complication of the sepsis syndrome, increasing in incidence as the severity of sepsis increases. Patients whose renal failure is sepsis related have a mortality of 75%. With sepsis, there is evidence of (usually local) infection with systemic signs of inflammation (↑temp, ↑HR). This may progress to sepsis syndrome if organ dysfunction ensues: typically there is confusion, oliguria, hypoxia, and acidosis. Full-blown septic shock implies hypotension refractory to volume resuscitation.

Causes of significant sepsis
- Gram-positive organisms
    - Staphylococci (including *S. aureus*, MRSA, and *S. epidermidis*) 20%–35%
    - *Streptococcus pneumoniae* 10%
    - Other gram-positive organisms 10%–20%
- Gram-negative organisms
    - *E. coli* 10%–25%
    - Other gram-negative organisms 5%–20%
- Others
    - Fungi (candida) 3%, viruses 3%, parasites (malaria) 1%–2%.

How sepsis becomes shock
Engulfed pathogens are lysed, liberating membrane products (classically lipopolysaccharide, LPS, or exotoxin), proteins, and DNA. These fragments are recognized by specific host receptors on cells (toll-like receptors) which → NFκ-B-dependent cell activation. Activated cells release proinflammatory mediators (IL-1, TNF, interferon), stimulating local and systemic host defense networks.

Systemically activated leukocytes modulate the immune response with increased local leukocyte recruitment into inflamed tissue. At the same time, anti-inflammatory pathways (negative feedback) are induced: inappropriate regulation of these pathways often leads to a deleterious prolongation of systemic inflammation.

Within inflamed tissue, and then systemically, endothelium up-regulates cellular adhesion molecules and tissue factor to encourage recruitment of effector cells. Inducible nitric oxide synthase generates large quantities of NO, and the integrity of intracellular tight junctions is compromised.

Clinically, this translates into the following:
- ↓Systemic vascular resistance (NO is a potent vasodilator and renders angiotensin II [AII] and adrenalin less efficacious.)
- ↑Capillary leak (tight junctions impaired)
- Local tissue injury (neutrophil recruitment with elastase release and oxidant burst)
- ↑Sympathetic activity
- Activation of the renin–angiotensin–aldosterone axis (AII as a vasoconstrictor, aldosterone to promote Na^+ retention, 📖 p. 294)
- Nonosmotic ADH (vasopressin) release (vasoconstrictor)

▶ Vascular smooth muscle becomes less sensitive to vasoconstrictors, so despite high circulating levels of adrenalin, angiotensin, and endothelin, the vascular tree remains (maximally) dilated.

The kidney in sepsis
Norepinephrine vasoconstricts the afferent arteriole, dropping the glomerular perfusion pressure → ↓GFR and Na^+ retention. High systemic NO levels → down-regulation of intrarenal NO production, altering RBF further, particularly in the metabolically vulnerable outer medulla. Inflammatory cells produce oxidants and proteases that injure renal endothelium (remember 20% of cardiac output is to the kidney), and a local coagulopathy → intraglomerular thrombus formation.

This → ↓O_2 delivery, and leads to ATN (as described 📖 p. 100).

Managing septic shock and ARF

Definitions

Systemic inflammatory response syndrome (SIRS)
- Temperature >38.5° or <35.0°C
- HR >90
- RR >20, pCO_2 <32 mmHg or the need for ventilation
- WCC >12 or <4 (or bands >10%).

Sepsis: SIRS +
- Positive cultures or local infection identified (e.g., cellulitis).

Severe sepsis: sepsis + one of the following:
- Skin mottling
- Capillary refill ≥3 seconds
- UO <0.5 mL/kg/h or the need for renal replacement therapy
- Lactate >2 mmol/L
- Altered mental status (or abnormal EEG)
- Plt <100 or DIC
- Acute lung injury (ARDS)
- Impaired cardiac function (echo or cardiac index measurement).

Shock: severe sepsis + one of
- MAP <60 mmHg (80 if known hypertensive) after 40–60 mL/kg NS or 20–30 mL/kg colloid
- Requiring norepinephrine >0.25 µg/kg/min or >5 µg/kg/min dopamine to maintain MAP >60 mmHg (or >80 if known hypertensive).

General priorities

There is an evidence base suggesting better mortality data for the following:

1. Early goal-directed therapy (maintain tissue perfusion):
   - Start volume resuscitation within 6 hours of diagnosis. Treat with boluses with careful monitoring.
   - Fill for target CVP 8–12 cm H_2O and MAP ≥65 mmHg.
   - Transfuse for Hct ≥30% if central SvO_2 (or $ScvO_2$) ≤70%.
   - Despite these measures, if central SvO_2 (or $ScvO_2$) remains ≤70% → dobutamine.
2. Culture and institute broad-spectrum antibiotics, and surgical treatment of localized infection (treat sepsis).
3. Insulin infusion for target glucose 80–110 mg/dl mmol/L (hyperglycemia impairs leukocyte function ± less well-understood effects?).
4. ♦ Hydrocortisone 50 mg IV q6h + fludrocortisone 50 µg po/NG daily if blunted adrenal response: random cortisol <15 µg/dL (415 nmol/L), or with cosyntropin no ↑ >9 µg/dL (250 nmol/L) above baseline (relative insufficiency).
5. Low tidal-volume ventilation 6–7 mL/kg is ideal BW (limits ventilator induced lung injury—barotrauma).
6. ♦ Drotrecogin-α (activated protein C) in high-risk (APACHE II score >24) patients without clinical improvement and no bleeding risk.

Renal priorities

Obviously, maintain independent renal function if possible.
- There are no convincing data to suggest that any particular vasopressor or volume expander is better or worse for the kidneys (norepinephrine is a reasonable first choice over dopamine. Use dobutamine if central venous oxyhemoglobin saturation continues <70% after resuscitation above.
- Avoid renoprotective strategies that lack an evidence base. (p. 122)—low-dose dopamine!

🔑 CVVH or CVVHD may be easier to use in critically ill patients, especially if the patient is on vasopressors, but has not been shown to be superior to intermittent HD regarding mortality in randomized trials.

🔑 "High-dose" CVVH or CVVHDF, aiming for a replacement or dialysate rate of 35–45 mL/kg/min, may improve outcomes.

🔑 A larger delivered hemodialysis dose (adequacy, Kt/V) may improve outcomes—the evidence is **not** conclusive. Most acute dialysis treatments do not reach the prescribed dose. Daily or more frequent hemodialysis may get around this problem to improve clearance as well as help with fluid management.

Two large trials, the ATN study in the United States and the RENAL study in Australia and New Zealand, are both large, multicenter, randomized trials looking at optimal renal replacement dosage in ICU patients with ARF. The ATN study will look at optimal HD and CVVHDF/SLED doses and the RENAL study will look at CVVHDF doses.

Calculating MAP

Mean arterial pressure is expressed as DBP + [SBP–DBP]/3.

Chapter 3

Chronic kidney disease

What is chronic kidney disease (CKD)? 152
Pathogenesis of CKD 154
Diagnosing CKD 156
Progression of CKD 158
Preventing progression: blood pressure 159
Preventing progression: other measures 160
Managing CKD 162
Complications of advanced CKD 164
Uremia 166
Anemia of CKD 168
Erythropoietin 170
Prescribing erythropoietin 172
Iron stores and iron therapy in CKD 174
Renal bone disease 1 176
Renal bone disease 2: physiology 178
Renal bone disease 3: clinical features 180
Renal bone disease 4: treatment 182
Hyperphosphatemia 184
Vitamin D analogues 186
Calcimimetics 188
Parathyroidectomy 190
Calciphylaxis 192
Cardiovascular disease in CKD 194
Pretransplant workup 196
Diet and nutrition in CKD 198
Malnutrition in CKD 200
Endocrine problems in CKD 202
Palliative treatment of advanced CKD 204

What is chronic kidney disease (CKD)?

Definition

The U.S. NKF-DOQI (National Kidney Federation—Kidney Dialysis Outcomes Quality Initiative) classification of chronic kidney disease (CKD) (Table 3.1) has rapidly been adopted internationally. It is both simple and useful, dividing CKD into five stages (Fig. 3.1), according to GFR.[1]

- Patients with a GFR >60 mL/min should not be considered to have CKD unless there is concomitant evidence of kidney damage, suggested by:
  - Abnormal urine findings (proteinuria, hematuria)
  - Structural abnormalities (e.g., abnormal renal imaging)
  - Genetic disease (e.g., APKD)
  - Histologically proven disease
- *Chronic renal failure* (CRF) is now an outmoded term denoting an irreversible decline in GFR.
- The exact prevalence of CKD in the general population is currently unknown. However, early stages of CKD appear common and represent a significant disease burden.
- Many cases of early and asymptomatic CKD are unrecognized and ∴ untreated.
- CKD prevalence increases with age.
- The most common identifiable causes are diabetes and vascular disease (including ↑BP).
- CKD is more common in many ethnic minorities.
- ▶ Most patients with CKD stages 1–3 do not progress to ESRD. Their risk of death from CV disease is higher than their risk of progression.

Table 3.1 NKF-DOQI classification of chronic kidney disease

CKD stage	GFR (mL/min/1.73 m² surface area)	Description
1	>90*	Normal renal function, but other evidence of kidney damage
2	60–89*	Mild reduction in renal function, with other evidence of kidney damage
3	30–59	Moderately reduced GFR
4	15–29	Severely reduced GFR
5	<15	End-stage, or approaching end-stage renal failure

* Early CKD is not diagnosed on GFR alone. There must also be evidence of chronic kidney damage (see below). Patients with a GFR of 60–89 mL/min, with no evidence of kidney disease, do not have CKD, but are classified as having a ↓GFR (± ↑BP).

---

[1] National Kidney Foundation (2002). *Am J Kidney Dis* **1**: S1–S266.

eGFR for diagnosis and management of CKD

- Cr has a nonlinear relationship with GFR. In early CKD, Cr may remain within the "normal" range and be misleading (📖 p. 29).
- eGFR is calculated from formulas that adjust the Cr for age, gender, and race (📖 p. 30).
- The most widely used is the MDRD equation, since it appears to be the most reliable and reproducible in individual patients.
- Normal GFR is ~100 mL/min/1.73 m^2, so eGFR roughly gives a percentage kidney function.
- CKD stages 1–5 are based on eGFR.

Cautions

- It is only an estimate (confidence intervals are wide; 90% of patients will have a GFR within 30% of their eGFR).
- eGFR is likely to be inaccurate at extremes of body habitus (malnourished, obese), as well as in pregnant ♀ and amputees.
- It is not validated under age 18.
- Race is only validated in Caucasians and blacks, though probably acceptable for use in South Asians.
- The MDRD equation tends to underestimate normal renal function.
- It is not validated if the GFR is rapidly changing.

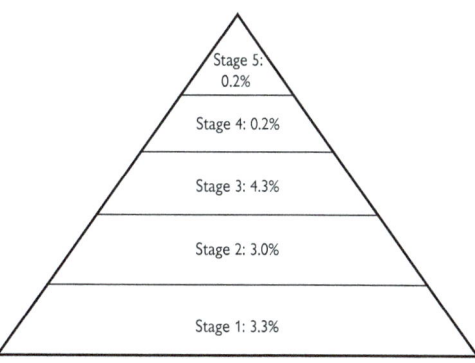

Fig. 3.1 The burden of chronic kidney disease in the U.S. population. Data are taken from the NHANES study in U.S. population.[1] ESRD represents just the tip of the iceberg—note the large numbers in stage 1–3 compared to 4 and 5. Early stages have significantly increased CV risk.

---

1 Coresh J, Astor BC, Greene T, et al. (2003). Prevalence of chronic kidney disease and decreased kidney function in the adult US population: Third National Health and Nutrition Examination Study. *Am J Kidney Dis* **41**(1): 1–12.

Pathogenesis of CKD

Causes of kidney disease
Accurate data on the causes of early CKD are scarce. Registry data focus on causes of ESRD. As only patients whose disease progresses (and who live long enough) reach dialysis or transplantation, it is difficult to extrapolate back to early CKD. Causes of ESRD in the United States are given below, though there is considerable variation worldwide.

Common causes of ESRD in the United States
- Diabetes (43%)
- Glomerulonephritis (21%)
- Interstitial nephritis/pyelonephritis (5%)
- Hypertension (25%)
- Polycystic kidney and hereditary disease (7%)

There is a tendency for renal dysfunction to progress. A series of interacting processes eventually results in the following:
- Glomerulosclerosis (glomerular scarring and obsolescence)
- Proteinuria
- Tubulointerstitial fibrosis.

Mechanisms
Raised intraglomerular pressure
- As nephrons scar and "drop out," remaining nephrons undergo compensatory adaptation, with ↑ blood flow per nephron attempting to "normalize" GFR (the Brenner hypothesis).
- ↑Glomerular capillary wall permeability is a feature of glomerular diseases.
- Renal vasodilatation may be an initiating event, with the glomerulus exposed to a higher capillary pressure.

Glomerular damage
- ↑ Intraglomerular pressure → ↑ wall stress and endothelial injury.
- ↑ Strain on mesangial cells → ↑ matrix deposition mediated (in part) by angiotensin II (AII) and cytokine release (TGF-β, PDGF).

Proteinuria
This may be due to an underlying glomerular lesion, or result from raised intraglomerular pressure. Protein or factors bound to filtered albumin (such as fatty acids, growth factors, or metabolic end-products) may lead to the following:
- Direct proximal tubular cell injury
- Local cytokine synthesis (→ recruitment of interstitial inflammatory cells)
- Profibrotic factors → interstitial scarring
- Transdifferentiation of tubular cells into fibroblasts.

Tubulointerstitial scarring

The degree of tubulointerstitial damage correlates better with long-term prognosis than glomerular damage. Proteinuria may itself be harmful to the tubulointerstitium, but chronic ischemic damage is also important: tissue oxygen tension is relatively low in the renal medulla, making tubules sensitive to hypoxic injury. Chronic ischemia occurs with:
- Damage to glomerular capillaries (glomerulosclerosis → altered peritubular perfusion)
- RAS activation → intrarenal vasoconstriction
- Intratubular capillary loss and increased diffusion distance between capillaries and tubular cells, leading to a vicious cycle of hypoxia.

Diagnosing CKD

▶ Always assume a ↓eGFR represents acute renal failure until proven otherwise. If uncertain, repeat within 5 days and refer as necessary.

Why is it important to identify patients with CKD?
- CKD predisposes patients to ↑CV risk. Modifying other CV risk factors (▶ ↑BP) is likely to ↓morbidity and mortality.
- Some patients will benefit from further investigation (e.g., renal biopsy).
- It may be possible to slow progression to ESRD.
- Complications of CKD (e.g., anemia and bone disease) can be identified and treated early.
- Those (relatively few) patients who will reach ESRD and require dialysis or transplantation need to be properly prepared.

Screening for CKD?
There is currently no evidence that screening of the general population for CKD saves lives or money. Screening should be targeted at those patients at most risk and repeated annually.

Who:
Patients with the following:
- Known CKD
- ↑BP
- Unexplained edema
- CHF
- Atherosclerotic disease (coronary, cerebral, peripheral)
- Diabetes mellitus
- Multisystem disease with possible renal involvement (e.g., SLE, myeloma)
- Bladder outflow obstruction, neurogenic bladder or diversion surgery; renal stone disease
- Chronic nephrotoxin use (e.g., NSAIDs, lithium, cyclosporin, ACEI, ARBs)
- Urologically unexplained hematuria
- Family history of kidney disease

How:
- Urinalysis for blood and protein (±PCR if positive)
- BP
- eGFR

Why is proteinuria so important?
- It is a marker of chronic kidney damage.
- It has prognostic value in the progression of CKD.
- It may itself cause progression of CKD (👁).
- It is a good surrogate treatment target.
- It is an independent CV risk factor.

The importance of BP

- Hypertension does not usually lead to significant renal disease. However, the prevalence of hypertension in the population is so high that hypertensive nephropathy remains a relatively common renal diagnosis (especially in black patients).
- Renal disease is a powerful risk factor for the development of hypertension (most patients with CKD have ↑BP).
- Blood pressure control slows progression of CKD.
- Any patient with hypertension should be examined for the presence of renal disease (UA, eGFR), and the BP should be regularly monitored in all patients with renal disease.

Detection and quantification of proteinuria (📖 p. 18)

- There is no need to perform 24-hour urine collections for quantification of proteinuria.
- If dipstick ≥1+, send a UA to exclude UTI, and send a sample (preferably early morning) to clinical biochemistry (ideally 2 samples, 2 weeks apart): Positive result:
  - Protein/creatinine ratio (PCR) ≥300 mg/gm of creatinine
  - Albumin/creatinine ratio (ACR) ≥30 mg/gm of creatinine
  - PCR is adequate in most instances. ACR is more sensitive for early disease screening in high-risk groups (e.g., those with diabetes).

Progression of CKD

Once CKD is established it tends to progress, regardless of underlying cause. Decline in GFR tends to be linear over time, unless clinical circumstances change. Progression of CKD is more often due to secondary hemodynamic and metabolic factors than to underlying disease activity.

Factors influencing progression of CRF

Nonmodifiable
- Underlying cause of kidney disease (tubulointerstitial disease tends to progress more slowly than glomerular disease)
- Race (progression faster in blacks)

Modifiable
- BP
- Level of proteinuria
- Plus:
  - Nephrotoxic agents
  - Underlying disease activity (e.g., SLE, vasculitis)
  - Further renal insults (superimposed obstruction, UTI)
  - Hypovolemia or intercurrent illness
  - Dyslipidemia
  - Hyperphosphatemia
  - Uncontrolled metabolic acidosis
  - Anemia
  - Smoking
  - Blood glucose control (if diabetic)

1. What can be done to prevent or slow down progression?
- Diagnose the cause of CKD.
  - This helps determine prognosis.
  - Is specific intervention or treatment possible?
  - History: check for systemic disease (e.g., DM, SLE, myeloma), lower urinary tract symptoms, stone disease, inherited renal disease; review all medications.
  - Examination: BP, hypovolemia, atherosclerosis, palpable bladder, stigmata of inflammatory disease.
  - Investigation: UA (hematuria and/or proteinuria may suggest a renal or systemic disease that might benefit from specific intervention), US renal tract (p. 38), renal biopsy (p. 634).

2. Influence mediators of progression
- BP (p. 159)
- Other factors (p. 160).

Preventing progression: blood pressure

Hypertension may be the cause or effect in CKD. Either way, it should be treated aggressively, as poor BP control causes (1) a more rapid decline in GFR (↑BP → ↑ glomerular filtration pressure and ↑ proteinuria → ↑ renal injury) and (2) ↑CV risk. BP targets are more stringent in CKD (and lower still for patients with proteinuria).

Blood pressure targets in CKD
- Without proteinuria (PCR <100 mg/mmol)
  - Treat at 140/90
  - Target 130/80
- With proteinuria (PCR >100 mg/mmol)
  - Treat at 130/80
  - Target 120/75
- Diabetes mellitus
  - Target 120/75

What drug?

Several studies have shown a beneficial preservation of renal function in proteinuric renal disease with use of ACEI and ARB. This may be "added value," over and above their antihypertensive effect. The evidence is not conclusive (especially for nonproteinuric CKD), but there is general consensus for first-line use. Putative mechanisms include the following:
- ↓ Efferent arteriolar tone → ↓ intraglomerular pressure and ↓ proteinuria.
- ↓ AII activity → AII-induced inflammation → ↓ fibrosis and scarring.
- ACEIs affect both angiotensin type 1 (A1) and type 2 (A2) receptors, but may not completely inhibit AII formation (📖 p. 342).
- ARBs block A1 receptors, but not A2.
- There is growing evidence that ACEI + ARB (dual blockade) is an effective therapeutic combination (📖 p. 344).

Antihypertensives in CKD: a suggested batting order

Expect to need ≥3 agents (warn patient that this is likely to be the case).
- First, limit Na⁺ intake and recommend other lifestyle measures (📖 p. 198).
- ACEI (especially if PCR >300 mg/dL)
- Loop diuretic (e.g., furosemide) if there is evidence of salt and water overload. Thiazide diuretics may be effective in early CKD.
- Add ARB if PCR remains >300 mg/dL.
- Dihydropyridine calcium channel blocker (e.g., nifedipine, amlodipine)
- β-blocker
- Centrally acting agent (e.g., clonidine)
- α-blocker (e.g., doxazosin)
- Vascular smooth muscle relaxant (e.g., minoxidil).

African-American patients may benefit from a different combination of drugs (📖 p. 321).

Preventing progression: other measures

Dyslipidemia

Experimental work suggests that hyperlipidemia accelerates ↓GFR. ✱ It is not yet clear whether treating dyslipidemia with statins limits progression (or ↓CV risk in CKD). However, lipid lowering is recommended for diabetics with CKD and for CKD patients with a history of myocardial events as secondary prevention.

- All the large studies of cholesterol lowering have excluded patients with CKD. The ongoing Study of Heart and Renal Protection (SHARP) has been designed to redress this issue.
- Current consensus is that dyslipidemia in CKD should be treated with statins even if the patient has no other CV risk factors.
- ⚠ Side effects are *more common* in CKD. Myalgia and a small rise in creatine kinase are common. ▶ More rhabdomyolysis is reported. Liver function abnormalities are also more common.
- Targets: In the absence of helpful evidence, these should be as for secondary prevention in the general population, e.g., total cholesterol <200 mg/dL, LDL <100 mg/dL.

Hyperphosphatemia

(See 📖 p. 184) Calcium phosphate deposition in the renal interstitium may contribute to progression of CKD, strengthening the argument for good control of the serum phosphate in these patients.

Acidosis

Acid in the nephron, experimentally at least, causes complement activation and interstitial damage. But there is no current evidence that administration of sodium bicarbonate slows CKD progression. Correction of acidosis is desirable for other reasons, however (📖 p. 165).

Anemia

It has been suggested that treatment with an erythropoiesis-stimulating protein (ESP) (📖 p. 170) may slow progression, but again, robust evidence is lacking.

Drugs, toxins, and infections

Once renal failure is established, remaining kidney function is highly susceptible to further (often irreversible) damage. Avoid the following:
- Hypovolemia
- Obstruction or recurrent urinary infection
- Nephrotoxins
  - Drugs (e.g., NSAIDS)
  - Radiocontrast (📖 p. 142).

Smoking

As well as increasing overall CV risk, tobacco consumption → ↓GFR in CKD. Patients should be strongly encouraged to quit smoking.

Diabetes

In patients with diabetic nephropathy, tight glycemic control *may* minimize the rate of decline of renal function (as well as prevent other CV complications).

Dietary protein restriction

In animal models, lowering protein intake protects against the development of glomerulosclerosis. Mediators appear to be ↓intraglomerular pressure and ↓glomerular hypertrophy. Nonhemodynamic effects, such as ↓TGF-β and ↓ matrix accumulation, may also be important. In humans, the benefit of dietary protein restriction remains controversial. Although progression may be retarded, a huge investment of effort is required on the part of the patient and dietetic staff. Long-term compliance is often poor. At present, optimal dietary treatment of patients with CKD is uncertain. 🖝 A reasonable regimen is an intake of ~0.8 to 1.0 g/kg of protein/day. Lower levels may risk malnutrition (particular in the context of either advanced CKD or nephrotic range proteinuria). Diabetic nephropathy *may* be more responsive.

Preventing progression—what's on the horizon?

The degree of tubular and interstitial damage is a better predictor of long-term renal prognosis than the severity of glomerular changes. So reducing scarring may slow declining GFR in progressive CKD. Experimental tubular injury may be reduced by the following:

- ACEIs (already shown in clinical practice to ↓ proteinuria) may ↓ tubular complement activation and ∴ interstitial inflammation.
- Experimentally, activation of the mineralocorticoid receptor → interstitial fibrosis and vascular changes. An ACEI or ARB may provide some protection against this. Additive mineralocorticoid receptor antagonism using eplerenone or spironolactone may provide additional benefit. Hyperkalemia would be a potentially dangerous complication of this strategy.
- Mycophenolate mofetil (MMF) may ↓ proteinuria (and renal scarring).
- Pirfenidone may inhibit, or even reverse, fibrosis in the interstitium, partly by suppressing TGF-β.
- BX471, a chemokine antagonist, appears to have an antifibrotic effect.

Managing CKD

General advice (all stages)
- Stop smoking.
- Reduce weight if obese.
- Encourage aerobic exercise.
- Check lipids and treat according to national guidelines.
- Avoid NSAIDs and other nephrotoxic drugs.
- Get vaccination against influenza and pneumococcus, hepatitis B, and, if patient is in need of a transplant, varicella zoster.

CKD stages 1–3
- ▶ Most of these patients will not progress to ESRD, so the emphasis should be on CV risk reduction.
- These stages can usually be effectively managed in a primary-care setting.
- Suggested criteria for referral to a specialist renal service are shown in Box 3.1.
- Stages 1–2: at least annual follow-up:
  - eGFR, urinalysis, and PCR
  - Meticulous BP control (📖 p. 159 for targets)
- Stage 3: at least 6-month follow-up:
  - eGFR, urinalysis, and PCR
  - Meticulous BP control (📖 p. 159 for targets).
  - If Hb <11 g/dL check ferritin, % saturation of transferin (start on po iron if <100 mg/dL. Or % saturation of transferin <20%), B_{12} and folate. Refer for IV iron ± EPO according to locally agreed-upon protocols (📖 p. 175).
  - Annual check of serum calcium, phosphorus, and parathyroid hormone (PTH) (stages 1 and 2)
  - Semiannual check of serum calcium, phosphorus, and PTH (stage 3).

CKD stages 4–5
- Refer to a nephrologist (▶ urgently if stage 5). Late referral of patients with advanced CKD is associated with poor outcomes.
- Full dietary assessment (📖 p. 198)
- Optimize calcium, phosphate, and PTH (📖 p. 182).
- Correct acidosis (📖 p. 165).
- Hepatitis B immunization
- Provide information on and discuss future treatments (dialysis, transplantation, or conservative/palliative treatment).

Box 3.1 When to refer to a nephrologist (varies by region)

- eGFR <30 mL/min/1.73 m^2
- eGFR <60 mL/min/1.73 m^2 **and any of the following:**
  - Progressive fall (>10 mL/min/m^2 in 2 successive years)
  - Microscopic hematuria
  - Proteinuria
  - >15% decline in eGFR with commencement of an ACEI or ARB (?renovascular disease)
  - Possible systemic illness (e.g., SLE, myeloma)
  - Hb <11 g/dL
  - Abnormal calcium or phosphate
  - PTH >70 pg/mL
  - Refractory ↑BP (150/90 despite 3 antihypertensive agents)
- eGFR >60 mL/min/1.73 m^2 **and** other evidence of renal disease/damage
  - PCR >300 mg/dL (or ACR >30 mg/dL)
  - Microscopic hematuria
  - Abnormal renal imaging
  - Family history of renal disease
- Other indications
- Suspected acute renal failure

CKD clinic

The transition from CKD to ESRD is a physically and psychologically demanding time. Such patients are best cared for in a multidisciplinary clinic (see ~6 weeks, more often in the later stages), with attention to the following:

- Ongoing measures to minimize rate of progression
- Dietary intervention
- Active management of complications (anemia, renal bone disease, acidosis, malnutrition)
- Predialysis counseling: choice of dialysis modality, individualized advice and support in the decision-making process
- Preparation for transplantation—education, identify potential living donors. Preemptive transplantation should be a goal.
- Formation of dialysis access (Referral to a surgeon at least 6 months prior to start of dialysis is preferable.)
- Access to palliative services for those who elect not to undertake dialysis treatment
- Timing initiation of dialysis—avoid symptomatic uremia.

Composition of the CKD clinic

- Nephrologist
- Specialist nurses (e.g., predialysis counseling, anemia management, pretransplant assessment, palliative care)
- Renal dietitian
- Vascular access surgeon
- Pharmacist
- Social worker.

Complications of advanced CKD

Fluid overload

Salt and water overload is usual in advanced CKD. However, as tubulointerstitial scarring progresses, loss of concentrating ability may → fixed (and often large) urine volumes and a relative salt-losing state (📖 p. 406). Such patients may be chronically hypo- rather than hypervolemic and require salt and water supplementation (e.g., $NaHCO_3$ 0.5–1.5 g tid and increased fluid intake).

Treating salt and water retention in CKD

▶ Careful clinical assessment of volume status
- Dietary salt restriction (📖 p. 199)
- Fluid intake restriction
- Start furosemide 40 mg od and titrate as necessary (maximum 250 mg daily).
- If there is a poor response, consider thiazide diuretic (metolazone 2.5–10 mg qd) for synergistic effect. ⚠ Diuresis may be brisk. Beware of ↓Na^+, ↓K^+, and volume depletion (consider admission).
- Monitor the following:
  - Daily weight—the best day-to-day guide of salt and water status. Ask patient to keep a diary of their weight at home. Weight loss should generally be ≤0.5–1 kg/day.
  - BP (especially postural ↓BP if overdiuresed)
  - Refractory volume overload may signal the need for renal replacement therapy.

Hyperkalemia

↓Na^+ delivery to the distal convoluted tubule → ↓ aldosterone-mediated Na^+/K^+ exchange and ↓K^+ excretion. ▶ ↑K^+ is a common and potentially fatal problem in advanced CKD, particularly in those treated with ACEIs or ARBs. Rapid rises in K^+ are generally more dangerous than gradual ones, as cell membrane stability is more vulnerable to acute changes.

What constitutes a worrying K^+ level?

It depends on the context and chronicity.
- 5.5–6.0 meq/L: Recheck routinely. Review medications. Arrange dietary advice.
- 6.1–6.5 meq/L: Recheck *urgently*. Review medications (withhold ACEI/ARB or add sodium polystryrene). Arrange dietary advice.
- >6.5 meq/L: ▶ Admit. See 📖 p. 199 for emergency management.

Measures to prevent ↑K⁺
- Dietary restriction (📖 p. 198)
- Diuretics: A loop diuretic (e.g., furosemide 40–160 mg qd) may promote urinary K⁺ loss (thiazides may be ineffective).
- Drug withdrawal or dose reduction if taking an ACEI or ARB. Review other contributory drugs (e.g., spironolactone, β-blockers, NSAIDS).
- Correct acidosis (see below).
- Add sodium polystyrene (15 g orally 1–4 times daily).
- Refractory ↑K⁺ may indicate the need for dialysis.

Acidosis (📖 p. 556).

Systemic effects of acidosis
- *Bone:* ↑ bone resorption and impaired mineralization, contributing to renal osteodystrophy (📖 p. 176)
- *Metabolism:* muscle weakness, fatigue, sense of ill health
- *Effects of respiratory compensation* (📖 p. 554): overventilation; may → symptoms of dyspnea ±exhaustion
- *Hyperkalemia:* Aldosterone-mediated exchange of H⁺ for K⁺ is enhanced in the collecting duct, → ↑K⁺. Acidosis also lessens K⁺ ingress via cell membrane Na⁺/K⁺ pumps.
- *Ionized calcium:* ↑ ionized (free) calcium (acidosis → ↓ albumin-bound fraction). ⚠ Correction of acidosis may → ↓Ca^{2+} and provoke tetany.
- *Nutrition:* Acidosis promotes catabolism by induction of proteolysis and resistance to growth hormone (→ malnutrition).

How to correct acidosis?
- Treat when venous HCO_3^- is <21 meq/L.
- Give $NaHCO_3$ 0.5–1.5 g/tid or sodium citrate 30 to 90 cc/day in three divided doses (start at low dose and titrate).
- ⚠ Na⁺ load may cause or worsen fluid overload. Consider concomitant loop diuretic.
- Refractory acidosis is an indication for dialysis.

Uremia

Uremia is the clinical syndrome caused by a substantial fall in GFR—it is *not* a result of ↑ blood urea concentration, but rather of failure to eliminate potentially toxic small and middle molecules. This leads to chronic inflammation and oxidative stress, with accumulation of metabolic end-products, accelerated atherogenesis, disruption of the immune system, and anemia. The retained compounds or toxins have multiple effects:
- Many remain unidentified.
- They are divided into "low" and "middle" molecular-weight molecules, by size (<500 D = low; >500 D = middle).
- Ur and Cr are routinely measured, but are not directly toxic. They act as markers for other LMW substances, including guanidines such as asymmetric dimethyl arginine (ADMA)—a potent inhibitor of nitric oxide synthase (NOS).
- Retained middle molecules include the following:
  - β_2-microglobulin (12,000 D)—a component of major histocompatibility complex (MHC) (the cause of dialysis-related amyloid)
  - Advanced glycation end-products (AGE)—products of nonenzymatic breakdown of sugars. Also retained in normal aging and diabetes. They are linked to atherogenesis and susceptibility to infection.
  - Complement factor D may activate the complement system and contribute to chronic inflammation in uremia.
  - Cytokines may maintain uremic chronic inflammation and malnutrition (short half-life suggests overproduction is more important).
  - Many, many others.
- ↑ Oxidant stress → ↑ oxidation products with ↓ antioxidant levels (in part due to impaired polyamine balance).
- Phosphate is retained, contributing to hyperparathyroidism, arteriosclerosis, and vessel calcification (→ ↓ arterial compliance, systolic hypertension, and diastolic dysfunction). (See p. 218).

See p. 167 for clinical manifestations of the uremic syndrome.

When to start dialysis

Current guidelines recommend commencing dialysis when
- GFR <15 mL/min with uremic symptoms (persistent nausea and vomiting, anorexia, malnutrition, volume overload, restless legs).
- GFR <10 mL/min whether symptomatic or not.
- Refractory hyperkalemia, acidosis, pulmonary edema, pericarditis, encephalopathy, and neuropathy are all (urgent) indications for dialysis (the aim should be to start dialysis *before* any of these are present).
- There is no clear evidence that an early start to dialysis confers a survival benefit.
- ▶ Preemptive transplantation is the treatment of choice of ESRD. Consider when GFR <20 mL/min.

Anemia of CKD

Erythropoietin (EPO) and the kidney

Red blood cell production is tightly regulated by a number of different growth factors. EPO is essential for the terminal maturation of erythrocytes, and differs from other growth factors in that it is produced by peritubular interstitial fibroblasts in the outer renal medulla and deep cortex of the kidney rather than the bone marrow. The kidney is ideally placed to regulate RBC production, as it is uniquely able to sense and control both O_2 tension *and* circulating volume (and differentiate between the two).

- Red cell mass is regulated by EPO.
- Circulating volume is regulated by salt and water excretion.
- The kidney maintains the Hb 12–14 g in normal conditions (maximizing tissue O_2 delivery).

Chronic kidney disease and renal scarring → ↓EPO synthesis, ↓RBC production, and anemia. This occurs in most forms of advanced CKD (eGFR <35 mL/min), with a few exceptions:
- Adult polycystic kidney disease
- Benign renal cysts
- Renal cell carcinoma.

In these instances, EPO may be overproduced.

Differential diagnosis of anemia in CKD patients

▶ EPO deficiency is not the only cause of ↓Hb in CKD.

Patients with CKD are susceptible to *all* other causes of anemia, so these should be actively sought in patients who appear disproportionately anemic or EPO resistant (p. 171):
- Iron deficiency (p. 174)
- Blood loss (GI tract, hemodialysis)
- Folate deficiency
- B_{12} deficiency
- Hemolysis
- Myelodysplasia
- Myeloma

EPO: mechanism of production

In states of normal O_2 tension, intracellular hypoxia-inducible factor 1 (HIF1) is inactivated by constitutive proline hydroxylation of one its two subunits (Fig. 3.2). This allows the α-subunit to be targeted by von Hippel–Lindau (VHL) protein for continuous protesomal degradation. In hypoxic conditions, α-subunit degradation does not occur, permitting full activation of functional HIF1 (and other) signaling pathways → EPO transcription. The renin–angiotensin system (RAS) also plays a role, with renin → ↑ EPO production (▶ an effect abolished by ACEI, hence their propensity to cause a mild fall in Hb).

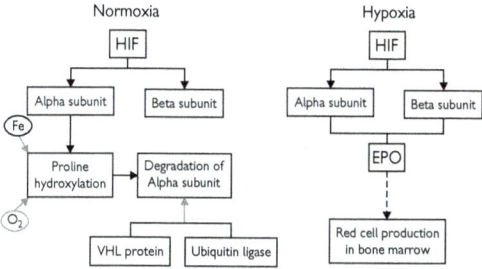

Fig. 3.2 Regulation of EPO production.

Erythropoietin

Recombinant EPO is a safe and effective means of maintaining Hb for most patients with CKD. Prior to its introduction, patients were almost invariably transfusion dependent, with all the attendant problems of iron overload, sensitization to foreign antigens (which had implications for future transplantation), and risk of blood-borne viral infection. EPO also has a number of beneficial nonhematological effects.

Nonhematological effects of EPO

- Enhanced quality-of-life scores
- Reduced fatigue
- Improved cardiorespiratory function and exercise capacity
- Reduction in LVH
- Improved cognitive function
- Improvement in sexual dysfunction
- Partial normalization of cortisol and carbohydrate metabolism
- Improved sleep quality

Who needs EPO?

Any anemic CKD patient, assuming other causes are unlikely or have been ruled out, needs EPO. Consider EPO when Hb <11 g/dL (local protocols may vary). Measuring EPO levels is expensive and rarely necessary.

Preparation for EPO therapy

- Have other causes of anemia been excluded, especially iron deficiency (📖 p. 174)?
- Is the patient likely to respond to EPO? Inflammatory cytokines associated with infection (or chronic inflammatory states) inhibit the effect of EPO. ▶ Treat these first. ↑CRP often predicts poor response.
- Is BP controlled? EPO tends to ↑BP. Severe ↑BP was not uncommon in the early days of EPO use (mechanism: vasoconstriction and enhanced adrenergic responsiveness), but has ↓ In incidence with refinement of treatment algorithms.

Which EPO?

There are two major preparations on the market:
- Epoetin-α (Epogen, Procrit)
- Darbepoetin-α (Aranesp®, Amgen)

Epoetin-α is given to hemodialysis patients intravenously with each treatment. Peritoneal dialysis patients receive Epoetin subcutaneously once weekly and CKD patients receive either Epoetin subcutaneously once every week to once every 3 weeks depending on response. Darbepoetin is a glycosylated form of Epoetin with a longer $t_{1/2}$ and can be given subcutaneously every 1–4 weeks depending on response.

EPO nonresponse

This is arbitrarily defined as a failure to reach target Hb, or the need for >500 IU/kg /week of EPO (or darbepoietin-α-equivalent) to maintain Hb at target.

▶ The most common cause is iron deficiency. Once this is excluded or treated, consider the following:
- Chronic blood loss (▶ particularly GI)
- Frequent hospitalization
- Infection or inflammation (measure CRP)
- Severe hyperparathyroidism (causes bone marrow fibrosis—check PTH)
- Aluminum toxicity (📖 p. 183)
- Hemoglobinopathies (Hb variants screen)
- B_{12} or folate or iron deficiency
- Occult malignancy
- Hemolysis (blood film, Coombs' test, haptoglobins, LDH)
- Inadequate dialysis (Kt/V, 📖 p. 219)
- Pure red cell aplasia (PRCA)
- Malnutrition
- Inadequate dosing
- Poor compliance?

Prescribing erythropoietin

Route of administration
- Either SC or IV (IV often used in hemodialysis patients, given at the end of a dialysis treatment)
- SC route ↓ dose requirements by ~25% (for EPO α and β, not darbepoietin).
- Rare reports of PRCA in patients treated with SC epoetin-α now appear to have been resolved.
- Patients can be taught to self-administer EPO at home using a range of user-friendly devices (EPO should be kept in a refrigerator).

Starting EPO
- ► Ensure that iron is replete (📖 p. 174).
- EPO-α A single weekly dose of 10,000 units/week—CKD
- EPO 50–150 units/kg IV three times a week—HD
- Darbepoetin-α has a typical starting dose of 0.45 µg/kg/week SC.
- To convert from EPO to darbepoietin ÷ total weekly dose by 200 and give once per week.
- Double the starting dose if there is clinical urgency and/or EPO resistance is likely.
  - Measure Hb and BP weekly at first.
  - If there is a rapid deterioration in BP, intensify antihypertensive medications (it is rarely necessary to withhold EPO).
  - Aim for ↑Hb of 1–2 g/dL/month until in target range (see Box 3.2).
  - ↑Dose monthly (~25% increments) if Hb rise is slow. Conversely, be prepared to ↓ dose if Hb rise is too rapid.
  - Iron stores are likely to rapidly deplete: ∴ monitor and replace as necessary.
  - Once in "steady-state," monitor Hb and iron stores every 1–3 months in predialysis patients and monthly in dialysis patients.
  - Check reticulocyte count in nonresponders (should ↑).

☞ Although higher targets have been sought as early fears about ↑thrombotic risks (and loss of vascular access in hemodialysis patients) were dispelled, it is now thought that overzealous correction (target Hb >13 g/dL) → increased mortality. Individualized targets are the likely future direction of EPO therapy.

Box 3.2 Target hemoglobin
- UK Renal Association: >10 g/dL. Upper limit is not specified.
- European guidelines: >11 g/dL (but not >14 g/dL). Aim for 11–12 g/dL if there is risk of CHF or ischemic heart disease.
- US K-DOQI guidelines: 11–12 g/dL.

Iron stores and iron therapy in CKD

▶ Giving EPO to an iron-deficient patient is a waste of time and money.

Iron deficiency is found in ~40% of patients with advanced CKD and high iron availability is required to maximize response to exogenous EPO. Patients are at risk of enhanced iron loss by various routes:
- GI bleeding (often subclinical)
- Multiple blood tests
- Hemodialysis itself (HD patients may lose up to 2 g of iron per year).

Monitoring of iron status is not always straightforward. Use ferritin and % saturation of transferrin.
- Ferritin
  - Target: 150–500 µg/L (i.e., well above the normal physiological range). Avoid >1000 µg/L.
  - Rationale: the cellular storage protein for iron. Plasma ferritin concentration usually reflects iron status.
  - Problems with interpretation: ferritin is an acute phase protein. If inflammation is present (▶ measure CRP simultaneously), a high or normal ferritin level may be misleading.
- Transferrin saturation (TSAT) >20%
  - TSAT = (serum iron/TIBC) x 100

Iron replacement
- Oral iron is not well tolerated (GI side effects) and compliance is generally poor.
- Medications that raise gastric pH decrease oral iron absorption.
- In many patients iron stores do not improve.
- Many units have developed policies based entirely on IV iron.

Predialysis
- Give iron orally.
  - If ferritin <100 µg/L or % saturation of transferrin <20 % start $FeSO_4$ 325 mg tid.
- Warn patients about GI intolerance. Oral iron should not be taken simultaneously with phosphate binders (📖 p. 175). If oral iron is poorly tolerated (or response inadequate), give IV iron.
- Start trial of oral iron for 4–6 weeks → recheck stores.

If on dialysis
- Give parenteral iron.

Monitoring
Iron stores and Hb should be measured every 1–2 months predialysis and monthly in dialysis patients.

Types of IV iron

- Iron dextran
  - Carries a risk of allergic reactions and anaphylaxis (0.6%).
  - A test dose should be given to new starters.
  - Resuscitation facilities should be available.
- Iron sucrose/sacharate (e.g., Venofer®)
  - Newer preparation
  - Risk of anaphylaxis appears to be minimal (0.05%). Test dose is unnecessary.
  - Typical dosing: predialysis (or CAPD): 200 mg weekly for 3 doses, then every 1–3 months. Hemodialysis: 100 mg/dialysis session for 10 doses (usually into the bubble trap)
- Sodium ferric gluconate (Ferrlecit®)
  - Anaphylaxis is rare. Test dose is unnecessary.
  - Typical dose: 125 mg IV with each dialysis for 4–8 doses

⚠ Iron overload should be avoided, particularly as free iron may cause oxidative tissue damage, increasing infections and cardiovascular risk. Unfortunately, no study in patients with ESRD has established a safe or toxic level of iron based on serum ferritin.

Renal bone disease 1

Definition
- Renal bone disease (osteodystrophy) is a heterogeneous disorder leading to diminished bone strength in patients with impaired kidney function.
- Virtually ubiquitous beyond CKD stage 3, its management represents a significant challenge.
- Uremic mineral metabolism (and its treatment) may have an impact on cardiovascular morbidity and mortality in CKD patients.

Classification (Fig. 3.3)
Osteodystrophy is a function of bone turnover, density, mineralization and architecture. Strictly speaking, bone biopsy with histological and histomorphometric assessment is required for diagnosis and classification. In practice, biopsies are very rarely performed (they are invasive, considerable expertise is needed to interpret them), and surrogate markers of bone turnover are (over) relied on (Table 3.2).

Secondary hyperparathyroidism (SHPT) ↑PTH causes increased bone resorption and formation ("high turnover" disease). Haphazardly organized, weakened bone results (classically osteitis fibrosa cystica).

Adynamic bone disease This represents a paucity of cells with decreased bone resorption and formation ("low turnover" disease). Pathophysiology remains poorly understood, but incidence has increased rapidly over the last two decades.

Mixed turnover disease is relatively common, as is evolution from one form to another.

Osteomalacia refers to a defect in mineralization. It is uncommon as an isolated finding and not helpful as a clinical description. It is generally related to a deficiency of $1,25(OH)_2D$, but aluminum intoxication and uremic acidosis are also risk factors.

Osteoporosis is usually defined in terms of bone mineral density (BMD) ∴ has little diagnostic meaning in the context of osteodystrophy, where low BMD can coexist with low- or high-turnover disease. DEXA scanning does not predict fracture risk in CKD.

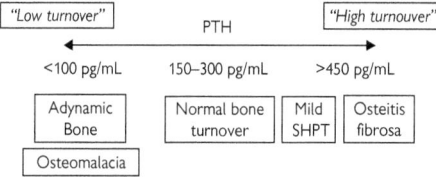

Fig. 3.3 The spectrum of renal bone disease. (Note: pg/mL = ng/L. For pmol/L multiply by 0.11.)

Table 3.2 Features of "high"- and "low-turnover" renal bone disease

	High turnover	Low turnover	
	Hyperparathyroid bone disease	Adynamic bone disease	Osteomalacia
Bone biopsy findings	↑Osteoblast and osteoclast activity	↓Osteoblast and osteoclast activity	↓Osteoblast and osteoclast activity
	Fibrosis	Thin osteoid seams	Widened osteoid seams
			Aluminum deposition
PTH	High	Low or normal	Usually low or normal
Alkaline phosphatase	Raised	Normal	Normal
Calcium	Variable	Often ↑	Normal or ↑
Phosphate	↑	Normal or ↑	Normal or ↑
DFO test*	Normal	Normal	Often elevated

* DFO test = desferrioxamine test: a noninvasive means of detecting aluminum overload.

Renal bone disease 2: physiology

If renal function is intact, concentrations of PO_4 and Ca^{2+} are maintained through interaction between PTH, $1,25(OH)_2D$ (calcitriol), and their three primary targets: bone, kidney, and GI tract.

Parathyroid hormone
PTH secretion (and parathyroid gland proliferation) is stimulated by ↓Ca^{2+}, ↓$1,25(OH)_2D$, and ↑PO_4. In most circumstances, ↓Ca^{2+} (acting via the parathyroid calcium-sensing receptor) overrides the other two. PTH acts on three fronts: (1) mobilizing skeletal calcium; (2) ↓ urinary Ca^{2+} + ↑urinary PO_4 excretion; and (3) ↑ renal production of $1,25(OH)_2D$ (in turn → ↑ intestinal Ca^{2+} and PO_4 absorption).

Vitamin D
Inactive vitamin D (from dietary sources and UV conversion in the skin) is metabolized in the liver to $25(OH)D$ and then converted to $1,25(OH)_2D$ by the renal 1α-hydroxylase enzyme. $1,25(OH)_2D$ alters gene expression by binding to an intracellular receptor (VDR) and exerts a number of important effects (Fig. 3.4).

Bone biology
Bone is not static, it continuously adapts to mechanical and metabolic requirements by a remodeling process centered around the coupling of osteoblastic formation and osteoclastic resorption. Multiple systemic hormones (including PTH and $1,25(OH)_2D$) and local growth factors (e.g., RANK/OPG) influence this process. Bone is the most important body reservoir of Ca^{2+} and PO_4.

The effect of renal failure

- Loss of functioning renal mass →
  - Phosphate accumulation
  - ↓$1,25(OH)_2D$ (→ ↓serum Ca^{2+})
- Secondary hyperparathyroidism (Fig. 3.5)
  - ↓Ca^{2+} + ↓$1,25(OH)_2D$ + ↑PO_4 → ↑PTH synthesis and release
  - Prolonged stimulation of parathyroid tissue → clonal proliferation of parathyroid cells (with areas of nodular hyperplasia)
  - These clones express less calcium-sensing receptor (CaR) and VDR.
  - Refractoriness to treatment is inevitable (termed tertiary or autonomous HPT).
  - In addition there is relative "skeletal resistance" to the effects of PTH (mechanism unclear).
  - Abnormal bone turnover results.
  - ↑PTH also has nonskeletal effects: LVH, cardiac fibrosis, extraskeletal calcification, peripheral neuropathy, impotence.

RENAL BONE DISEASE 2: PHYSIOLOGY 179

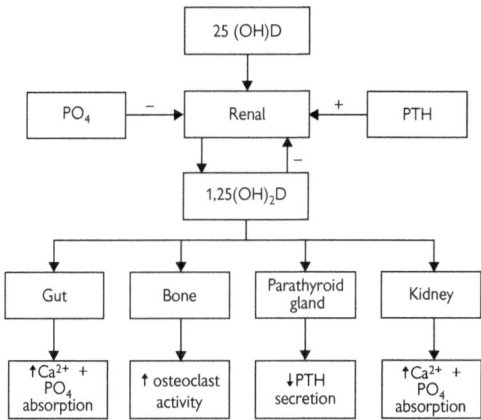

Fig. 3.4 Overview of vitamin D metabolism.

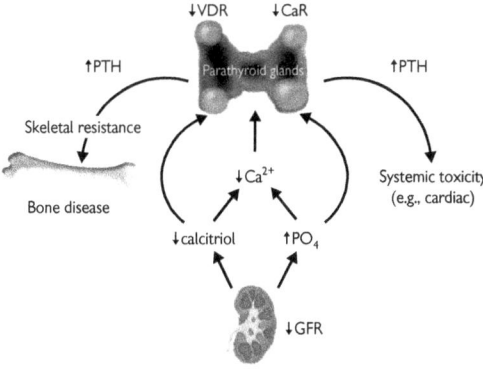

Fig. 3.5 The pathogenesis of secondary hyperparathyroidism (SHPT).

Renal bone disease 3: clinical features

Secondary hyperparathyroidism (SHPT)
- It is usually asymptomatic.
- Clinical sequelae occur late (with significant biochemical and histological disease), including:
  - Bone pain and arthralgia
  - Muscle weakness (especially proximal)
  - Pruritis (cutaneous calcium phosphate deposition)
  - Bony deformity (e.g., resorption of terminal phalanges)
- ↑ fracture risk (hip fracture risk ~5x in dialysis patients)
  - Mortality following fracture rises ~2.5x.
- Marrow fibrosis contributes to anemia and poor response to EPO therapy.

Adynamic bone disorder (ABD)
- It is usually asymptomatic.
- There is probably no ↑fracture risk.
- Adynamic bone buffers calcium poorly; ↑Ca^{2+} is common.
- Aluminum-related low-turnover bone disease is often painful.

Cardiovascular risk
- ▶ Poor control of serum PO_4, calcium phosphate product (CaxP), and PTH are all associated with ↑CV morbidity and mortality.
- ↑CaxP is associated with soft tissue, vascular, and cardiac calcification.

Diagnosis
No one marker is perfect, so a clinical data set is used (Table 3.2).

Biochemical
- Check Ca^{2+}, PO_4, and PTH at least every 3 months (more often if treatment changes are made) in CKD stages 4 and 5, and annually in stage 3.
- PTH: The ability of serum PTH to predict high- and low-turnover disease is actually quite poor, though improves at extremes of PTH (>450 pg/mL: high-turnover disease, <100 pg/mL: low-turnover disease).
- Calcium: ↓ in untreated SHPT (though rises with vitamin D analogue and calcium-based phosphate binder treatment); often ↑ in ABD.
- Phosphate: raised.
- Alkaline phosphatase: ↑ in SHPT (a marker of bone formation—others, e.g., osteocalcin, are also elevated).

Radiology
The availability of PTH measurements means X-rays are rarely necessary.
- SHPT: subperiosteal bone resorption (distal and middle phalanges of hands and feet), osteosclerosis (→ "rugger jersey spine" on lateral film).
- ABD: generally normal.

PTH assays

- In addition to intact PTH (PTH 1–84), which acts on its targets via the classical PTH-1 receptor, most commonly used assays also detect other biologically active fragments (e.g., 7–84) of the hormone.
- These N-terminally truncated peptides appear to exert an inhibitory influence on bone cells (probably via a distinct C-PTH receptor) and could be a contributory factor to skeletal PTH resistance.
- A new generation of assays, more specific for "whole" PTH, has been developed and is likely to attract increasing attention as their clinicopathological validation progresses.

Factors contributing to adynamic bone disease

- Low PTH
- Overtreatment with vitamin D
- ↑ Calcium intake
- Diabetes mellitus
- ↑ Age
- Aluminum accumulation
- Acidosis
- CAPD
- Corticosteroid therapy

Renal bone disease 4: treatment

Goals
- Keep serum Ca^{2+} and PO_4 within the normal range.
- Keep bone turnover and strength as near normal as possible.
- Keep serum PTH appropriate to the above objectives.
- Prevent the development of parathyroid hyperplasia.

The standard treatment package comprises:
- Measures to ↓ serum PO_4:
  - Dietary PO_4 restriction
  - Removal through adequate dialysis
  - Oral phosphate binders (prevent absorption)
- Measures to ↑ serum Ca^{2+} and suppress PTH synthesis and secretion:
  - Calcium salts (e.g., $CaCO_3$); also act as phosphate binders
  - Vitamin D analogues (e.g., calcitriol, alfacalcidol, paricalcitol)
- Measures to suppress PTH synthesis and secretion directly:
  - Calcimimetic agents

Therapeutic targets
- Guidelines developed by the NKF-K/DOQI[1] reflect that renal osteodystrophy and its treatment may be associated with a modifiable increase in cardiovascular risk.
- Much more rigorous targets for calcium, phosphorus, and PTH than previously are advocated (see below).
- Suggested phosphate levels at CKD stages 3 or 4 are similar to the normal physiological range, with only a minor concession at stage 5.
- The target for PTH is also close to normal in patients up to stage 3 CKD.
- In stages 4–5, target PTH is 3–6× the upper limit of normal, reflecting observational data that suggest normal bone turnover is most likely to be achieved in uremic bone when PTH is modestly elevated ♦.

CKD stage	GFR (mL/min)	PTH (pg/mL)	Calcium (mg/dL)	Phosphorus (mg/dL)
3	30–59	35–70	8.5–10.2	2.7–4.6
4	15–29	70–110	8.5–10.2	2.7–4.6
5	<15 or dialysis	150–300	8.4–9.5	< 5.5

- Data confirming that achieving these goals will have a significant impact on mortality is awaited.
- Currently, practice falls well short of meeting these targets.

1 National Kidney Foundation (2003). K-DOQI™ clinical practice guidelines for bone metabolism and disease in chronic kidney disease. *Am J Kid Dis* **42**: S1–201.

Aluminum toxicity

History
In the 1970–80s, clusters of dialysis units reported patients with aluminum toxicity. Investigation found high geographic concentrations in dialysate water to be responsible, and improved purification techniques eliminated this route of exposure. Aluminum-containing phosphate binders were left as the main source.

Presentation
Aluminum toxicity (→ ↓PTH secretion, ↓ mineralization, and ↓ osteoblastic activity) previously accounted for the majority of low-turnover pathology. There is also EPO-resistant anemia, encephalopathy, and neurotoxicity.

Current practice
Aluminum-containing phosphate binders should be avoided (use for <4 weeks and in those with limited life expectancy are possible exceptions). If extended use is necessary, aluminum levels should be monitored. Serum aluminum should be <20 µg/L (0.7 µmol/L) in dialysis patients. Levels >60 µg/L (2.2 µmol/L) suggest aluminum overload. Sequential levels may detect the development of overload in at-risk patients. However, serum aluminum is not a reliable indicator of overall body content, and a desferrioxamine (DFO) stimulation test may be required (→ rise in aluminum level after IV DFO). Symptomatic patients may benefit from regular DFO chelation treatment.

Hyperphosphatemia

Control of phosphate

Phosphate control is the weak link in the therapeutic approach to SHPT.

Dietary restriction (📖 p. 199)
- Phosphate is contained in almost all foods (especially meats, milk, eggs, and cereals).
- It is difficult to balance dietary phosphate restriction against adequate protein intake (recommended levels of daily dietary protein provide 30–40 mmol of phosphate).

Phosphate binders (Table 3.3)
- These are taken a few minutes before a meal to bind phosphate in the gut. The amount taken is proportional to size of meal and serum PO_4 (usually 1–3 tablets).
- None are particularly potent and ∴ large amounts are needed.
- The most effective binder is one that the patient will take—demanding regime + unpalatable tablets = poor compliance (>50% dialysis patients do not take their binders regularly).
- They should not be taken at the same time as iron supplements.
- Aluminum hydroxide is the prototype binder and remains the most effective. ⚠ Aluminum toxicity (skeletal and neurological) restricts use (<4 weeks).
- Calcium-containing phosphate binders (CCPB) have been the mainstay.
  - They not only bind PO_4 but help correct $\downarrow Ca^{2+}$ (and suppress PTH).
  - ☞ Patients receiving CCPBs are in positive calcium balance. CCPBs have ∴ been implicated as a cause of vascular calcification (and adverse CV outcome).
  - CCPBs should ideally be restricted to 1500 mg elemental calcium/day.
  - Avoid use if there is low-turnover disease (PTH <150 pg/mL).
- Non-calcium-, non-aluminum-containing binders, e.g., sevelamer hydrochloride (Renagel®) and lanthanum carbonate (Fosrenol®), allow calcium and aluminum to be avoided.
  - Both are extremely expensive. Others are likely to be developed.
  - They are no more effective than CCPBs.
  - Efficacy in preventing CV morbidity and mortality is unproven.
  - Sevelamer may lead to less hypercalcemia and is associated with slower progression of coronary calcification.
  - Sevelamer lowers LDL cholesterol and may provide additional CV risk modification.

Adequate dialysis
- Dietary intake of phosphate exceeds daily removal by dialysis.
- A significant amount of phosphate is in the intracellular compartment, so significant rebound occurs post-HD treatment. CAPD is more efficient at PO_4 removal than hemodialysis.
- Poor PO_4 control may be an indication for more frequent dialysis.
- Daily dialysis regimens can control phosphate with no binder requirement (supplementation may be necessary!).

Table 3.3 Phosphate binders

Binder	Advantages	Disadvantages	Examples
Calcium-based binders	Inexpensive. Help correct Ca2+ and suppress PTH. Calcium acetate has a smaller calcium load per equivalent phosphate-binding dose.	Calcium load may predispose to vascular and soft tissue calcification.	Calcium carbonate • Tums® (500 mg calcium) • Calcichew® (500 mg calcium) • Os-cal 500® (500 mg calcium) • Tums EX® (300 mg calcium) Calcium acetate Phoslo® (250 mg calcium)
Aluminum based	Cheap. Very effective	Risk of aluminum toxicity. Need to monitor levels. Short-term use only	Alucaps® • Al(OH)$_3$ 475 mg Amphogel® (liquid)
Sevelamer HCl	Avoids calcium and aluminum	Expensive. GI intolerance. Large doses needed. Long-term outcome data not yet available. Causes a mild metabolic acidosis	Sevelamer hydrochloride (Renagel®) • 1–3 800 mg tablets with each meal
Lanthanum	Avoids calcium and aluminum	Expensive. Long-term consequences of administration unknown (no toxicity in short-term studies). Role in clinical practice not yet established	Lanthanum carbonate (Fosrenol®) • 750–3000 mg/day in divided doses

One strategy is to use multiple binding agents to achieve a normal phosphate, with each binder used at a different meal. This avoids excessive calcium administration and ameliorates the cost of newer binders.

Vitamin D analogues

The other mainstay of SHPT treatment, Vitamin D, requires 1α-hydroxylation at the level of the kidney for activity. This is pharmacologically bypassed by using the 1α-hydroxylated vitamin D analogues calcitriol or alfacalcidol (1α-calcidol) or paracalcitol.

Nutritional vitamin D deficiency

In CKD stages 3–4, screening for nutritional vitamin D deficiency is recommended when PTH >70 pg/mL (serum 25-hydroxyvitamin D <30 ng/mL). Treatment with ergocalciferol 50,000 U monthly × 6 [25 (OH)D 16–30 ng/mL], 50,000 U weekly × 4 weeks then 50,000 U/month × 5 months [25 (OH)D 5–15 ng/mL], 50,000 U weekly × 12 weeks then 50,000 U/month × 3 months [25 (OH)D < 5 ng/mL].

Treatment

- ▶ *Control serum phosphate first.*
- Start with a low dose (0.25 μg/day calcitriol, or 2.5 μg doxercalciferol 3x/week, or paricalcitol 2 μg 3x/week orally) and increase as necessary over several months.
  - CKD stage 3: treat elevated PTH to target of 35–70 pg/mL
  - CKD stage 4: treat to target 70–110 pg/mL
  - CKD stage 5: treat to target 150–300 pg/mL

Monitoring
Monitor serum Ca^{2+}, PO_4, and PTH (monthly initially). Avoid ↑Ca^{2+} and PTH oversuppression.

Side effects and toxicity
↑Ca^{2+} and ↑CaxP frequently complicate treatment. More than just a therapeutic inconvenience, this has implications for bone turnover (↑ adynamic bone disease), soft tissue and vascular calcification, and CV morbidity and mortality.

Newer vitamin D analogues

- Much attention has been given to the development of vitamin D analogues with less propensity toward hypercalcemia.
- Many have shown potential in the experimental setting and a few are available for clinical use (e.g., paricalcitol).
- Advantages over calcitriol and alfacalcidol remain unproven, though there may be marginal benefits.
- ◆ One large cohort study has suggested a possible survival advantage for those patients treated with paricalcitol.
- A therapeutic trial may be warranted in patients prone to ↑Ca^{2+}.
- Paricalcitol is given IV on dialysis (0.04–0.1 μg/kg).
- Further randomized, prospective studies are awaited.

Vascular calcification

- There has been increasing recent appreciation that vascular calcification, previously considered relatively benign, might predict or even contribute to uremic CV risk.
- Identification and quantification have been facilitated by advances in radiological techniques, particularly electron-beam CT (EBCT).
- There are two types:
  - Intimal (within atherosclerotic plaques)
  - Medial (medial wall—"Mönckeberg's sclerosis")
- Both occur in CKD patients:
  - Calcium content of atherosclerotic plaques from HD patients is greater than that in age-matched controls.
  - Medial calcification causes arterial stiffness (→ diastolic dysfunction → ↑ morbidity and mortality).
- An association between calcification and oral calcium intake has called into question the future role of both calcium-containing phosphate binders and vitamin D analogues ♦*.
- This may be simplistic; a new paradigm that departs from the traditional view of ↑CaxP promoting passive soft tissue calcification is emerging:
  - Evidence: (1) spontaneous vascular calcification in mice carrying specific gene deletions; (2) recognition of certain previously "bone-specific" regulatory proteins in calcified arteries; (3) the ability of several stimuli (including inorganic phosphate and uremic serum) to provoke calcification in vascular smooth muscle cells.
  - Hyperparathyroidism, phosphate loading, ↑BP, abnormal glucose metabolism, ↑ lipids, and natural inhibitor deficiencies are all likely to play a role in addition to calcium and vitamin D intake.
- This integration of bone and vascular biology is yielding novel treatments—e.g., the bone morphogenetic protein BMP-7 has been shown to have efficacious effects in animal models of vascular calcification and bone disease.
- Some advocate routine screening for vascular calcification with quantification if possible (e.g., aortic calcification on abdominal X-ray, pulse-wave velocity studies, EBCT).

Calcimimetics

The calcium sensing receptor (CaR)

First cloned in 1993, the CaR is constitutively expressed across multiple cell types and credited with roles in many aspects of cell function. Its main purpose is the control of extracellular Ca^{2+} concentration and regulation of steady-state PTH secretion.

Calcimimetic agents

- These are small molecules that bind to the parathyroid CaR and mimic the effect of ↑ extracellular Ca^{2+}:
  - Type I includes Ca^{2+} itself and other cationic compounds. They directly activate the CaR.
  - Type II includes not strictly agonists, but allosteric modulators that ↑CaR sensitivity to ambient Ca^{2+}.
- Calcimimetics ↓PTH with a simultaneous ↓ in serum Ca^{2+}.
- Parallel reductions in PO_4 and CaxP are also seen. In this respect they differ importantly from other available treatments (Table 3.4).
- Side effects include upper GI intolerance (10%–15%), and mild ↓Ca^{2+} is frequent (though rarely problematic). Despite the ubiquitous distribution of the CaR, CNS, cardiac, and other side effects have not been noted.
- Evidence for clinical efficacy in HD patients has increased (and data are emerging for predialysis and CAPD). It is hoped they will facilitate improved compliance with national Ca^{2+}, PO_4, and PTH targets.
  But
- These agents are extremely expensive.

Role

More data are needed to decide where the need is greatest.
- From a biochemical standpoint, therapy (vitamin D sterol or calcimimetic) can be chosen according to the clinical phenotype of the patient (Table 3.5).
  - The "vitamin D phenotype": the SHPT patient in whom serum Ca^{2+}, PO_4, and CaxP product are all low-normal or subnormal. Vitamin D therapy is usually effective in bringing biochemical parameters to target. Risk of ↑Ca^{2+} or ↑PO_4 is relatively low.
  - The "calcimimetic phenotype": potentially more difficult to treat. Here SHPT is accompanied by a high-normal or frankly elevated Ca^{2+}, often with ↑PO_4 and CaxP product. Treatment with vitamin D will ↓PTH, but aggravate ↑Ca^{2+} and ↑PO_4.
- Vitamin D and calcimimetics work well together. Their modes of action at the level of the parathyroid are different and effects on PTH suppression appear additive. Calcimimetics may ↓ serum Ca^{2+}, "making room" for the use of vitamin D analogues.

Dosing: cinacalcet (Sensipar®)

Oral: Initial dose is 30 mg once daily, increased incrementally (60 mg, 90 mg, 120 mg, 180 mg) as necessary to maintain target PTH. Hypocalcemia may require dose reduction.

Table 3.4 Relative actions of current treatments on calcium, phosphorus, CaxP, and PTH concentrations

	Calcium-based binder	Calcium-free binder	Vitamin D sterols	Calcimimetics
PTH	↓↓	↓	↓↓↓	↓↓↓
Calcium	↑↑	↔ or ↑	↑	↓
Phosphorus	↓↓	↓↓	↑	↓
CaxP	↓ or ↑	↓	↑	↓

Table 3.5 Clinical phenotypes frequently encountered in CKD patients

	Calcium	Phosphorus	CaxP
"Vitamin D phenotype"	Low-normal or low	In target	In target
"Calcimimetic phenotype"	High-normal or high	Above target	High

Parathyroidectomy

▶ An elevated PTH alone is not an indication for parathyroidectomy.

Indications
- Tertiary or autonomous hyperparathyroidism is a failure of hyperplasic, overactive glands to suppress adequately in response to optimal medical therapy
- Manifests clinically as ↑PTH (usually >800 pg/nL) with persistent ↑Ca^{2+}
- PO_4 and alkaline phosphatase are usually raised.
- If calcium is low or normal, ↑PTH indicates SHPT and further medical treatment is necessary.
- Calcimimetic therapy (📖 p. 188) may prove to have a role in reducing the need for parathyroidectomy and may be an alternative in those in whom surgery has failed, is refused, or is deemed too high risk.
- Inappropriate parathyroidectomy may have deleterious consequences for the skeleton (→ low-turnover disease).

Preoperative considerations
Imaging: isotope scans (e.g., MIBI) allow localization of the parathyroid glands prior to surgery and identify ectopic (e.g., retrosternal) tissue.

Ear, nose, throat (ENT): All patients should have their vocal cords visualized preoperatively—there is a risk of damage to the recurrent laryngeal nerve during surgery, so preexisting problems need documentation.

Prevention of "hungry bone syndrome": High-dose vitamin D for a few days preoperatively may help prevent rapid and severe falls in Ca^{2+} postoperatively (calcium influx into bone).

Postoperative considerations
Hemorrhage: This is rare, but may cause tracheal compression. Monitor drains carefully.

Hypocalcemia may be profound in the days following surgery. Check Ca^{2+} 2–4 hours postoperatively, then 12 hours for 2–3 days. Give calcitriol 0.5–4.0 μg/day with oral calcium (1–3 g in divided doses). If serum Ca^{2+} falls below 7.5 mg/dL or tetany develops, administer IV calcium (see 📖 p. 542 for regimen) and continue oral vitamin D.

PTH is measured postoperatively to ensure success.

Parathyroidectomy technique

The amount of parathyroid tissue removed at operation can be varied.

Partial parathyroidectomy Parathyroid tissue is deliberately left behind in an attempt to avoid the consequences of absent PTH (principally ABD). Unfortunately, further autonomous PTH secretion often necessitates repeat (and technically more difficult) surgery.

Total parathyroidectomy with reimplantation Parathyroid tissue is implanted into an extraparathyroid site (usually the arm). This tissue is then more easily accessible if recurrent hyperparathyroidism develops. Unfortunately, parathyroid regrowth in the neck remains common.

Total parathyroidectomy This is attempted removal of all parathyroid tissue; it is currently the favored technique. Serum calcium is subsequently maintained with calcitriol or alfacalcidol. Regrowth of islands of parathyroid cells is not uncommon. Serum PTH will ↑ with time.

Radiological ablation Ultrasound localization and ablation through ethanol injection has met with variable success.

Calciphylaxis

Definition
Calciphylaxis (calcific uremic arteriolopathy) is a small-vessel vasculopathy involving mural calcification with intimal proliferation, fibrosis, and thrombosis. It occurs predominantly in individuals with renal failure and results in ischemia and necrosis of skin, soft tissue, visceral organs, and skeletal muscle.

Incidence
First described in 1962 and considered rare until recently, its incidence is 1%, with a prevalence 4% of ESRD patients. Mortality is 80% at 1 year (almost always due to sepsis).

Presentation
- *Painful* erythematous livedo reticularis-like skin patches that ulcerate. Panniculitis and secondary infection follow.
- Two patterns are recognized: (1) ulcers on the trunk, buttocks, or thighs (over adipose tissue), and (2) ulceration on the extremities.
- Not just the skin is affected—it may also occur in arterioles supplying other organs (lung calcification on the chest X-ray is common).
- Bone scans show ↑ uptake over lesions.
- Skin biopsy is characteristic.

Risk factors
- Uremia (though also seen post-transplantation, and in primary HPT)
- ↑ Calcium phosphate product
- ↑ PTH
- Vitamin D analogue use
- Race (Caucasian)
- ♀ > ♂
- Obesity (BMI >30)
- Warfarin use
- Protein C or S deficiency
- Diabetes mellitus
- Malnutrition.

Treatment
⚠ No treatment is of proven benefit.
- Scrupulous wound care
- Aggressive treatment of sepsis
- Lower CaxP: avoid calcium-based binders, daily hemodialysis, lower dialysate Ca^{2+}
- Parathyroidectomy *may* help if ↑PTH and ↑CaxP
- Stop warfarin
- Bisphosphonates, hyperbaric oxygen, sodium thiosulphate are under study
- Steroids are probably of no benefit (⚠ sepsis).

Renal bone disease management summary

SHPT
- Check calcium, phosphate, and PTH at least every 3 months (more often if treatment changes made) in CKD stages 4 and 5, and annually in stage 3.
- In CKD stages 3 and 4, if PTH >70 pg/mL measure serum 25-hydroxyvitamin D and consider replacement if <30 µg/L.
- Control serum phosphate with a combination of diet, phosphate binders, and adequate dialysis.
- Once phosphate is controlled, add paricalcitol, or doxicalciferol or calcitriol, titrating the dose up, aiming for a target PTH according to CKD stage and a serum calcium in the lower half of normal range.
- Uncontrolled SHPT: Review diet and intensify phosphate binder and vitamin D therapy if possible. Consider paricalcitol and cinacalcet if high calcium limits further vitamin D treatment.
- If ↑Ca^{2+}, switch to non-calcium-containing binder and consider lowering dialysate Ca^{2+}.
- Parathyroidectomy is the last resort if medical management is unsuccessful.

ABD
- Aim to increase PTH-driven bone turnover.
  - Reduce or stop calcium-containing binders and vitamin D analogues (aim for serum Ca^{2+} in the low-normal range).
- Lowering the dialysate calcium concentration (HD and CAPD: 1.0 mmol/L) may help ↓Ca^{2+} and ↑PTH.
- Excluded significant aluminum deposition, if applicable.
- Exogenous PTH (pulsatile administration) and calcimimetics may prove to have an anabolic role in ABD, as circadian PTH release is thought necessary for normal bone formation.

Cardiovascular disease in CKD

Patients with early CKD are at increased risk of CV disease—most will die a CV death before progressing to ESRD. Those starting RRT often do so with a high CV disease burden; dialysis patients are ~20x more likely to die from CV causes than the general population. A cardiac cause of death is implicated in >40% of deaths at ESRD. Several factors contribute.

Traditional cardiovascular risk factors more common in CKD

- Hypertension (almost always present) and left ventricular hypertrophy (LVH)
- Diabetes (common cause of CKD)
- Dyslipidemia
- Physical inactivity

Risk factors common in (or unique to) uremia

- Arteriosclerosis and diastolic dysfunction
- Albuminuria
- Volume overload
- Oxidant stress and inflammation
- Malnutrition
- Accumulation of advanced glycosylation end-products
- Left ventricular hypertrophy
- Hyperparathyoidism, calcium overload, and metastatic calcification
- Anemia
- Myocardial fibrosis and possible abnormal myocyte function
- Nitric oxide/endothelin derangement
- Carnitine deficiency
- Hyperhomocysteinemia

Of 100 patients with an eGFR <60 mL/min ~1% will progress to ESRD each year. However, there is a 10% death rate (mainly CV disease), so after 10 years, 8 patients will require RRT, 27 will have "smoldering" CKD, and 65 will be dead.

▶ An estimated 8,000,000 people in the U.S. have an eGFR <60 mL/min.

Managing risk factors

All CKD patients are at high risk of CV events. Microalbuminuria itself is an independent risk factor for cardiovascular outcomes, possibly because it is a marker of generalized endothelial dysfunction. Interventions should include the following:
- Lifestyle advice re: smoking, diet, obesity, exercise
- Meticulous BP control
- Management of lipids, usually with a statin
- Glycemic control (if diabetic)
- ☙ Good evidence for the benefit of such interventions in CKD patients is lacking—advice is currently based on extrapolation from the nonrenal population.

Acute coronary syndrome (ACS) in CKD

▶ CKD is a significant predictor of mortality in ACS patients. ACS may present atypically (silent ischemia, hypotension, collapse) in patients with advanced CKD. Typical chest pain and ST elevation are uncommon in dialysis patients. CKD patients with an ACS should receive standard management, but with some provisos:
- LVH (and strain) can complicate ECG interpretation.
- Cardiac enzymes:
  - CK may be nonspecifically elevated in CKD.
  - Troponin levels may not be helpful. Troponin T, and to a lesser extent troponin I, are often elevated in CKD (and may be independent markers of CV risk). ▶ A significant ↑ level in the right context is likely to be a true positive (especially if rising).
- CKD and dialysis do not contraindicate thrombolysis. Recent renal biopsy, line insertion (especially if accidental arterial puncture), uncontrolled ↑BP (>200/110), or uremic pericarditis might. Percutaneous coronary intervention may be preferable in these circumstances.
- Platelet function is deranged in uremia: aspirin and clopidogrel carry a greater bleeding risk than in the general population. Studies on these agents have generally excluded patients with renal disease. The consensus is to administer them, unless bleeding risk is particularly high.
- Glycoprotein IIb/IIIa inhibitors require dose reduction.
- Low molecular-weight heparins require dose adjustment if eGFR <30 mL/min (→ 50% standard dose). Unfractionated heparin may be safer.
- Fluid status should be optimized: overloaded patients should be diuresed or dialysed.
- Correct anemia. Tranfuse if necessary (on dialysis if fluid overload or hyperkalaemia). Aim for Hb 11–12 g/dL.
- β-blockers (⚠ may need dose reduction), statins, calcium channel blockers, and nitrates can be administered as usual.
- Hypotension peri-MI or ACS may cause ↑Cr in the CKD patient (→temporary or permanent dialysis dependence).
- Hemodialysis in the context of an ongoing ACS may be dangerous (⚠ hemodynamic instability, arrhythmia). Treat in a high-dependency environment. CRRT (📖 p. 128) may be preferable.

Coronary angiography in the renal patient

☙ Angiography and emergency angioplasty may be the treatment of choice in the renal patient with ACS. However,
- Ensure adequate hydration and give NAC if time permits (📖 p. 143).
- Minimize contrast dose if possible.
- These renoprotective measures apply equally to dialysis patients who retain significant residual renal function.
- Restenosis rates *may* be higher in CKD patients.
- Even with these attempts at renoprotection, a decline in renal function may follow intervention. ▶ Measure daily UO and SCr until stable, and optimize fluid balance.

Pretransplant workup

CKD patients considered fit for potential transplantation merit cardiovascular workup, as early post-transplant mortality is 50% cardiac. Prior to listing any potential recipient, adequate screening is required (Table 3.6).

Recommended screening tests
- No test is ideal. Coronary angiography is sensitive and specific but invasive and carries the risk of contrast nephropathy (📖 p. 142).
- Less invasive screening tests (exercise stress test, thallium/sestamibi radionuclide imaging, dobutamine stress echocardiography) are relatively insensitive in this population (high pretest probability of significant disease).

Screen according to risk
- Coronary angiography has been suggested for all "high-risk" patients, defined as any patient with significant CKD who has one or more of the following:
  - History of ischemic heart disease
  - ECG compatible with ischemic heart disease
  - Diabetes mellitus
  - Peripheral vascular disease
- Duplex US assessment of iliac and carotid arteries is also desirable.
- "Medium-risk" patients (age >50, smokers, history of hypertension, prolonged duration of CKD, first-degree relative with CAD or dyslipidemia) should have noninvasive assessment followed by angiography if the results are positive or inconclusive (sensitivity of these tests is low, so threshold for angiography should also be low).
- "Low-risk" patients (nonsmokers, age <50, nondiabetic, no clinically overt CV disease) do not require cardiac screening.

Intervention
Revascularization for clinically significant coronary lesions is recommended. Early studies suggested that angioplasty was less effective than bypass grafting. However, the introduction of stents (and more recently drug-eluting stents) is likely to have changed the risk/benefit ratio—further studies are awaited.

Uremic cardiomyopathy

This is probably not the result of one specific uremic toxin but of a combination of factors:
- ↑*Arterial stiffness:* ↑ phosphate → vascular smooth muscle cell transdifferentiation into osteoblast-like cells, causing vascular medial calcification. This leads to arteriosclerosis, ↓ arterial compliance, and ↑ pulse pressure. This is analogous to the arterial changes seen in the elderly, but prematurely. The result is ↑ cardiac workload and worsening LVH and diastolic dysfunction.
- *Cardiac fibrosis:* Local and systemic angiotensin II and PTH → ↑ cardiac stiffness, myocyte injury, and diastolic and systolic dysfunction.
- *Anemia:* → ↑ LVH and ↑ cardiac work.
- *Myocyte dysfunction:* Myocyte contractility is reduced, possibly as a result of changes in intracellular bioenergetics.

Table 3.6 Pretransplant investigations

Age <50 nondiabetic	Age 50–60 nondiabetic	Age >60 nondiabetic	Diabetic
History	History	History	History
Examination	Examination	Examination	Examination
ECG	ECG	ECG	ECG
Chest X-ray	Chest X-ray	Chest X-ray	Chest X-ray
Tissue typing	Tissue typing	Tissue typing	Tissue typing
Virology*	Virology*	Virology*	Virology*
Patient information	Patient information	Patient information	Patient information
Surgical assessment	Noninvasive cardiac testing	Noninvasive cardiac testing	Noninvasive cardiac testing (possible angiography)
	Leg arterial Doppler imaging	Carotid Doppler imaging	Carotid dopplers
	Surgical assessment	Leg arterial Doppler imaging	Leg arterial dopplers
		Surgical assessment	Post-micturition bladder US
			Surgical assessment

* Virology: hepatitis B & C, HIV, CMV, EBV, varicella-zoster (± HTLV 1 & 2).

Diet and nutrition in CKD

Dietary advice is extremely important in the management of CKD and the maintenance of broader health in CKD patients.

Measurement of nutritional status
▶ No single parameter should be considered in isolation.

Assessment should include the following:
- History and examination to identify ongoing medical problems that may limit nutritional intake—psychosocial issues may be important.
- *Dietary interview or diary*: quantitative intake of nutrients
- *Subjective global assessment (SGA)* is a simple scoring (subjective and objective) made on history and examination. It is well validated in CKD, and powerful enough to predict outcome.
- *Anthropometric measurements* include body mass index, skin-fold thickness, estimated percent weight loss, and mid-arm muscle circumference.
- *Serum albumin* reflects not only protein intake but is also susceptible to changes with inflammation or infection. It is a strong predictor of future mortality in new starters on dialysis.
- *Adequacy of dialysis*: Inadequate dialysis is a common contributing factor to malnutrition (uremic toxins are anorectic and proinflammatory). Dialysis adequacy (pp. 221 and 242) should be assessed in conjunction with the normalized protein catabolic rate (nPCR), which is a measure of the rate of urea formation (p. 219). When any patient is in steady state, urea formation correlates with protein intake and protein breakdown.

Fluid restriction
- CKD stages 4–5: Fluid and salt restriction is often important to prevent volume overload.
- On dialysis: When the urine output drops, fluid restriction is vital to minimize weight gains. Aim for weight gains of 1–1.5 kg or less/day. In an anuric patient, this means a fluid restriction of 750–1000 mL. This must be combined with salt restriction.

Protein intake
- Intake averages ~80 g/day in the developed world, although requirements may be only 50 g.
- A low-protein diet may slow the progression of renal failure in patients with CKD (p. 161). Set against this is the danger of paients reaching dialysis with significant malnutrition. Most units advocate no more than *moderate* protein restriction. Daily protein targets:
  - 0.8 g/kg/day for CKD stages 3–5
  - 1.2 g/kg/day when on dialysis
- Protein sources include meat, fish, eggs, milk, nuts, pulses, and beans.

Carbohydrate intake
- Adequate energy intake is essential for patients with CKD, especially those undergoing protein restriction.
- Target 30–35 kcal/kg/day.
- The source is mainly complex carbohydrates, some from mono- or polyunsaturated fats. Dovetailing a diabetic diet with a renal diet can be difficult.
- Examples include sugar, jams, marmalade, and specialist high-energy renal drinks.

Phosphate restriction (see also 📖 p. 184)
- The kidney is the main route of phosphate excretion. Current guidelines suggest a restriction of dietary phosphate of 0.8–1g/day if
  - serum phosphate >4.6 mg/dL in CKD stages 3–4 *or*
  - serum phosphate >5.5 mg/dL in CKD stage 5 *or*
  - ↑PTH.
- Prescribe phosphate binders if dietary restriction alone fails (📖 p. 184).
- Phosphate-rich foods include all protein-containing foods, making phosphate restriction difficult to achieve. Examples include milk, cheese, custard, yogurt, ice cream, cola, chocolate drinks, beer, liver, baked beans, dried peas, and beans (e.g., chick peas), nuts, whole-grain products, bran cereals, and many convenience foods.

Potassium restriction
- Typical intake is ~50–120 mmol/day. With failing renal function, potassium excretion falls, making potassium restriction necessary (especially in patients taking an ACEI or ARBs).
- K^+-rich foods include dairy products, potatoes (baked, chips, and crisps), some fruits (bananas, grapes, dried fruit, fresh pineapple), fresh fruit juice, tomatoes, sweet corn, mushrooms, chocolate, and coffee.

Salt restriction
- Typical intake is ~9–12 g.
- This is a vast excess over physiological needs.
- Salt restriction is helpful if ↑BP ± volume overload (helps reduce thirst and hence fluid intake). Aim for an intake of <5–6 g/day.
- Na^+-rich foods include cheese, salted butter and margarine, salted meat (bacon, ham), tinned meat, vegetables and soups, packaged meals.

There are several resources on the Internet that can help patients and their families understand and adjust to these dietary restrictions. The nutrition section of the National Kidney Foundation (U.S.) Web site is a good starting point (www.kidney.org)—even containing a complete cookbook.

Malnutrition in CKD

Malnutrition is common in CKD (affecting up to 50% of dialysis patients) and a powerful predictor of survival. Contributors include the following:
- Anorectic uremic toxins (leptin)
- Chronic low-grade inflammation
- Dietary restriction (low-protein diet)
- Medication (phosphate binders, iron)
- Dialysis itself (especially CAPD, where protein losses into the dialysate may be 1–2 g/L, or ~10 g/day: this would be considered a nephrotic range if lost in the urine!).

Managing malnutrition in the CKD patient
- Assess the severity of malnutrition (p. 198).
- Measure current nutritional intake.
- Address correctable factors:
  - ▶ Correct underdialysis (e.g., change modality, improve access).
  - Seek and treat occult infection.
  - Investigate and treat gut problems or gastroparesis.
  - Define and intervene if there are psychosocial problems.
- Consider dietary supplements; a wide range are available. Renal-specific oral supplements are low in potassium/phosphate and are concentrated (limiting the volume of fluid given).
- Overnight nasoenteral (or PEG) feeding may be beneficial in more severe cases of malnutrition when adequate oral intake cannot be maintained.
- IDPN = intradialytic parenteral nutrition. Given on dialysis, it provides amino acids, glucose, and lipids. It is not a substitute for oral supplements, but can deliver ~1500 kcal/session (of which ~500 kcal is lost in dialysate!). It can be a useful adjunct if the patient is able to manage 50% of the desired daily intake by mouth.
- Amino acid–containing PD solutions (Nutrineal®) may offer benefit in malnourished PD patients ✒.
- Total parenteral nutrition (TPN) should be reserved for those who cannot be fed enterally. Electrolyte quantities (particularly potassium, phosphate, and magnesium) should be reduced and monitored daily.
- ✒ Appetite stimulants and anabolic agents are of uncertain benefit:
  - Growth hormone (costly)
  - Megestrol acetate (A progesterone) 625 mg once daily.

Inflammation in CKD

Patients with CKD have ongoing low-grade inflammation, with ↑ acute-phase proteins (CRP, ferritin), ↑ inflammatory cytokines, hypoalbuminemia, and hypercholesterolemia. Contributors include:
- Repeated infections
- Oxidant stress (decreased levels of antioxidants, increased oxidative and carbonyl stress)
- Accumulation of AGE products
- Arteriosclerosis and abnormal endothelial function
- Malnutrition (both a cause and an effect of chronic inflammation)

Protein–energy malnutrition may coexist—there is increasing evidence that chronic inflammation and oxidant stress increase metabolic demands and predispose to malnutrition. The triad of malnutrition, inflammation, and accelerated atherosclerosis has been labeled the *MIA syndrome*. A vicious cycle may commence, often culminating in death from cardiac disease. This may account for the apparent paradox that patients on dialysis with a higher body mass index tend to survive longer.

Endocrine problems in CKD

Thyroid function
Tests may be difficult to interpret as thyroid-binding globulin is lost in the urine if heavy proteinuria, causing a ↓ in measured T4. Clinical assessment and measurement of T3 and TSH may be necessary for correct interpretation.

Adrenal axis function
Addison disease is difficult to diagnose in the context of CKD, especially in dialysis patients, as the characteristic electrolyte changes may be masked by renal dysfunction and dialysis. Suspect this if there is persistent hypotension (or postural hypotension). Many renal patients have received corticosteroid therapy, with consequent steroid-related side effects (📖 p. 370).

Sexual dysfunction (♀)
Reduced libido is frequent. Comorbidity (vascular disease, diabetes) and concomitant drug treatment may be relevant. Altered body image and self-perception may also play a role, as may depression and anxiety. Offer counseling. ► Anemia contributes to reduced libido and should be corrected. Disturbances in menstruation and fertility are common. Amenorrhea is virtually ubiquitous at ESRD. Gynecological assessment is often helpful. Pregnancy in CKD and dialysis is discussed in Chapter 10.

Sexual dysfunction (♂)
Erectile dysfunction is common. It may be multifactorial (arterial disease, neuropathy, psychological factors, side effects of drug treatment). Where possible, treat the underlying cause. Testosterone deficiency is not uncommon in dialysis patients and should be corrected with replacement therapy. Sildenafil (Viagra®) is effective, but should be avoided in patients on nitrates and those with significant coronary artery disease or hypotension. Vacuum devices or penile implants may be useful, especially if there is a physical cause for impotence.

Hyperprolactinemia
Elevated circulating prolactin concentrations, secondary to increased secretion and decreased clearance, are common in advanced CKD. Causes include galactorrhea (♀) and gynecomastia (♂). Bromocriptine may normalize levels. The contribution of ↑ prolaction to sexual dysfunction in both sexes is unclear.

Early menopause
This is not associated with CKD per se, but may occur in patients treated with cyclophosphamide or other cytotoxic agents.

Growth retardation

Resistance to growth hormone (GH) is an important consequence of advanced CKD. Although circulating GH levels are normal (or elevated), resistance to its action causes growth retardation in children and muscle wasting in adults. This resistance is the consequence of multiple defects in the GH/IGF-1 axis: GH receptor expression is down-regulated, as is activity of the downstream JAK/STAT signal transduction pathway. IGF-1 (a major mediator of GH action) expression and activity are also significantly reduced. Growth delay can now be treated with recombinant GH. Other contributors to growth retardation are steroid therapy, malnutrition, and renal osteodystrophy.

Palliative treatment of advanced CKD

The decision not to have dialysis
- Patients who start dialysis with significant comorbidity and functional dependence typically only survive a few months—months that may be filled with hospital admissions, painful illnesses, and unpleasant procedures.
- For such patients, continuing supportive care without commencing dialysis may allow a better quality of life with little or no reduction in life expectancy.
- The decision whether to commence dialysis at ESRD is ultimately made by the patient (assuming the patient has the capacity). The renal team has a duty to ensure that this decision is as informed as possible, by explaining the implications of withholding dialysis and the pros and cons of commencing it. Family members should also be involved.
  - The process cannot be rushed. A decision not to accept dialysis should be made over time, and be consistently held.
  - Patients may (and often do) change their minds (in either direction).
  - If severely uremic, a patient may be unable to be involved in the decision-making process.
  - It can often be difficult to determine whether debility is uremic in origin (and ∴ potentially reversible), or secondary to preexisting comorbidity.
  - Patients referred late have no time to go through the predialysis counseling process and may be denied the opportunity to make informed decisions about their care.

Symptomatic management of ESRD
As uremia advances, so do uremic symptoms (📖 Chapter 1). However, with prompt symptomatic treatment, patients can feel reasonably well and remain active until the very end of life. Many units now run a service specifically for such patients, concentrating resources and care to include:
- Physical and social support—patients may become increasingly reliant on family members ± other careers. District nurses, social workers, home care teams, physiotherapists, and occupational therapists can be involved as required.
- Diet: anorexia is common. Megestrol acetate (A progesterone) 625 mg once daily may stimulate appetite. Check for oral candida and if present, treat with fluconazole 50–100 mg daily. Harsh dietary restrictions may be inappropriate and can be relaxed.
- Taste disturbance: try zinc 220 mg orally once daily.
- Nausea and vomiting: consider conventional antiemetics (e.g., compazine 25–50 mg tid, metoclopramide 5 mg tid, haloperidol 0.5–2.0 mg daily). If dyspeptic symptoms: PPI (e.g., lansoprazole 30 mg daily). Constipation may be contributory: use laxatives early.
- Confusion (usually a late development): check for reversible causes (e.g., ↓Na^+, ↑Ca^{2+}, constipation, drug toxicity).
- Seizures are rare: manage acutely with benzodiazepines.
- Skin: dry skin, pruritis and excoriation are common. Control ↑PO_4 and SHPT (often the cause), use emollients (e.g., MimyX Cream, Lubiderm with Menthol), and try antihistamines, as they may give some relief

- (e.g., cetirizine 5 mg orally each day). If symptoms are localized try capsaisin 0.025% cream (SE: burning sensation).
- Acidosis: may cause dyspnea and exhaustion. Consider $NaHCO_3$ or sodium citrate (0.5–1 meq/kg/day). Avoid sodium citrate in patients taking aluminum-containing phosphate binders as citrate enhances aluminum absorbtion.
- Dyspnea: if there is pulmonary edema consider diuretics, bronchodilators, ?O_2; give advice on sleeping position.
- Anemia: transfusion, IV iron, EPO
- Anxiety and depression (▶ these are common and should be actively investigated): lorazepam 0.5–1 mg orally, opiates, SSRIs (e.g., citalopram 20 mg od).
- Restless legs: correct anemia and iron deficiency. Gabapentin 200–300 mg 3x/week following HD, Carbidopa/Levodopa 25 mg/100 mg ½ tablet each day.
- Pain control: as in all palliative care, the WHO "analgesic ladder" should be used with gradual escalation of drug potency.
  - Acetominophen in therapeutic doses is safe and effective in uremia.
  - NSAIDs are usually contraindicated (they worsen remaining renal function).
  - Opioids are often required in the terminal stages (see Box 3.3).
- Psychological support: this is a terminal illness, and patients need appropriate support.

Withdrawal of dialysis

- As with the decision not to start dialysis, the decision to withdraw it should be made by the patient with the help and support of the multidisciplinary team.
- Withdrawal means that death will probably occur within a few days if the patient has no significant residual renal function. The decision to withdraw may be prompted by a catastrophic medical event (e.g., a CVA, loss of vascular access). Less often, it is the culmination of a number of smaller events that has, in the view of the patient, had unacceptable consequences for their quality of life.
- ⚠ Depression should be looked for and treated, as it may be influencing the decision.
- The decision to withdraw dialysis should be made over a period of time, and be held consistently.

Care of the dying patient

- The patient should be able to die peacefully and with dignity, in a place of his or her choice, surrounded by loved ones. This requires planning, so that care at home, in a hospice, or in the hospital can be arranged at short notice.
- Critical pathways may facilitate management of the last few days of life.
- Family support: Before death, family members may be involved in the physical care of the patient, and need support and help. At the time of death and afterwards, help should be available to cope with the grieving process (this will need to be culturally appropriate).

CHAPTER 3 **Chronic kidney disease**

Box 3.3 Prescribing opioids in renal failure

These are effective, but use with caution. Opiates accumulate and may cause significant side effects (e.g., drowsiness, confusion, respiratory depression, twitching, and seizures). Consider the following:

- Tramadol (50 mg tid po) for mild-to-moderate pain not controlled by nonopioids.
- Oxcodone 5 mg 4 hourly (titrate dose up daily if necessary).
- Fentanyl transdermal patch (25 µg/hr) for stable severe pain. This is equivalent to 8–16 mg hydromorphone or 60–120 mg morphine. Increase dose when oral opiate dose reaches this level.
- Avoid meperidine, as breakdown products are active metabolites that are renally excreted.

Chapter 4

Renal replacement therapy

A brief history of renal replacement therapy (RRT) 208
Introduction 210
Hemodialysis (HD) 212
Dialysers and membranes 216
HD prescription 218
Variables in the dialysis prescription 220
Vascular access 222
Complications of vascular access 224
Acute HD complications 226
Peritoneal dialysis (PD) 228
Types of PD 230
PD fluids 232
Prescribing PD 234
Peritonitis 236
Other complications 240
PD adequacy 242
Ultrafiltration failure 244
The well PD patient 246
Basic transplantation 248
Compatibility 250
Pretransplant assessment 252
Living donor transplantation 254
Pretransplant management 256
The transplant operation 258
Post-transplant management 260
Principles of recipient management 262
Immunosuppression 264
Surgical complications 266
Graft dysfunction 268
Acute rejection 270
Chronic allograft nephropathy (CAN) 272
Post-transplant infections 274
Cytomegalovirus (CMV) 276
BK virus nephropathy 278
Post-transplant malignancy 280
Expanding the donor pool 282
Kidney–pancreas transplantation 284

A brief history of renal replacement therapy (RRT)

In the last 40 years it has become possible to keep ESRD patients alive.

1861	Term *dialysis* first coined
1913	First "artificial kidney" built and used in animals
1923	First human peritoneal dialysis (PD)
1924	First human hemodialysis (HD)
1933	First (unsuccessful) cadaveric kidney transplant
1946	PD used to treat ARF
1947	First cadaveric kidney transplant. The patient had pregnancy-related ARF. The graft was placed externally (on arm) and lasted 6 days (and ARF had resolved).
1948	First dialysis in the United States
1948	Kolff–Brigham dialyser developed—a major technological advance
1948	HD used to treat ARF in the Korean War
Early 1950s	Cadaveric transplants for CRF (into thigh with ureterostomy); no immunosuppression—all rejected within 6 months
1954	First successful monozygotic twin transplant*
1959	Nonmonozygotic twin transplant (with whole-body irradiation as immunosuppression)
1959	Intermittent PD, with repeated abdominal puncture, described
1960	Peter Medawar and Franc Burnet receive Nobel Prize for describing principles of immunologic rejection
1960	Scribner shunt—the first access device enabling repetitive use
1960	First long-term HD patients (Seattle)
1962	6-mercaptopurine used successfully for immunosuppression
1963	Steroids and azathioprine used with greater success
1964	First home HD patients
1966	Cross-matching introduced
1966	Forearm arteriovenous fistula (AVF) developed
1967	First successful liver and heart transplants
1968	Tenckhoff PD catheter introduced
1975	Hemofiltration introduced
1976	Continuous ambulatory peritoneal dialysis (CAPD) introduced
1976	Introduction of cyclosporin—1-year graft survival dramatically improves
1977	Continuous AV hemofiltration described
1982	First kidney pancreas transplant
1990	*Joseph Murray awarded Nobel Prize for his pioneering transplant work.

Introduction

Normal functioning kidneys
- remove excess salt, water and acid.
- remove or regulate other electrolytes (e.g., K^+, Ca^{2+}, Mg^{2+}, PO_4).
- remove waste products of metabolism (Ur and Cr measured routinely, but many others).
- make EPO.
- Produce 1-α hydroxylase that activates vitamin D.

Dialysis acts as surrogate for all but the last two of these (which can be achieved pharmacologically). Even at best, it is only partially effective. Transplantation completely replaces normal kidney function and should be regarded as the optimum treatment of ESRD. Transplanted patients survive longer and have a better quality of life. However, not everyone is fit for transplantation—ESRD patients are often frail with appreciable co-morbidity, especially vascular disease.

Facts and figures

The number of people receiving RRT worldwide is expected to double over the next 10 years. Eventually it will reach "steady state"—the number of patients starting dialysis = those leaving through transplantation, withdrawal, or death. Throughout the world there are wide variations in treatment rates for patients with ESRD (Table 4.1). These variations are explained (partly) by demographic factors (ethnic populations → ↑ incidence of CKD).

In 2004 there were 104,364 incident ESRD patients in the United States, with 90% on HD, 7% on PD, and 3% undergoing transplantation. The 2004 U.S. Renal Data Service (USRDS) renal registry data showed the following:
- Diabetes is the most common etiology of ESRD, accounting for nearly 50% of incident patients. Hypertension (HTN) and glomerulonephritis (GN) are the second and third most common etiologies, repectively.
- Patients over age 65 represent the fastly growing segment of the ESRD population.
- Annual mortality of ESRD patients in the United States is 24% per year.

Resources
- Total Medicare expenditures for ESRD = $18.5 billion
- Average cost of HD $67,000, Average cost of PD $49,000
- Transplantation is the most cost-effective form of RRT.

Morbidity and mortality

In the United States the most common etiologies of death among dialysis patients are cardiac, septicemia, and cerebrovascular disease.

Table 4.1 RRT treatment rates by country[1]

Country	New patients starting treatment (pmp)	Overall number of patients (pmp)
United States	336	1403
Germany	184	919
Greece	163	812
Belgium (Dutch speaking)	160	855
Spain (Catalonia)	146	1022
Denmark	138	679
Italy	136	835
Austria	136	750
Sweden	124	735
New Zealand	119	655
Wales	105*	641*
Scotland	101	644
Netherlands	100	639
Australia	97	633
Norway	94	606
England	91*	547*

* Estimate from partial coverage of UK Renal Registry.

1 From the UK National Service Framework for renal services, Part 1. Available at www.doh.gov.uk/NSF/renal.

Data sources: US Renal Data Service, ERA-EDTA Registry, UK Renal Registry, ANZ Data, Quasi-Niere, Italian Registry of Dialysis and Transplantation (RIDT).

Hemodialysis (HD)

What is HD?
- During dialysis blood is exposed to dialysate (a solution containing physiological concentrations of electrolytes) across a semipermeable membrane.
- Pores in the membrane allow small molecules (e.g., Ur [MW = 60 Da], Cr [113 Da]) and electrolytes, but not larger ones (e.g., plasma proteins [albumin 60,000 Da, IgG 140,000 Da]) or blood cells to pass through.
- Concentration differences across the membrane allow molecules to diffuse down a gradient. This allows waste products to be removed and desirable molecules or ions (e.g., HCO_3) to be replaced.
- Water can be driven through the membrane by hydrostatic force (ultrafiltration [UF]).
  - By varying the pressure gradient across the membrane (trans-membrane pressure, or TMP) the amount of water removed can be controlled.
  - In addition to a means to remove water (~1–4 L) that has accumulated between dialysis sessions (ingestion of fluid and foods and byproduct of metabolism) UF can also be used as a means of solute clearance by convection (see Hemofiltration below).

Hemofiltration (HF)
- In addition to *diffusion*, fluid shifts across the dialysis membrane also allow solutes to cross by *convection* (termed *solute drag*). This underlies the technique of hemofiltration.
- Because large volumes of fluid must cross the membrane to enable significant solute removal, physiological fluid *replacement* is mandatory to avoid hypovolemia.
- During routine HD, HF is used only as a means of removing fluid that has accumulated between sessions ∴ no fluid replacement is necessary.
- In continuous techniques (p. 128), HF plays a more prominent role. It may also be combined with diffusion in *hemodiafiltration* (see Box 4.1).

What is required for hemodialysis?
- Vascular access (in-dwelling venous catheter, arteriovenous fistula, or arteriovenous graft p. 222): large volumes of blood must be removed from the patient, exposed to a dialysis membrane, and then returned.
- Anticoagulation (p. 220) prevents blood clotting in the extracorporeal circuit (usually with heparin).
- Dialysis membrane (p. 216): must be as biocompatible as possible, with an adequate surface area and permeability to facilitate solute clearance and ultrafiltration.
- Dialysate (p. 216) needs to be of sufficient purity and containing the required concentration of electrolytes.
- Effective control and safety mechanisms (p. 214) are blood and dialysate flow, TMP, temperature, and detection of blood leaks or air.

Box 4.1 Hemodialysis and hemofiltration

Hemodialysis
- Solute clearance is by diffusion (mainly).
- Dialysate is required.
- Diffusion is maximized by maintaining high flow rates of blood and dialysate and by pumping the two through the dialyser in countercurrent directions.
- Larger MW (>20 KDa) molecules are generally pozorly removed.
- HD is usually administered intermittently (e.g., 4 hours, 3×/week).

Hemofiltration
- Solute clearance is by convection (mainly).
- HF is achieved by generating a TMP across the membrane.
- No dialysate is required.
- Large volumes need to be filtered to achieve adequate solute clearance. This would cause hypovolemia unless replacement fluid is administered (usually pre-prepared 5–10 L bags).
- HF removes larger MW (30–50 KDa) molecules (e.g., vitamin B_{12} and β_2-microglobulin) more efficiently than dialysis.
- Continuous (24-hour) HF is associated with greater hemodynamic stability and often favored for RRT in an ICU setting (p. 126).

Hemodiafiltration
- This combines HD and HF to get the best of both modalities.
- Use is growing in many outpatient dialysis facilities.
- It is set up as for HD, but with a higher TMP to produce a significant ultrafiltration.
- Both dialysate and replacement fluid are required.
- "Online" generation of replacement fluid is now available in some centers—fluid is produced from ultrapure water and dialysate within the dialysis machine itself. This ↓ cost and dispenses with the need for unwieldy bags of fluid in the dialysis unit.

HD apparatus

Principle
Blood is removed from the patient, anticoagulated, pumped through a dialyser, and then returned to the patient (Fig. 4.1). Within the dialyser blood and dialysate (flowing in opposite directions) are separated by a semipermeable dialysis membrane.

Dialysate
- This is a solution of purified water, Na^+ (132–150 mmol/L), K^+ (usually 1.0–3.0 mmol/L), Ca^{2+} (1.0–1.25 mmol/L), Mg^{2+}, Cl^-, dextrose, and buffer.
- Purified water is generated in a treatment plant (involves microfilters, activated carbon, deionization, and reverse osmosis).
- AAMI standards for water purity are <2 EU/mL endotoxin, <200 cfu/mL microbial count.
- H^+ ions have a low plasma concentration and are not removed by dialysis. Buffer (alkali equivalent) is ∴ added to dialysate.
- Bicarbonate is now preferred to acetate as a buffer.
- HD machines either mix dialysate concentrate, buffer, and water for the individual patient, or this is done centrally before distribution around several machines.

Alarms and monitors
These will stop the blood pump and clamp lines if the situation demands.
- Air detectors, located distally in the venous circuit, prevent air emboli.
- Pressure monitors:
  - Arterial → detect ↓ pressure secondary to poor access flow and line disconnections.
  - Venous → detect ↑ pressure secondary to resistance to venous return (usually represents an access problem).
  - Dialysate outflow pressure → monitor TMP (to vary UF rate).
- Dialyser integrity
- Temperature
- Conductivity
  - Electrical conductivity is used to monitor proportioning of dialysate to water.
  - Many machines use conductivity to enable changes to Na^+ concentration ("Na^+ profiling") (p. 226).

Newer machines
- Blood volume monitoring: Hematocrit (Hct) in the arterial line is used as a surrogate for blood volume (↓plasma H_2O → ↑Hct). This monitoring is used to fine-tune UF and BP control.
- Access recirculation measurements: ensures that the same small volume of blood is not dialysed repetitively.
- Delivered Kt/V: Ur concentration in the dialysate outflow line or dialysate conductivity is used to calculate delivered dialysis dose.

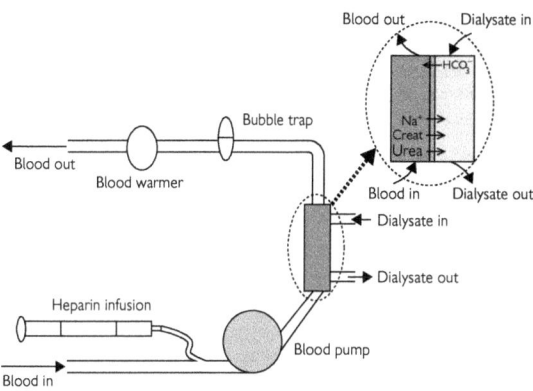

Fig. 4.1 The HD circuit.

Apparatus
- Blood pump: usually a roller "peristaltic" pump
- Bubble trap: traps air → ↓risk of air embolism
- Heparin (📖 p. 214): The HD machine is primed with heparinized saline and further heparin is administered as an infusion or intermittent bolus into the arterial side of the extracorporeal circulation.
- Blood flow rate: usually 200–500 mL/min
- Dialysate flow rate: usually 600–800 mL/min
- Heaters: Dialysate and blood are kept at 37°C.
- Dialyser: a rigid polyurethrane shell (~30 scm long) containing hollow fibers (capillaries) of dialysate membrane. This arrangement maximizes the available surface area for dialysis (0.5–2.1 m^2). Two ports each allow blood and dialysate to enter and exit. Priming volume is ~50–100 mL. To reduce cost, dialysers are often resterilized and used again.
- Dialyser efficiency depends on membrane thickness, pore size, and dialyser structure. Efficiency of solute clearance is measured as KoA (mass transfer urea coefficient), provided for each dialyser by the manufacturer. KoA varies from 300 to 1100 (>600 = high-efficiency dialyser, requiring higher blood and dialysate flows).

Dialysers and membranes

Biocompatibility
- Dialysis membranes are not inert. They can activate complement and inflammatory cascades (→ short and long-term complications).
- A biocompatible membrane is one that elicits the minimum inflammatory response in patients exposed to it.
- Improved biocompatibility may →
  - ↓ hypersensitivity reactions
  - Less intradialytic ↓BP
  - Slower loss of residual renal function
  - Improved nutrition
  - ↓ amyloid deposition
  - ↓ morbidity and mortality (♦)

Cellulose membranes (e.g., Cuprophan®)
- The original membrane and least biocompatible
- Largely superseded by synthetic membranes

Modified cellulose membranes (e.g., Cellulose acetate)
This type is more biocompatible.

Synthetic membranes (e.g., Polysulfone®, polyamide, polyacrylnitrile)
- Recently developed
- Most biocompatible
- More permeable than cellulose membranes:
  - Solute clearance is similar to that of cellulose membranes.
  - ↑β_2-microglobulin clearance

High vs. low flux
High-flux membranes are usually synthetic membranes with a large pore size → enhanced clearance of middle and large molecules. ♦ They may lead to better outcomes.

Surface area
↑Dialyser surface area (usually 0.5–2.1 m^2) → ↑ delivered dialysis.

HD prescription

Intermittent HD places exacting demands on a patient. As it only partially replaces renal function, fluid and dietary restrictions remain of paramount importance.

Dialysis can be considered adequate if it provides relief of uremic symptoms and controls acidosis, fluid balance, and serum K^+. It should also allow a feeling of physical and psychological well-being.

Aspects of dialysis adequacy

- *Solute clearance.* Small molecule clearance is relatively easy to measure (see Box 4.2). Aim to achieve a target Kt/V of >1.2 or URR >65%.
- *Blood pressure and fluid balance.* As a general rule, ↑BP in a dialysis patient should be treated by ↓ "dry weight" (i.e., postdialysis weight). This should be the weight at which salt and water balance is optimal. Oligoanuric patients (most chronic HD patients) need to restrict their interdialytic salt and fluid intake to achieve this, aiming for weight gains of 1–2.5 kg (maximum) between sessions. Targets:
    - Predialysis BP <140/90
    - Postdialysis BP <130/80
    - Preferably without use of antihypertensive agents
- *Nutrition.* Blood Ur levels depend on the rate of production as well as rate of excretion. ⚠ A low predialysis Ur may reflect poor nutrition rather than good dialysis. Targets:
    - Serum albumin >35 g/L
    - nPCR >1.0 g/kg/day (see Box 4.2)
    - Acceptable anthropometric measures
- *Clearance of other molecules:*
    - "Middle" molecule clearance is thought to be important to prevent the long-term complications of dialysis. β_2-microglobulin is the most used marker.
    - Phosphate clearance is also important, and appears to correlate more with hours of dialysis than rate of small molecule clearance.
- *Quality of life and life expectancy.* There is a trade-off to be made between the number of hours spent on the machine (∴ ↑ dialysis dose) and quality of life. For patients with a limited life expectancy, the latter may be a more important consideration.

Box 4.2 Measuring dialysis adequacy

In the 1980s, the National Cooperative Dialysis Study (NCDS) established timed average Ur concentration as a determinant of morbidity and mortality on HD. Subsequent mathematical analysis of this data has led to the development of urea kinetic modeling (UKM) as the accepted method of measuring small solute clearance.

Kt/V is a measure of Ur clearance where
- K = dialyser urea clearance
- t = time on dialysis
- V = volume of distribution of Ur (estimated from patient size)

The *single-pool Kt/V* assumes that at the end of dialysis, the concentrations of intracellular and extracellular Ur are equal:

$$spKt/V = -\ln[Upost/Upre - 0.008t] + [4 - 3.5\, Upost/Upre] \times UFvol/wt\ post$$

Upre = urea predialysis; Upost = urea postdialysis;
UFvol = volume removed on dialysis

The *two-compartment model* acknowledges that in reality it takes time for Ur to be redistributed postdialysis and that the extracellular Ur concentration is lower than the intracellular one. An equilibrated Kt/V or eKt/V can be calculated from the spKt/V.

A simpler measurement of Ur clearance is the *urea reduction ratio* (URR), which does not take account of the amount of fluid removed by ultrafiltration. It is thus less accurate, but has been shown to correlate with outcome:

$$URR = (1 - Upre/Upost) \times 100$$

Normalized protein catabolic rate (nPCR)
This is a measure of Ur generation, which reflects nutritional status. It can only be reliably used in patients who are "stable" when Ur generation will broadly reflect protein intake. It is felt that patients require an nPCR >1.0 g/kg/day. nPCR of <0.8 g/kg/day is associated with higher mortality.

Residual function
When HD is first commenced, residual renal function may contribute greatly to the total amount of solute clearance (Kru). This is usually calculated with a 24-hour urine collection. Residual function tends to diminish quickly on HD (→ repetitive ↓BP ± bioincompatibility) (📖 p. 216).

Variables in the dialysis prescription

- *Number of sessions per week.* Less than three sessions usually means inadequate dialysis (unless there is significant residual renal function). Daily (or nocturnal) dialysis delivers excellent biochemistry and quality-of-life scores, but is only practical in a few enthusiastic (and well resourced) centers with equally enthusiastic patients. Most patients dialyse three times per week.
- *Number of hours per session.* As above, the more the better, though there are diminishing returns as the number of hours is increased. Control of BP, phosphate, and middle molecule clearance are easier to achieve with longer hours.
- *Blood flow.* Higher blood flow rates = more dialysis if all else is equal. A blood flow rate of <250 mL/min is suboptimal. Thus inadequate access = inadequate dialysis.
- *Dialyser size and type.* The larger the surface area of the dialyser, the greater the delivered dose of dialysis per unit time. High-flux dialysers have larger pore sizes, and are able to deliver enhanced middle molecule clearance per unit time if blood flows are adequate. Studies have yet to show long-term benefits.
- *Hemodiafiltration* may deliver enhanced middle molecule clearance, phosphate clearance, hemodyamic stability, and ($\bullet$*) life expectancy.
- *Dialysate composition and flow rate.* The concentrations of Na^+, K^+, Ca^{2+} and HCO_3^- may be altered in the dialysate. Higher flows may enhance clearance.

Anticoagulation

The extracorporeal circuit will usually clot without anticoagulation.

Aim: Minimize risk of dialyser clotting the blood, while minimizing risk of bleeding complications in the patient.

Heparin is usually used, with a bolus of 1000–5000 units (~50 U/kg) at the start of dialysis given into the "arterial" side of the extracorporeal circuit, followed by an infusion of 1000–1500 units/h, stopping 15–60 min before the end of the session. This is usually monitored by measurement of activated clotting time (ACT) on the dialysis unit. Normal: 90–140 s, target 200–250 s (baseline +80%). Intermittent boluses according to ACT can also be given.

Patients at ↑ bleeding risk are given "tight reduced" or no heparin, accepting the increased risk of clotting. Heparin-induced thrombocytopenia (HIT) is a rare complication associated with long-term heparin use. LMW heparin can also be used as anticoagulation for dialysis. It is usually given as a single-dose pretreatment, but is much more expensive than unfractionated heparin. Prostacyclin (infused IV at 4–8 ng/15 kg/min) and citrate (complex administration protocol!) are alternatives, especially if bleeding risk is high.

Ensuring adequate small solute clearance is delivered

Kt/V
US DOQI guidelines suggest a single pool Kt/V >1.4 (target) and Kt/V> 1.2 (minimal) for patients dialysed 3x/week, equating to a URR of ~65%. The landmark HEMO study compared two target Kt/V levels. Patients with a target Kt/V of 1.2 had no difference in mortality or cardiac events compared to those with a Kt/V of 1.6.

Residual renal function should always be taken into account.

Prescribed versus delivered Kt/V
Most guidelines suggest monthly measurement of Kt/V. Online methods of measuring Kt/V are provided on modern dialysis machines (often using Na^+ clearance to estimate urea clearance).

If Kt/V fails to meet target, options are to:
- Improve vascular access: if flows are poor, or if there is access recirculation, it will be hard to improve clearances.
- Increase blood flow or use larger needles—this is beneficial if access is reasonable.
- Increase dialyser size—this has a modest impact.
- Increase dialysate flow.
- Increase dialysis time or frequency—this has major benefit.

Computer modeling software can help decide which elements of the prescription require modification to improve Kt/V.

⚠ HD adequacy is multifaceted. Achieving a desired Kt/V does not necessarily lead to optimal dialysis.

Vascular access

Reliable vascular access is the cornerstone of HD therapy and timely planning of access creation is a major facet of CKD care. Roughly 25% of all admissions in the dialysis population relate to access failure or other complication and remain an important source of morbidity and mortality.

- *Arteriovenous fistula (AVF)*. This is the optimal form of vascular access. It requires the surgical anastamosis of an artery and a vein, either at the wrist (radiocephalic) or elbow (brachiocephalic, brachiobasilic) (Fig.4.2). If suitability of veins is in doubt, then vascular mapping with US is desirable. Maturation for 6–8 weeks (minimum) is required prior to needling (∴ advance planning crucial).
- *Polytetrafluoroethylene (PTFE) graft*. This is second best. A synthetic graft is interposed between an artery and a vein (Fig. 4.2), requiring a larger operation than AVF creation. This type of graft is necessary if veins are inadequate to fashion an AVF (e.g., DM, previous phlebotomy or cannulation). Lower-limb (femoral loop) sites are possible in addition to upper-limb sites. The graft is useable within days, but thrombosis and infection (usually necessitating removal) are problematic. Half-life is shorter than with AVF.
- *Tunneled (and cuffed) dialysis catheter*. A dual-lumen (or two single-lumen) venous catheter(s) is placed in a central vein (internal jugular or subclavian; femoral is less common). The catheter is available for immediate use and usually left in situ for 1–3 months (occasionally longer). It is a useful bridge until an AVF matures. Blood flows (300–450 mL/min) are lower than for an AVF or graft.
- *Temporary dialysis catheter* (📖 p. 632). This is for immediate use (ARF). Internal jugular, subclavian, or femoral catheters should ideally be left in situ ≤2 weeks (femoral: <5 days). This catheter has a much higher infection risk than that of other forms of access.

Principles of vascular access monitoring

- Poor access flow: inadequate arterial inflow, venous stenosis, intra-access thrombosis, poor needle positioning
- Normal blood flow is 800–2000 mL/min (graft >AVF). Poor flow → poor dialysis and ↑risk of thrombosis.
- Measuring flow:
  - Venous pressures: measured while on dialysis. High (or rising) pressures (>200 mmHg at 200 mL/min pump speed) may indicate venous obstruction (examine for evidence of collateral venous enlargement).
  - Serial measurements of flow can be made with US dilution techniques. Flow <600 mL/min or 25% decrease from baseline predicts significant stenoses and impending thrombosis.
  - Further investigations: Doppler US, fistulography (± balloon angioplasty).

Fistula care: what every doctor and patient should know

- Dialysis access is extremely precious.
- Arm veins should be preserved in predialysis patients (no IVs or phlebotomy between elbow and wrist).
- Cannulation should only be carried out by a trained operator (usually a dialysis nurse, ideally the patient).
- Technique: avoid using the same site repetitively (→ false aneurysm formation).
- *Never* put a BP cuff on a fistula arm.
- Do not use a fistula to take blood.
- Hypotension → ↑ thrombosis risk.
- ↑Hct (too much EPO) predisposes to thrombosis. Keep within the recommended guidelines, and at the lower end of these if patient is at risk.
- A clotted fistula or graft requires immediate attention (time to declotting is a major determinant of success).

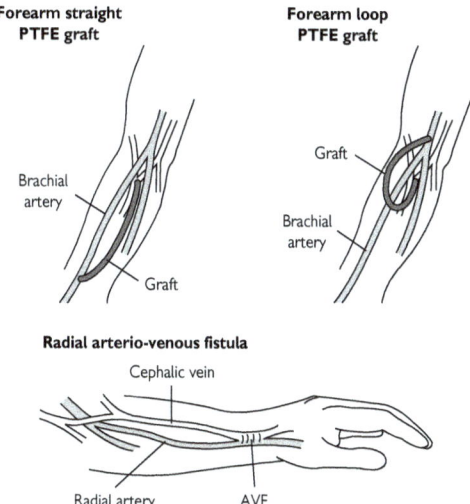

Fig. 4.2 Permanent vascular access for hemodialysis. Reproduced with permission from Levy J, Morgan J, and Brown E (2004). *Oxford Handbook of Dialysis*, 2nd ed. Oxford: Oxford University Press.

Complications of vascular access

Lines

▶ Infection
- Mortality secondary to sepsis is 100- to 300-fold higher in dialysis patients compared to the general population.
- Fever in an HD patient with a line = line sepsis until proven otherwise.
- Infection of temporary lines is extremely common (15%–60% insertions). Risk ↑ with duration of use. For tunneled lines, 3–4 episodes per 1000 catheter days (0.7–1.5 episodes/year) is common.
- Causes: ~70% → *Staph. aureus* (⚠ MRSA) or *Staph. epidermidis*. Gram-negative organisms are more common with femoral catheters.
- Sterile insertion technique (📖 p. 632) and meticulous nursing care are mandatory.
- Eradication of *Staph.* carriage may ↓incidence (e.g., nasal Mupirocin cream).

Clinical features
- The patient usually presents with fever, rigors, ± ↓BP while on dialysis. They may also have nausea and vomiting, diarrhea, and confusion.
- Examination and investigation
  - The line often appears innocent, but check for an erythmatous or purulent exit site (→ swab for C+S). Is there a tunnel infection?
  - General exam: Look for stigmata of endocarditis, chest signs, and other sources of infection.
  - Blood cultures are from the line and peripheral vein.
  - CRP
  - Get a chest X-ray if there are chest signs.

Treatment
- Start antibiotics empirically if there is fever >38°C, rigors, or ↓BP.
  - Give vancomycin 10–20 mg/kg (usually 1 g) + gentamicin 1–2 mg/kg IV and measure levels daily (↓ quicker in patients with significant residual function). Third-generation cephalosporins are an alternative to gentamicin. Tailor therapy to culture results. Vancomycin is not efficiently removed by HD, gentamicin is.
  - Continue for at least 2–6 weeks.
- If the patient is hemodynamically stable, you may change the line over a guide wire 48 hours after initiation of antibiotics. Remove line if ↓BP (some advocate immediate removal in all cases).
- If there is persistent fever or ↑CRP, consider metastatic infection: infective endocarditis, arthritis, osteomyelitis, epidural abscess.
- Avoid inserting new lines until sepsis is cleared ("in–out" femoral lines for each dialysis session may be necessary).

Other line complications
- Thrombosis. Instill thrombolytic agent tPA 1 mg/mL to the internal lumen and leave for 4–24 hours.
- Catheters may → central venous stenosis, preventing subsequent catheter placement and compromising AVF maturation and flow. This may lead to SVC obstruction, with swollen arms, chest wall, breast, and face. Multiple collateral veins may be visible. Balloon angioplasty ± stent insertion may be successful, but recurrence is common.

▶ Clotted fistula or grafts

- No thrill or buzz = thrombosis (ensure that the patient knows this).
- Arrange urgent declotting. This may be radiological (physical declotting or local thrombolysis) or surgical in the first instance (local policies differ).
- Check electrolytes. Insert a temporary line if dialysis is required.
- The longer time between thrombosis and declotting, the less chance of success (especially for AVF).
- Prevention.
  - Grafts: There is some evidence for dipyridamole ± aspirin. Warfarin may have a limited role in selected patients.
  - AVF: There is no evidence of benefit for any agent.

Other complications of fistulas and grafts

- Infection: Fistulas rarely become infected beyond a superficial cellulitis. PTFE infection is not uncommon. It may be occult, causing weight loss, EPO resistance, and failure to thrive. Antimicrobials are rarely successful and management usually involves surgical removal.
- Aneurysm or pseudoaneurysm formation may occur at needling sites, especially if sites are not rotated. Surgery may be necessary.
  - Bleeding from an infected or aneurysmal AVF or graft is a much feared complication (proceeds under arterial pressure!).
  - ▶ Wear a gown, gloves, and goggles. Apply direct pressure to the bleeding site and obtain immediate surgical consultation. Establish wide-bore IV access, check clotting, cross-match blood.
- Distal ischemia or steal syndrome: Flow through the fistula or graft may compromise distal blood supply. Cold or numb peripheries are common, but may → infarction or ischemic pain. AVF ligation or graft removal may be necessary.
- Excess flow may → large ↑ in cardiac output with cardiac decompensation. "Banding" an AVF may ↓ flow.
- Extravasation: blood leakage into the soft tissues. This can cause rapid limb swelling, hemodynamic compromise, compartment syndromes, secondary infection, and access thrombosis.

Acute HD complications

Intradialytic hypotension
- ↓BP requiring intervention occurs during 10%–30% of treatments.
- Pathogenesis is complex, but in essence, fluid removal on dialysis → contraction of the intravascular compartment, compensatory vasoconstriction, and compartmental fluid shifts.
- Patients at risk include those with the following:
  - Large fluid gains (removal of >1.5 L/day)
  - Poor LV function
  - Antihypertensive therapy
  - DM
  - Autonomic dysfunction
  - Sepsis
  - Hypoalbuminemia

Management (see Table 4.2)
- Place patient's head down, stop UF, and give 100 mL bolus of saline.
- Exclude cardiac cause (ischemia, arrhythmia, pericardial effusion).
- Provide education on importance of salt and water restriction.
- Reassess postdialysis ("dry") weight—is it too low?
- Omit antihypertensive agents on the day of dialysis.
- Try longer dialysis hours, enabling slower fluid removal, or daily dialysis (often impractical)
- ↓ dialysate temperature.
- UF profiling: isolated UF before dialysis
- Na^+ profiling—start with high-dialysate Na^+ and gradually reduce.
- Drugs: Midodrine, a peripherally acting vasoconstrictor (α_1 agonist) appears to be of benefit in selected patients. Give orally predialysis.
- Blood volume monitoring (p. 214).

Table 4.2 Acute HD complications

Complication	Cause	Management
Air embolism	Air in dialysis circuit	Clamp lines. Give O_2. Place head down in L lateral position
Arrhythmias	Multifactorial	Check electrolytes, cardiac investigation
Blood loss	Bleeding tendency, heparin	↓ heparin
Chest pain	Angina, ↓BP, air embolism	Address cause
Cramps	Volume contraction ±↓ osmolality, ↓Mg, ↓ carnitine	↑ osmolality (e.g., 25 mL 50% dextrose). Stop dialysis
Hemolysis	Dialysate is contaminated or too warm	Clamp lines. D/C dialysis
Hypoxemia	Bioincompatibilty (p. 559), lactate buffer	Synthetic dialyser, HCO_3^- buffer
Nausea, vomiting, and headache	Unknown (?minor disequilibrium syndrome p. 126)	Analgesia

Chronic HD complications

Dialysis falls well short of providing the clearance of native kidneys. As the number of years on dialysis ("dialysis vintage") increases, the consequences of this shortfall become more apparent:
- Loss of access sites
- Renal bone disease (p. 176)
- Dialysis arthropathy: Accumulated β_2-microglobulin deposits in joints, causing pain and carpal tunnel syndrome. HDF and other methods that improve middle molecule clearance may be of benefit.
- Chronic inflammation: HD is associated with chronic activation of inflammatory cascades (→membrane bioincompatibilty, repeated episodes of clinical/subclinical infection, ↑ advanced glycation end-products, ↑ oxidative stress, and malnutrition). Effects may be:
  - Malnutrition (a vicious cycle develops)
  - Poor EPO response
  - Accelerated vascular and cardiac disease (p. 194)
  - ↑ Susceptibility to infection
  - ↑ Mortality
- Quality of life (QOL): Transplanted dialysis patients report greatly improved QOL scores. HD makes great physical and psychological demands on both patients and their families.

Peritoneal dialysis (PD)

PD is the dialysis modality of approximately 100,000 patients worldwide. It is generally accepted that patient survival on PD compared to that on HD is similar. In fact, these modalities should be seen as complementary, offering different advantages that individuals may benefit from at different times in their dialysis history—the so-called integrated dialysis care approach.

Physiology and concepts

The semipermeable dialysis membrane of the peritoneum comprises the capillary endothelium, supporting matrix, and the peritoneal mesothelium. Fluid and solute move between the fluid-filled peritoneum and blood through what is known as the "three-pore model" of PD.

- *Large pores* (20–40 nm) allow macromolecules such as proteins to be filtered between compartments (effectively via venular or lymphatic absorption).
- *Small pores* (4–6 nm) are responsible for the transport of small solutes such as sodium, potassium, urea, and creatinine.
- *Ultrasmall pores* (<0.8 nm) transport water alone and are likely to be aquaporins.

The net movement of solutes such as urea then depends on
- Net diffusion through small and convection through large pores
- Total volume of dialysate infused
- Net fluid ultrafiltration (or absorption).

Effective peritoneal surface area

Peritoneal capillary endothelium is the predominant barrier to peritoneal solute transport. However, at any one time, not all capillaries are equally perfused and not all are close enough to the mesothelium (and thus dialysate) for effective dialysis. The "effective peritoneal surface area" then varies (e.g., with peritonitis, or changing dialysate volumes). Increasing the effective peritoneal surface area allows faster rates of small solute transfer, but not necessarily better dialysis—by increasing dissipation of glucose, UF might ↓ (p. 229).

Ultrafiltration (UF)

The net movement of water (UF) relies on the presence of a high intraperitoneal osmotic gradient (generated by glucose) or oncotic gradient (generated by glucose polymers such as icodextrin). Opposing fluid movement into the peritoneum is any absorption of dialysate via lymphatics (especially if ↑ intraperitoneal hydrostatic pressure from patient posture or high instilled PD volumes).

The osmotic gradient is usually generated by glucose and depends on
- The glucose concentration of the dialysate
- A patient's blood glucose
- The rate of absorption of glucose itself from PD fluid

UF is optimized by
- Ensuring normoglycemia (relevant for diabetics).
- Adjusting the tonicity of the PD solution (glucose concentration).
- Altering the duration of each dialysis dwell.
- Adjusting dwell volumes; an ↑ often (but not always) leads to ↑UF.

As an alternative to glucose-based solutions, glucose polymers (such as icodextrin) are poorly absorbed and metabolized slowly—these PD solutions provide a sustained *oncotic* gradient over longer dwells and permit ↑UF, particularly for high transporters (p. 234).

↑ dwell volumes of dialysate may maintain the glucose gradient for longer, but ↑ intraperitoneal pressure may ↑ lymphatic return. Also, ↑volume might increase effective peritoneal surface area, with more rapid absorption of glucose, lessening the glucose gradient.

Types of PD

Intermittent PD was originally developed for the treatment of ARF where HD facilities were not available (📖 p. 212). Rapid exchanges over a 24-hour period are repeated two or more times a week (Fig. 4.3). For cost reasons, the peritoneal catheters used for treatment of ARF are often different from those used for patients with ESRD.

Continuous ambulatory PD (CAPD) consists of three to five exchanges with dwell times of 4–10 hours in 24 hours, usually performed by the patient connecting and disconnecting the PD catheter to dialysate bags. A nighttime exchange can be performed by machines (such as Quantum®). Advantages include simplicity and flexibility—the timing of the exchanges can be adjusted to times convenient for patients, although dwells less than 3 hours are generally discouraged.

Automated PD (APD) uses an automated machine to perform exchanges at night while the patient is sleeping. The machine is usually programmed to perform at least four exchanges over 8 hours (can be more depending on individual tolerance). At the end of the overnight exchanges, the machine can be programmed to leave the patient "dry" during the day (nighttime intermittent peritoneal dialysis [NIPD]). Alternatively, the machine can perform a "last fill," leaving PD fluid in the peritoneum. Patients may then perform a further exchange during the day (either manually or using the APD machine—continuous cycling peritoneal dialysis [CCPD]).

Tidal APD has the machine programmed to only partially drain out PD fluid at the end of any dwell during the nightly cycles ("75% tidal" indicates that the machine will stop draining fluid out when 75% of the expected drain has been extracted). Although efficiency of dialysis is reduced, it is useful for patients whose sleep is disturbed through discomfort experienced when "dry."

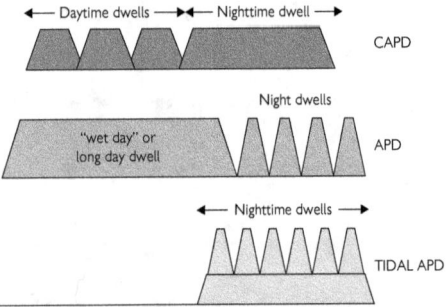

Fig. 4.3 Types of peritoneal dialysis (PD). Reproduced with permission from Levy J, Morgan J, and Brown E (2004). *Oxford Handbook of Dialysis*, 2nd ed. Oxford: Oxford University Press.

CAPD technique

Disconnect, flush-before-fill Y-systems are now the norm (Fig. 4.4). The connectology has been refined over the years to minimize peritonitis through touch-contamination. At the time of an exchange, the patient connects a Y-shaped set with a sterile drain bag and a fresh dialysate bag. Patients are taught to make this connection using sterile techniques, although various assist devices are available to aid patients with dexterity or visual problems (e.g., UV Flash Compact®). After the waste dialysate is drained into the empty bag, the Y-connector is flushed (theoretically flushing away any contaminating bacteria in this portion of the giving set) using a small volume of fresh dialysate. The remaining dialysate is infused into the patient's abdomen.

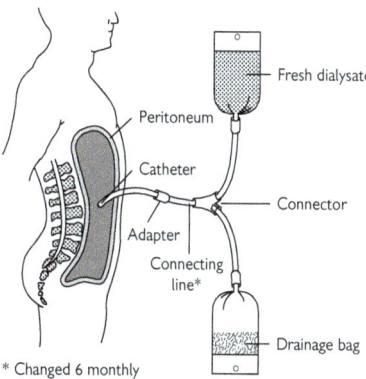

* Changed 6 monthly

Fig. 4.4 "Disconnect" PD system. Reproduced with permission from Levy J, Morgan J, and Brown E (2004). *Oxford Handbook of Dialysis*, 2nd ed. Oxford: Oxford University Press.

PD fluids

Peritoneal dialysate needs to remove uremic toxins and fluid, normalize electrolytes, and correct acidosis. Ideally, fluid should be compatible with long-term peritoneal health. Each CAPD bag has a volume of usually 2 L. The contents of each dialysis bag is designed with the above in mind:
- Volume: This is usually 2 L, but 1.0, 2.5, or 3 L, 5 L, and 6 L bags are also available.
- Glucose concentration: There are three standard concentrations, 1.5%, 2.5%, and 4.25% (osmolality 346, 396, and 485 osm).
- Sodium: Na^+ 132 meq/L (although lower concentrations may improve salt and thus water removal)
- Electrolytes: Calcium ranges from 3.5 meq/L to 1.5 meq/L magnesium.
- Buffer: Lactate is widely used at 35 meql/L (rapidly converted in the liver to bicarbonate).

Newer solutions may contain the following:
- Bicarbonate rather than lactate as the buffer
- Icodextrin rather than glucose as colloid to achieve UF
- Amino acids as a nutritional supplement that also lacks the toxicity of glucose (see below).

A number of newer peritoneal dialysis solutions have been developed and are approved in Europe. Of the ones listed above, only Icodextrin-based dialysis solutions are available in the Unites States. Others are likely to become available over the next several years.

Biocompatible solutions

PD fluid is sterilized through heat treatment. During this process, at the pH of lactate-based glucose solutions, glucose-degradation products (GDP) and advanced glycation end-products (AGE) are formed. These are believed to damage the peritoneal membrane: AGE exposure correlates with fibrotic changes. Thus, more "biocompatible" solutions have been developed with this in mind.

One solution depends on a twin-bag system: heat sterilization of the compartment containing glucose (at very low pH) generates very low levels of GDP and AGE. The second compartment contains the acid-buffer—e.g., predominantly bicarbonate in the case of Physioneal® or lactate in the case of Balance®. Definitive evidence that use of these solutions lead to improved clinical outcome is awaited, although retrospective analysis of registry data suggested the patient survival was better in the group treated with biocompatible solutions.

Other solutions that rely on molecules other than glucose to provide the osmotic gradient have no GDP or AGE. In this respect, they can be considered biocompatible.

Commercially available solutions in the United States
- Baxter
  - Dianeal®—glucose/lactate containing
  - Extraneal—icodextrin
- Fresenius
  - Staysafe®—glucose/lactate in single compartment
  - Staysafe Balance®—glucose/lactate in twin-bag system.

Prescribing PD

Aim for "adequate" dialysis with as little impact on the patient's social or psychological well-being. Dialysis adequacy (📖 p. 219) and UF failure (📖 p. 229) are discussed elsewhere.

The concept of "transporter" status

High concentrations of glucose generate an osmotic gradient across the peritoneal membrane. During the dialysis dwell, glucose is absorbed → ↓ glucose concentration and dialysate osmolality within the peritoneum. The rate of glucose dissipation correlates with the rate at which creatinine equilibrates across the peritoneal membrane and can change over time (termed the "transport" status of the patient) and can be measured during a peritoneal equilibration test (PET, 📖 p. 243).

"High" transporters allow rapid movement of urea and other small molecules across the peritoneal membrane (through small pores, 📖 p. 229). But glucose is also rapidly absorbed, ↓ the gradient: thus UF at the end of a CAPD dwell is likely to be low. So a high transporter often has difficulty achieving adequate small solute clearance.

- High transporters are particularly suitable for APD (frequent short dwells maximize UF and total solute removal).
- Low transporters benefit less from very short dwells on APD. Introducing a fifth PD exchange may be preferable (either manually or using an automated machine to deliver a single exchange at night, 📖 p. 230).

Most patients start CAPD on four (1.5% dextrose) PD bags. If this fails to provide adequate UF, one exchange is changed to a higher glucose concentration bag or Extraneal®. Further increases in glucose concentration may be necessary to achieve adequate dialysis and UF.

Avoiding glucose exposure

High peritoneal glucose exposure over time (often years) predicts the development of UF failure, and causality has been suggested. An alternative to glucose in the dialysate is icodextrin (Extraneal®).
- Icodextrin is a 20-glucose polymer with potent colloidal effects.
- It is usually used for the longest dwell (overnight in CAPD, daytime dwell in APD).

Particularly suited to high transporters, icodextrin is absorbed into the lymphatics, so the osmotic gradient is maintained even in high transporters (reflection of rate of movement across small pores).

⚠ Increasing the volume of each exchange can increase intraperitoneal pressure and adversely affect UF.

Based on individuals' membrane transport characteristics (PET 📖 p. 243), computer software can be used to predict small solute clearance and UF. These can be particularly useful when responding to falling UF or solute clearance.

Peritonitis

Peritonitis is (one of) the major complication(s) of PD, leading to significant morbidity and mortality. Repeated episodes of peritonitis might also accelerate peritoneal membrane failure, requiring transfer to hemodialysis. The incidence of peritonitis has declined from about 3 episodes per patient per year in the 1980s to 0.6–0.7 episodes per patient per year (or roughly 1 episode every 18 months); this is attributed to improved patient education and better catheter technology. The disconnect "flush-before-fill" system has also been an important advance.

Clinical features

These include abdominal pain, nausea, and vomiting. "Cloudy" PD effluent is highly suggestive. High fever and being systemically unwell with signs of an ileus, and peritonism can also occur. Diagnosis:
- PD fluid for microscopy and Gram stain. It should have a dwell time of 4 hours or more, with >100 WBC/mm^3 (>50% neutrophils).
- Culture PD fluid (discuss with microbiology) and blood
- CBC (↑WBC).

Patients should be taught to report cloudy effluent as soon as it is seen. Abdominal pain can be very severe. Rapid peritoneal flushing can improve symptoms, but samples from the original cloudy bag should be sent for microscopy, Gram stain, and culture.

▶ Always consider other causes of peritonitis (e.g., perforation, strangulated hernia).

Bacteriology
- Gram-positive cocci, 45%–75% (coagulase-negative staphylococci, *Staph. aureus*) These are often introduced after touch contamination of the connections, or catheter exit site infections. Colonization of catheter biofilms can lead to recurrence of peritonitis and necessitate catheter exchange.
- Gram-negative organisms, 15%–25% (*Pseudomonas*, coliforms). These are usually of bowel origin. Air in the peritoneum is common and may not indicate bowel perforation. Suspect perforation if there are mixed gram-negative organisms on culture.
- Culture is negative or "no growth" (ideally, positive cultures in >85%).
- Mycobacterial infections, 1% (TB), should be considered in patients with culture-negative peritonitis not responding to empiric antibiotic therapy. Smears of PD effluent are rarely positive for acid-fast bacilli and diagnosis is usually made on culture (6 weeks) or at laparoscopy or laparotomy with confirmation on peritoneal biopsy.
- Fungal, 3% (usually *Candida* spp.), peritonitis is infrequent but has a poor prognosis. It often follows recent antibiotic therapy in at-risk patients.

Allergy
Allergic peritonitis is well described, often found with newly prescribed icodextrin solutions (although it can occur with glucose-based solutions). In general, the elevation of WBC is modest and the proportion of eosinophils in PD effluent can be high (>10%). This type does not respond to antibiotics. Withdrawal of icodextrin usually helps.

Complications of peritonitis

- *Relapsing peritonitis* is a second episode of peritonitis with the same organism within 4 weeks of completing antibiotic therapy. It is our practice to consider a second episode of culture-negative peritonitis as a relapse if it fulfills the temporal relationship. Prolonged antibiotics (particularly for relapses secondary to staphylococcus) are required.
- *Antibiotic treatment failure.* You need to exclude abscess formation if there is no response to protocol antibiotic therapy. PD catheters should be removed and laparotomy considered, especially if other intra-abdominal pathology is suspected. CT of the abdomen is useful for diagnosis and drainage of infected encysted fluid.
- *Acute and chronic UF failure.* Vasodilatation as a result of inflammation may lead to ↑ glucose absorption, reduced glucose gradient, and impaired UF. Repeated bouts of peritonitis can lead to long-term changes in peritoneal membrane structure and function, causing chronic UF failure.
- *Malnutrition.* Peritoneal protein loss through the inflamed peritoneum can be very high. Anorexia and prolonged ileus can exacerbate nutritional status further.

Treatment

Empiric antibiotic therapy should be initiated in cases of definite peritonitis without awaiting results of culture. Many protocols exist and are influenced by local experience—contact your microbiologist. The International Society of Peritoneal Dialysis recommends
- gram-positive cover with vancomycin or a cephalosporin +
- gram-negative cover with an aminoglycoside or third-generation cephalosporin.

In the United States, despite concerns over the development of vancomycin resistance, most units use vancomycin-based regimens. Protocols differ from unit to unit, but as an example:
- Vancomycin 2 g IP on day 1, with a further dose on days 5–7 depending on trough vancomycin levels +
- either gentamicin 0.6 mg/kg IP daily (adjusted against trough gentamicin levels on days 3–5) or, alternatively, to spare residual renal function (defined in terms of UO) from aminoglycoside nephrotoxicity, ceftazidime 1 g IP daily.

Once the culture result and sensitivities are known:
- If gram-positive: continue weekly vancomycin. If S. *aureus*, add in rifampicin 300 mg po bid. Stop gentamicin/ceftazidime.
- If gram-negative: continue ceftazidime or gentamicin. Although concerns about aminoglycosides affecting residual renal function exist, this is not borne out by evidence. It is our practice to administer ceftazidime if UO >100 mL/day, and gentamicin if patient is functionally anuric (<100 mL/day). Stop vancomycin.
- If culture is negative: continue both, doses adjusted according to trough drug levels.
- If there is mixed gram-negative growth: add in metronidazole and consider laparotomy (suspect bowel perforation).
- Treat for 14–21 days.

▶ Mupirocin ointment administered to the catheter exit site can prevent not only exit site infection but also S. *aureus* peritonitis. Gentamicin cream may be as effective against S. *aureus* and prevent pseudomonal peritonitis as well.

Special considerations for APD

Even in the absence of peritonitis, long day dwells may be "misty." However, because cycling times may be short, cloudy overnight dialysate is less common than with CAPD. Moreover, in some cases, PD effluent is directly drained into a sink. Thus, it is important for APD patients to recognize potential symptoms of peritonitis and to perform a dwell of at least 2 hours (for inspection and sampling of fluid for M, C+S) when such a diagnosis is in doubt. Treatment also requires some technique modifications. One option is to convert patients to CAPD for the duration of the episode. Alternatively (and we believe, preferably), give antibiotics as above into the last dwell on the machine (first ambulatory dwell).

Catheter exit site infection

This presents as a purulent and/or bloody discharge from an exit site, often associated with erythema, or pain. Crusting alone is not indicative of an acute exit site infection. *Causes* are usually S. *aureus*, *Pseudomonas*.

The use of prophylactic topical exit site ointment (with mupirocin or gentamicin) reduces such infections. Reducing nasal carriage of S. *aureus* also reduces exit site infections.

Treatment
- Swab for culture and confirm that PD fluid is clear.
- If there is only erythema and crusting, increase local care to twice daily.
- If there is purulent drainage and culture is positive, adjust therapy once culture result and sensitivities are known.
- Topical antibiotics are not appropriate.
- Empiric therapy: start cephalexin 500 mg bid or clarithromycin 500 mg bid.
- Gram-positive organisms: continue cephalexin or clarithromycin depending on sensitivities. Treat for 14 days. If S. *aureus* is confirmed, add in rifampicin 300 mg bid.
- Gram-negative organisms: ciprofloxacin 500 mg po bid for 14 days. If *Pseudomonas*, treat with IP ceftazidime as for PD peritonitis.

Trauma to the exit site increases the likelihood of infections. Increasing the frequency of exit site care (to daily or twice-daily dressings) is often advocated during infections. Crusts or scabs should not be forcibly removed and the exit site in general should be protected from trauma (that includes dressings that immobilize the catheter, thereby preventing pulling on the exit site).

A tunnel infection is defined as erythema and/or tenderness over the subcutaneous catheter pathway, ± intermittent discharge from the exit site. Diagnosis of tunnel infection can be confirmed by ultrasound examination. Treatment usually involves removing the catheter, as peritonitis is a common complication.

Other complications

Drainage problems

This should be differentiated from UF failure. Catheter flow problems can present with either slow drainage (drainage takes >15–20 min under gravity) or incomplete drainage: high residual volume measured on PET or when the drain volume is less than the infused volume of a "rapid" exchange. Causes include the following:
- Constipation.
- Catheter occlusions (external kinking, thrombus and omental wrapping)
- Fluid leaks into subcutaneous tissue from hernia or insertion site.

Inflow problems can also occur, for many of the same reasons. In addition, if the catheter tip is trapped in a small area of intra-abdominal adhesions, inflow can be limited. Careful history and examination should be sufficient to determine most causes. Plain kidney-ureter-bladder (KUB) imaging can be performed to exclude catheter malposition and constipation.

Most drain problems can be improved without surgery:
- Laxatives (regular senna and lactulose, or sorbitol)
- Intracatheter heparin locks (e.g., 500 units as a lock, or 500 units/L in exchanges)
- Thrombolytics such as TPA infused down the catheter
- Endoluminal brushes

If surgical repositioning is required, it is often useful to perform an omentectomy (and adhesolysis if appropriate).

Peritoneal leaks

Dialysate may leak down the catheter tunnel into the subcutaneous tissues or externally via the exit site. A patent processus vaginalis may allow PD fluid to track into the scrotum, mimicking a hernia or hydrocele. Small diaphragmatic hernias may permit PD fluid to enter the pleural space.

Clinically, local edema ± skin peau d'orange appearance may signify a subcutaneous leak. Fluid leaking from the exit site can be dipsticked for glucose to confirm that it is glucose-rich dialysate. Similarly, pleural taps or aspirates from hydroceles can be tested for glucose. If in doubt, perform CT peritoneogram. Our protocol is to infuse 100 mL of non-ionic contrast into a 2 L PD bag and drain in 1 L. Perform CT 1–2 hours thereafter.

Leaks around the catheter often heal with temporary (2–4 weeks) discontinuation of PD (which may require temporary HD). We restart PD using smaller volumes to reduce intra-abdominal pressure. If leaks recur, the PD catheter can be repositioned with a new insertion site. Hernias should be repaired in a standard manner. APD with a dry day (NIPD) can be particularly successful to minimize recurrence.

Sclerosing encapsulating peritonitis (SEP)

SEP is a feared complication of long-term PD therapy with very poor prognosis. The incidence is about 0.9%, usually in PD patients at an average of 65 months from the initiation of PD. The peritoneal cavity becomes encased in fibrous tissue, with bowel wall thickening and peritoneal calcification. It is thought to be multifactorial in origin, with prior severe peritonitis, foreign-body reactions to plasticizers on catheters, and long-term PD using less biocompatible solutions all suggested as being pathogenic.

Clinically
- Symptoms of intermittent bowel obstruction
- Poor UF or UF failure
- Malnutrition is frequent.

Symptoms may occur after peritonitis, or even after stopping PD.

Investigation of choice is CT of the abdomen, demonstrating peritoneal thickening and calcification with entrapped bowel loops. Peritoneal biopsy is diagnostic.

Treatment

This is limited, and based on anecdotal evidence:
- Stop PD.
- Use renal transplantation if possible.
- Trial of immunosuppression (e.g., rapamycin) is a therapeutic option.
- Tamoxifen has also been suggested to be effective in case reports.
- Surgery may be associated with a high risk of perforating bowel.

PD adequacy

The absence of uremic symptoms and volume overload does not imply dialysis adequacy. Other imprecise criteria for adequacy include the folollowing:
- Patient quality of life (e.g., by subjective global assessment scoring)
- Improved biochemistry and correction of anemia
- Adequate nutrition.

Formally, the delivered dose can be measured by calculating weekly clearance for urea (Kt/V) (📖 p. 219) and creatinine (CCr).
Although there is a minimum threshold of dialysis clearance to maintain good health, increasing the dialysis dose beyond this does not appear to improve survival. The most powerful predictor of patient survival on PD is not dialysis adequacy but the presence of residual renal function.

With these provisos, the current U.S. and U.K. PD adequacy guidelines are as follows:
- US K/DOQI
  - CAPD: weekly Kt/V > 2.0 and CCr 50–60 L/week per 1.73 m^2 (depending on transport status)
  - APD: weekly Kt/V > 2.1 and CCr 63 L/week per 1.73 m^2
- UK Renal Association
  - CAPD: Kt/V > 1.7 and CCr 50 L/week per 1.73 m^2
  - Recommends aiming for higher targets for high average and high transporters (📖 p. 234) and APD patients.

How to improve a low Kt/V / CCr

CAPD
Review transport status (📖 p. 234):
- If high or high average transporter, consider converting to APD.
- If low or low average transporter, ?↑ dwell volume or add fifth exchange.
- Increasing dialysate osmolality to increase the drain volume will also improve total clearance.

APD
- Consider introducing daytime dwell(s).
- Optimize cycle duration in accordance with patient transport status (short cycles for high transporter). This might necessitate increasing the total duration of APD.

Increasingly, preserving residual renal function and controlling salt and water balance in PD patients is seen as a vital measure of technique success. If there is meaningful UO, consider the following:
- ACE inhibitors as renoprotective agents.
- Avoid nephrotoxins (NSAIDs, contrast, *perhaps* aminoglycosides).
- Diuretics to better achieve salt and water balance.

The peritoneal equilibration test (PET)

This is an assessment of peritoneal membrane transport function; the ratio of dialysate and plasma creatinine concentrations (D_{cr}/P_{cr} ratio) after a 4-hour dwell is a measure of solute equilibration. High and low transporters are defined to be $D_{cr}/P_{cr} > 0.8$ or < 0.5 ($\pm$ 1 SD), respectively.

Since glucose absorbed from the dialysate is very quickly metabolized, the D/P ratio for glucose is meaningless. Instead, the fraction of glucose absorbed from the dialysate at 4 hours is compared with the initial dialysis solution (D/D_0). This is also a useful indicator of transport status.

A PET is also a useful objective assessment of ultrafiltration. However, a UF volume <400 mL after modified PET using a 4.25% glucose dwell is more specific for UF failure.

Ultrafiltration failure

PD patients with fluid overload are either noncompliant with a realistic fluid restriction or have inadequate UF (Fig. 4.5). Inadequate UF might be the result of inappropriate dialysis prescription or the failure of an appropriate prescription to drain adequate volumes; the latter is *UF failure*.

Patients are asked to achieve a dry weight through fluid restriction and use of hyperosmolar PD bags. However, setting accurate dry weights is difficult in PD, so aim to adjust the dialysis prescription for adequate fluid removal (sum of UO and net UF). As a general rule, aim for a target of 1 L/day. If the patient is anuric (UO <100 mL/day), minimum daily UF should be 750 mL.

General rules for better fluid removal are as follows:
- Consider a modified PET to differentiate UF failure from other cases of fluid overload. Calculating D_{cr}/P_{cr} ratio can also help diagnose the cause of UF failure (📖 p. 243).
- Evaluate the residual volume during PET: a "normal" residual volume is up to 200–250 mL. Higher volumes might suggest catheter-related drainage problems (also check drain time for the PET test).
- Exclude mechanical problems (📖 p. 240).
- Avoid long dwells (>4 hours) with low glucose concentrations.
- Use icodextrin instead of glucose for the longest dwell.
- If the patient is on APD, consider an additional short day exchange.

Causes
- High transporter status (often seen in long-standing PD patients)
- If it is not high transporter, consider the following:
  - Leaks
  - Reduced effective peritoneal surface area from peritoneal adhesions
  - Increased lymphatic absorption
  - Aquaporin deficiency or failure (indicated by loss of sodium sieving during modified PET).

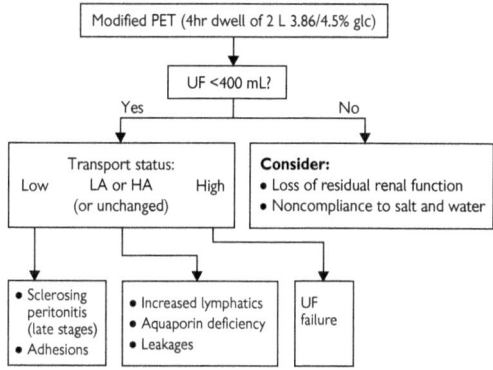

Fig. 4.5 Diagnosing causes for hypervolemia in PD.

The well PD patient

For adequate dialysis maintain residual renal and peritoneal membrane function.
- Dialysis adequacy should be measured in terms of clearance of small solute clearance (including Kt/V and CCr) and nutritional parameters.
- Aim for normotension by good salt and water removal—generally by achieving minimum daily fluid removal of 750 mL.
- Preserving residual renal function (basically, UO) makes the above goals easier to achieve and may improve outcomes (an argument for use of ACE inhibitors and avoidance of NSAIDs).

Increments in patients' transport status (p. 234) make maintaining good UF and small solute clearance difficult without onerous dialysis regimens. High intraperitoneal glucose concentrations and exposure to GDP or AGE are suggested to hasten peritoneal membrane changes, so use of solutions low in GDPs such as twin-bag "physiological" solutions or icodextrin and amino acid solutions *may* be desirable ().

Complications

Minimize peritonitis and exit site infections through education about good technique. This includes teaching patients to identify and present themselves for early treatment. Monitor nutritional status closely. Early stages of sclerosing peritonitis may be reversible and early diagnosis relies on a high index of suspicion.

Social rehabilitation

Rehabilitation is also extremely important for individual PD patients and should encompass adapting the timing of PD exchanges or APD to the working environment (perhaps negotiating a dedicated area at the workplace, or delivery of solutions to the workplace). Travel (either within the same country or abroad) improves patients' sense of well-being and should be supported. Support for the other family members including children and spouse should not be overlooked.

Basic transplantation

Practical transplant immunology

Histocompatibility and allorecognition

The immune response to a transplanted kidney is determined by an array of cell surface proteins, encoded by a group of histocompatibility genes known as the major histocompatibility complex (MHC). The MHC presents fragments of "non-self" proteins to T lymphocytes to initiate an immune response.

In humans the MHC genes encode a polymorphic group of proteins called the human leukocyte antigens (HLA).
- Class I HLA includes HLA-A, HLA-B, and HLA-C, present on most cell surfaces. Antigens associated with class I molecules are recognized by cytotoxic CD8+ T lymphocytes, which become activated.
- Class II HLA consists of HLA-DR, HLA-DQ, and HLA-DP and is generally only present on antigen-presenting cells (APCs) such as macrophages and renal mesangial and dendritic cells. Class II antigens are recognized by CD4+ T lymphocytes, leading to their clonal expansion. Activated CD4+ cells release cytokines that activate CD8+ cells.

Each individual inherits an allele from each parent (a haplotype).

The recognition of transplanted antigens by recipient T cells is by *direct* and *indirect* pathways (Fig. 4.6).
- Direct pathway: Donor APCs present foreign peptides to recipient cytotoxic CD8+ T lymphocytes, leading to their activation. This pathway is largely responsible for early rejection. Donor APC can also present proteins to recipient CD4+ T-helper lymphocytes, leading to their activation.
- Indirect pathway: Donor proteins shed from cell surfaces or donor cells engulfed by recipient APCs are presented to recipient CD4+ T- helper lymphocytes.

The binding of a T cell to an APC leads to the initiation of the immune reaction. This process requires three distinct steps, or "signals" (Fig. 4.7):
- Signal 1: Binding of APC MHC molecule to the T-cell receptor (TCR) leads ↑ intracellular calcium → activation of calcineurin. Calcineurin activates NFAT → release of IL-2, but only in the presence of signal 2.
- Signal 2: Binding of complementary costimulatory pathway molecules present on APC and T lymphocytes (e.g., B7:CTLA4, ICAM:LFA1, etc.) → activation of tyrosine kinase, which together with signal 1 leads to induction of IL-2 and other T-cell activation genes.
- Signal 3: Signals 1 + 2 → induction of cytokine and cell activation genes (principally IL-2) which bind their receptors → clonal proliferation.

If signal 1 occurs without the subsequent signal 2, then activation of the T cell does not occur and instead *apoptosis* may occur. This process may lead to donor-specific tolerance and is the subject of intensive research.

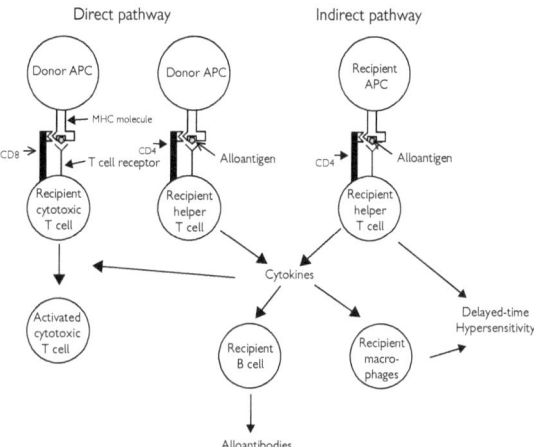

Fig. 4.6 Direct and indirect recognition of transplanted antigens.

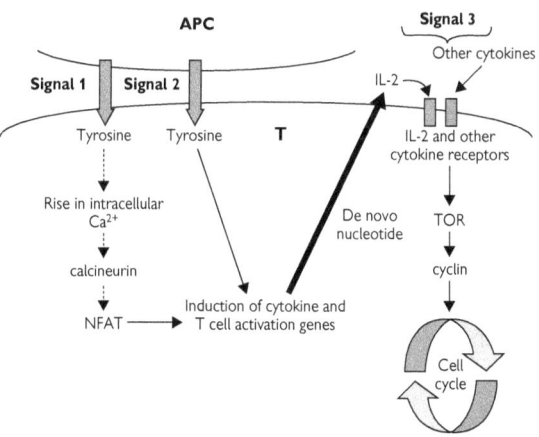

Fig. 4.7 T-cell activation (TOR = target of rapamycin).

Compatibility

Matching donor to recipient

Four areas need to be considered:
- Blood group
- Tissue type (HLA)
- Antibodies
- Donor: recipient characteristics.

Blood group

ABO antigens are expressed on endothelial cells in the kidney and naturally occurring anti-blood group antibodies develop at 6 months of age.

▶ The same rules apply for transplantation and blood transfusions, i.e., group O are universal donors and group AB, universal recipients. ABO-incompatible transplants are generally avoided.

Tissue typing

The most clinically relevant HLA antigens are HLA-A and HLA-B (class I) and HLA-DR (class II). The degree of mismatch between the donor and recipient is usually quoted at these three loci, i.e., HLA-identical donors have a 0,0,0 mismatch, whereas those pairs that share 1 HLA-A, 1 HLA-B, and 1 HLA-DR have a 1,1,1 mismatch. Minor HLA antigens exist, but their clinical impact is small. Benefits of a well-matched graft include:
- Lower acute rejection rates
- Better long-term graft survival
- Fewer subsequent anti-HLA antibodies
- Lower incidence of delayed graft function.

The effect of matching on acute rejection is less evident in the modern era of immunosuppression. The impact of matching on long-term survival, however, is still relevant (Fig. 4.8).

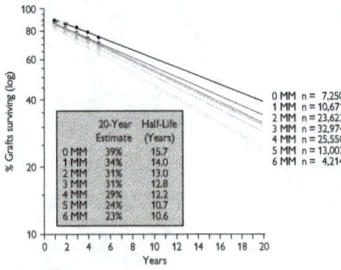

Fig. 4.8 Percent survival HLA A+B+DR mismatches (MM): first cadaver kidney transplants 1985–2003. From the Collaborative Transplant Study (www.ctstransplant.org). Used with permission.

Each mismatched HLA antigen is likely to initiate an immune response, which is especially important if repeat transplantation is ever required. Recipients may develop anti-HLA antibodies or memory T cells against mismatched antigens, "forbidding" organs with these antigens from being used in a given recipient.

Panel-reactive antibodies (PRA)
PRA is the individual response to a notional pool of antigens in a local population (i.e., all the antigens weighted for frequency). Patient sera is incubated with lymphocytes from a panel of representative donors and complement: PRA is expressed as the percentage of donor wells with cell lysis (45% PRA should imply recipient antibodies against 45% of the most commonly occurring antigens in that population). The higher a patient's PRA, the more likely a positive cross-match (p. 253) at the time of transplantation.

Anti-HLA antibodies
Patients are "sensitized" to develop anti-HLA antibodies when previously exposed to non-self HLA antigens. Both direct and indirect pathways → B-cell activation and anti-HLA antibody production.

Sensitization events
- Previous transplant (degree of mismatching important: 0,0,0 less likely to be sensitized)
- Pregnancy
- Blood transfusion.

▶ The presence of circulating donor-specific anti-HLA antibodies at the time of transplantation → hyperacute rejection.

Anti-HLA antibodies may disappear with time, and desensitization protocols aim to remove preformed antibodies prior to transplantation (p. 252).

Donor characteristics
Donor and recipient should be as closely "biologically" matched as possible; for instance, kidneys from elderly donors do not, on average, last as long as those from younger donors and may sensitize younger recipients to subsequent (better-matched) grafts. Unfavorable donor characteristics include the following (these are not absolute—use of marginal kidneys is one means of expanding the overall donor pool):
- ↑BP or DM
- Prior donor viral hepatitis or intravenous drug use (IVDU)
- Donors with systemic sepsis or certain malignancies at brain death
- "Non-heart beating" donors have an increased incidence of delayed graft function (itself a predictor of poor outcome).

Recipient characteristics
- It may be technically difficult to implant a kidney from a large donor into a small recipient
- A small donor (e.g., pediatric) to a large recipient may not transplant enough nephron mass.
- Large recipient polycystic kidneys may limit placement of a new organ (native nephrectomies may be necessary).

Pretransplant assessment

Medical (see p. 196)
Potential recipients should be fit to undergo surgery and long-term immunosuppression.
- Cardiac: ischemic heart disease should be treated. High-risk patients (e.g., DM) are usually screened with thallium scans or angiography (p. 196).
- Vascular: ?peripheral vascular disease
- Malignancy: at least 2, preferably 5, years disease-free (depends on histology)
- ♂: PSA (age >50), ♀: cervical smear, mammography
- No evidence of occult infection (?CRP)
- Obesity (BMI >30 at ↑surgical risk)
- Thrombosis history: exclude thrombophilia (→ ↑ risk of graft loss)
- Bladder: LUTS or recurrent UTIs require urological assessment.
- HIV and hepatitis B + C are not necessarily contraindications to transplantation.
- Compliance
- Reassess fitness every 1–2 years if patient is on transplant waiting list.

Immunological
- Tissue type for HLA matching
- Regular determination of PRA and anti-HLA antibody status
- Cross-match:
  - On the day of transplant
  - Detects preformed anti-donor HLA and non-HLA antibodies that predict hyperacute rejection
  - Either cell-dependent cytotoxicity assay (CDC—recipient sera incubated with donor lymphocytes + complement) or flow cytometry
  - Positive cross-match → abandon transplant
- Patients at high immunological risk usually require heavier immunosuppression.

High immunological risk
- Patients receiving their second or subsequent transplant
- Patients having lost a previous transplant to rejection
- African-American recipients
- Patients with historic donor specific anti-HLA antibodies
- Patients with a high PRA.

Cross-matching

Prior to successful transplantation, any anti-donor antibodies need to be identified to exclude hyperacute humoral rejection and immediate graft failure. This is done by mixing recipient serum (containing potential anti-donor antibody) with donor cells (expressing HLA). A number of tests can be used to detect antibody–antigen interactions:

The complement-dependent cross-match (CDC)
- Once recipient serum and donor T cells are combined in a multi-well tray, complement is added (with dye, see below).
- Sensitivity can be increased by adding goat anti-human light-chain antibody (which binds recipient antibody → improved antibody cross-linkage and fuller complement activation).
- Cell death (by complement-dependent killing) is identified by adding a dye that binds exposed DNA (i.e., loss of membrane integrity) under fluorescence.
- Transplanting across a positive CDC predicts hyperacute rejection.

Flow cytometry
- More sensitive than CDC. A flow-cytometer mixture is prepared of the following:
  - Donor lymphocytes
  - Anti-CD antibodies (e.g., CD3 identifies T cells, CD19 B cells)
  - Recipient serum
  - Anti-Fc antibodies (directed against the Fc component of Ig) tagged with a fluorescent dye
- Flow cytometry readouts allow specific cells to be grouped (e.g., all T cells), and the intensity of dye fluorescence (i.e., binding of anti-Fc to antibodies bound in turn to HLA on cells) qualifies positivity.
- A positive T-cell cross-match (but not necessarily B cell) → rejection.

Donor-specific antibodies (DSA)
- A powerful and sensitive tool for detecting anti-donor antibodies (DSA).
- Donor tissue type is described conventionally.
- Latex beads containing commercially prepared, implanted specific HLA antigens when mixed with recipient serum allow detection of recipient antibodies (often at very low titer) to specific antigens.

Living donor transplantation

▶ Living donor transplantation is the treatment of choice for ESRD.

Advantages
- It has better graft and patient survival than cadaveric transplantation—regardless of genetic relationship and HLA mismatch.
- ▶ Preemptive transplantation (prior to dialysis) → best outcome of all.
- Prolonged dialysis is avoided while waiting for transplantation. Time on dialysis may be a risk factor for poorer transplant outcome.
- Closer HLA matching might be possible.
- It expands the overall donor pool.
- Surgery can be scheduled electively.
- There is minimal ischemic damage to graft (∴ ↓delayed graft function).
- There is less potent immunosuppression (possibly).
- It has psychological benefits (better compliance, sense of well-being).

Disadvantages
- Stress to donor (and family)
- Perioperative donor morbidity (wound problems, DVT) and mortality (~1 in 3000)
- ✴ Later development of donor ↑BP, proteinuria, or CKD (mean donor CrCl at 25 years ~72% of that prior to nephrectomy)
- It is difficult to guarantee "freely given" consent. ?coercion. Potential donors should be assessed in isolation from recipients and allowed to withdraw (without explanation) at any stage.

Assessment of a potential live donor
1. Willing to donate? → information and discussion
2. ABO compatibility
3. HLA typing and cross-matching (recipient against donor)
4. Medical evaluation
   - History, clinical exam
   - Urine: dipstick, micro and ACR
   - U+E, Cr, eGFR
   - CBC, clotting, LFTs, bone ± Hb electrophoresis (?sickle cell trait)
   - Fasting glucose ± glucose tolerance test (if fasting value >100 mg/dL, ↑BMI, or family history of type 2 DM)
   - PSA (♂>50 years of age)
   - ECG, chest X-ray
   - GFR
   - HIV, hepatitis serology, CMV, EBV
5. Donor anatomy: CTA/MRA ± angiography (?multiple renal arteries)
6. Informed consent
7. Donor nephrectomy: laparoscopic techniques (→ less invasive, smaller scar, ↓ hospital stay, more appealing to donors) increasingly popular
8. Donors should be followed up (and outcome data collected).

Absolute and relative contraindications to live donation

- Age <18 or >75 years
- Hypertension (BP >140/90 or on antihypertensive medication)
  - Donation may still be possible if BP is well controlled and estimates of overall CV risk are low.
- BMI >30–35 kg/m^2
- Type 2 DM, abnormal glucose tolerance, previous gestational DM
- Malignancy
- Other significant comorbidity
- Microalbuminuria or overt proteinuria
- Recurrent renal stone disease
- Other significant renal disease
  - Microscopic hematuria: donation may still be possible (need urology workup [p. 20] and renal biopsy)
- ↓GFR (<70 mL/min, though some age-related flexibility)
- Transmissible infection (HIV, hepatitis)

Pretransplant management

Types of donors

Cadaveric (CAD) This is the most common form of transplant in the United States. Organs are retrieved from donors certified as brainstem dead. After consent (either as an advance directive from a donor, or from the family) is confirmed, organs are perfused and harvested, and cold-stored for transport.

An organ distribution network (UNOS) is required that selects potential recipients from differing centers according to tissue type. Kidneys are allocated locally, then regionally, and then nationally. The best immunological match is usually offered the kidney. The kidney is then transported from harvesting to transplanting center. However, there is a significant and growing organ shortfall: the transplant waiting list is increasing rather than decreasing, and waits for organs are lengthening.

Non-heart beating (NHB) Organs are retrieved following circulatory arrest. The inevitable delay between circulatory arrest and perfusion results in a period of warm ischemia (p. 250). Delayed graft function is common and long-term graft survival may be shorter.

Living donors (LD) (p. 254) This is the most common donor type in many countries. The donor may be related or unrelated, though there is generally an established emotional relationship between the pair (spouse or good friend). Altruistic ("good Samaritan") donation refers to the allocation of a live donor kidney to an appropriate patient on the cadaveric waiting list (with donor–recipient anonymity). ☞ The purchase of organs is illegal.

Before surgery

- NPO with insulin sliding scale if patient is diabetic
- Document full donor details, including the following:
  - Age, gender, and cause of death
  - Associated comorbidity and complications
  - Hemodynamic stability
  - Renal function (Cr) at harvesting ("perfusion")
  - Whether L or R kidney, and any anatomical anomalies or surgical damage
- Full history and examination of potential recipient, including the following:
  - Any recent ill health
  - Current effort tolerance, and date of last cardiac assessment
  - Quality of peripheral (groin and distal) pulses
  - Any thrombotic events or risk
  - Estimate native UO

- Document tissue type and mismatch
- CMV status of donor and recipient (p. 262)
- Discuss the surgery with the patient
- Plan immunosuppression:
  - Stratify risk (immunological, and nonimmunological, p. 264).
  - Document current and historical PRA (p. 264).
  - Prescribe immunosuppression to local protocols.
- Ensure that the patient is adequately dialysed preoperatively (and limit anticoagulation if on hemodialysis).

The transplant operation

Cadaveric donor issues
Meticulous management of brain-dead potential donors is critical for the viability of harvested organs. Important issues:
- Respiratory: adequate ventilatory support and treatment (often prophylactic) of infection
- Hemodynamic: volume resuscitation ±inotropes/pressor agents
- Endocrine: Diabetes insipidus (↓vasopressin secretion), adrenal insufficiency, and thyroid dysfunction are all common (an empirical cocktail of steroids, vasopressin, and tri-iodothyronine is often administered).

Retrieval
- Takes place in operating room. Several retrieval teams (heart–lung, liver, renal) are often present.
- Both kidneys are harvested, with each (usually) sent to a different center.
- Along with the kidney, the renal artery (on a cuff of aorta), the renal veins (with a cuff of IVC), and the ureter (with periureteral tissue) are removed.
- The kidneys are perfused with a physiological solution (e.g., Marshall's or University of Wisconsin) and placed on ice for transport.

Warm ischemic time: period between circulatory arrest and start of cold storage (should be close to zero).

Cold ischemic time: period of cold storage before transplantation.

Recipient operation
- The kidney is examined "on the bench," with particular attention paid to the arterial anatomy (accessory arteries cannot be sacrificed as there is no collateral supply).
- Graft implantation is heterotopic, usually into the right iliac fossa.
- Native kidneys are not removed.
- Vascular anastamoses are end-to-side to the iliac vessels (usually external iliac).
- An implantation biopsy may be taken (especially if donor is marginal).
- The ureter is joined to the recipient bladder. A submucosal tunnel or oversew of bladder muscle prevents reflux. A JJ stent is often placed (removed cystoscopically at ~12 weeks).
- A drain is usually left in the perirenal space.

Intraoperative CVP is maintained at >10 cmH$_2$O with saline (± albumin). Mannitol (or frusemide) is often given as the vascular clamps are released.

Post-transplant management

After surgery
▶ Talk to the surgeon and review the intraoperative notes: are there any technical or anesthetic complications? How was the BP and fluid balance in the operating room? Was induction immunosuppression given as prescribed? Is there immediate urine output?

Fluid balance
- CVP line (⚠ chest X-ray) and urinary catheter (→ protects the ureteric anastomosis; leave in situ for 3–5 days) are usual.
- Maintain accurate fluid input/output charts. Check daily weights.
- UO is a good indicator of adequate graft function (⚠ beware of confusion with residual renal function).
- Drain volumes: if excessive, send fluid for electrolytes and Cr to exclude urinary leak.
- There is minimal evidence for routine use of renal dopamine (📖 p. 122).
- Immediate transplant function may result in brisk diuresis. Nevertheless, significant fluid weight gain occurs.
- Keep volume replete with IV saline. Typical regimen:

CVP (cmH$_2$O)	IV fluid replacement
<5	UO + 100 mL
6–10	UO + 60 mL
11–15	UO + 30 mL
>16	UO only + reassess clinically

Analgesia
- Avoid NSAIDs.
- Patient-controlled analgesia (PCA) is favored (⚠ opiate accumulation, especially if patient is anuric).

Graft assessment
- Immediate (⚠ postoperative ↑K$^+$ especially if UO poor)
- Examine patient and ensure that blood supply to feet is good and symmetrical.
- Assess graft perfusion as soon as feasible:
  - DTPA/MAG-3 perfusion scan
  - Doppler US
  - ▶ This is particularly important with delayed graft function, or if there is an abrupt tail-off in UO, to exclude a vascular event. In those passing good quantities of urine and clearing biochemically, graft assessment is not as pressing.

- Daily U&E, CBC, LFT, bone
  - ↓ phosphate is often an early sign of tubular function and may precede a fall in Cr.
  - Expect a fall in Hb (blood loss, hemodilution).
- Daily blood glucose (steroids and calcineurin inhibitors [CNIs] may → hyperglycemia)
- Therapeutic levels: cyclosporin, tacrolimus, rapamycin
- Lymphocyte subsets in those receiving anti-T-cell antibody induction
- Protocol transplant biopsy? (some centers).

General measures
- NPO until advised by surgical team
- Chest physiotherapy
- DVT prophylaxis—TED stockings, LMW heparin
- Consider osteoporosis prophylaxis (steroid-induced bone loss occurs early—there is good evidence for beneficial effect of bisphosphonates):
  - IV pamidronate 1 mg/kg rounded up or down to 60 mg or 90 mg within 48 hours and repeated on 30 day
  - Oral weekly alendronate or risedronate
- CMV prophylaxis (p. 277), especially if CMV– recipient or CMV+ donor
- Pneumocystitis prophylaxis (co-trimoxazole 480 mg bid)
- ☞ Tuberculosis prophylaxis if previous infection or high-risk population—evidence is poor (isoniazid 100 mg od + pyridoxine 10 mg od)
- Nystatin lozenges for prophylaxis against oral candida while on high-dose corticosteroids.

Principles of recipient management

Early: discharge to 12 weeks
- See frequently (weekly).
- CBC, U/A, Cr, electrolytes, LFT
- ANY rise in creatinine needs further attention and perhaps investigation (p. 268).
- Immunosuppression—optimize levels: too low → rejection; too high → graft dysfunction (calcineurin inhibitors)
- If at risk for CMV infection (p. 276)—weekly CMV viral load
- BP, PCR, and urine culture
- Blood glucose (de novo post-transplant diabetes).

Intermediate: 3 months to 1 year
Less frequent clinic visits: weekly → biweekly → monthly. During this period the focus is on the following:
- Monitoring graft function (⚠ CNI toxicity, rejection, obstruction)
- Monitoring immunosuppression
- Surveillance for infections
- Modifying long-term CV risk (BP, lipids).

Late: beyond 1 year
Clinic visits monthly are eventually reduced to every 3–4 months. The main focus during this period is:
- Monitoring graft function (⚠ chronic allograft nephropathy)
- Cardiovascular health
- Skin malignancies
- Post-transplant lymphoproliferative disease (PTLD)
- Osteoporosis
- If applicable, managing complications of chronic graft dysfunction (anemia, calcium, phosphate and hyperparathyroidism, nutrition).

Immunosuppression

Calcineurin inhibitors: cyclosporin, tacrolimus (FK506)

These agents disrupt T-cell signal 1 (📖 p. 248). They have a narrow therapeutic window ∴ monitor levels (trough). They are available in oral and IV (one-third of oral dose) form. Toxicity:
- Renal vasoconstriction → ↓GFR
- Aggravate delayed graft function (📖 p. 268)
- Renal fibrosis and scarring (→CAN ● 📖 p. 272)
- ↑BP
- ↑K⁺, ↓Mg²⁺, ↑urate
- Thrombotic microangiopathy
- Post-transplant DM (especially tacrolimus)
- Cosmetic—virilization, hirsuitism, gum hypertrophy (especially cyclosporin)
- Others: ↑LFTs, dyslipidemia, coarse tremor.

⚠ Inducers (rifampicin, phenytoin) and inhibitors (erythromycin, fluconazole) of cytochrome P450 → altered drug levels → rejection or toxicity. Rapamycin should be used with caution with calcineurin inhibitors (↑ levels 2- to 3-fold).

Antiproliferatives

Rapamycin (sirolimus) inhibits TOR (target of rapamycin), a regulatory kinase involved in cytokine-dependent cell proliferation. It is given orally and has a long half-life (no IV preparation). Toxicity includes delayed graft function, myelosuppression, thrombotic microangiopathy, delayed wound healing, pneumonitis, and proteinuria.

Mycophenolate mofetil (MMF) is a prodrug; it is rapidly converted to active mycophenolic acid (MPA) to inhibit de novo purine nucleotide synthesis (→ ↑ lymphocyte proliferation). It is given po or IV. Toxicity includes nausea, bloating, diarrhea, mouth and esophageal ulceration, and myelosuppression. Both tacrolimus and rapamycin ↑ active MPA levels.

Azathioprine is metabolized to a purine analogue that competitively inhibits purine synthesis to ↓T-cell activation. It is given po and IV (half oral dose). Toxicity includes myelosuppression and hepatitis.
⚠ *Allopurinol* should be used with great caution with azathioprine. Consider transfer to MMF.

Corticosteroids inhibit cytokine-regulated lymphocyte signaling, and chemokine-driven lymphocyte homing to areas of inflammation. They are given po or IV. Toxicity includes DM, osteoporosis, and ↑BP. They are used to prevent and treat rejection.

Antibodies

- Monoclonal (OKT3) and polyclonal (ATG) antibody therapy directed against CD3 used to deplete T cells in high immunological risk patients in the peritransplant period (📖 p. 252) and to treat severe rejection. This therapy has a profound immunosuppressive effect.

- Monoclonal antibodies directed at CD25, the IL-2 receptor expressed on activated T cells (daclizumab, basiliximab). These prevent activation and clonal expansion. They are well tolerated and replace T-cell-depleting agents as induction therapy.
- IV immunoglobulin (IV Ig) is occasionally used to treat rejection and increasingly in desensitization regimens (p. 282).
- Alemtuzumab (Campath-1H® is a humanized anti-CD52 lymphocytic (both T and B cells) monoclonal antibody increasingly used in induction protocols. Administration may allow a reduction in maintenance immunosuppression, but long-term outlook data are awaited.

Dosing recommendations and target levels

- These are *not* absolute, and practice varies widely between centers.
- Cyclosporin (Neoral®): 7.5–10 mg/kg/day in two divided doses against trough levels. Depends on center, immunological risk, and nephrotoxicity. There are no absolutes; however, as guidance:
  - 150–200 ng/mL <3 months
  - 125–175 ng/mL 3–12 months
  - 75–150 ng/mL >12 months
- Tacrolimus (Prograf®): load as 0.15 mg/kg/day in two divided doses, aiming as guidance for:
  - 7–15 ng/mL <3 months
  - 5–10 ng/mL >3 months
- Azathioprine:
  - 1.5 mg/kg/day in single dose
- Mycophenolate mofetil:
  - CellCept® 1 g bid or 500 mg qid (↑1.5 g bid if high risk)
  - Myfortic® 720 mg bid
  - ↓ starting dose by 50% if on tacrolimus or sirolimus
  - Mycophenolate acid levels are measurable and can be useful as there is much interindividual variation in pharmacokinetics.
- Sirolimus (rapamycin, Rapamune®)
  - 6 mg daily ↓ to 2–4 mg of trough levels of 8–10 ng/mL

If converting po to IV, the cyclosporin and tacrolimus dose should be divided by 3 (i.e., 33% oral). Dose equivalence for MMF or azathioprine.

Biologicals
- Anti-CD25 antibodies:
  - Basiliximab 20 mg IV on day 0 and day 4
  - Daclizumab 1 mg/kg/dose IVI on day 0, and then for 1–4 further at 2-week interval doses
- Anti-thymocyte globulin (ATG) or OKT3 as per local protocol; they differ widely. Such agents are directed against CD3, and → profound T-cell depletion. They are usually given with hydrocortisone and chlorpheniramine to minimize side effects (fever, arthralgia, myalgia). Monitor lymphocyte subsets (number of CD3+ cells) for response to therapy.

Surgical complications

Early

Anastamotic leak
This presents abruptly after transplant as evolving hemorrhagic shock (hypotension, tachycardia, poor perfusion, oliguria and ↓Hb). Urgent reexploration is usually indicated.

Renal arterial and venous thrombosis or occlusion
This complication occurs in 0.5%–2% of transplants. Risk factors include:
- Complex vascular anastomoses
- Donor vascular disease
- Recipient thrombophilia (▶ polycythemia, anti-phospholipid antibodies)
- Recipient sickle cell disease (→ pretransplant exchange transfusion to ↓sickle Hb + graft warmed prior to reperfusion).

Symptoms present (usually) within the first week. Suspect thrombosis/occlusion if there is sudden ↓UO, macroscopic hematuria, pain (often severe), graft tenderness, or swelling.

Investigations include urgent Doppler US and isotope perfusion scan.

Management is with surgical exploration (disappointingly, this is rarely successful).

Urinary leak
This may occur (in 1%–3%) anywhere along the transplant urinary tract, but most commonly at the fresh vesicoureteric anastamosis. It may occur as a complication of transplant biopsy.

It is often silent, but may be painful (as the collection of irritant urine expands) ± scrotal/labial swelling. UO may taper off, or drain sites drain (or leak) ↑ volumes of fluid.

Investigation includes ↑ serum Cr (resorbed urinary creatinine) and biochemical analysis of fluid (which will differentiate the collection from a lymphocele, which resembles serum).

Management: Isotope scanning will prove urinary extravasation. Catheterize the bladder. Generally reimplantation is required (though short-term drainage may offer benefits in distal leaks).

Lymphocele
Graft implantation interrupts the pelvic lymphatics. This may result in a collection of lymph around the transplant (~10% of transplants).
- Usually small and uncomplicated
- May become large enough to obstruct the kidney or iliac veins
- May become secondarily infected
- May cause DVT
- More common in those treated with sirolimus
- Diagnosis is by US.

Indications for drainage include discomfort, obstruction, or infection. Drainage is usually carried out percutaneously. Recurrent lymphoceles may need surgical intraperitoneal "marsupialization" for long-term drainage.

Wound infection
Contributing factors include uremia, corticosteroid use, sirolimus use, diabetes, and obesity. Causative organisms are usually gram positive.

Late

Renal artery stenosis
Transplant renal artery stenosis may occur early with a poor anastamosis, or later with atheromatous buildup at the origin of the transplant renal artery.

Patients present with ↓GFR, poor BP control, salt and water retention ± ACEI-related transplant dysfunction. Suspect stenosis with progressive transplant dysfunction and worsening scarring on biopsy in the right clinical setting.

Investigation includes Doppler US, angiography (± angioplasty and stenting).

Ureteric stenosis
This occurs in 1%–5% of transplants. It arises in the distal ureter, usually including the vesicoureteric anastomosis. Causes include:
- Marginal blood supply (which is common, the ureter is supplied from some distance by the transplant renal artery, ∴ ↓ blood supply → ureteric ischemia and fibrosis).
- BK virus (📖 p. 278) is increasingly recognized as an important cause.
- There are rarely secondary urothelial tumors.

Investigation: US will show a hydronephrosis and allows placement of a nephrostomy to decompress the system. Once placed, antegrade examination with contrast can be performed.

Management includes ureteroplasty, JJ stenting, and surgical reimplantation. Occasionally a native ureter is mobilized and anastomosed to transplant pelvis as surgical reconstruction.

Bladder dysfunction
Transplantation may reveal bladder outflow obstruction, or bladder nerve, or muscle failure. Examine for a palpable bladder, consider urodynamic studies, and arrange for pre- and postmicturition US of the bladder.

Graft dysfunction

Classification
- Delayed graft function occurs in the immediate post-transplant period. It is unusual with living donors, but is affects ~30% of cadaveric grafts.
  - Of these, 50% will recover by day 10.
  - 33% will recover between days 10 and 20.
  - 10%–15% will recover after this
  - 2%–15% will not function: primary non-function
- Early graft dysfunction is in the first 3 months post-transplant.
- Late graft dysfunction is after 3 months.

Delayed graft function (DGF)
- Definition:
  - Need for more than one post-transplant dialysis
- Importance:
  - Affects long-term graft survival
  - Associated with acute rejection
- Usually ATN occurs histologically (📖 p. 100), as hyperacute rejection is rare in the contemporary immunosuppressant era. Once early surgical complications have been excluded (📖 p. 266), the differential includes the following:
  - ATN
  - Early rejection
  - Thrombotic microangiopathy
  - Recurrent glomerulonephritis (▶ FSGS)
- Investigations include U/A, electrolytes Bun/creatinine, Hb, Plt count, blood film, and LDH, as well as drug levels. Check donor-specific antibodies. Isotope perfusion scan, US → transplant biopsy (usually on day 3–5 if there is a high immunological risk or day 7 if not).
- Management depends on the cause.

Table 4.3 Risk factors for delayed graft function

Donor	Recipient
Non-heart-beating donor	Black race
Inadequate perfusion/cold storage	Vascular disease
Long cold ischemia time (>24 h)	Intraop/postop ↓BP
Preharvest ATN	Highly sensitized (PRA >50)
↑BP, vascular disease	Calcineurin inhibitors
Older donor (>55)	
Marginal donors[1]	

1 Marginal donors include those with ↑BP or diabetes.

Calcineurin inhibitors and early ATN

Only reduce the dose if consistent with clinical findings—otherwise repeat it. If cyclosporin or tacrolimus trough levels are beyond target, suggest the following:
- Reduce by 10%–25% total daily dose.
- If there is ongoing DGF, biopsy to exclude other causes.

Early graft dysfunction
- Initial graft function, but ↑Cr within the first 3 months
- Major causes:
  - ▶ acute rejection (p. 270)
  - CNI nephrotoxicity
  - Thrombotic microangiopathy
  - Obstruction
  - Recurrent disease (?proteinuria, nephritic urine sediment)
  - Infection (p. 274)
- Investigation: US, drug levels, transplant biopsy.

Late graft dysfunction
- Pre- and postrenal causes must be excluded.
- Chronic allograft nephropathy and recurrent disease (p. 272).

Thrombotic microangiopathy

- Associated with both cyclosporin and tacrolimus
- Pathogenesis is unclear, but involves direct endothelial toxicity, ↓prostacyclin synthesis, vasoconstriction, platelet aggregation, and thrombosis.
- May occur <1 week to >5 years
- Often this is an unexpected finding on transplant biopsy following ↑Cr.
- Occasionally there is ↓Plt, red cell fragmentation, and ↑LDH.
- Exclude antiphospholipid syndrome and CMV disease.

Optimum management is unclear: ↓ or stop CNI. Conversion to rapamycin *may* be desirable. Plasma exchange is uncertain.

Acute rejection

▶ Treat suspected rejection immediately.

Introduction
Acute rejection is defined as a sudden deterioration in graft function associated with specific immunopathological changes as categorized according to histological criteria (▶ Banff classification, Table 4.4).
- Modern immunosuppressive regimes have reduced the incidence of early acute rejection to 10%–20%.
- <10% of patients experience rejection after 1 year (often associated with noncompliance).
- Kidneys that recover still have a 10% ↓ in 1-year survival. Rejection also has a negative impact on long-term graft survival.
- Classical presentation of fever, painful graft, and oligoanuria is now rare. Acute rejection usually presents with asymptomatic ↑Cr.

Hyperacute rejection
This is virtually eradicated by ABO- and cross-matching. Circulating preformed, donor-specific anti-class I HLA antibodies bind to endothelial cells, activating complement and clotting cascades → vascular thrombosis within 3 days of transplant. Graft loss is inevitable.

Acute cell-mediated rejection
- This is the most common form of rejection (~90%).
- Typically it occurs 1–12 weeks post-transplantation.
- It is asymptomatic—there may be fever, graft tenderness, and ↓UO.
- Histologically, tubulointerstitial and vascular infiltration cause distinguished (prognostic) implications:
  - Cellular: a mature lymphocytic (but usually not neutrophilic) infiltrate of the parenchyma, with interstitial edema. Tubular architecture may be disrupted and infiltrated by lymphocytes (tubulitis).
  - Vascular: ± above findings, lymphocytic infiltration is under the arterial endothelium, with endothelial cell injury (± stromal hemorrhage).
- First-line treatment consists of IV methylprednisolone (0.5 or 1 g/day IVI in 100 mL 0.9% NaCl for 3 days).
- Maintenance immunosuppression should be increased, ± switched to more potent agents.
- Response is expected within 5 days, with a ± 75% response rate.
- If refractory or severe (→ vascular involvement), use ATG, or OKT3.

Humoral or antibody-mediated rejection

This type of rejection occurs within 1–3 weeks. Anti-HLA antibodies fix complement within the graft → endothelial injury. It may also occur as a late event.

- It may contribute in part to ~4%–20% of all acute rejection.
- Histology:
  - Neutrophils marginating in peritubular capillaries, arterial inflammation → fibrinoid necrosis of arterioles
  - C4d is diagnostic (a complement degradation product derived from classical pathway activation); stains positive in peritubular capillaries.
- Measure circulating donor-specific anti-HLA antibodies (DSA) by ELISA. Positive titers are highly suggestive in the right clinical context.
- Treatment is controversial:
  - Plasma exchange (remove anti-donor antibodies) and IV Ig (anti-idiotypic effect) is increasingly reported as successful.
  - Many still advocate anti-CD3 antibodies if there is concurrent cell-mediated rejection (as is often the case).
  - Some recommend rituximab (anti-CD20 antibody).
- There is a high risk of graft loss (~40%) if patient is C4d positive.

The revised Banff criteria

Rejection is usually classified by the Banff criteria (Table 4.4).

Table 4.4 Banff criteria

Borderline		↑ Immunosuppression
IA	Moderate tubulitis (>4 MC in >25% of sample)	Optimize immunosuppression levels
IB	Severe tubulitis (>10 MC in >25% of sample)	Switch to more potent drug (→ Tacro, MMF, sirolimus) Pulse corticosteroids If unresponsive, consider anti-T-cell therapy
IIA	Mild → moderate arteritis in one or more vessel	
IIB	Severe arteritis (>25% ↓ in luminal area)	
III	Transmural arteritis with fibrinoid necrosis and perivascular inflammation	Switch to tacrolimus Anti-T-cell therapy
Antibody-mediated		Switch to tacrolimus Anti-lymphocyte therapy Consider IV immunoglobulin ± plasma exchange Rituximab

MC, mononuclear cells.

Chronic allograft nephropathy (CAN)

Both immunological and nonimmunological factors play a role in graft dysfunction and loss beyond the first 3 months (Table 4.5). CAN is a histological term used to describe the appearances found with progressively declining graft function. At 2 years post-transplant, 70%–90% of grafts will show features of CAN.

Histology

Characteristic histological changes include focal tubular atrophy, interstitial fibrosis, and arterial narrowing. Some have tried to distinguish CNI toxicity from rejection (in practice this is often difficult).

- Rejection is more likely (under-immunosuppressed):
  - Cellular infiltrates → subclinical rejection (i.e., unchanged Cr).
  - There is presence of a chronic transplant glomerulopathy (capillary wall double contours, mesangial widening, mesangiolysis, secondary FSGS).
  - C4d staining ± donor-specific antibodies
- CNI toxicity is more likely (overexposure to CNI) with the following:
  - Nodular hyalinosis within arterial walls
  - Stripe fibrosis

Clinically

Usually, deteriorating eGFR (months → years) is accompanied by ↑BP and proteinuria. It is analogous to CKD in native kidneys.

Prevention and treatment

- The optimal treatment remains unclear. Data from centers performing protocol biopsies suggest that subclinical rejection is a frequent early finding and predicts subsequent CAN. ☞ This in turn suggests that using more potent early immunosuppression may limit the development of CAN; however, this result may come at the price of more infection and malignancies.
- CNI toxicity should be remediable, by one of the following:
  - CNI avoidance immunosuppression
  - Early CNI withdrawal.

Table 4.5 Contributors to chronic graft failure

Alloantigen dependent	Alloantigen independent
▶ Chronic rejection	▶ CNI toxicity
• Poor HLA matching	• Delayed graft function
• Prior sensitization	• Prolonged cold ischemia
• Donor specific antibodies	• Reduced nephron number
• Inadequate immunosuppression	• ↑Donor age, ↑BP, ↑lipids
	• CMV disease, BK nephropathy

- MMF may have antifibrotic effects independent of immunosuppression. Regimes using low or no CNI and MMF may offer advantages.
- Similarly for sirolimus, treat with CNI avoidance or early withdrawal.
- ☞ Use of MMF or sirolimus may slow progression of CAN (i.e., treatment and not just prevention).
- Control BP with ACEI ± ARB.
- Treat hyperlipidemia.

Recurrent and de novo glomerulonephritis (GN)

Recurrence of original disease following transplantation affects ~10%–20% of patients and accounts for up to 8% of graft failures at 10 years.

	Recurrence rate	Graft loss
Primary FSGS	~40%	>50%
IgAN	~40%	~20%
Membranous	<10%	~25%
MCGN I	~20%	~33%
MCGN II	>90%	~30%
Diabetic nephropathy	~100%	<5%

MCGN I, II: mesangiocapillary glomerulonephritis type I, type II.

- Primary FSGS may recur within days of transplantation, with torrential nephrotic syndrome and graft dysfunction (from ATN). Plasma exchange has been used with variable success.
- The most common de novo form of GN post-transplant is membranous nephropathy.

Transplanted Alport's patients may rarely develop de novo anti-GBM antibodies and a rapidly progressive crescentic glomerulonephritis as donor α5 type IV collagen is recognized as non-self.

Post-transplant infections

Transplant recipients are immunosuppressed and, as such, susceptible to a wide variety of infectious pathogens (Fig. 4.9). Generally, the aim is to prevent predictable infections (that occur at often predictable times post-transplant) if possible. Such strategies might include the following:
- Perioperative broad-spectrum antibiotics
- Co-trimoxazole (*Pneumocystis carinii* pneumonia [PCP], UTI)
- ❦ Isoniazid (TB in high-risk recipients)
- Valganciclovir/ganciclovir (CMV in at-risk recipients).

Timing of infection

Infections in the first month
- Standard postoperative infections are related to the procedure itself—see surgical complications (📖 p. 266).
- Urinary tract infection is common. Anuric dialysis patients often have small-capacity dysfunctional bladders, and in-dwelling urinary catheters or ureteric stents contribute further. If a UTI is recurrent, get US transplant + bladder pre- and post-micturition. A plain abdominal X-ray may detect a retained stent or calculi (transplant or native kidneys).
- Other bacterial infections include chest, wound, and lymphocele infections, *C. difficile*.
- Donor → recipient bacterial infections (usually *S. aureus* or gram- negative organisms).

1 to 6 months
- Viral infections: cytomegalovirus (CMV), herpes simplex virus (HSV), shingles, Epstein–Barr virus (EBV)
- Opportunistic infections: *Listeria, Aspergillus, Pnemocystis carinii*.

Beyond 6 months
- Chronic viral infection: BK nephropathy, EBV-driven PTLD.

General management issues

▶ When treating these infections
- Use dose reductions for GFR: watch Cr carefully.
- Look for drug interactions, particularly antimicrobials that may induce or inhibit cytochrome P450 and thus modify immunosuppressant levels; watch CNI trough levels carefully.

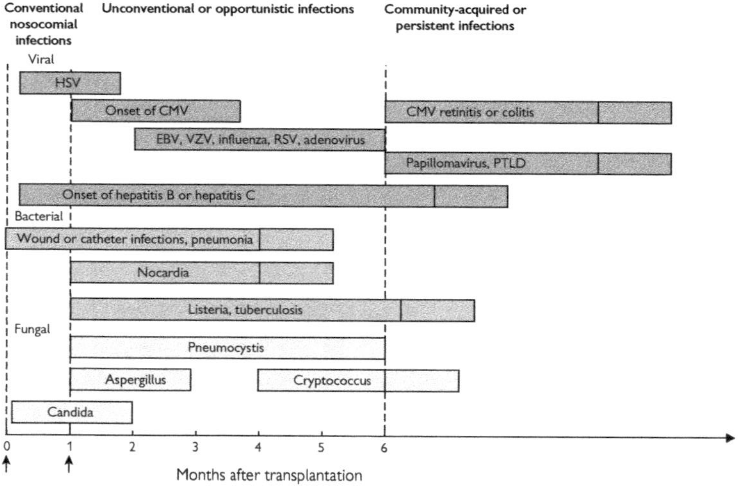

Fig. 4.9 Sequence of post-transplant infection. Adapted with permission from Davidson AMA, Cameron JS, Grunfeld J-P, et al. (eds.) (2005). *Oxford Textbook of Clinical Nephrology*, 3rd ed. Oxford University Press.

Cytomegalovirus (CMV)

▶ CMV is the most important infectious complication of renal transplantation.

CMV is a DNA (herpes type) virus that infects about 40%–50% of the normal population. Previous exposure is reflected by anti-CMV IgG positivity (measured routinely in all donors and recipients: CMV-naïve patients who receive a kidney from a CMV-positive donor are most at risk) (see Table 4.6).

Clinical features
- Can be asymptomatic (CMV viremia)
- Fever, malaise, neutropenia, ↓Plt (CMV disease)
- Hepatitis, pancreatitis, pneumonitis, chorioretinitis, invasive GI disease (esophagitis, gastritis, colitis, perforations), graft dysfunction (tissue invasive disease)
- Usually occurs 1–4 months post-transplant
- △ CMV causes further host immunosuppression (predisposing to secondary invasion—PCP and fungi).
- ☙ CMV may be a risk factor for rejection.
- Detection is by polymerase chain reaction (PCR) for viral DNA:
  - Quantitative PCR >500 copies/mL implies viremia (laboratory assays vary).
  - Most will be symptomatic >3000 copies/mL.
- Cytopathic viral inclusions may also be identified on tissue samples (colon, kidney, esophagus, etc.).

Treatment
- If there is tissue-invasive disease use IV ganciclovir for 10–14 days. If WCC is low, stop MMF or azathioprine. Relapses are not infrequent. Dose as follows:
  - eGFR >70   5 mg/kg bid
  - eGFR 50–69   2.5 mg/kg bid
  - eGFR 25–49   2.5 mg/kg daily
  - eGFR 10–24   1.25 mg/kg daily
  - eGFR <10, dialysis 1.25 mg/kg 3/week (after HD)
- An alternative, particularly if there is viremia without tissue-invasive disease, is to use oral valganciclovir:
  - eGFR >60   900 mg od
  - eGFR 40–59   450 mg od
  - eGFR 25–39   450 mg alternate days
  - eGFR 10–24   450 mg twice weekly
  - eGFR <10, dialysis Use IVI ganciclovir
- Monitor quantitative CMV PCR weekly.

Prophylaxis

There are two strategies:
- Universal prophylaxis for all "at-risk" patients immediately post-transplant
- Preemptive therapy—quantitative PCR is used for surveillance to detect early disease.

If detected, consider reduction in immunosuppression. Valganciclovir (dose as above) is used for effective prophylaxis in the post-transplant period (for 6 months).

Table 4.6 Risk of CMV according to serological status

Donor CMV status	Recipient CMV status	Risk
Negative	Negative	Low
Positive	Negative	High
Negative	Positive	Medium
Positive	Positive	Medium
Either donor and/or recipient CMV positive and treatment with ATG/OKT3		High

BK virus nephropathy

This disease is also known as polyoma virus–associated nephropathy. BK virus is a polyoma virus (with a prevalence of ~70% in adults) recently recognized as a significant pathogen in renal transplantation. First described in the late 1990s, allograft disease secondary to infection with BK species affects between 3% and 5% of transplant recipients. The virus achieves latency in tubular cells, and infection may → graft failure (although most cases are asymptomatic). BK virus nephropathy appears to be related to the intensity of immunosuppression.

Clinically
BK virus nephropathy presents as follows:
- Sterile pyuria ± hematuria
- ↑Cr secondary to lymphocytic infiltration of the allograft (⚠ difficult to distinguish from cellular rejection)
- Ureteric ulceration or stenosis → strictures, transplant hydronephrosis
- Hemorrhagic cystitis.

Diagnosis
Urine cytology: Infected tubular cells are shed into the urine—so-called decoy cells are present in 90% of infected patients (>10 decoy cells/hpf is suggestive of disease). Blood PCR for BKV is the most specific technique available, though not necessarily an indication to treat—*a renal biopsy is required*.

▶ The characteristic finding is a tubulointerstitial nephritis with mononuclear cell infiltrates, and viral inclusion in tubular cells. Confirm BK virus using immunohistochemistry (see Fig. 4.10).

Treatment
- It is unsatisfactory, and many will lose their grafts.
- Generally, aim for reduction of immunosuppression.
- There is no clear evidence for the use of antivirals, but cidofovir 0.25–1 mg/kg/dose (every 2 weeks) for 1–4 doses may be of benefit. Cidofovir is nephrotoxic.

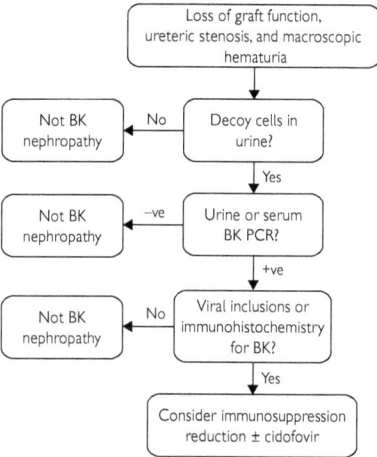

Fig. 4.10 BK virus investigation and treatment algorithm.

Post-transplant malignancy

Skin

Approximately 50% of transplant recipients 20 years post-transplant have (or have had) a skin cancer, usually squamous cell carcinomas (SCC) but also basal cell carcinomas. Skin type, human papilloma virus, and sun exposure appear to be risk factors for the development of SCC.

▶ Advocate sun protection at all times, and seek regular skin review. Kaposi sarcoma occurs more frequently in recipients from endemic areas, with human herpes virus 8 implicated.

Post-transplant lymphoproliferative disorders (PTLDs)

The PTLDs include the following:
- Non-Hodgkin's lymphomas (90%), of recipient B-cell origin
- Myeloma (4%)
- Hodgkin's disease (2.5%)

PTLD occurs in 1%–5% of renal transplant recipients, occurring more frequently in those more heavily immunosuppressed. Diagnosis occurs at two peaks: 12–18 months post-transplant, and then again at >5 years out. Primary infection with EBV infection is often implicated—EBV becomes immortalized in B cells, and may → unregulated proliferation and resistance to apoptosis.

▶ Primary EBV infection after transplantation ↑ risk for PTLD by 10- to 76-fold. Early PTLD tends to be EBV positive and later PTLD less so. Presentation is variable, ranging from a viral-type illness to specific evidence of organ dysfunction:
- PTLD occurs in unusual sites and is often extranodal.
- Fever is common, as is malaise.
- The transplant itself may be infiltrated.
- GI: pain, bleeding, diarrhea, obstruction
- Hepatitis, meningeal involvement, retroperitoneal disease
- There may be ↑ lymphocyte count and LDH.

There is a strong correlation between histological appearance and the response to treatment: polyclonal polymorphic types respond to treatment much better than monotypic monoclonal PTLD.

With EBV-positive B-cell PTLD, patients may respond to gradual reduction of immunosuppression without the need for chemotherapy. This process can be tailored by measuring EBV-specific T-cell subsets (their appearance with reduction of immunosuppression may herald regression of tumor). ☞ From this observation, there is now interest in infusing EBV-directed cytotoxic T lymphocytes (CTL) as treatment for PTLD. Rituximab is being used in tumors that express CD20.

Cervical and vulval carcinoma
Post-transplant ♀ are more likely to develop these, and should be screened regularly using cervical smear screening and examination.

Solid tumors
There is a slight ↑ risk of many solid tumors in transplant recipients, but specific screening programs for recipients are not merited. Tumors of the native kidneys or anogenital region are much more common in the transplant than the general population.

Expanding the donor pool

Sensitized patients (those with preformed antibodies against a variety of common antigens) may wait for prolonged periods to be offered a well-matched cadaveric transplant, and may find living donation contraindicated by a positive cross-match. As a result, there has been a resurgence of interest in anti-HLA antibody removal prior to transplantation and in other schemes that may increase the number of available organs.

Transplanting across a positive cross-match

Once a suitable living donor is identified, the aim is to remove antibodies prior to transplant:
- Plasma exchange removes circulating antibodies (including anti-HLA).
  - Antibody removal is often a temporary phenomenon.
  - Transplantation occurs once a recipient is "anti-donor antibody" negative.
- IV immunoglobulin has a more sustained effect on antibody levels.
  - It may be used successfully on patients waiting for a cadaveric transplant.
  - High-dose IV Ig is given against serial DSA (p. 253).
  - The mechanism of action is not fully elucidated. It probably involves anti-idiotype along with immunomodulatory type actions.
- Patients receiving such treatments are at ↑ risk of humoral rejection post-transplant (p. 270).

Transplanting across blood groups

Blood group O individuals are universal donors and AB universal recipients. Until fairly recently, transplantation was only carried out in blood group–matched pairs or according to "transfusion rules." This is no longer the case. Blood group A patients can be grouped as A1 and A2: those with A2 express much lower amounts of A antigen on cell surfaces and can be considered blood group O if the recipients have no or low levels of circulating anti-A antibodies. Anti-blood group antibody removal is also being increasingly performed. Using techniques such as plasma exchange or immunoabsorption, these antibodies can be removed prior to transplantation. Again, rejection rates are higher.

Live donor exchange schemes

Such schemes are gaining in popularity: if a patient has a live donor, but for ABO or immunological reasons the transplant cannot go ahead, donors and recipients agree to swap pairs (see Fig. 4.11). Donor nephrectomies are carried out simultaneously to prevent a particular donor from backing out after their relative has received a kidney.

Xenotransplantation

Research continues in this area. Natural antibodies responsible for hyperacute rejection have been identified. Concern remains regarding the possible transmission of viral pathogens to humans.

Example of live donor exchange scheme

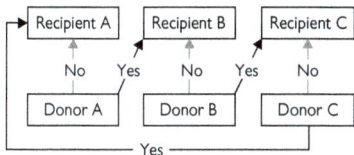

Fig. 4.11 Donor A is unable to donate to recipient A for immunological reasons. The same is true of the pairs B and C. Using an exchange scheme, donor A donates to recipient B, donor B to recipient C, and donor C to recipient A.

Kidney–pancreas transplantation

Transplantation is the treatment of choice for diabetic patients with ESRD. In addition to kidney transplantation alone, options are:
- Combined kidney–pancreas transplantation (80%)
- Pancreas (cadaveric) after kidney (living donor) transplantation (20%)
- Islet cell transplantation (see Box 4.3).

Benefits
- Pancreas transplantation corrects the glycemic state (HbA1c falls to normal), leading to improved quality of life (freedom from both insulin and dialysis).
- Prevention of progression of diabetic complications (and possibly partial reversal ●→)
- Beneficial effect on lipids
- Survival is comparable to that for live kidney transplant alone.

Selection criteria
- Type 1 DM with stage 5 CKD
- Age <50 years (usually)
- Sufficient CV reserve (ejection fraction >50%, no uncorrected IHD)
- Established diabetic complications.

Surgical technique
There are two options:
- Bladder drainage. The kidney is transplanted into the left iliac fossa and exocrine secretions of the pancreas routed into the bladder via a duodenal cystotomy. Metabolic complications include:
  - Acidosis (HCO_3 depletion) and Na^+ loss (→ relative hypotension requires sodium bicarbonate administration (e.g., 2 g qid)
  - Calcium bladder stones (alkaline urine)
  - Chemical cystitis/urethritis
  - Reflux pancreatitis
- Enteric drainage: Exocrine secretions drains into bowel. This results in fewer metabolic complications and is now generally preferred.
- Pancreatic venous drainage; two options:
  - Into systemic circulation (→ no first-pass metabolism ∴ hyperinsulinemia → ? ↑ risk of atherosclerosis)
  - Into portal circulation (more physiological, no hyperinsulinemia).
- Immunosuppression. Steroids, tacrolimus, and MMF
- Rejection rates are low and can be detected by renal dysfunction (and biopsy of the renal allograft).
- There is more morbidity in the first year (length of hospital stay doubles compared to that for kidney transplant alone).
- There is a 20%–30% chance of laparotomy during the post-transplant period.
- Fungal infection is more common than after kidney transplant alone.
- There is 85% and 70% 1- and 5-year pancreas survival after simultaneous pancreas–kidney tranplantation (higher kidney survival).
- Post-transplant hyperglycemia is caused by graft dysfunction, de novo type 2 DM (steroids), and recurrent autoimmune injury.

Box 4.3 Barriers to successful islet cell transplantation

Islet cell transplantation shows promise, but early excellent results have proved difficult to sustain. Reasons for this include:
- Immune-mediated destruction (highly immunogenic)
- Insufficient islet cell mass (more than one donor needed)
- Drug toxicity (CNIs and steroids are toxic to islet cells)
- Recurrent transplantation is often necessary.

Chapter 5

Hypertension

Hypertension facts and figures 288
What is hypertension? 290
Pathogenesis 292
BP measurement 298
Clinical assessment 300
Classification of hypertension 302
Treatment thresholds 304
Lifestyle measures 306
Secondary hypertension 308
Primary hyperaldosteronism 310
Specific causes of hyperaldosteronism 312
Other "hyperaldosteronism" syndromes 314
Other causes of secondary hypertension 316
Drug management of hypertension 318
Drug treatment of hypertension 320
Clinical trials in hypertension 324
The ASCOT study 330
Diuretics 332
β-blockers 336
α-blockers 338
Calcium channel blockers (CCBs) 340
ACE inhibitors (ACEIs) 342
Angiotensin II receptor blockers (ARBs) 344
Other antihypertensives 346
Resistant hypertension 348
Hypertensive urgencies and emergencies 350
Assessing urgencies and emergencies 352
Management of urgencies and emergencies 354
Orthostatic hypotension 356

Hypertension facts and figures

Epidemiology

The World Health Organization (WHO) identifies hypertension as the *single most important* preventable cause of premature death in developed countries. It is the most common indication for prescription drug therapy.

- NHANES data from 1999 to 2000 indicate an incidence of 29%–31% in the 18-year and older population
- Approximately one-third of those in middle age and two-thirds in old age are hypertensive.
- It occurs in association with other CV risk factors rather than isolation.
- Significant underdiagnosis and treatment remain common. The *"rule of halves"*:
  - Half of those with ↑BP have not been diagnosed.
  - Half of those who have been diagnosed are not on treatment.
  - Half of those receiving treatment do not have adequate control.

Classifying hypertension

Essential hypertension is a heterogeneous genetic and environmental condition.

Secondary hypertension implies ↑BP is secondary to an underlying disorder. It accounts for ~5%–10% of cases (📖 p. 308).

Hypertension facts and figures

- Systolic blood pressure (SBP) ↑ with age until the eighth decade.
- Diastolic blood pressure (DBP) ↑ up to age 50, after which it stabilizes or ↓ slightly.
- DBP is the best indicator of CV risk <50 years of age. With ↑ age there is a shift to SBP (then pulse pressure) as the principal predictor.
- Reduction in SBP of 20 mmHg systolic or DBP of 10 mmHg is associated with reductions in death from stroke and IHD of ~50% (slightly more in younger patients, slightly less in older ones). This is consistent down to 115/75—there is no clear threshold below which further reduction in BP is no longer beneficial.
- Nonpharmacological strategies (i.e., lifestyle measures) have been shown to ↓BP.
- Antihypertensive drug treatment not only ↓BP, but also ↓complications.
- Patient education is paramount: ↑BP is an asymptomatic condition and benefits of treatment may not be immediately apparent to the patient.

Major cardiovascular risk factors

- Hypertension*
- Smoking
- Obesity (BMI ≥30)*
- Physical inactivity
- Dyslipidemia*
- Diabetes mellitus (DM)*
- Albuminuria or GFR <60 mL/min
- Age (♂ >55 years, ♀>65 years)
- Family history of premature CV disease (♂ <55 years, ♀<65 years)

* Components of the metabolic syndrome.

Target organ damage (TOD)

- Heart: LVH, IHD, LV dysfunction, and CHF
- Brain: stroke, transient ischemic attack (TIA), and vascular dementia
- Chronic kidney disease
- Peripheral arterial disease
- Retinopathy.

SBP, pulse pressure, and CV risk

SBP
- Historically DBP was thought to be the best predictor of CV disease.
- Now it is clear that SBP has a continuous independent relationship with stroke and IHD risk.
- It can be difficult to get SBP to target, particularly in the elderly.

Pulse pressure (PP) and risk
- A wide PP (SBP minus DBP) more accurately predicts adverse CV outcome than SBP or DBP.
- PP appears to be a marker of arterial stiffness.
- PP may identify those with SBP at particular risk.
- The majority of trial data is for SBP and DBP, so the major guidelines are based on these rather than PP.

What is hypertension?

BP variation in a population follows a normal distribution, so an arbitrary cutoff point defines abnormal (Fig. 5.1). Normal BP varies among races, the sexes, with age, and even throughout the day. Even if an arbitrary definition of ↑BP could be agreed upon, it would differ depending on the population studied.

Important prognostic differences in systolic vs. diastolic hypertension have only recently been recognized, with systolic pressure (and partial pressure) now thought to be more important in predicting risk.

Perhaps the most useful definition, then, is the following:
Hypertension is a level of blood pressure that places an individual at increased risk of cardiovascular events.

▶ An individual whose BP is just below that cutoff has a virtually identical CV risk to that of an individual whose cutoff is just above it.

The great apes do not get hypertension, nor do present-day hunter-gatherer populations (with a similar diet and lifestyle to that of our ancestors). There is something about our *environment* and *diet* that predisposes to hypertension. Genes and genetics are relevant, but insufficient in isolation.

Important principles in pathophysiology

BP = cardiac output (CO) × systemic vascular resistance (SVR)

The final common pathway in chronic hypertension is increased SVR. The earliest event in the development of hypertension is usually a rise in CO. Increased CO causes an increase in wall/lumen ratio in resistance vessels (to normalize wall stress). This leads to a sustained rise in SVR, and causes chronic hypertension. Cardiac output is usually *normal* in those with *established* hypertension.

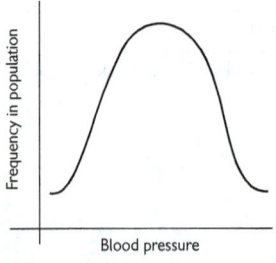

Fig. 5.1 Distribution of BP in any population: the cutoff for defining "high" BP is arbitrary.

WHAT IS HYPERTENSION?

Central role of the kidney
- Sodium excretion depends on renal perfusion pressure (the Guyton hypothesis). So ↑ renal perfusion → pressure natriuresis. In hypertension this curve is pushed to the right (see Fig. 5.2).
- Monogenic (rare!) forms of ↑BP suggest that tubular ion transport mechanisms are important mediators of blood pressure control.
- There is much redundancy in control of BP. Many neuroendocrine systems contribute to it in overlapping and interlocking ways. And any or all of these may lead to abnormal blood pressure.

Salt intake and blood pressure

A high dietary salt intake is an important but not absolute condition for the development of hypertension. The Intersalt trial showed that populations with a low intake of dietary sodium have a low prevalence of hypertension—essential hypertension is seen mainly in societies with a salt intake >6 g/day. Modest reduction in salt intake for people on a typical Western diet results in a BP drop of 5.3/3.7 mmHg in hypertensive patients and 1.9/1.1 mmHg in normotensive individuals. If salt intake were reduced over many years, the population benefits might be substantial.

"Salt-sensitive hypertension" is said to occur when BP varies with salt intake. In most people the renal pressure natriuresis curve is steep (a small ↑ in BP → to a large ↑ in salt excretion). If this curve is shallow, then BP will vary with salt intake. This occurs in patients with CKD, but also in others with more subtle disruption of renal tubuloglomerular feedback (📖 p. 618). It is more common in African-American and obese patients.

In societies in which salt is consumed in vast excess of physiological requirements, to have a blood pressure sensitive to salt intake may predispose to hypertension.

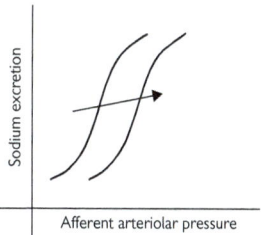

Fig. 5.2 In the normotensive individual, salt balance is maintained at a normal BP. The slope of the curve is very steep, such that dietary salt loading does not significantly alter BP. In hypertensive individuals the curve is shifted to the right, though it remains parallel. Thus, on a normal sodium diet, salt balance is maintained, but at a higher BP. In salt-sensitive individuals the rightward shift is accompanied by a depression of the slope (not shown). Thus, not only is the BP set point on a normal diet elevated, but the BP also increases in response to dietary salt loading.

Pathogenesis

Genetics

Inheritance is not Mendelian. No one gene is responsible.

Blood pressure levels are similar among close relatives (even those with "normal"-range BP), suggesting alleles on several different genes may have an effect on BP.

Rare monogenic causes of hypertension (see Box 5.1) have been identified using linkage analysis in afflicted families. Defects in these genes may also be important in *essential* hypertension (gene defects coding the β and γ subunits of the epithelial Na^+ channel (linked to Liddle's syndrome) are associated with BP variations in the general population. Research focus has been on likely culprit genes (especially the angiotensinogen gene). Our understanding remains far from complete.

Genes that have been associated with essential hypertension include:
- ACE polymorphisms (I/I and I/D phenotypes associate with salt-sensitive hypertension)
- α-adducin polymorphisms. A cytoskeletal protein that regulates ion transport in the renal tubule. Polymorphisms may relate to salt sensitivity, diuretic sensitivity, and essential hypertension.
- 11 β-hydroxysteroid dehydrogenase (GG phenotype correlates with salt sensitivity)
- AT-1 receptor gene. In experimental studies AT-1a +/+ mice have higher blood pressures than –/– mice. Clinical relevance is unknown.

Box 5.1 Rare single gene causes of hypertension

Liddle's syndrome Mutations affect the epithelial sodium channel (ENaC). This syndrome is autosomal dominant, with ↑BP characterized by ↓ renin, ↓ aldosterone, and ↓K^+ (📖 p. 538).

Glucocorticoid-remediable aldosteronism (📖 p. 310)

Syndrome of apparent mineralocorticoid excess (📖 p. 312)

Pregnancy-associated hypertension A gene defect → partial activation of the mineralcorticoid receptor by progesterone (rare).

Pheochromocytoma may occur with one of the following:
- Multiple endocrine neoplasia type 2A: mutations in the RET proto-oncogene. Autosomal dominant, pheochromocytoma, medullary thyroid carcinoma, and hyperparathyroidism
- Von Hippel–Lindau (VHL) disease: mutations in the VHL tumor suppressor gene, autosomal dominant. This disease presents with adrenal pheochromocytomas, renal cell carcinomas, and cerebellar and retinal hemangioblastomas.
- Neurofibromatosis type 1 (NF1): mutations in the NF1 tumor suppressor gene, autosomal dominant. Patients present with pheochromocytomas, multiple neurofibromas, café-au-lait spots, and Lisch nodules of the iris.

The renin–angiotensin system (RAS)

This system plays a central role in salt and water homeostasis, and BP control. Abnormalities in the RAS affect blood pressure, and the system is a therapeutic target (ACE inhibitors, AII receptor blockers, 📖 pp. 342 and 344). In the juxtaglomerular apparatus, granular cells synthesize and release renin. Renin converts inactive angiotensinogen into angiotensin I, which in turn is converted by angiotensin-converting enzyme (ACE) in the lungs to active angiotensin II (AII). AII binds two receptors, AT-1 and AT-2 (see Box 5.2).

Renin release is mediated by
- ↓ afferent arteriolar (i.e., renal perfusion) pressure of any cause
- Sympathetic nervous system activation (granular cell β_1-receptors)
- ↓ Na^+ delivery to the distal tubule (sensed by the macula densa)
- Prostacyclin, adrenocorticotropic hormone (ACTH).

Increased renin

Increased renin occurs in renal artery stenosis, renal cell carcinoma (RCC), benign reninoma (very rare), and other renin-secreting malignancies (also very rare).

▶ Many patients with essential hypertension have ↑ plasma renin levels *not* related to any of the above, nor of any therapeutic use.

Angiotensin
Circulating AII binds vascular receptors, but *locally released* AII works at tissue level in a paracrine fashion. Levels in tissue have no correlation with systemic levels, but may correlate better with disease pathogenesis.

Box 5.2 Actions of angiotensin II

- Arteriolar vasoconstriction (and venules to a lesser extent)
- Efferent renal arteriolar vasoconstriction
- Aldosterone secretion
- Epinephrine (adrenalin) release
- Smooth muscle hypertrophy
- Increased reabsorption of sodium in PCT
- Inhibits renin release (negative feedback loop)
- Renal mesangial cell growth and matrix expansion
- Myocardial growth and matrix expansion
- Stimulates thirst and ADH release.

Most effects are mediated by the angiotensin type 1 (AT-1) receptor. The role of AT-2 receptors remains unclear, but angiotensin binding may regulate vasodilatory, proliferative, and apoptotic effects of AII.

Aldosterone

Aldosterone synthesis occurs mainly in the zona glomerulosa of the adrenal cortex and is tightly regulated by the RAS, or by electrolyte imbalance: ↑K^+ or ↓ salt intake → aldosterone synthesis. Aldosterone acts at the collecting duct to promote Na^+ retention and K^+ excretion (📖 p. 626). Cortisol *also* activates the mineralocorticoid receptor—so aldosterone-sensitive tissues contain high levels of 11-β hydroxysteroid dehydrogenase 2 (this converts cortisol to cortisone, which is incapable of activating the receptor), and this protects the mineralocorticoid receptor from states of high circulating cortisol.

Extrarenal actions of aldosterone
- Paracrine action in nonepithelial tissues (brain, heart, epithelium)
- Associated with vascular inflammation and cardiac fibrosis. The same may be true of other nonvascular tissues
- Activates profibrotic and growth factors in other tissues (including the kidney)

Arterial stiffness

Arterial pressure depends in part on the compliance of conduit arteries. Stiff arteries are less able to dampen a surge in pressure in systole, so systolic pressure is higher. A stiffer artery will also conduct a pulse wave more rapidly. Normally, the pulse wave is reflected back from the small vessels, arriving back at the heart during diastole. If conducted more rapidly, the reflected pulse wave may reach the heart during systole, further ↑ systolic pressure, and ↓ diastolic pressure. Coronary artery perfusion, which occurs predominantly during diastole, may be affected.

The more common causes of reduced compliance (or ↑stiffness) include:
- Ageing: Loss of elastin, calcification of arterial walls, lipid deposition, and defective endothelial function all contribute.
- Diabetes: ↑ arterial stiffness is accelerated (even if ↑BP is absent), as nonenzymatic glycosylation of connective tissue and high insulin levels ± activation of the sympathetic nervous system alter compliance.
- Chronic kidney disease, and especially ESRD: Oxidant stress, impaired endothelial function, abnormal lipid profile, calcification of the arterial wall (exacerbated by disordered calcium, phosphate and PTH), and a variety of putative uremic toxins are thought important (📖 p. 144).

⚠ Increased arterial stiffness and pulse wave velocity are *independent predictors* of all causes of mortality and cardiovascular morbidity and mortality in patients with hypertension.

Endothelial dysfunction and nitric oxide

↑BP is associated with impaired endothelium-dependent relaxation of the vessel wall. A number of factors influence endothelial function:
- Nitric oxide (NO)
  - → relaxation of vascular smooth muscle. NO is released by endothelium in response to shear stress (i.e., blood flow).
  - Endogenous NO synthase (eNOS) → continuous normal basal release. Inducible NOS (iNOS) → high concentrations of NO in response to inflammatory cytokines.
  - ↓ NO has been reported in hypertensive patients (+ their offspring).
- Oxidative stress: Free radicals scavenge NO, forming potentially toxic byproducts. Radicals themselves (such as superoxide, O_2^-) are potent vasoconstrictors.
- Prostaglandins: Prostacyclin (PGI_2) is released by endothelial cells in response to shear stress and has a synergistic effect on tone with NO.
- Angiotensin II is a vasoconstrictor and also contributes to free-radical generation and to endothelin release.
- Endothelins are a potent vasoconstrictor, opposing the actions of NO. They also cause renal Na^+ retention, ↑ aldosterone, vascular smooth muscle cell proliferation, cardiac hypertrophy, and fibrosis. Their causal role in hypertension is unclear.

Sympathetic nervous system (SNS)

Activation of the SNS is clearly linked with acute hypertension—chronic activation may have a role in the genesis of long-term hypertension in those with a genetic predisposition. SNS activation causes the following:
- ↑ in stroke volume (via α-1 and -2 receptors)
- ↑ in heart rate (via β-1 receptors)
- ↑ in systemic vascular resistance (via α-1 receptors)
- Activation of the RAS (via β-1 receptor-mediated renin release).

Other factors

- Insulin resistance has a clear relationship with hypertension:
  - Fasting insulin levels correlate with BP in insulin-resistant patients.
  - Relatives of those with ↑BP are more likely to have insulin resistance.
  - Insulin resistance predicts the subsequent development of ↑BP.
  - Mechanisms may include SNS activation and Na^+ retention.
- Natriuretic peptides, including:
  - ANP (atrial natriuretic peptide). It is released by atrial tissue in response to stretch, i.e., volume overload.
  - BNP (brain natriuretic peptide). It was first discovered in the brain but synthesized and secreted by ventricular myocardium.
  - Urodilatin. It has a similar structure to ANP but is confined to the kidney. It is synthesized in distal tubular cells, causing natriuresis.

The natriuretic peptides are secreted in response to volume overload, leading to a compensatory natriuretic effect. Other effects include vasodilation, modulation of vascular smooth muscle function, and control of the RAS system. Their role in the pathogenesis of hypertension is less clear. In experimental studies, defects in natriuretic peptide production cause salt-sensitive hypertension.

BP measurement

Clinic

The mercury sphygmanometer remains the gold standard, although semi-automated devices are increasingly popular. Validation and maintenance are vital.

Procedure
- No coffee, strenuous exercise, or smoking just before measurement.
- Sit the patient in a quiet room for 5 min.
- Measure with the patient sitting and support the arm at heart level.
- The cuff bladder should encircle ≥80% of the upper arm. The standard adult bladder is 12 × 26 cm (some consider 12 × 35 cm standard).
  - Cuff too large → underestimation
  - Cuff too small → overestimation
- In elderly or diabetic patients, check for orthostatic hypotension by repeating after 2 min standing.
- Use Korotkoff phase I (appearance) for SBP and phase V (disappearance) for DBP. If phase V goes to zero, use phase IV (muffling).
- Take two measurements 1–2 min apart and read to the nearest 2 mmHg.
- Measure in both arms. If there is a significant difference, use the arm giving the higher value for subsequent readings.
- Don't round up or down to preconceived values (observer prejudice).
- Document the time of measurement in relation to medication.

Home

Wrist monitors are not as accurate as upper-arm devices and not recommended. Explain the device to patients, and ensure that it is used properly.
- Pros include involving patients in their own management (? better compliance), allowing multiple readings on different days, and reducing the "white coat" effect (p. 299). ▶ Home readings predict target organ damage.
- Cons include many monitors being inaccurate and poorly maintained. Measurements are not taken under standardized conditions.

Clinic readings demonstrably correlate with CV risk.

Ambulatory BP monitoring (ABPM)

ABPM provides a measure of BP during "normal life"—it may correlate better with CV risk and TOD (♦*). It presently complements rather than replaces standard measurements. Tell the patient to refrain from strenuous exercise, straighten their arm during measurement (this is tricky if driving), and to keep a concurrent diary, e.g., sleep times. BP is measured at repeated intervals (commonly every 30 min), throughout the day and night. SBP and DBP can be plotted over time, with most devices providing average day, night, and 24-hour pressures (Fig. 5.3).

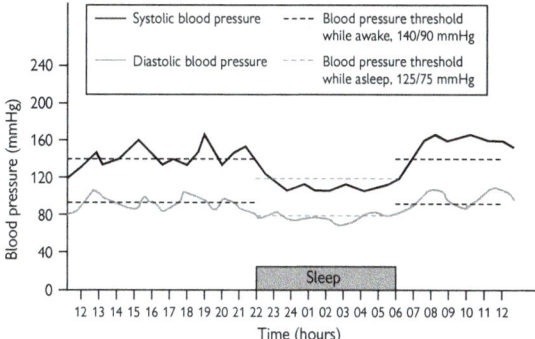

Fig. 5.3 Example of variation in daytime and nighttime BP.

ABPM readings and interpretation

	Normal	Abnormal
Daytime	<135/85	>140/90
Nighttime	<120/70	>125/75
24 hours	<130/80	>135/85

A relatively high nocturnal BP (blunted nocturnal hypotension or "dipping") without a fall of <10/5mmHg, may indicate an adverse prognosis.

Potential indications for ABPM
- Unusual clinic BP variability, or other discrepancies in readings
- Hypertensive clinic values but hypotensive symptoms
- Possible "white coat" hypertension (first and last hours ignored)
- Evaluation of real or apparent drug resistance
- Investigation of autonomic dysfunction.

"White coat" hypertension (isolated clinic hypertension)

- Clinic BP is consistently elevated, but ABPM readings are normal.
- Consider this when BP appears elevated but there is no TOD.
- The anticipation of BP measurement → alerting reaction → ↑BP.
- This can result in normotensive patients being diagnosed with hypertension. It also occurs in treated hypertensive patients.
- Prevalence ↑ with age and is higher for milder forms of hypertension.
- It may be a precursor of sustained hypertension.
- It may in itself confer ↑CV risk (☞not in all studies).

Clinical assessment

History and examination
- Duration of elevated BP. Previous monitoring, treatment, and control
- Other CVD risk factors
  - Cigarette smoking
  - Obesity (BMI ≥30 kg/m^3)
  - Physical inactivity
  - Dyslipidemia
  - Diabetes mellitus (DM)
  - Microalbuminuria or e-GFR <60 mL/min
  - Age (>55 for men, >65 for women)
  - Family history of premature CV disease
- Is there anything to suggest secondary hypertension (📖 p. 308)?
  - Young age (<30 years, especially if non-obese and Caucasian)
  - Sudden-onset hypertension
  - Recurrent episodes of "flash" pulmonary edema
  - Acute renal failure with initiation of ACEI or ARBs
  - Sudden deterioration in BP control
  - New-onset hypertension after age 65
  - Severe or "resistant" (≥3 drugs) hypertension
- Are there other contributory factors?
  - Drugs
  - Excess alcohol intake
  - Sleep apnea
  - History of thyroid disease
  - Use of oral contraceptives
  - Excess salt intake
  - Environmental stress
- Is there target organ damage?
  - Heart: LVH, angina, or prior MI, CHF, history of coronary revascularization
  - Brain: stroke or TIA
  - Peripheral vascular disease
  - Fundi: hemorrhages, exudates, or papilledema (retinopathy grades I and II have little prognostic value)
  - Renal impairment or proteinuria
- Previous drug treatment and side effects
- Contraindications to specific drugs, e.g., bronchospasm
- Family history: ↑BP, stroke, diabetes, ↑ lipids, renal disease, premature IHD.

Investigations

Routine
- Urinalysis (?protein ± blood)
- Renal function profile (and eGFR)
- Blood glucose—preferably fasting
- Lipid profile—preferably fasting
- ECG for LVH (±LV strain—higher risk) and evidence of IHD

Optional
- Echocardiogram
- Uric acid (↑in the metabolic syndrome)
- Hb and Hct
- Microalbuminuria
- Vascular US
  - Plaque detection
  - Measurements of intima media thickness
  - Pulse wave velocity to estimate large-artery compliance.

Classification of hypertension

Drawing up guidelines is easy; transferring them into clinical practice isn't.
- **Prehypertension** (systolic 120–139 mmHg or diastolic 80–89 mmHg
  - Greater prevalence of traditional cardiovascular risk factors
  - Higher cardiovascular risk
  - Patients without DM, CKD, end-organ damage, or CV disease are treated with nonpharmacologic treatment.
- **Grade 1** (SBP: 140–159 and/or DBP: 90–99 mmHg)
  - Encouraged lifestyle measures
  - Initial drug choice: thiazide-type diuretic. May also consider ACEI, ARB, BB, CCB, or a combination.
- **Grade 2** (SBP ≥160 or DBP ≥100 mmHg)
  - Encouraged lifestyle measures
  - Usually requires two drugs to control
  - Consider thiazide and ACEI, ARB, β-blocker, calcium channel blocker (CCB).

Hypertension emergencies
- ▶ Significant elevation in blood pressure associated with acute target end-organ damage (encephalopathy, angina, myocardial infarction, pulmonary edema, eclampsia, stroke, head trauma, life-threatening arterial bleeding, papilledema or aortic dissection) requires immediate hospitalization and treatment with parenteral therapy.

Hypertensive urgency
- Severe hypertension usually with DBP >120 mmHg and not associated with end-organ damage
- No proven benefit from rapid reduction in BP
- Need initiation of combination oral therapy or titration of existing medications.

Isolated systolic hypertension (ISH)
- Traditionally defined as SBP >160 with DBP <90
- JNC 7 defines upper limit of SBP as 140 mmHg (see Table 5.1)
- Generally occurs in older patients
- ISH is associated with 2–4x increase in risk of MI, LVH, CKD, and cardiovascular mortality.
- Thiazide diuretic is the preferred first agent.

Table 5.1 JNC 7 classification of BP

Category	Systolic blood pressure (mmHg)	Diastolic blood pressure (mmHg)
Optimal blood pressure	<120	<80
Pre-hypertension	120–139	80–89
Grade 1 hypertension (mild)	140–159	90–99
Grade 2 hypertension (moderate to severe)	≥160	≥100
Isolated systolic hypertension	>140	<90

If SBP and DBP fall into different categories, the higher value is taken.

There are several important sources of guidelines for the classification and treatment of hypertension:
- The Joint National Committee on Prevention, Detection, Evaluation, and Treatment of High Blood Pressure (JNC) (USA)
- The British Hypertension Society (BHS)
- The WHO/International Society for Hypertension
- The National Kidney Foundation—Kidney Disease Outcomes Quality Initiative (NKF/K-DOQI) (hypertension in the context of renal disease).

All draw on the results of large, randomized, controlled trials and meta-analyses to formulate their recommendations. All are available online.

Treatment thresholds

Aim for a target of
- <140/80 mmHg
- <130/80 mmHg if DM, CKD, or cardiovascular disease.

There is now little evidence to support the J-shaped curve hypothesis—i.e., generally, the lower the BP the better.

Suggested indications for specialist referral
- Urgent treatment needed
  - Accelerated hypertension (severe hypertension with grade III–IV retinopathy)
  - Particularly severe hypertension (220/120 mmHg)
- Renal disease
- Associated with CHF
- Possible secondary hypertension
- Resistance to treatment (≥3 drugs)
- Multiple drug intolerances
- Multiple drug contraindications
- Other situations
  - Unusual blood pressure variability
  - Possible white-coat hypertension
  - Hypertension in pregnancy

Lifestyle measures

Lifestyle changes can ↓BP, ↓ drug requirement, and improve CV risk (see Table 5.2). They may also ↓ the incidence of hypertensive complications (☛unproven). Clear advice should be provided to all patients, as well as those with a high-normal (pre-hypertensive) BP or positive family history.

Low-sodium diet
This diet ↓BP in both normotensive and hypertensive patients, enhancing the latter's response to drug therapy. Usual Na^+ intake is in the range of 150–200 meq/day; ↓ to <100 meq/day (~2.3 g of Na^+ or 6 g NaCl) by avoiding salt in cooking, salt on the table, processed foods (including many breads, stock cubes, "ready meals," numerous breakfast cereals, and pre-prepared sauces). Cook with natural ingredients. If necessary, refer patient to a dietitian. Note: 1 g of Na^+ contains 44 meq, 1 g of NaCl contains 17 meq of Na^+; 5 g of NaCl ~ 1 teaspoon.

⚠ Low Na^+ salt substitutes often contain KCl, ∴ avoid in renal patients.

Weight loss
Obesity (BMI ≥30 kg/m^2) is fuelling the increasing incidence of ↑BP and type 2 DM. Weight reduction improves BP, even without dietary Na^+ restriction, and has beneficial effects on insulin resistance, lipids, LVH, and diabetic control.

Healthy eating
The Dietary Approach to Hypertension Trial (DASH), though short, showed impressive reductions in BP. The diet is rich in fruit and vegetables, provides high amounts of K^+, Mg^{2+}, and Ca^{2+}, limits intake of total and saturated fats, and (moderately) restricts Na^+ intake (3 g/24 h).

The DASH eating plan can be downloaded at: www.nhlbi.nih.gov/health/public/heart/hbp/dash

Exercise
Brisk walking for 30 min ≥5 ×/week has been shown to ↓ the risk of DM by >50% and reduce BP by up to 10 mmHg. Even mild exercise is beneficial. Isometric (weight training, etc.) and strenuous exercise tend to ↑BP and are best avoided until BP is under control.

Alcohol
Patients who consume >2 drinks/day have a 1.5–2× increase in the incidence of hypertension compared to that in nondrinkers. The relationship between alcohol consumption and hypertension is linear and greatest when alcohol consumption >5 drinks/day.

Caffeine
Caffeine is an adenosine receptor antagonist (→ vasoconstriction). More than 5 cups of coffee/day is undesirable. Caffeine is also present in tea and cola drinks. Recommend decaffeinated alternatives.

Stress management
Meditation, cognitive therapy, biofeedback, and muscle relaxation are some examples of stress management. A modest, if variable, response has been seen in some studies. More studies are needed.

Table 5.2 Lifestyle interventions for BP reduction

Intervention	Recommendation	Expected SBP reduction (range)
Weight reduction	Maintain ideal BMI (20–25 kg/m^2)	5–10 mmHg per 10 kg weight loss
DASH eating plan	Consume diet rich in fruit, vegetables, and low-fat dairy products with reduced content of saturated and total fat	8–14 mmHg
Dietary sodium restriction	↓ dietary sodium intake to <100 mmol/day (<2.3 g sodium or <6 g sodium chloride)	2–8 mmHg
Physical activity	Undertake regular aerobic activity, e.g., brisk walking for ≥30 min most days	4–9 mmHg
Alcohol	♂ <21 units/week ♀ <14 units/week	2–4 mmHg

Additional lifestyle measures that ↓CV disease risk

- Stop smoking. This does not ↓BP, but will improve overall CV risk. Quitting before middle age returns life expectancy to near that of life-long nonsmokers.
- Reduce total fat intake.
- Replace dietary saturated fats with monounsaturated fats.
- Increase consumption of oily fish.

Secondary hypertension

This probably accounts for ~5%–10% of all cases of ↑BP, although the true prevalence remains unknown. It is more common in the subgroup of "resistant" hypertension. History, examination, and routine investigation along with a high index of suspicion should identify those in need of specialist assessment. The diagnoses are important to make, as curative treatment is available for many. Diagnostic clues are shown in Table 5.3.

Classification

1. **Renal disorders** (📖 p. 159 for ↑BP in CKD)
   - Renal parenchymal disease: acute/chronic GN, tubulointerstitial disease, adult polycycstic kidney disease (APKD), obstructive uropathy
   - Renovascular disease (📖 p. 412)
   - Renin-producing tumors (📖 p. 312)
   - Genetic diseases affecting tubular transport (Liddle syndrome, 📖 p. 538). These are very rare.

2. **Endocrine disorders**
   - Excess mineralocorticoid (📖 p. 310–311): primary aldosteronism, apparent mineralocorticoid excess, congenital adrenal hyperplasia, licorice ingestion, ectopic ACTH secretion, exogenous mineralocorticoids—e.g., fludrocortisone, pseudohyperaldosteronism
   - Others, including pheochromocytoma, Cushing's syndrome, hypothyroidism, hyperthyroidism (↑SBP), hyperparathyroidism, acromegaly, or the carcinoid syndrome.

3. **Drugs**
   - Estrogen-containing contraceptives, sympathomimetics (cold cures), glucocorticoids, NSAIDS (and COX-2 inhibitors), cyclosporin, monoamine oxidase inhibitors, amphetamines, cocaine, sodium bicarbonate.

4. **Pregnancy** (📖 p. 574)
   - Pregnancy-induced hypertension, preeclampsia and eclampsia.

5. **Miscellaneous**
   - Coarctation of the aorta (↓renal perfusion)
   - Obstructive sleep apnea
   - Increased intracranial pressure or spinal cord injury
   - Acute LVF and intravascular volume overload (IV fluids!)
   - Hyperdynamic circulation (systolic hypertension):
     —Anemia
     —Fever
     —Thyrotoxicosis
     —Aortic regurgitation
     —AV fistulas
   - Acute intermittent porphyria
   - Alcohol withdrawal.

Table 5.3 Diagnosis and treatment of secondary hypertension

Condition	Diagnostic clue	Further investigation
Primary renal disease	• ↑C_r • Proteinuria ± hematuria	• Renal US (?APKD) • Renal biopsy
Renovascular hypertension	• ↑C_r • Acute ↑C_r post ACEI/ARB • Renal asymmetry on imaging • Flash pulmonary edema • Abdominal bruit	• CT angiogram • MRA • Duplex US • ± Formal angiography
Primary aldosteronism	Hypokalemia (rarely → muscle weakness, polyuria, arrhythmias)	• Plasma aldosterone/renin ratio • Urinary aldosterone excretion • Saline infusion test
Apparent mineralo-corticoid excess	• Mainly children • ↑BP, ↓K^+, ↓ renin • Aldosterone not ↑	↑ ratio of THF to THE in urine (see text)
Pheochromocytoma	Paroxysmal symptoms (headache, palpitations sweating)	Urinary or serum total and fractionated catecholamines
Thyroid disease	Hypo- and hyperthyroidism are associated	Thyroid function
Hyperparathyroidism	Serum Ca^{2+} ↑	Serum i-PTH
Cushing's syndrome	• Corticosteroid therapy • Cushingoid appearance (central obesity, striae bruising, etc.), muscle weakness, hyperglycemia, oligomenorrhea	• Urinary cortisol excretion • Dexamethasone suppression tests
Coarctation of the aorta	• Midsystolic murmur (precordium → back) • Weak femoral pulses • Radiofemoral delay • BP in arms ↑, BP in legs ↓	• CT or MRA • ± aortography
Obstructive sleep apnea	Snoring, daytime somnolence, morning headache, obesity (large collar size)	• Sleep observation with pulse oximetry • Formal polysomnography
Acromegaly	↑ sweating, headaches, fatigue, arthralgia, change in shoe or ring size, change in appearance, hyperglycemia	• ↑IGF-1 • Failure to suppress GH to <2 mU/L post 75 g oral glucose load

Primary hyperaldosteronism

This condition includes disorders of autonomous aldosterone hypersecretion with suppressed renin levels. Aldosterone acts on the distal tubule to ↑ renal Na^+ retention (with ↑ urinary K^+ and H^+ loss), increasing total body Na^+ content and driving hypertension. Primary hyperaldosteronism is thought to account for ~0.1% of the hypertensive population (possibly an underestimate, some say 1%–10%) and is the most common endocrine disorder leading to secondary hypertension.

Clinical and biochemical findings vary widely. It is often asymptomatic, but may present with ↓K^+, metabolic alkalosis, and mild ↑Na^+ (which helps distinguish it from essential BP treated with diuretics, where Na^+ is usually low-normal). If severe, ↑K^+ → tetany, myopathy, and nephrogenic diabetes insipidus (polyuria and nocturia).

Causes of primary hyperaldosteronism

- Conn's syndrome (aldosterone-producing adrenal adenoma), ~70%
- Bilateral adrenal hyperplasia, ~30%
- Glucocorticoid-remediable aldosteronism
- Aldosterone-producing adrenal carcinoma (↑↑ aldosterone and ↓↓K^+—may also produce cortisol and sex steroids)

Diagnosis

- Measurement of K^+ has been considered a screening test, but only 50%–80% have ↓ K^+ early on (↓↓ underdiagnosis).
- Document renal K^+ wasting (urinary K^+ >30 meq/day).
- Plasma aldosterone concentration/plasma renin activity (PAC/PRA) ratio (Fig. 5.4)
  - This is a commonly used diagnostic test. Unregulated aldosterone secretion → suppressed renin production and ↑ aldosterone/renin ratio (ARR).
  - See Box 5.3.
- Normal, 4–10
- Hyperaldosteronism, 30–50
- Must know lower limit of lab for plasma renin, 0.6 or 0.1?
- PAC >20 and PAC/PRA >30, 90% sensitivity and specificity for diagnosis of aldosterone-producing adenoma
- Confirmatory testing
  - High Na^+ diet for 3 days (120 meq/day—ask your dietician) then measure 24-hour urinary aldosterone secretion. Adequate salt loading can be confirmed by urinary Na^+ >250 meq/24 h. IV N saline (2 L/day) is an alternative salt load. The normal response will be suppressed aldosterone secretion ∴ lack of suppression can be used to confirm the diagnosis.
  - ⚠ May precipitate ↓K^+ in normokalemic patients who were previously on a low-salt diet.

- Fludrocortisone suppression test: 0.2 mg bid for 2 days. Administration of fludrocortisone further suppresses PRA without suppressing plasma aldosterone below a threshold value. A PAC >5 on day 3 is a positive test.
- Adrenal CT and MRI are used to localize tumors (>1.5 cm).
- Adrenal venous sampling is occasionally necessary—the distinction between an adenoma and hyperplasia is important because of the role of surgery in the former.

General principles of treatment

Use spironolactone (a competitive antagonist of the mineralocorticoid receptor p. 335) at initially 50–100 mg (most patients will require 100–200 mg/day) (side effects include gynecomastia, impotence, menstrual irregularities, and GI upset). Eplerenone is an alternative. Add amiloride 5–20 mg if ↓K^+ persists. Other antihypertensive agents may also be required. Do surgical resection if there is adenoma: 70% of patients are normotensive at 1 year (poorer results in some series—especially if BP is longstanding). Some argue for a trial of spironolactone in all cases of resistant hypertension (p. 348).

Box 5.3 Doing a PAC/ PRA : the nuts and bolts

- Time: 0700–0900
- Posture: upright
- Potassium: normalize first with supplements, as ↓K^+ suppresses aldosterone
- ⚠ Discontinue all drugs influencing RAS (β-blockers, ACEI, ARB, diuretics) for a washout period of 2 weeks (6 weeks for spironolactone). The "cleanest" drugs are α blockers—e.g., doxazosin.
- Result: aldosterone (ng/dL)/plasma renin activity (ng/mL/h) >30–50. The ↑ the ratio the more likely the diagnosis.

Specific causes of hyperaldosteronism

Primary hyperaldosteronism

Glucocorticoid remediable aldosteronism (GRA)
GRA is very rare and is autosomal dominant. A chimeric aldosterone synthase/11β-hydroxylase is ectopically expressed in the adrenal fasciculata. ACTH → stimulates enzyme activity → normal cortisol production + aldosterone excess (→ volume expansion and ↑BP). GRA presents with ↑BP at a young age, along with a family history (early hemorrhagic stroke in some pedigrees). Diagnosis is now confirmed with genetic testing. Dexamethasone → suppression of ACTH secretion → ↓ enzyme activity → ↓aldosterone production.

Congenital adrenal hyperplasia (CAH)
In CAH there are inherited enzymatic defects (autosomal recessive) in cortisol production. Clinical features depend on the enzyme affected, but result from (1) ↓cortisol synthesis and (2) ↑ACTH-driven steroid production. Two forms (of six) are associated with mineralocorticoid excess and ∴ ↑BP.
- 11β hydroxylase (CYP11B1) deficiency, presenting in childhood; ♀ are virilized and ♀ are sexually precocious.
- 17α hydroxylase (CYP17) deficiency. This is extremely rare. It presents with ↑BP, ↓K^+, and hypogonadism—often at puberty.

Secondary hyperaldosteronism

This results when aldosterone hypersecretion occurs secondary to ↑circulating renin levels—often in response to renal hypoperfusion. ↑Renin → ↑ circulating AII, ↑ peripheral resistance, and ↑BP (often severe). Associated secondary hyperaldosteronism → ↑ tubular Na^+ reabsorption (∴ ↓K^+). Causes include the following (see Fig. 5.4):
- Renal artery stenosis
- Renal infarction, e.g., atheroemboli
- Cirrhosis (vasodilatation → ↓ effective circulating volume)
- CHF (falling CO → ↓ effective circulating volume)
- Nephrotic syndrome
- Renal trauma (so-called Page kidney)
- Renin-secreting tumors (see Box 5.4).

Box 5.4 Renin-secreting tumors

These tumors are very rare. Renin-secreting tumors of the juxtaglomerular cells → angiotensin-induced ↑BP. They present with severe ↑BP, ↓K^+ (↑urinary K^+ excretion), ↑ renin, ↑AII, and ↑ aldosterone.

Diagnosis is with MRA, CT, and angiography (tumor blush).

Treatment is with ACEI and ARBs, which effectively ↓BP. Surgery may be curative.

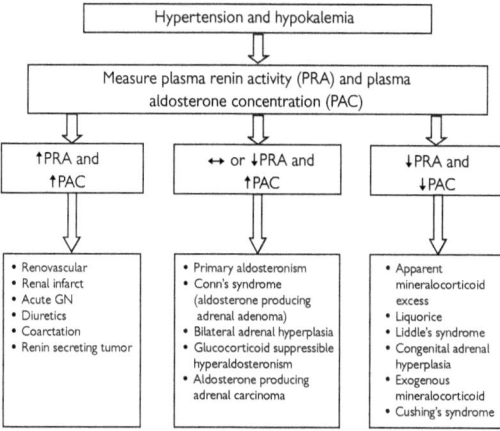

Fig. 5.4 Diagnostic algorithm for hyperaldosteronsim.

Other "hyperaldosteronism" syndromes

Other mineralocorticoids may occasionally be the cause of a clinical syndrome very similar to that seen with ↑ aldosterone, namely ↑BP, ↓K^+ with alkalosis. Crucially, both renin and aldosterone are suppressed. Causes include the following:
- Apparent mineralocorticoid excess
- Congenital adrenal hyperplasia
- Licorice ingestion
- Ectopic ACTH secretion
- Exogenous mineralocorticoids; e.g., fludrocortisone.

Apparent mineralocorticoid excess

<1% hypertensives This condition is autosomal recessive, presenting in childhood. There is an inactivating mutation in 11β-hydroxysteroid dehydrogenase 2 (11βHSD2). The mineralocorticoid receptor (which has an equal affinity for cortisol and aldosterone) is protected from ongoing cortisol stimulation by 11βHSD2, which metabolizes cortisol → cortisone (relatively inactive). As cortisol is present at 100-fold concentrations compared to those of aldosterone, absence or inhibition of this enzyme allows cortisol to flood the receptor, → chronic activation.

Diagnosis ↑ ratio of urinary tetrahydrocortisol (THF + 5α-THF) (metabolite of cortisol) to tetrahydrocortisone (THE) (metabolite of cortisone).

Treatment Block the mineralocorticoid receptor (spironolactone) or suppress ACTH secretion (dexamethasone, suppresses endogenous cortisol synthesis, but does not activate the mineralocorticoid receptor).

Glycyrrhizinic acid in licorice can bind the 11βHSD2 enzyme, creating a state of apparent mineralocorticoid excess. Look out for it in herbal preparations.

"Pseudoaldosteronism"

This is caused by abnormalities of renal tubular transport rather than elevated renin or aldosterone. The electrolyte abnormalities mimic those seen with ↑ aldosterone, hence the name. See 📖 p. 538. Causes include the following:
- Liddle syndrome
- Bartter syndrome (normotensive)
- Gitelman syndrome (normotensive).

Other causes of secondary hypertension

Cushing's syndrome

↑BP is very common, affecting ~80%. A 24-hour urinary cortisol excretion is a reliable diagnostic test (normal cortisol excretion is 10–55 µg/day). Diagnosis is confirmed by a 2-day low-dose dexamethasone suppression test (0.5 mg every 6 hours for eight doses) or an overnight suppression test (1 mg at 2300h). In the 2-day test, urinary cortisol excretion >27 nmol (10 µg) per day on day 2 indicates Cushing's syndrome, as does plasma cortisol >140 nmol/L (5 µg/dL) at 0800h in the overnight test. Serum ACTH concentrations, a long dexamethasone suppression test ± corticotrophin releasing hormone (CRH) stimulation test, and adrenal/pituitary imaging will help distinguish different forms of the syndrome (Cushing's disease is most common, with overproduction of ACTH by the pituitary gland).

Pheochromocytoma

This condition is very rare (<0.1% hypertensives). Adenoma (rarely carcinoma) of adrenal medulla → oversecretion of catecholamines (adrenaline → ↑HR and contractility, noradrenaline → ↑SVR). It can arise in extra-adrenal chromaffin tissue (e.g., paraaortic ganglia). Most patients have ↑BP most of the time, although symptoms (including pallor, palpitations, anxiety, angina, headache, sweating, and nausea) may be paroxysmal. Postural ↓BP is also seen, with occasional fulminant presentation. The sensitivity and specificity of various screening tests are shown in Table 5.4. Many centers use 24-hour urine catecholamines ×3 (acidified container). MIBG scanning may localize the tumor and metastases (~10% malignant). It is often large and periadrenal ∴ visible on US or CT. Treatment is with α- and β-blockade prior to surgery.

Table 5.4 Sensitivity and specificity of screening tests for pheochromocytoma

Test	Sensitivity (%)	Specificity (%)
Plasma metanephrines	99	89
Plasma catecholamines	85	80
Urinary catecholamines	83	88
Urinary metanephrines	76	94
Urinary vanillymandelic acid	63	94

Reproduced with permission from Pacak K (2001). Recent advances in genetics, diagnosis, localisation and treatment of phaeochromocytoma. *Ann Internal Med* **134**: 315–29.

Coarctation of the aorta

This is a rare cause of secondary ↑BP in children and young adults, occurring in ♂ > ♀. It represents <1% of congenital heart disease. A ridge extends into the aortic lumen just distal to the left subclavian artery. Often asymptomatic, it may be diagnosed after CV examination (mid-systolic murmur, radiofemoral delay, ↑BP [arms > legs]), or chest X-ray (aortic "3-sign" from pre- and post-stenotic dilatation and posterior rib notching). If undetected in childhood, it presents with cardiac failure in middle age and prognosis is then poor.

Diagnosis is with CT, MRA, or aortography.

Treatment is surgical. BP correction is age dependent (>90% in childhood).

Drug-induced hypertension

📖 p. 308.

Obstructive sleep apnea (OSA)

The number of diagnosed and treated patients with OSA is rising rapidly. ↑BP, which may be difficult to treat, is commonly associated and may be related to disease severity (though obesity and other comorbid factors may contribute more). Treatment of OSA improves BP.

Treatment includes weight reduction, alcohol avoidance, correction of airway obstruction, oral prosthetic devices, CPAP, and uvulopalato-pharyngoplasty.

Thyroid disease

Hypothyroidism may influence the RAS and is associated with ↑DBP. Hyperthyroidism is associated with an ↑ basal metabolic rate (BMR), ↑SBP, and a wide PP.

Drug management of hypertension

- The primary goal of treatment is to achieve a ↓ in long-term CV morbidity and mortality risk.
- Patients will accrue benefit even if they do not achieve target BP.
- The benefits of BP lowering therapy are primarily determined by the level of BP control rather than class of drug used to achieve it ☙. This is an important issue—the difference in cost between older (β-blockers and thiazides) and newer (CCBs, ACEI/ARBs) drugs is considerable.
- In general, the lower the BP the better.
- Most patients will require ≥2 drugs to attain target.
- Combination medications have a role.
- Compliance is improved with once-a-day formulations.
- Explain the benefits of drug treatment as well as possible side effects.
- Marked interindividual variation in drug responses reflects heterogeneity in the pathogenesis of ↑BP. Profiling patients according to their hypertensive phenotype with a view to individualizing drug therapy has proved difficult (exceptions: the elderly and ethnic groups).
- Drug withdrawal might be possible if other lifestyle interventions are undertaken and prove successful.
- Once BP is adequately controlled, provide at least twice-yearly review for monitoring.
- The four major groups are equally well tolerated. They are prescribed in ~ equal amounts in primary care, though costs vary considerably.
  - Thiazide diuretics (📖 p. 332)
  - β-blockers (📖 p. 336)
  - ACEI and ARBs (📖 p. 342–345)
  - Calcium channel blockers (CCBs)
  - α-blockers are not recommended as first line (📖 p. 338)
- ☙ The benefits are probably the same regardless of the initial agent you use. It depends which guideline you follow. JNC 7 recommends thiazides as first-line agents.
- When considering which agent for which patient, it is useful to consider *compelling indications* (Table 5.5) and *compelling contraindications*. There are other less definite pros and cons that will be assigned different importance by different prescribers.

Table 5.5 Compelling indications influencing initial choice of antihypertensive

	Diuretic	β-blocker	ACEI	ARB	CCB	Aldosterone antagonist
CHF	X	X	X	X		X
Post-MI		X	X			X
High-risk CAD	X	X	X		X	
Diabetes	X	X	X	X	X	
CKD			X	X		
Recurrent stroke prevention	X		X			

Data from Chobanian AV, et al. (2003). The Seventh Report of the Joint National Committee on Prevention, Detection, Evaluation, and Treatment of High Blood Pressure: the JNC 7 report. *JAMA* **289(19)**: 2560–72.

Drug treatment of hypertension

Algorithms

Guidelines for treatment of hypertension are based on clinical trials. Current recommendations incorporate 1) the degree of BP elevation and 2) the presence or absence of other comorbid conditions.

JNC 7

If BP is not within range following lifestyle modification, antihypertensive medications are indicated. The Seventh Report of the Joint National Committee on Prevention, Detection, Evaluation, and Treatment of High Blood Pressure (JNC 7) divides initial therapy recommendations based on presence or absence of comorbid conditions.

Comorbid conditions that would influence initial antihypertensive medication choice would include CHF, post-myocardial infarction, high risk of coronary artery disease, diabetes, chronic kidney disease, and recurrent stroke prevention.

Absent these comorbid conditions, JNC 7 suggest a thiazide-type diuretic as initial therapy for patients with stage 1 hypertension.

Patients with stage 2 hypertension usually require combination therapy to control hypertension. JNC 7 suggests a thiazide-type diuretic plus ACEI, or ARB or ß-blocker or CCB.

Special situations

Hypertension in African Americans

The prevalence of ↑BP and complications such as CHD, stroke, and renal disease is higher in African Americans than in other ethnic groups.

There is evidence of differential BP-lowering efficacy of particular drugs within some ethnic groups. Black people, in general, suffer with low-renin hypertension, so agents (ACEI, ARB, and β-blockers) that suppress renin production may not be effective, especially when used as monotherapy. However, they may be effective in combination with other agents, especially diuretics and CCBs.

Hypertension in the elderly

CHD and stroke remain the major killers over age 65, with BP being the most common treatable risk factor.

SBP ↑ with age. DBP ↑ to age 60, plateaus, and then falls. This leads to an age-related increase in PP and isolated SBP. BP variability also increases ∴ more measurements are desirable prior to treatment. ↑BP in the elderly is ∴ a major public health issue. Hypertension occurs in two-thirds of patients over age 65.

Clinical trials have shown that older people benefit just as much, if not more, from intervention as younger patients.

The elderly are more prone to orthostatic hypertension (→ falls → fractures), so treatment may need to be titrated to the standing value. Other lifestyle interventions still apply. Low-renin hypertension is the norm, so begin treatment with a thiazide or CCB. Second line, ARBs are demonstrably more effective than β-blockers.

Hypertension in diabetes mellitus (see p. 443).

Hypertension in CKD (see p. 157).

Hypertension in pregnancy (see p. 576).

Oral contraceptives, HRT, and BP

Oral contraceptives
- The combined oral contraceptive (OC) modestly ↑BP in a minority of women (~1%). Occasionally elevations may be severe. The rise in BP may not become apparent for several months or even years after OC introduction. The mechanism(s) of ↑BP remain uncertain, and it has not been possible to identify women at particular risk. OC use is also associated with ↑ stroke and MI risk.
- BP should be measured prior to OC use and at least every 6 months thereafter.
- Progesterone-only pills have not been associated with ↑BP and are recommended for women with both OC-induced ↑BP and preexisting ↑BP. In those women wishing to remain on OC, antihypertensive medication should be given early consideration.
- For older women (age >35), with higher CV risk (e.g., smokers), nonhormonal forms of contraception are preferable.

Hormone replacement therapy (HRT)
- HRT use is not associated with ↑BP and its use is not contraindicated in preexisting hypertensives.

Clinical trials in hypertension

The benefits of lowering BP are supported by one of the most authoritative evidence bases in clinical medicine. The foundation of this evidence base is the prospective, randomized clinical trial.

Trial designs
- Duration rarely >5 years
- End points
  - All-cause mortality
  - Cause-specific morbidity and mortality (usually CAD ± stroke; more recently, CHF).
  - The "composite primary end point" has emerged (i.e., a combination of events), because trials seldom have sufficient power to examine specific outcomes.
- Early trials compared active therapy with placebo, often among patients with severe ↑BP. Consequently, they had ↑ power and could be conducted on a relatively small scale. Such trials became unethical as the benefits of BP lowering became apparent.
- Modern "head-to-head" trials tend to assess whether drug classes offer advantages over others (drug companies are desperate to demonstrate benefits "beyond BP lowering") (see Table 5.6).
- BP differences between treatment arms now tend to be minimal, resulting in ↓ study power and requiring ↑ patient numbers.
- Contemporary treatment objectives also influence trial design—most patients now require multiple drugs to achieve target.
- Most patients at high CV risk will receive concomitant treatment with aspirin ± a statin, further diminishing trial power.
- Trials are hugely expensive.
- The data from clinical trials are often pooled for meta-analysis. This provides increased power to examine drug-specific effects.

Controversies
- Do specific classes of drugs offer benefits for CV disease prevention beyond the expected benefits of BP lowering?
  - There are marked drug-specific differences in their effect on CV structure and function as well as metabolic end points. The relevance of these effects on longer-term outcomes remains unknown.
  - Could certain classes of drugs be potentially harmful with specific outcomes?
- With regard to study design, can treatment be solely measured in terms of CV events, or is the real aim to prevent the evolution of a destructive disease process?
- Clinical trials rarely run for more than 5 years, while life expectancy in middle-aged hypertensives is 20–30 years.

Meta-analysis of BP-lowering trials: the BPLTTC

The Blood Pressure Lowering Treatment Trialists Collaborative (BPLTTC) is an international alliance of the principal investigators of the largest trials of antihypertensive regimes. The project is based at the George Institute for International Health, a department of the University of Sydney.

Its objective is to address questions concerning safety and outcome with specific drug classes. To achieve this, data from recent trials are pooled and subjected to meta-analysis (∴ providing the necessary statistical power to examine drug specific effects).

Their most recent analysis, published in 2003*, incorporated data from 29 randomized, controlled trials involving ~160,000 patients, with a mean duration of follow-up of 2.0 to 8.0 years (>70,000 patient years). The mean age was 65 years (52% ♂, 48% ♀).

Conclusions
- Treatment with any of the commonly used regimens ↓ the total risk of major CV events.
- Larger reductions in BP produce larger reductions in risk.
- ACEI and diuretics β-blockers are more effective at preventing heart failure than regimes based on CCBs. Other differences in regimes beyond BP lowering are less certain (including for stroke).

* Turubull F, et al. (2003). Lancet 362: 1527–35. www.thegeorgeinstitute.org/bplttc

Table 5.6 Recent major trials in hypertension

Study acronym	Full name	Purpose
AASK	African American Study of Kidney Disease and Hypertension *JAMA* (2002); **288**: 2421–31	To determine whether lowering BP below recommended CV goals or particular agents slowed the progression of hypertensive renal disease (GFR 20–65 mL/min). Patients received ramipril or amlodipine, with both compared to metoprolol.
ALLHAT	The Antihypertensive and Lipid Lowering Treatment to Prevent Heart Attack Trial *JAMA* (2002); **288**: 2981–97	The largest double-blind, randomized trial of hypertensive patients (n = 42,418). Hypothesis: fatal CAD and nonfatal MI would be lower in patients randomized to "new" drugs (ACEI and CCBs) than in those taking a thiazide.
ANBP-2	The Second Australian National Blood Pressure Study *N Engl J Med* (2003); **348**: 583–92	To compare outcomes with an ACEI (mainly enalapril) and a diuretic (mainly hydrochlorothiazide) among elderly patients with ↑BP (open label)
ASCOT	The Anglo-Scandinavian Outcomes Trial *Lancet* (2005); **366**: 895–906	To compare the effects on CAD of a β-blocker ± diuretic ("old-fashioned") vs. a CCB ± ACEI ("modern") in patients with ↑BP A second arm (*Lancet* 2003; **361**: 1149–58) compared atorvastatin with placebo for ↑ lipids in hypertensive patients.
HOPE	Heart Outcomes Prevention Evaluation Study *N Engl J Med* (2000); **342**: 145–53	To compare ramipril to placebo for prevention of CV events in patients with evidence of atherosclerotic CV disease who were on standard therapy (~50% nonhypertensive).

Results	Comments
AASK: Ramipril was superior in ↓ rate of decline. The amlodipine arm was stopped early because of worse outcomes.	Showed (surprisingly) that the level of BP attained did not affect the rate of decline of renal function.
ALLHAT: A Doxazosin arm was stopped early (median 3.3 years follow-up) after interim data suggested an ↑ risk of combined CAD events. The main finding was that thiazides, CCBs, and ACEI all provide similar protection from CAD. Thiazides appeared superior to CCBs and ACEIs in preventing some adverse CV outcomes. CCBs are not associated with excess CV deaths—a concern in previous studies.	General conclusion: thiazide diuretics are unsurpassed in preventing the major complications of ↑BP. They are also well tolerated and inexpensive. They became the initial drug of choice in many guidelines. Criticisms: (1) designed in an era of monotherapy, (2) many conclusions drawn on the basis of secondary end points, (3) randomization deprived some patients with CHF of their diuretic, (4) old-fashioned treatments were used for step up (e.g., clonidine, reserpine).
ANBP-2: Similar BP control was observed in both arms. The ACEI group had an ↓ incidence of nonfatal CV events (benefits restricted to ♂).	Apparently at odds with the findings of ALLHAT, though the study designs were very different.
ASCOT: Stopped early (median follow-up 5.4 years) because of superior results in the CCB/ACEI arm for several secondary end points, including all-cause mortality and new-onset DM (primary end points were nonfatal MI and fatal CHD). Atorvastatin treatment resulted in a significant ↓ in the incidence of stroke.	Unique in its focus on combination therapy. Good press for CCBs after a lot of bad press. Likely to reignite concerns regarding new-onset DM with diuretics + β-blocker. Has been the catalyst for an early review of current guidelines.
HOPE: Ramipril decreased the combined relative risk of MI, stroke, or CV death by 22%.	Provided considerable impetus to the "beyond-BP-lowering" hypothesis. There were important BP differences between the groups that probably accounted for the results (and led cynics to dub it the "HYPE" trial).

Table 5.6 (Contd.)

Study acronym	Full name	Purpose
HOT	Hypertension Optimal Treatment Study *Lancet* (1988); **351**: 1755–62	To assess the relationship of major CV events with three target DBPs (≤90, ≤85, or ≤80 mmHg) Also whether low-dose aspirin, in addition to ↓ BP therapy, ↓ CV events
INSIGHT	Intervention as a Goal in Hypertension Treatment. *Lancet* (2000); **356**: 366–72	To compare CV events in high-risk hypertensive patients treated with nifedipine or amiloride + hydrochlorothiazide
LIFE	Losartan Intervention for Endpoint Reduction in Hypertension *Lancet* (2002); **359**: 995–1003	To compare the long-term effects of losartan with atenolol on CV mortality and morbidity in hypertensive patients with LVH
NORDIL	The Nordic Diltiazem Study *Lancet* (2000); **356**: 359–65	To evaluate the potential preventative effects of diltiazem on CV morbidity and mortality compared to a β-blocker ± diuretic
PROGRESS	Perindopril Protection against Recurrent Stroke Study *Lancet* (2001); **358**: 1033–40	To investigate whether perindopril, alone, or in combination with indapamide, influenced stroke recurrence (~50% patients nonhypertensive)
STOP-2	The Swedish Trial in Old Patients with Hypertension-2 *Lancet* (1999); **354**: 1751–6	Patients aged 70–84 were assigned to either an ACEI, a dihydropyridine CCB, or a "conventional" therapy (β-blocker ± diuretic)
SYST-EUR	Systolic Hypertension—Europe *Lancet* (1997); **354**: 757–64	To investigate whether antihypertensive treatment in elderly patients with isolated SBP could ↓CV events (primarily stroke). Participants received placebo or nitrendipine (with enalapril and hydrochlorothiazide added if needed).
VALUE	Valsartan Antihypertensive Long-term Use Evaluation *Lancet* (2004); **363**: 2022–31	To investigate whether, for the same level of BP control, valsartan is more effective than amlodipine in ↓CV events

Results	Comments
HOT: Achieved BPs were 144/85, 141/83, and 140/81. The lowest incidence of CV events occurred at DBP 83 mmHg. The benefit of progressive BP reduction was most marked in patients with DM. Aspirin caused a further significant ↓ in CV events (due entirely to a ↓ in MIs).	Defined a new optimal BP target (DBP 83 mmHg). Further reductions did not ↑CV events (i.e., did not support the "J-curve" hypothesis).
INSIGHT: Both regimens resulted in equivalent BP control and outcomes.	The diuretic group needed significantly more add-on antihypertensive medications. Less new-onset DM was seen in the CCB group.
LIFE: BP control was identical between the two groups. Primary events were fewer, the incidence of new-onset DM lower, and LVH regression greater for losartan than for the β-blocker.	One interpretation: the benefits of losartan extend beyond its BP-lowering effects. Another: apparent benefits of losartan are actually due to negative effects of atenolol.
NORDIL: There were no differences in the incidence of the primary end point (a composite of all stroke, MI and other CV events). Secondary analysis indicated a ↓ in the incidence of stroke in the CCB group.	One of the few studies to evaluate a non-dihydropyridine CCB. The protection against stroke probably reflected better BP control in the CCB group.
PROGRESS: Those on perindopril had a significant ↓ in recurrent stroke	Often cited as evidence for the "beyond-BP-lowering hypothesis" for ACEI, but the improved stroke outcome was probably driven by the more pronounced ↓ in BP in the combined perindopril + diuretic arm.
STOP-2: No difference in primary end points among the three arms. ACEIs were associated with a lower risk of MI and CCF than that for those treated with a CCB.	Suggested newer and older drugs are generally equivalent.
SYST-EUR: Stopped early because of a 42% ↓ in stroke in the active arm. Cardiac events were also reduced, but not significantly.	Also suggested that CCBs may have a protective role in vascular dementia.
VALUE: There were no differences between treatment groups in CV morbidity or mortality.	Good BP control in groups underscored the importance of achieving target BP, whatever the agent(s) used.

The ASCOT study

The Anglo-Scandinavian Cardiac Outcomes Trial (ASCOT) is a large, multicenter study[1] that is likely to change the drug management of hypertension. For many years the consensus was that reductions in mortality or morbidity were due to BP lowering rather than any specific drug class. This was reflected in national and international guidelines. Drug effects "beyond blood pressure lowering," particularly affording cardiovascular protection, had been claimed in many studies over the last 10–20 years, but flawed study designs had called into question the validity of the results.

ASCOT appears to have changed this—robustly designed, the trial has already led to a redraft of the UK BHS/NICE Guidelines (published June 2006). The BP-lowering arm is discussed here (a lipid-lowering arm showed significantly fewer cardiovascular events in those patients treated with a statin and was also stopped early).

Study design
- 19,257 patients from the UK and Scandinavia
- Age 40–79 years
- Patients all had hypertension + at least three other cardiovascular risk factors.

Treatment regimens
- Treatment arm 1: calcium channel blocker (amlodipine) ± ACEI (perindopril)
- Treatment arm 2: β-blocker (atenolol) ± thiazide diuretic (bendroflumethiazide)
- α-blocker (extended-release doxazosin) added if BP did not reach target

Target BP
The target was 140/90 (130/80 for patients with diabetes). Most patients achieved this (mean 2.2 agents).

Median follow-up
Median follow-up was 5.5 years (<2% patients were lost to follow-up).

Results
The primary end point was fatal coronary heart disease or nonfatal MI. The trial was stopped early when the data-monitoring group reported significantly more events in the atenolol-based group.

A 10% reduction in the primary end point was seen in the amlodipine ± perindopril group ($p = 0.1$, so not statistically significant). However, this group also had:
- ↓ all-cause mortality (11%)
- ↓ cardiovascular mortality (24%)

---

1 Dahlof B, Sever PS, Poulter NR, et al. (2005). Prevention of cardiovascular events with an antihypertensive regimen of amlodipine adding perindopril as required versus atenolol adding bendroflumethiazide as required in the Anglo-Scandinavian Cardiac Outcomes Trial-Blood pressure Lowering Arm (ASCOT-BPLA): a multicentre randomized controlled trail. *Lancet* **366**: 895–906.

- ↓ all coronary events (13%)
- ↓ fatal and nonfatal strokes (23%)
- ↓ new-onset diabetes (30%).

When the primary end point was adjusted to include coronary revascularization (in line with changing clinical practice during the period of data collection), a significant reduction was observed (14%) in the amlodipine ± perindopril group.

BP lowering was better in this group (by 2.7/1.9 mmHg). However, further analysis, matching patients with similar BP, suggested continued benefit in the amlodipine/perindopril group,[2] ∴ BP control is unlikely to be the whole reason for the benefit.

Significance of ASCOT

ASCOT is set to shape future guidelines and clinical practice. The likelihood is that
- ACE inhibitors (or ARB) ± calcium channel blockers will be recommended for first-line use except in specific situations.
- Thiazide diuretics may be an alternative first line in the elderly, but second line in younger age groups.
- β-blockers can no longer be recommended as first line. This has proved to be the case in the recently revised BHS/NICE Guidelines in the UK—others may follow.

---

[2] Poulter NR, Wedel H, Dahlof B, et al. (2005). Role of blood pressure and other variables in the differential cardiovascular event rates noted in the Anglo-Scandinavian Cardiac Outcomes Trial-Blood Pressure Lowering Arm (ASCOT-BPLA). *Lancet* **366**: 907–13.

Diuretics

See also 📖 p. 532

Diuretics work by directly inhibiting the Na^+ transporters and channels mediating renal Na^+ reabsorption.

Efficacy depends on active secretion of the diuretic into the proximal nephron, such that high concentrations are achieved at sites of action along the tubule. Renal insufficiency impairs proximal secretion → relative diuretic resistance. Higher doses may still be effective, but risk ↑ toxicity.

The Na^+ and volume loss associated with diuretics is initially accompanied by the activation of vasoconstrictor mechanisms (including RAS). This ↑ SVR and attenuates their antihypertensive effect. Over a period of days, SVR falls through poorly understood mechanisms and antihypertensive effects become sustained. This is one of the reasons that diuretics and ACEI/ARBs are a good combination (see Fig. 5.5).

Thiazide and thiazide-like diuretics

Examples
- Thiazide: hydrochlorothiazide
- Thiazide-like: chlorthalidone, indapamide.

Mechanism
- Compete with both Na^+ and Cl^- to block the Na^+–Cl^- cotransporter in the distal convoluted tubule (DCT) (normally responsible for 5%–7% of filtered Na^+ reabsorption).
- ↑Na^+ delivery to distal nephron → ↑Na^+/K^+ exchange and, indirectly, ↑H^+ excretion: hypokalemic metabolic alkalosis often results.
- Blocking the Na^+–Cl^- cotransporter ↑Ca^{2+} reabsorption (mechanism unknown). Thiazides ∴ have a role in renal stone disease and exert a protective effect in osteoporosis.
- Thiazide-like agents differ in several of their actions including duration of action, channel-blocking activity, and inhibitory influence on carbonic anhydrase. The implications for clinical practice are uncertain.

Role
- Effective, good evidence base, and inexpensive
- Introduced in 1957, they are still the first-line antihypertensive in several guidelines.
- ↑ plasma half-life and sustained renal actions make them preferable to loop diuretics as antihypertensives (except in special situations 📖 p. 334).

Problems
- Hypokalemia (dose dependent)
- Impaired glucose tolerance (especially when used with a β-blocker)
- Small ↑ in LDL cholesterol and triglycerides
- Small ↑ in serum urate
- Efficacy ↓ in those taking NSAIDS
- Avoid if history of gout
- Avoid if taking lithium (↑ risk of lithium toxicity).

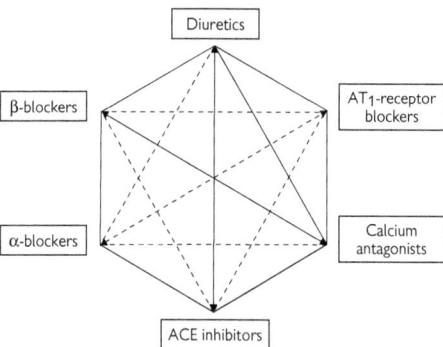

Fig. 5.5 Possible combinations of different classes of antihypertensive agents. The most rational combinations are represented as thick lines. From 2003 ESH/ESC Guidelines for the management of arterial hypertension (*Journal of Hypertension* (2003); **21**: 1011–13). Used with permission.

Loop diuretics

Examples
Furosemide, bumetanide.

Mechanism
- They block the type 2 $Na^+K^+2Cl^-$ (NKCC2) cotransporter in the thick, ascending limb of loop of Henle (which is usually responsible for 15%–20% of filtered Na^+ reabsorption).
- Tubuloglomerular feedback would normally act to compensate by a ↓ in GFR, but this is dependent on an identical (∴ inhibited) co-transporter in the macula densa.
- As for loop diuretics, hypokalemic metabolic alkalosis may result.
- Initial Na^+ and volume loss may be compensated for by Na^+ retention during the latter part of the dosing interval, with amelioration of BP-lowering efficacy. Twice-daily dosing (at least) is ∴ required.

Role
Loop diuretics are more potent natriuretics than thiazides, but less effective BP-lowering agents. They have little place in the routine management of ↑BP, except in patients with CHF (with volume overload), renal impairment (with volume overload), or some other edematous state (e.g., cirrhosis).

Potassium-sparing diuretics

Examples
Amiloride, triamterene.

Mechanism
- They block the epithelial Na^+ channel (ENaC) expressed in the late DCT and collecting duct.
  - ENaC plays a central role in the control of urinary Na^+ reabsorption, ECF volume homeostasis, and BP regulation.
  - Several hormones, including aldosterone, vasopressin, angiotensin II, insulin, and endothelin, regulate ENaC activity.
  - Liddle syndrome (📖 p. 538) is caused by activating (gain of function) mutation(s) in ENaC.
- K^+ absorption is tightly coupled with ENaC Na^+ absorption. Drugs blocking ENaC ∴ cause K^+ retention. They also have Mg^{2+}-sparing effects.

Role
Potassium-sparing diuretics are not first-line agents. They are useful adjuncts to limit ↓K^+ and ↓Mg^{2+} with other diuretics. ↓K^+ may actually ↑BP and is associated with insulin resistance, DM, arrhythmias, and sudden death.

Amiloride may be used to prevent ↓K^+ and ↑BP associated with excess glucocorticoids or mineralocorticoids (📖 p. 310) and in patients with Liddle syndrome.

Problems
Watch for hyperkalemia! Cautions include renal impairment (especially in DM), combination with β-blockers, ACEI/ARB or spironolactone. The incidence of ↓K^+ when amiloride is co-prescribed with a thiazide or loop diuretic is very low.

Mineralocorticoid antagonists

- RAS activation is associated with worse outcomes in patients with CHF and ↑BP.
- Plasma aldosterone levels correlate with mortality in CHF and with LVH in hypertensive patients.
- Patients with primary hyperaldosteronism appear to have worse CV outcomes.
- Aldosterone activates mineralocorticoid receptors in the heart, vasculature, and brain. Adverse consequences of activation include endothelial dysfunction, myocardial fibrosis, myocyte hypertrophy, vascular injury, and centrally mediated elevations in BP.
- Pharmacological blockade of mineralocorticoid receptors ↓LVH and microalbuminuria in hypertensive patients.
- Administration in severe CHF has been associated with a ↓ in mortality (RALES study).
- Although ACEI and ARBs ↓ aldosterone production, with chronic use levels return toward normal.
- Spironolactone and eplerenone are mineralocorticoid receptor antagonists.
    - Spironolactone has long been used in the treatment of conditions associated with secondary hyperaldosteronism and volume expansion such as cirrhotic ascites.
    - Eplerenone is more selective for the mineralocorticoid receptor than spironolactone and may be better tolerated.
- These agents may also have an antihypertensive role in patients with "resistant" hypertension in whom undiagnosed primary hyperaldosteronism may be more common than currently appreciated ♦.

Adverse effects include gynecomastia (common), GI upset, impotence, and ↑K^+ (⚠ caution with ACEI and ARB, especially if there is renal impairment).

β-blockers

These agents are competitive inhibitors of catecholamines at β-adrenergic receptors. Many are available, with marked interdrug differences in pharmacodynamic and pharmacokinetic properties. In general, these characteristics influence clearance and the side-effect profile rather than efficacy.

Examples
See Table 5.7.

Mechanism
This remains a matter of debate. See box below.

> *Putative BP-lowering mechanisms of β-blockers*
> - ↓Cardiac output
> - ↓Renin release
> - ↓Plasma volume
> - ↓Vasomotor tone
> - ↓Peripheral vascular resistance
> - Improved vascular compliance
> - Resetting of baroreceptor levels
> - Effects on prejunctional β-receptors: ↓ noradrenaline release
> - ↓Pressor response to catecholamines with exercise and stress
> - Direct CNS effect

Role
β-blockers are useful if there is concomitant angina, post-MI (↓mortality risk), arrhythmias, or hyperdynamic circulation. Carvedilol, metoprolol, and bisoprolol have been shown to reduce morbidity and mortality in patients with stable CHF. Labetolol is useful in pregnancy (p. 574) and when parenteral treatment of hypertension is necessary (p. 355). β-blockers are probably less effective in African-American patients and in the elderly.

Problems
- Avoid in obstructive airways disease, marked bradycardia, AV node disease.
- They can cause lethargy, impaired concentration and memory, vivid dreams, hallucinations, depression (CNS effects may be more prominent with lipid-soluble agents), deterioration in peripheral vascular disease, and Raynaud's symptoms.
- Metabolic effects
  - ↓HDL-cholesterol and ↑ triglycerides
  - ↑ likelihood of new-onset DM, particularly when combined with a thiazide. Avoid this combination in high-risk patients: strong family history of T2DM, impaired glucose tolerance, clinically obese (BMI >30), or of South Asian or Afro-Caribbean origin (combination leads to ~1 new DM case for every 250 patients treated per year).
  - They worsen glycemic control and hypoglycemic awareness in T1DM (worse with nonselective agents).
- Combined with diltiazem or verapamil β-blockers may cause slowing of SA node ± negative inotropic effect.

Table 5.7 Examples of β-blockers

	β₁-selectivity[a]	Intrinsic sympathomimetic activity[b]	Membrane stabilizing activity[c]	α-blocking activity[d]	Major route of elimination[e]
Acebutolol[1]	+	+	+		Renal
Atenolol[1]	++				Renal
Bisoprolol	++				Both
Carvedilol			++	+	Hepatic
Celiprolol		+		+	Both
Labetolol				++	Hepatic
Metoprolol[1]	++				Hepatic
Nadolol[1]					Renal
Nebivolol	+			+	Renal
Oxprenolol[1]					Hepatic
Pindolol[1]		++	+		Both
Propranolol			++		Hepatic
Sotalol[2] ⚠			†	+	Renal
Timolol[1]					Hepatic

1 A combination tablet with a thiazide diuretic is available. Atenolol is also available combined with a CCB.

2 ⚠ Sotalol is not licensed for use in hypertension. †Sotalol has class III antiarrhythmic properties and can prolong the QT interval.

β-blockers differ in terms of their β₁ selectivity, intrinsic sympathomimetics activity (ISA), membrane-stabilizing activity (MSA), α-adrenergic blocking ability, and pharmacokinetic properties.

a β₁-selectivity: These agents have less effect on β₂-receptors and are therefore relatively cardioselective. This applies at lower doses only. Theoretically an advantage in patients with obstructive airways disease, these agents should still be regarded as a contraindication. They may not block arteriolar β₂-receptors, which is an advantage in T1DM with hypoglycemia.

b Intrinsic sympathomimetic activity (ISA): partial agonist activity at β₁-receptors, β₂-receptors, or both. Identified as slight cardiac stimulation, inhibited by propranolol. These agents cause less bradycardia and AV node slowing, are possibly less negatively inotropic, and have less effect on peripheral vascular resistance. They appear to have a better lipid profile. It is unclear if these represent an overall advantage (or disadvantage).

c MSA: These agents have a quinidine or local anesthetic–like effect on the cardiac action potential. They are usually seen above therapeutic levels and ∴ are apparent in overdose.

d α-blocking activity: antagonistic properties at both α- and β-adrenergic receptors. This causes a reduction in peripheral and coronary vascular resistance. The benefit of carvedilol in heart failure is not dependent on this property.

e Water-soluble agents are predominantly excreted via the kidney and have a longer half-life. ⚠ Dose reduction is often necessary in renal impairment. Lipid-soluble agents mainly undergo hepatic excretion. They are usually shorter acting (requiring bid or tid dosing) and responsible for more CNS side effects (they cross the blood–brain barrier).

α-blockers

α-adrenoceptors participate in the regulation of vascular tone by the sympathetic nervous system (SNS) and play a role in the genesis of ↑BP and other CV disorders.

Examples
- Selective $α_1$-antagonists: doxazosin, prazosin, terazosin
- Unselective $α_1$- and $α_2$-antagonists: phentolamine, phenoxybenzamine.

Mechanism
- $α_1$-receptors are postsynaptic. Norepinephrine → ↑ intracellular Ca^{2+} flux → ↑ smooth muscle contraction → vasoconstriction. Selective $α_1$-blockade causes ↓SVR and BP with little or no effect on heart rate or cardiac output. α-blockers are essentially vasodilators.
- $α_2$-receptors are presynaptic. Stimulation → ↓ norepinephrine release.
- Nonselective and $α_1$- and $α_2$-antagonists were developed first.
- In normotensive patients with normal sympathetic tone and vascular resistance, α-blockers have minimal BP-lowering effect.

Role
- Their antihypertensive effect is only modest when used as single agents. Effects are additive with other antihypertensive classes.
- The ALLHAT study (see Box 5.5 and 📖 p. 326) provided bad press for α-blockers.
- In light of the above, they are not considered first (or even second) line.
- They have favorable lipid effects (↓ total cholesterol, LDL, triglycerides; ↑HDL).
- They are safe and effective in renal insufficiency.
- BP-lowering effect is independent of age, race, and gender.
- Nonselective α-blockers are useful in the management of pheochromocytoma (📖 p. 316).

Problems
Prazosin has a short half-life, causing first-dose (and postural) ↓BP, which is generally less of a problem with longer-acting agents. Dizziness can persist (even without demonstrable postural ↓BP). Use caution with sildenafil (Viagra®), tadalafil, and vardenafil (→ rapid ↓BP). Stress that incontinence is aggravated in ♀. α-blockers can cause fluid retention (∴ good combined with a diuretic).

Box 5.5 α-blockers and ALLHAT (📖 p. 326)

The doxazosin limb was stopped early (3.3 years follow-up, ~9000 patients) because of a 25% ↑ incidence of CV disease (mainly CHF; there was no difference in primary end points—fatal and nonfatal MI) compared to the thiazide group. As a result, α-blockers have fallen in popularity with guideline authors and prescribers alike. However, (1) SBP was higher in the doxazosin arm, and (2) randomization deprived many patients with CHF of diuretics, β-blockers, or ACEI, disadvantaging the α-blocker group.

β-blockers remain a good component of multiple drug regimens for moderate to severe ↑BP and are particularly useful in ♂ with concomitant prostatic disease. Avoid their use with coexisting CHF.

α-blockers and bladder outflow symptoms (see 📖 p. 515)

- Lower urinary tract symptoms (LUTS) associated with BPH and obstruction are common in ♂ over age 60.
- Bladder emptying involves relaxation of α_1-receptor-mediated smooth muscle contraction in the bladder neck and prostate.
- α_1-receptors are integral to the bulbospinal pathways from the brainstem → lumbosacral cord, which inhibit reflex urination.
- α-blockers relieve the symptoms of outflow obstruction and decrease the need for surgery.
- Newer α-blockers, e.g., tamsulosin (Flomax®), are "uroselective," acting on the α-receptor subtypes α_{1a} and α_{1b}, within the bladder neck and prostate, with limited effect on systemic BP.
- α-blockers are effective, with >60% of patients reporting improvement. Medical therapy is now common and transurethral resection of the prostate (TURP) rates are in decline.
- α-blockers are the best monotherapy for symptom relief of LUTS.
- In patients with moderate to severe symptoms and demonstrable prostatic enlargement, combination therapy of an α-blocker and 5α-reductase inhibitor (blocks conversion of testosterone → dihydrotestosterone), e.g., finasteride, provides effective symptom relief and retards disease progression.

Calcium channel blockers (CCBs)

Examples
- Dihydropyridine (vasodilating) CCBs: nifedipine, amlodipine, felodipine, isradipine, nicardipine, nisoldipine
- Non-dihydropyridine (cardiac active) CCBs: diltiazem, verapamil

Mechanism
- They block voltage-dependent L-type Ca^{2+} channels → ↓ calcium entry into smooth muscle cells → ↓ smooth muscle contraction → ↓ vascular resistance → arterial vasodilatation.
  - Dihydropyridines are more selective at Ca^{2+} channels in vascular smooth muscle cells and ∴ more powerful vasodilators.
  - Non-dihydropyridines block Ca^{2+} channels in cardiac myocytes and ↓cardiac output. They have antiarrhythmic properties via the AV node (verapamil > negative inotrope and chronotrope than diltiazem).
- Other CCB effects include ↓ aldosterone release, ↓ growth and proliferation of vascular smooth muscle cells, anti-atherogenic in animal models.
- They moderately ↑Na^+ excretion via natriuresis. ↓BP effect is not augmented by dietary Na^+ restriction (unlike other classes).
- CCBs undergo first-pass metabolism to some degree. Most are short acting and ∴ require multiple dosing regimens or a slow-release delivery system.

Role
- The BP-lowering effect is equivalent to that of most other drug classes. Among CCBs, antihypertensive properties are roughly equivalent.
- CCBs can be combined with all other classes (⚠ avoid diltiazem or verapamil with β-blockers—cardiac effects are additive).
- They are a good choice in patients with concomitant angina.
- They are effective in low-renin ↑BP (i.e., black or elderly patients)
- There are no adverse effects on lipids.
- ↓BP effect is not blunted by NSAIDs.
- The ASCOT trial (📖 p. 330) has elevated their status.

Problems
- Flushing, tachycardia, or headache occurs, especially with short-acting agents.
- Dose-dependent peripheral edema occurs with dihydropyridine CCBs. This is not due to fluid retention (∴ diuretic unresponsive) but secondarily to mismatched arteriolar and venous vasodilatation.
- Gum hypertrophy occurs with dihydropyridine CCBs.
- Avoid use in systolic LV impairment (especially non-dihydropyridine)
- CCBs have many drug interactions—these are worth checking before prescribing CCBs. Grapefruit juice inhibits cytochrome P450 CYP3A and ↑ the bioavailability of several dihydropyridine CCBs.

- Several trials have suggested that CCBs are not as effective protection against hypertensive or diabetic renal disease as ACEI or ARBs and are ∴ not first line in this situation.
- Verapamil use is often accompanied by constipation.

⚠ Early formulations of some dihydropyridines (e.g., capsular or sublingual nifedipine) had a rapid onset of action, unpredictable BP-lowering effect accompanied by reflex sympathetic stimulation, tachycardia, and RAS activation. These agents have no place in the management of hypertension.

ACE inhibitors (ACEIs)

Examples
Captopril, , enalapril, fosinopril, lisinopril, quinapril, ramipril, trandolapril.

Mechanism
- Block conversion of angiotensin I → angiotensin II (AII) by angiotensin-converting enzyme (ACE). The resulting ↓ in AII → vasodilatation and ↓BP.
- AII has many actions potentially detrimental to the CV system (📖 p. 286).
- Alternative pathways of AII production, e.g., chymases and other tissue proteases, are unaffected.
- In the short term, ACEIs reduce AII levels, but with chronic treatment they return to normal ("AII escape"). Other mechanisms of BP lowering are ∴ thought to be active. Possibilities:
    - ↑ bradykinin → ↑ nitric oxide ± ↑PGI$_2$ (→ vasodilatation).
    - ↑ angiotensin-(1–7), a peptide that is antagonistic to AII.
    - ↓ sympathetic nervous system activity.
    - Direct effect on endothelial function and vascular remodeling
- ACEIs can be subdivided according to their affinity for tissue ACE. It is possible that lipophilic compounds with high tissue affinity (e.g., ramipril, quinapril) exert greater influence on endothelial function and provide CV benefits independent of BP lowering ✦.
- Increasing the dose of an ACEI does not generally alter peak effect, but extends duration of response. Many patients benefit from a second daily dose.

Role
- Comparable BP lowering to other classes (but no better).
- Cardioprotective and renoprotective ∴ good choice if: CHF, post-MI, DM, chronic renal failure (especially proteinuric) or LVH.
- Patients at high risk of CV disease may have improved survival when treated with ACEI (independent of BP reduction ✦).
- Synergistic effects when used in combination with diuretics (diuretics → Na$^+$ depletion → RAS activation → AII dependent (and ∴ ACEI responsive) ↑BP. Also ameliorate diuretic induced ↓K$^+$ (↓AII induced aldosterone release).
- Also suitable for combination with β-blockers, α-blockers and CCBs (ASCOT study likely to promote the latter 📖 p. 330). Insufficient evidence at present to recommend routine combination with ARB.
- Relatively ineffective monotherapy in certain groups with low renin ↑BP; e.g., blacks, though response highly variable (↓Na$^+$ diet increases efficacy). Generally effective in the elderly.
- Documenting plasma renin activity or ACE gene polymorphisms to 'individualize' therapy is not useful—neither predict response.
- Lack adverse metabolic effects.

Problems
- *Renal insufficiency* is much feared by clinicians. If glomerular filtration pressure is dependent on AII-driven efferent arteriolar tone (e.g., volume depletion, renal artery stenosis, CHF), then ACE inhibition may cause a precipitous decline in GFR.
- ⚠ *Precautions*: Ensure that patient is volume replete, ask those on diuretic therapy to take the first dose before retiring to bed. Check UA and renal function profile before commencing treatment and 5–7 days thereafter. Expect (and allow) an ↑ in Cr of ≤20% or a ↓ in eGFR of 15%.
- *Hypotension*: Acute falls in BP occur with ACEI when RAS is activated, e.g., overdiuresis, CHF, accelerated hypertension. This is rare when therapy is initiated in uncomplicated hypertensive patients (admission to hospital for ACEI introduction was commonplace in the 1980s). Postural hypotension is actually comparatively uncommon.
- *Hyperkalemia* is unusual unless there is renal impairment ± other drugs causing ↑K^+ (e.g., amiloride, spironolactone, β-blockers).
- *Cough* is common (5%–40%, ♀ > ♂) and generally resistant to all measures except drug withdrawal (↑ bradykinin ± other vasoactive peptides; e.g., substance P → cough reflex activation).
- *Angioneurotic edema* is rare. It occurs more among blacks than in Caucasians, is also bradykinin mediated and potentially fatal. Stop the ACEI and avoid use for life.
- ↓ *Erythropoietin secretion* may cause or worsen anemia.
- *Pregnancy* is contraindicated.
- *Rash and altered taste* occur mainly with captopril.

Angiotensin II receptor blockers (ARBs)

Examples
These include candesartan, irbesartan, losartan, valsartan, eprosartan, olmesartan, and telmisartan.

Mechanism
- Developed more recently than ACEIs, ARBs essentially block the vasoconstrictive action of AII on smooth muscle.
- There are two AII receptor subtypes:
  - AT_1 mediates (1) vasoconstrictor effects of AII and (2) AII-induced growth in the myocardium and arterial wall.
  - AT_2 function is less well understood. It is expressed at high levels in fetal tissues, with ↓ expression after birth. It is probably responsible for many of the proliferative effects of AII.
- There are two major differences between ACEIs and ARBs:
  - ACEIs ↓ activity of AII at both AT_1 and AT_2 receptors. ARBs only ↓AT_1 activity, with no effect on AT_2.
  - ACE is a kininase, so ACEIs lead to ↑ kinins. Kinins are responsible for some ACEI side effects (especially cough), but may also mediate some of their beneficial effects, including BP lowering and ↑ insulin sensitivity.
- AII blockade leads to ↑ renin, ↑ angiotensin I, and ↑AII, though this accumulation does not appear to overwhelm receptor blockade.

Roles
- ARBs have BP-lowering effect similar to that of ACEIs and other main classes.
- As with ACEIs, ARBs are synergistic with diuretics.
- Evidence is growing that ARBs have similar benefits to those of ACEIs in conditions other than ↑BP, such as CHF (Val-HeFT and CHARM studies) and post-MI (VALIANT).
- Several major trials (IDNT, IRMA-2, RENAAL) have demonstrated renoprotection with ARBs in nephropathy associated with T2DM.

Problems
- Generally well-tolerated, ARBs have a similar side-effect profile to that of ACEIs.
- There is less cough than with ACEIs (as kinin mediated), though angioedema has been reported.
- Altered taste
- ARBs are contraindicated in pregnancy.

Combined ACEIs and ARBs

- There is good theoretical rationale for using them in combination:
  - ACEIs do not completely block the formation of AII (other tissue proteases are involved).
  - ARBs are selective for the AT_1 receptor, leaving AT_2 receptor exposed to ↑AII.
  - With ACEIs, ↓AII → ↑ renin release, eventually returning AII towards baseline ("AII escape").
- Combination therapy is effective in LV dysfunction (Val-HeFT and CHARM studies).
- There is growing evidence to support their combined use in proteinuric renal disease (e.g., COOPERATE).
- ON-TARGET is a large study aiming to compare the effects of telmisartan, ramipril, and their combination on CV mortality in high-risk patients. It should be completed in 2007.
- There is insufficient evidence at present to recommend combination therapy for the hypertension treatment.

Other antihypertensives

With the exception of methyldopa and clonidine, these drugs are rarely seen in the routine treatment of ↑BP. They are still widely used around the world, as generic formulations mean lower costs in many instances.

Centrally acting agents

Methyldopa
This agent is metabolized to a methyl-norepinephrine, a false neurotransmitter that (1) displaces norepinephrine from α-adrenergic receptors, preventing smooth muscle contraction, and (2) stimulates adrenergic receptors in the central vasomotor centers, inhibiting sympathetic outflow. There is a large dose range (250 mg–3 g daily) and it remains widely used to treat hypertension in pregnancy (📖 p. 574). In nonpregnant patients it is best given with a diuretic.

Problems include a positive Coombs' test in 20% (though overt hemolytic anemia is rare), dry mouth, edema, drowsiness, febrile illness, and depression. Avoid use in liver disease.

Clonidine
Clonidine stimulates adrenergic receptors in the central vasomotor centers, inhibiting sympathetic outflow. A clonidine suppression test is occasionally used in the diagnosis of pheochromocytoma (📖 p. 316).

Problems include dry mouth, sedation, and depression. It is associated with severe rebound ↑BP (which may require treatment with parenteral α-blockers).

Direct acting vascular smooth muscle relaxants

Hydralazine and minoxidil
These agents ↓ arteriolar resistance. The consequent ↓ peripheral resistance and BP causes reflex sympathetic activation with tachycardia and palpitations. This can be offset with a β-blocker.

Problems include flushing, headache, and palpitations. Avoid use in ischemic heart disease. These agents cause Na⁺ and water retention (especially minoxidil) ∴ give with a diuretic. Hydralazine can cause a lupus-like syndrome, particularly in slow acetylators. Minoxidil causes hirsutism and has been associated with pericardial effusions in the dialysis population. Hydralazine's metabolites accumulate in renal failure ∴ avoid; minoxidil is OK.

Antihypertensives on the horizon

Endothelin antagonists
The endothelins are a group of potent vasoconstrictor peptides produced in many different tissues. ET-1 is the predominant endothelin secreted by the endothelium, where it acts in a paracrine fashion. Several antagonists are under investigation and it is hoped they will prove reno- and cardioprotective as well as antihypertensive. Bosentan is already licensed for use in primary pulmonary hypertension.

Vasopeptidase inhibitors
These agents inhibit both ACE and neutral endopeptidase, a membrane-bound metalloprotease involved in the enzymatic degradation of natriuretic (📖 p. 296) and various other peptides (including angiotensin II). Several are in development (e.g., omapatrilat). The Achilles heal appears to be the frequency of angioedema.

Renin inhibitors
These are another means of antagonizing RAS. Effects may prove additive to ACEIs and ARBs.

Resistant hypertension

This condition is relatively common—in up to 20%–30% of study populations in clinical trials, usually as a consequence of poorly controlled SBP (Fig. 5.6). Compliance is often a central issue in apparent resistance, underlying the importance of a good physician–patient relationship.

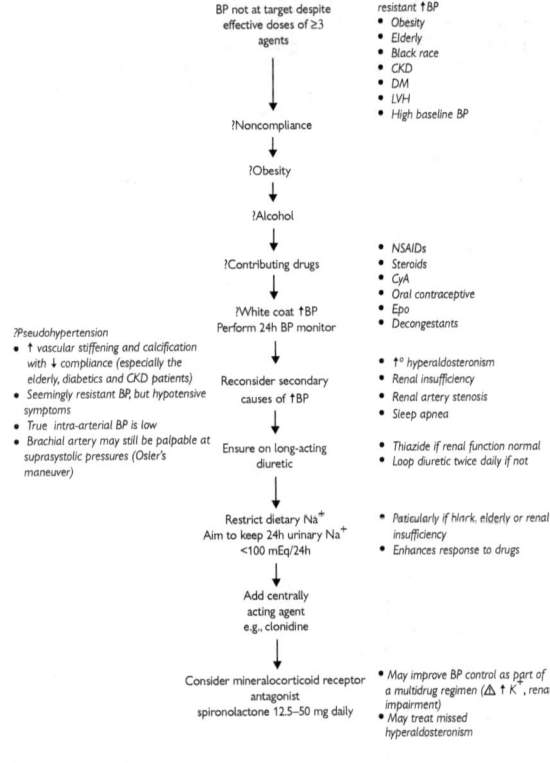

Fig. 5.6 Pathophysiology of resistant hypertension.

Hypertensive urgencies and emergencies

Definitions
- ▶ Hypertensive crises are classified as *emergencies* or *urgencies* based on the presence or absence of progressive target organ dysfunction.
- *Emergencies* include severe ↑BP associated with acute target end-organ damage (encephalopathy, angina, myocardial infarction, pulmonary edema, eclampsia, stroke, head trauma, life-threatening arterial bleeding, papilledema, or aortic dissection) requires immediate hospitalization and treatment with parenteral therapy.
- *Urgencies* include severe ↑BP *without* evidence of acute or progressive target organ dysfunction.
- The term *malignant hypertension* was coined before antihypertensive therapy improved an appalling prognosis (1-year mortality ~90%). It is a syndrome of ↑BP with progressive target organ damage and papilledema. Pathologically, arteriolar fibrinoid necrosis is characteristic.
- *Accelerated hypertension* was applied to the scenario of retinal hemorrhages and exudates without papilledema. The distinction from malignant hypertension is unhelpful, as both carry an identical prognosis.
- There is no threshold of BP above which malignant hypertension
- develops. DBP ranges from 100 to 180 mmHg; SBP, 150–290 mmHg.
- ▶ Severity is not determined by the BP alone—it is the clinical context and degree of target organ dysfunction.
- Malignant hypertension affects <1% of the hypertensive population, but the hypertensive population is large. ♂ > ♀ are affected.
- Essential hypertension accounts for ~2%–30% of episodes in
- Caucasians, but ~80% in African Americans.
- Renal disease (intrinsic and renovascular) accounts for most of the rest. Other previously unrecognized forms of secondary BP may also be responsible.
- The duration of hypertension prior to the development of a malignant phase may range from days to years.

Pathophysiology (see Fig. 5.7)
Vascular autoregulation
Autoregulation describes the ability of organs to maintain their perfusion regardless of BP. ↑BP causes distal arteriolar vasoconstriction, protecting end organs from hypertensive mechanical stress. Hypertensive emergencies are associated with a failure of this process, resulting in transmission of ↑BP to the microvasculature, where mechanical trauma → endothelial injury → ↑ vascular permeability → leakage → platelet and fibrin deposition → fibrinoid necrosis. Release of catecholamines and vasopressin also contributes.

Endocrine and paracrine mediators, including the renin–angiotensin system (RAS), are activated with ↑ AII, leading to further vasoconstriction and ischemia. Volume depletion due to pressure natriuresis stimulates further renin release and worsens ↑BP. A vicious cycle of vasoconstriction and worsening ↑BP ensues.

Pathological changes

Vascular lesions are due to endothelial injury and consist of myointimal proliferation and fibrinoid necrosis, with subendothelial lipid deposition and hyaline thrombi. Vascular smooth muscle hypertrophy and collagen deposition contribute to medial thickening, which, with cellular intimal proliferation, results in the "onion skin" appearance of small vessels with luminal narrowing (Fig. 5.8). Ischemia or infarction of end organs may occur. These changes are particularly seen in the kidney, with proliferative endarteritis of the interlobular arteries, fibrinoid necrosis of the afferent arteriole, and glomerular ischemia (± tubulointerstitial damage).

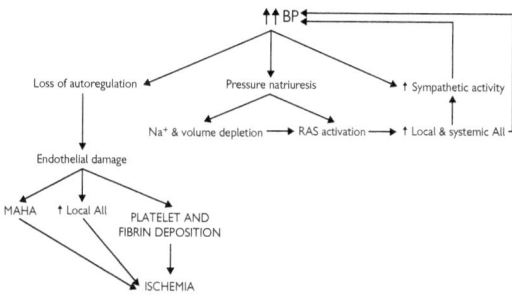

Fig. 5.7 The pathophysiology of malignant hypertension. MAHA, microangiopathic hemolytic anemia. Redrawn with permission from *Acute Renal Failure in Practice*, Imperial College Press.

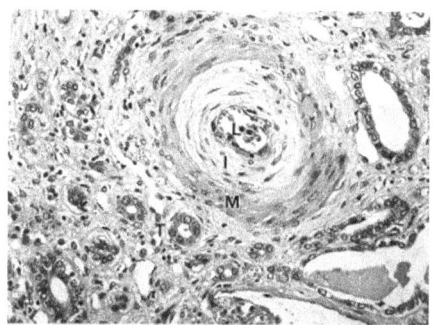

Fig. 5.8 Proliferative endarteritis of an interlobular artery in malignant hypertension. I, arterial intima showing gross proliferative change and "onion-skin" appearance; L, severely narrowed arterial lumen; M, arterial media; T, tubular atrophy and interstitial fibrosis. Reproduced with permission from Davison AMA, Cameron JS, Grunfeld J-P, et al. (eds) (2005). *Oxford Textbook of Clinical Nephrology*, 3rd ed. Oxford: Oxford University Press.

Assessing urgencies and emergencies

How does the BP compare to previous readings?
- 160/100 may be sufficiently high to cause acute target organ damage (TOD) in a previously normotensive patient.
- A patient with long-standing hypertension may tolerate a higher BP without any evidence of acute TOD.

Clinical assessment
- ▶ Assess degree of target organ involvement.
- *Urgency* is ↑BP without acute or progressive TOD.
- *Emergency* is ↑BP with acute or progressive TOD.

Is there evidence of target organ damage?

Acute TOD
▶▶ *Manage as an inpatient as an emergency.*
- Neurological symptoms: at risk for hemorrhagic or thrombotic stroke, encephalopathy (altered consciousness, fits, focal signs)
- LV dysfunction
- Acute renal failure (send UA and renal function profile)
- Chest pain ⚠ Acute coronary syndrome → MI or **aortic dissection**. Perform ECG, and check pulses. If in doubt get CT of aorta.
- Visual symptoms ± *either* grade III *or* IV hypertensive retinopathy
- Pancreatitis due to hemorrhagic infarction (rare)

What medication has the patient been on until now?
- Continue current medication, adding in further treatment as necessary.
- Check adherence to medication (recent noncompliance is very common in this situation). ⚠ Beware of precipitating hypotension by restarting multiple antihypertensives in the previously nonadherent patient.
- ⚠ Remember to check for recreational drug use (cocaine, amphetamines).

Symptoms and signs
- *BP*: no pathognomic values. Usually >220/140 (range: DBP 100–180 mmHg, SBP 150–290 mmHg). Check the BP in both arms, look for missing pulses, bruits, or an abdominal aortic aneurysm.
- *Eyes*: visual disturbances (35%–60%): patients often present to ophthalmology.
- *Neurological*: headache (60%), dizziness (30%), neurological deficit—e.g., hemiparesis, cortical blindness (<10%). Encephalopathy (from cerebral edema) is uncommon—confusion, seizures, and coma.
- *Renal*: ARF (30%).
- *Cardiovascular*: dyspnea secondary to LV dysfunction (~10%), chest pain (~4%).

Hypertensive retinopathy

Grade 1: arterial narrowing (tortuosity, "silver wiring" are subjective)
Grade 2: AV nicking
Grade 3: hemorrhages and exudates
Grade 4: papilledema

Investigations
- *Urinalysis:* proteinuria (can be nephrotic range—send PCR ± 24-hour collection), hematuria, cellular casts (red cell casts may indicate parenchymal renal disease)
- *Renal function profile*
  - *Serum creatinine:* ↑ secondary to acute (or acute on chronic) renal failure
  - *Potassium:* ↓K^+ (secondary hyperaldosteronism → hypokalemic alkalosis; renin and aldosterone are both raised in malignant hypertension), ↑K^+ (secondary ↑ to ARF) also possible
- *CBC:* microangiopathic hemolytic anemia: ↓Hb, ↓ platelets, red cell fragments, ↓ haptoglobins, ↑ESR
- *ECG (± echocardiogram):* LVH, ischemia, MI
- *CT brain:* if ↓GCS or neurological signs
- *Renal biopsy:* a prognostic (rarely diagnostic) renal biopsy may be necessary.

Secondary hypertension?
Some conditions require specific management. Consider list in Box 5.6.

Box 5.6 Causes of hypertensive emergencies
- Essential hypertension
- Renal parenchymal disease
  - Glomerulonephritis
  - Tubulointerstitial disease
- Systemic diseases
  - Systemic sclerosis
  - HUS/TTP
  - SLE
  - Antiphospholipid syndrome
  - Vasculitis
- Renovascular disease
  - Atheromatous
  - Fibromuscular hyperplasia
- Preeclampsia/eclampsia
- Coarctation
- Endocrine
  - Conn syndrome
  - Pheochromocytoma
  - Cushing's syndrome
- Drugs
  - Cocaine
  - Amphetamines
  - Ecstasy
  - MAOI interactions
  - Erythropoietin
  - Cyclosporin
  - Tacrolimus
- Tumor related
  - Renal cell cancer
  - Lymphoma

Management of urgencies and emergencies

Hypertensive urgency
▶ *Severe uncontrolled hypertension (>120 diastolic BP) with no evidence of acute TOD*
- If there is no acute TOD, the patient does not require admission.
- Start with a single agent (e.g., amlodipine 5 mg daily). Aim for diastolic BP 100–110 mmHg at first. Recheck BP after 24–48 hours.
- If still uncontrolled, use a double dose of amlodipine to 10 mg daily.

Recheck after every 2–3 days until BP is at the desired level. Further suggested order (titrate doses up, then add in another agent):
- Atenolol 25–100 mg daily
- Ramipril 2.5–10 mg daily (⚠ watch SCr and K+ carefully to exclude RAS)
- Furosemide 40–120 mg 12–24 hours (especially if renal failure) or Losartan 50 mg q24h, titrate to 100 mg q24h
- Doxazosin (use long-acting preparation) 4–8 mg daily.

Hypertensive emergency
▶ Severe uncontrolled hypertension with acute TOD
- Oral agents usually provide gradual and controlled ↓ in BP (Table 5.8).
- *Use the same order as for hypertensive urgencies.*
- Too rapid ↓BP may → cerebral infarction or worsening renal failure.
- Aim for a diastolic BP of 100–110 mmHg over 24–36 hours.

When to use IV antihypertensives
- Hypertensive encephalopathy
- Aortic dissection
- Acute LV dysfunction or cardiac ischemia
- ▶ Need intensive monitoring, ideally with arterial line.

Aim for 160/100 mmHg during the first 24 hours, or 20%–25% drop in MAP[1] over 4 hours. You will need to lower rate faster (to lower target) if there is aortic dissection.
- Labetalol 20 mg IV stat (can be repeated ×2 within 10–15 min), then infusion of 0.5–2 mg/min
- Sodium nitroprusside 0.25–10 µg/kg/min, with dose increase of 0.5 µg/kg/min every 5 min until response.

Once BP is within the target range, transfer to oral agent and wean IV infusion down over 4–8 hours.

Prognosis

Without effective treatment, 1-year mortality is ~90%; with treatment it is <10%. Many patients who develop renal insufficiency will recover renal function, even if they are initially dialysis dependent, though this may take several months.

---

1 MAP estimated as DBP + [SBP—DBP]/3.

Table 5.8 Drugs used in hypertensive emergencies

Drug	Route and dose	Comment
Calcium channel blockers	- Oral - Start with amlodipine 5–10 mg or nifedipine XL 30 mg	- NEVER use rapid-release formulations. - Nimodipine used post-subarachnoid hemorrhage
β-blockers	- Oral - Useful second line (e.g., atenolol 50 mg daily)	- SE: bronchospasm
ACE-inhibitors	- Oral - Start with low dose (e.g., ramipril 2.5 mg or captopril 6.25 mg) and titrate up	- May cause rapid fall in BP - Treatment of choice in scleroderma crisis
Diuretics	- Oral/IV - Frusemide 40–120 mg 12 h	- Beware of volume-depleted patients
α-blockers	- Oral - Doxazosin ER 4 mg 12 h (up to 8 mg 12 h)	- Useful second or third line because of titration range
Labetolol	- IV - Up to 2 mg/min as infusion or 20–80 mg bolus every 10 min	- Safe in pregnancy. Used in eclampsia - SE: bronchospasm, LVF, heart block
Esmolol	- IV - 250–500 µg/kg/min - Initial bolus of 0.5–1.0 mg/kg	- Very short half-life - SE: bronchospasm, LVF, heart block
Sodium nitroprusside	- IV - Start 0.25–10 µg/kg/min (↑ 0.5 µg/kg/min every 5 min until response) Range 0.25–10 µg/kg/min	- Potent, rapid-acting, vasodilator - Requires close monitoring (?arterial line) and light-resistant delivery equipment - SE: nausea, vomiting, thiocyanate accumulation (especially if renal impairment)
Nitrates (NTG)	- IV - 10–100 µg/min	- Familiar - SE: headache, tachycardia, vomiting
Hydralazine	- IV - 5–10 mg bolus, repeated after 1 h. Infusion: start 200–300 µg/min, maintenance 50–150 µg/min	- Arterial vasodilator used in eclampsia - SE: Na^+ and water retention, headache, tachycardia, vomiting
Phentolamine	- IV - 5 mg repeated as necessary	- Pheochromocytoma - SE: tachycardia, dizziness, flushing, nausea
Fenoldopam	- IV - 0.1–0.3 µg/kg/min	- Newer agent—a dopamine-1 agonist and peripheral arterial vasodilator. Also ↑ urine flow and both Na^+ and K^+ excretion ∴ attractive with renal impairment - SE: headache, tachycardia, flushing

Orthostatic hypotension

This is a frequent clinical problem, particularly in the elderly. It is generally defined as a 20/10 mmHg (symptomatic) fall in BP within 5 min of assuming an upright posture. Symptoms include weakness, dizziness, visual disturbance, presyncope, blackouts, and falls. (See Fig. 5.9).

Normal response
Standing → splanchnic and lower-limb blood pooling → ↓ venous return → ↓cardiac output → ↑BP → reflex sympathetic and parasympathetic activation → ↓peripheral vascular resistance → ↑venous return → cardiac output → ↑BP.

Causes of orthostatic hypotension

- Hypovolemia
- Drugs
- Autonomic dysfunction
  - ↓ Baroreceptor sensitivity (in elderly)
  - Pure autonomic failure
  - Multiple system atrophy (Shy-Drager syndrome)
  - Parkinson disease
  - Diabetes mellitus
  - Amyloidosis
  - Postural tachycardia syndrome (POTS)
  - Paraneoplastic autonomic dysfunction
- Endocrine disorders
  - Addison syndrome
  - Hypoaldosteronism
  - Pheochromocytoma
- Miscellaneous
  - Paroxysmal syndromes
    —Micturition syncope
    —Cough syncope
  - Varicose veins
  - Carcinoid syndrome
  - Mastocytosis

Volume depletion
This requires exclusion in all cases.

Antihypertensive drugs
These are a frequent culprit. Other drugs include nitrates, opiates, tricyclic antidepressants, and alcohol.

Pure autonomic failure
This is characterized by orthostatic ↓BP with a static heart rate, ↓ sweating, impotence, nocturia, constipation, anemia, and supine ↑BP. Symptoms are slowly progressive and often worse early in the morning and postprandially. It is associated with ↓ levels of plasma noradrenaline and degeneration of postganglionic neurons (with Lewy body inclusions).

Multiple system atrophy
This is a progressive neurodegenerative condition of unknown etiology. It occurs in ♂ > ♀, over age 50. Autonomic dysfunction (often first symptom) is accompanied by combinations of extrapyramidal, pyramidal, and cerebellar dysfunction.

Postural tachycardia syndrome (POTS)
POTS is relatively common, at age <40, ♀ > ♂. The etiology is uncertain, but abnormalities of autonomic regulation are implicated. The presence of tachycardia distinguishes it from autonomic failure. Often there is little or no fall in BP. Tilt-table testing is diagnostic.

Decreased baroreceptor sensitivity in the elderly
Mild postural ↓BP in the elderly is associated with abnormal responses to baroreceptor reflexes such as tilting; it may be associated with ↑mortality.

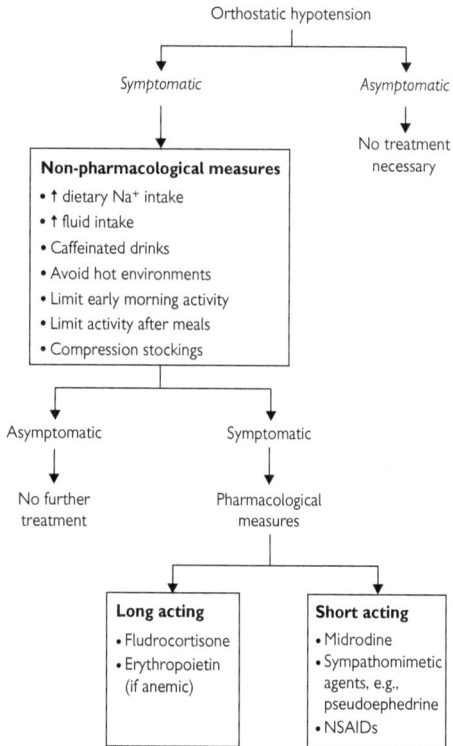

Fig. 5.9 Treatment of orthostatic hypotension. Reproduced with permission from Jordan J, et al. (1998). Am J Med **105**: 116–24.

Chapter 6

Diseases of the kidney

Approaching glomerular disease 360
Histology of glomerular disease 362
Focal and diffuse glomerulonephritis 364
Approaching focal and diffuse glomerulonephritis 366
General principles of management of focal and diffuse
  glomerulonephritis 367
Immunosuppressive management of glomerulonephritis 368
IgA nephropathy 372
Management of IgA nephropathy 374
Postinfectious glomerulonephritis 376
Membranoproliferative glomerulonephritis (MPGN) 378
Hereditary nephropathies 380
Other forms of glomerulonephritis 382
The nephrotic syndrome 384
Minimal change nephropathy 388
Membranous nephropathy (MN) 390
Focal and segmental glomerulosclerosis (FSGS) 394
Treatment of FSGS 396
Thrombotic microangiopathy (TMA) 398
Thrombotic thrombocytopenic purpura (TTP) 400
Hemolytic-uremic syndrome (HUS) 401
Management of HUS, TTP, and TMA 402
Tubulointerstitial diseases 404
Chronic tubulointerstitial diseases 406
Analgesic nephropathy 408
Renovascular disease 410
Management of ARAS 412
Other renovascular diseases 414
Adult polycystic kidney disease (APKD) 416
Complications of APKD 418
Other cystic kidney diseases 420
Urinary tract infections (UTIs) 422
Reflux nephropathy 428
Nephrolithiasis 430
Investigating recurrent stone-formers 432
Acute renal colic 435

Approaching glomerular disease

Glomerulonephritis (GN) is classified by clinical presentation, histological appearances (Fig. 6.1), or etiology (e.g., lupus or post-streptococcal GN).

By clinical syndrome
- Asymptomatic urinary abnormalities (📖 p. 360)
- Focal and diffuse glomerulonephritis (📖 p. 364)
- Nephrotic syndrome (📖 p. 384).

These may all be accompanied by ↑BP ± renal impairment.

Asymptomatic urinary abnormalities
Such abnormalities are common and usually detected on routine urinalysis for unrelated problems. A positive dipstick for hematuria or proteinuria should always be repeated (e.g., after 72 hours). A trace to positive on dipstick may be spurious.

Microscopic hematuria
Dipstick analysis is very sensitive but nonspecific. If persistent, arrange urine microscopy to confirm hematuria (defined as >3 RBC/hpf on 2/3 AM urine specimens) and to examine red cell morphology. Dysmorphic RBCs, acanthocytes, or RBC casts imply glomerular bleeding (📖 p. 52).

Dipstick positive proteinuria
Always repeat dipstick analysis. Transient proteinuria is not uncommon, especially in concentrated urine.

Possible causes of "benign proteinuria"
- Orthostatic (postural)
- Vigorous exercise
- Febrile illnesses and infectious diseases
- Congestive heart failure.

Arrange for urine microscopy to exclude pyuria or casts, and culture to exclude infection. Proteinuria can be quantified on spot samples (urine protein/creatinine ratio [PCR], 📖 p. 18) or by 24-hour urine collection.

Hematuria and proteinuria
This combination usually requires referral and further investigation to exclude an early glomerular lesion. Repeat dipstick to confirm findings and if positive, check spot urine PCR.

Helpful investigations (📖 p. 366)
- Urine microscopy for RBC morphology
- Quantify proteinuria
- BUN, Cr, electrolytes, albumin
- US kidneys.

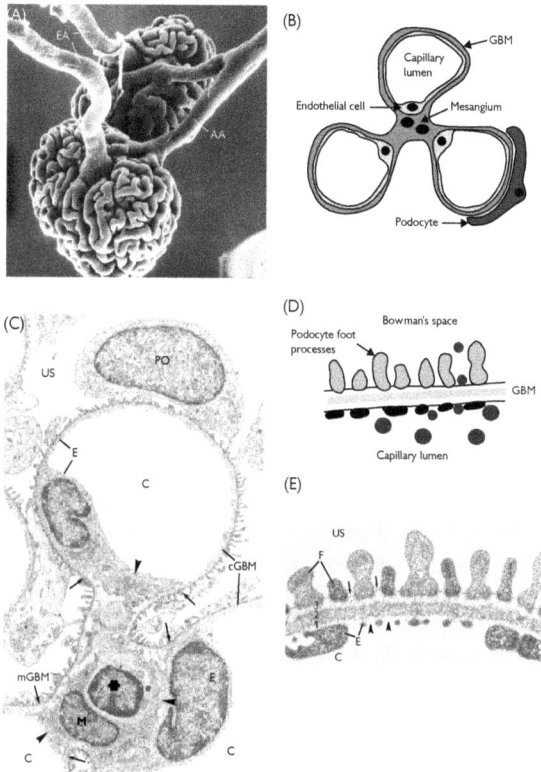

Fig. 6.1 (A) Glomerular vessels. AA = afferent arteriole; EA = efferent arteriole. (B) Cartoon of glomerular capillaries. GBM = glomerular basement membrane. (C) Electron microscopy of glomerular capillaries. C = capillary; E = endothelial cell; cGBM = capillary GBM; mGBM = mesangial GBM; PO = prodocyte; US = ultrafiltration space. (A–C) Reproduced with permission from Davison AMA, Cameron JS, Grunfeld J-P, et al. (2005). *Oxford Textbook of Clinical Nephrology*. Oxford: Oxford University Press. (D) Cartoon of glomerular filter. (E) Electron microscopy of glomerular filter: F = prodocyte foot process.

Histology of glomerular disease

Renal tissue is sampled at renal biopsy (📖 p. 634) and prepared for the following:
- Light microscopy: various histochemical stains, e.g., H+E, periodic acid–Schiff (PAS), Jones silver stain, Masson's trichrome. This is useful for morphology, chronicity, and diagnosis.
- Immunohistochemistry: immunofluorescence and immunoperoxidase staining. It is used to localize immunoglobulins or complement fractions within glomeruli by use of fluorescein-labeled antibodies. Their nature and pattern of staining are characteristic for certain GNs.
- Electron microscopy is useful for examining glomerular deposits and cell and membrane structure.

When examining a preparation of renal cortex, many glomeruli (10–30 on average) are sampled. The following descriptive terms are then used (Fig. 6.2):
- Focal or diffuse? *Focal* lesions affect some (<50%) of the sampled glomeruli, but not all. *Diffuse* lesions involve most (>50%) if not all of the glomeruli.
- Segmental or global? *Segmental* lesions affect *part* of an affected glomerulus, while global lesions involve most of any tuft.
- Proliferative or not? *Proliferative* lesions describe an increase in local cell number. For instance, an increase in mesangial cells ("mesangial proliferative") is a feature of IgA nephropathy.
- Crescentic or not? Glomerular parietal epithelial cells (lining Bowman's capsule) proliferate in response to local inflammatory and procoagulant signals, with fibrin deposition and adhesions filling some or all of Bowman's space.
- Matrix or membrane? Look for an expansion of *matrix* produced by mesangial cells as found in IgA nephropathy, or an increase in glomerular basement *membrane* (GBM) width (and thus capillary wall thickness) as found with immune deposits.
- Necrosis or sclerosis? *Necrosis* refers to fresh cell death as a result of ongoing injury, while *sclerosis* reflects a scarred glomerulus or glomerular segment.

As an example:
Focal and segmental glomerulosclerosis affects some glomeruli, but not all, and only part of any affected tuft. The disease leads to scarring within glomeruli.
Diffuse proliferative crescentic glomerulonephritis affects most glomeruli, with hypercellularity (increased cell number) and the formation of crescents in Bowman's space.

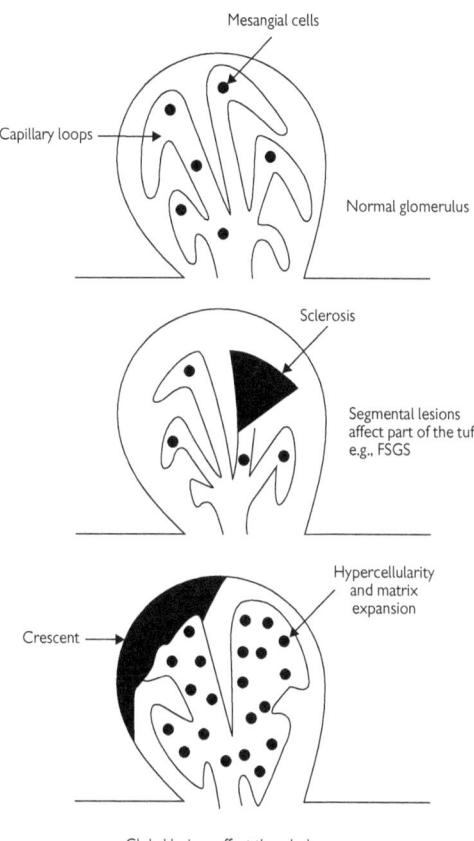

Fig. 6.2 Defining terminology used in describing glomerulonephritis.

Focal and diffuse glomerulonephritis

The underlying pathology is glomerulonephritis. It may present (rapidly) as:
- Impaired renal function
- Hematuria and proteinuria
- Oliguria with signs of fluid retention.

It is a spectrum of disease with a variety of etiologies marked by a common site of primary injury: the glomerulus. Onset may be insidious, with urinary abnormalities alone, or fulminant, with a rapidly progressive crescentic GN and acute renal as well as other organ failure. Patients who have these diseases are often described as having a urinalysis with a nephritic pattern, referring to dysmorphic RBCs and/or RBC casts with variable degrees of proteinuria.

Mechanisms of glomerular injury

The injury leading to most GN is immunologically mediated (Fig. 6.3), with loss of tolerance to autoantigens provoking both arms of the immune system (cellular and humoral). These antigens may be native to the glomerulus itself (occurring normally within the tuft, e.g., the GBM in anti-GBM disease), circulating antigens, or antigen–antibody complexes that become localized in glomerular structures.

Antigen–antibody binding may then fix and activate complement (forming immune complexes [ICs]) or recruit inflammatory cells, causing injury that differs depending on the site of the IC (e.g., IgA-containing complexes in the mesangium activate these cells leading to IgA nephropathy). Local complement activation and recruited neutrophils, and macrophages generate oxidant species and proteases, inflammatory cytokines, growth factors, vasoactive factors, and procoagulants.

Damage to and activation of surrounding cells and matrix then leads to the changes seen on histology: hematuria, proteinuria, and impairment of glomerular filtration. This damage is determined by the location of the ICs, complement fixing properties of the immunoglobulins, in situ vs. passive trapping of ICs, number of ICs formed, and host responses to such ICs. Cellular immunity may add to or cause further structural changes in the glomerulus (especially true of pauci-immune GN, where localized ICs play no role).

Resolution from inflammation may return an inflamed glomerulus to normal, or, if the healing phase is poorly regulated, may lead to cellular dropout, scarring, and CKD.

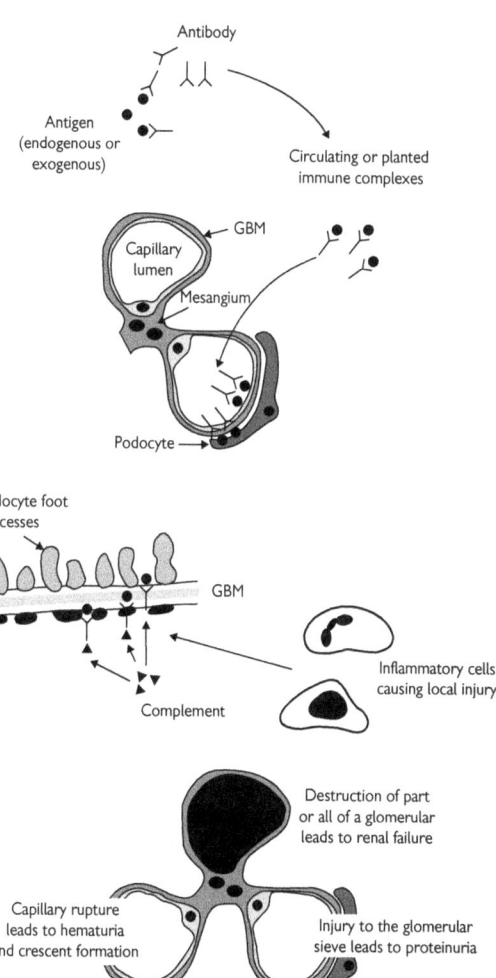

Fig. 6.3 An example of an immune complex–mediated GN.

Approaching focal and diffuse glomerulonephritis

Causes of an acute nephritic syndrome
- IgA nephropathy and Henoch–Schönlein purpura
- Lupus nephritis
- Postinfectious GN
- Anti-GBM disease
- ANCA-positive small-vessel vasculitis and idiopathic pauci-immune GN
- Idiopathic crescentic GN
- Membranoproliferative GN.

Investigations
- Dipstick urine for hematuria, proteinuria
- Urine microscopy for RBC morphology ± casts. RBCs originating from the lower urinary tract are usually normal in appearance. Bleeding from glomerular capillaries means RBCs traverse the tubules and are exposed to osmotic stress, and lysed cells release enzymes that deform RBCs. Dysmorphic RBCs ± acanthocytes (thorn-like spicules on the RBC membrane) may be seen. RBC casts may be present.
- 24-hour proteinuria is variable (may be <1 g/day, but also may be in the nephrotic range).
- BUN, Cr, electrolytes, Ca, PO_4, LFTs.
- Acute phase markers (ESR, C-reactive protein).
- Check rapidly progressive glomerulonephritis lab screen and/or myeloma screen with urinary light chains.
- US kidneys.
- Renal biopsy.

General principles of management of focal and diffuse glomerulonephritis

Sodium and fluid restriction
▶ It is vital to correctly assess volume status.
- Fluid overload ± pulmonary edema often complicates oliguric GN—limit sodium intake ~88 mEq/day (~2 g/day).
- Set oral intake at 1000 mL/day (adjusted according to volume status and UO).
- Diuretics may promote a natriuresis: use loop diuretic, e.g., furosemide 40–400 mg/day po or IV titrated against response and renal function.
- Rarely, dehydration may be present, in which case increased oral intake or volume resuscitation with IV NS may be needed.

Review volume status and monitor weight daily, and chart input and output to plan the following day's fluid balance. An in-dwelling catheter is required only in very ill patients when accurate urine output cannot be recorded.

Control BP
↑BP may be significant and is usually volume-related. Aim for target BP of ≤130/80. ACEI or ARBs offer theoretical advantages in the control of ↑BP secondary to renal disease, due to their antifibrotic and antiproteinuric effects, but their use may precipitate further decline in renal function if there is ARF:
- Use diuretics as above.
- Use step-wise add-on, e.g., β-blockers ± calcium channel blockers.
- ACEI (e.g., ramipril) ± ARB—titrate up from low dose with daily increments—is the first choice once renal function stabilizes.

Dialysis if required according to standard indications (📖 p. 126)
Dialysis may be needed early in cases of ARF secondary to GN: plan ahead for insertion of dialysis access.

Other supportive measures
Other general measures include treatment of infection, adequate nutrition, and management of the other organ complications often associated with systemic diseases causing GN.

Specific therapies: immunosuppression
This is almost always tailored to a histological diagnosis, so renal biopsy is usually indicated as soon as feasible.
  See under particular diagnosis, and "Starting immunosuppression," 📖 p. 368.

Immunosuppressive management of glomerulonephritis

Starting immunosuppression

❶ Treatment of glomerulonephritis often involves aggressive therapies in the short term to improve long-term renal and patient survival. The initial goal is to achieve *induce remission* prior to altering therapy to *maintain* remission. When starting a drug, the dictum of "first do no harm" always applies. These medications have many side effects; you must determine the potential risk/benefit ratio for use.

Monitor toxicity

⚠ CBC, BUN, Cr, electrolytes, LFTs weekly at induction of therapy.

Preventing drug toxicity

- Address with patients the risks of abrupt steroid withdrawal and the need to increase dose with stress (intercurrent illness or anesthesia).
- Prophylaxis against gastric irritation using proton pump inhibitors (PPIs) or H_2 receptor antagonists by convention (evidence is poor).
- Offer prophylaxis against PCP with trimethoprim/sulfamethoxazole for duration of cyclophosphamide therapy (800 mg/160 mg qd or 3 times/week).
- Warn diabetics and those with impaired glucose tolerance to monitor blood sugars closely, and inform their physicians.
- In those at high risk for tuberculosis (e.g., previous TB, recent exposure, patients from endemic areas), consider primary prophylaxis with isoniazid + pyridoxine (evidence is poor).
- Steroid-induced bone demineralization is an early event (within the first months of treatment). Prescribe calcium (1300 mg/day) and vitamin D_3 (800 IU/day) containing preparations. Consider bisphosphonate use (e.g., risedronate SR 35 mg weekly or alendronate SR 70 mg weekly) in those at risk (if >5 mg prednisolone/day for >3 months) to prevent osteoporosis. Many bisphosphonates require 50% dose reduction with CKD.
- Treat steroid-exacerbated hyperlipidemia with HMG-CoA reductase inhibitors (statins). CKD and microalbuminuria increase the risk for cardiac events.

Commonly used drugs

Induction brings about disease remission. Maintenance obviously maintains remission.

Prednisone (I, M)
- To induce remission, use either as high dose po (1 mg/kg/day) or by IV pulse (0.5–1 g/day for 3 days).
- Steroids are also used to maintain remission at lower doses. They act as a potent anti-inflammatory agent, modulating both B- and T-cell-mediated immunity, as well as inhibiting the effector function of both monocytes and neutrophils through regulation of cytokine-driven responses. ▶ Ensure bone and gastric prophylaxis in those at risk, and monitor diabetics for impaired glucose tolerance or worsening glycemic control.

Cyclophoshamide (I)
Use either orally (1–2.5 mg/kg/day) or as IV pulses (0.5–1 g/m² BSA), depending on disease and renal function. This is an alkylating cytotoxic agent that impairs cellular DNA replication, leading to decreased T-cell proliferation and increased cell death, altering inflammatory states. Use in remission is less common with alternative medications available.

Using IV cyclophosphamide
- Body surface area is calculated as $\sqrt{(\text{height (m)} \times \text{Wt (kg)}/3600)}$.
- Advise patient about risks (📖 p. 370).
- Check WBC at day 10–14 and every 2 weeks.
- Ensure prophylaxis vs. PCP with trimethoprim/sulfamethoxazole 160/480 mg qd or three times per week for duration.
- Protect the bladder with vigorous oral fluids, and 1 L NS 2–4 hours before cyclophosphamide infusion. Give intravenous mesna (dose equal to cyclophosphamide dose), half before infusion and half 2 hours after infusion.
- Antiemetics as ondansetron 4–8 mg IV 30 minutes pre- and 4–8 hours post-infusion + dexamethasone 10 mg po at 4 hours after infusion.

Cyclosporine (I, M) is given orally in two divided doses. This is a calcineurin inhibitor that limits IL-2-driven nuclear transduction and thus T-cell activation.

Tacrolimus *is another calcineurin inhibitor increasingly used for similar indications.*

▶ Monitor GFR over longer term for signs of calcineurin inhibitor nephrotoxicity.

Azathioprine (M) is given orally in a single daily dose. An antiproliferative pro-drug, it is metabolized to 6-mercaptopurine, restricting lymphocyte proliferation through inhibition of folate-dependent DNA synthesis.

⚠ Avoid or stop allopurinol as it may precipitate profound leukopenia.

Mycophenolate mofetil (I, M) is given orally in two or three divided doses. It is an antiproliferative drug that inhibits lymphocyte expansion and antibody production. It promotes T-cell-programmed cell death and decreases cell–cell interactions.

Rituximab (I) is an anti-CD20 monoclonal antibody directed against a B-cell surface marker, resulting in widespread B-cell and antibody depletion over time. Rituximab shows promise in treatment of lupus nephritis and other GNs, but it is best used in centers with specialist expertise. It is given weekly (375 mg/m^2) for 4 treatments.

Important side effects
❶ All immunosuppressants predispose to infection by nature.

Prednisone
Insomnia, psychosis, weight gain, ↑BP, impaired glucose tolerance, dyslipidemia, poor wound healing, osteoporosis/aseptic necrosis, and gastritis.

Cyclophosphamide
- Leukopenia, and ↑ risk of infection, especially herpes zoster. Dose is reduced for WBC <3500.
- Gonadal toxicity (discuss loss of fertility prior to starting treatment—in ♀, measure LH/FSH before therapy, and limit total exposure)
- Hemorrhagic cystitis → longer-term bladder cancer (⚠ use mesna if giving IV, and have a low threshold for investigating new hematuria in those previously exposed).
- ⚠ Oral cyclophosphamide is more toxic to the *ovaries* and *bladder* than the IV form, particularly if >10 g cumulative dose is used.
- Nausea and vomiting if given IV.
- Teratogenic.
- Can cause SIADH.
- Rarely hepatitis, cardiomyopathy, pulmonary fibrosis.

Azathioprine
GI side effects (anorexia, nausea, vomiting), myelosuppression, hepatotoxicity (check WBC, LFTs by day 14–21 after starting drug). There is a long-term risk of skin cancers.

MMF
Myelosuppression. GI effects such as nausea and diarrhea in particular are not uncommon—divide dose to tid rather than bid, or reduce drug dose. MMF is teratogenic. There may be an increased risk of lymphoproliferative disease.

Cyclosporine (C) and tacrolimus (T)
Nephrotoxicity, ↑BP (C>T), neurotoxicity (severe headaches, seizures, tremor), hirsutism (C), gum hypertrophy, dyslipidemia, diabetes (T>C), gout (C), thrombotic microangiopathy, squamous cell skin cancer and ?lymphoproliferative disease, among others. Multiple drug interactions change levels.

Tapering steroids

Prednisone is the most widely used oral corticosteroid. Its use in renal disease is usually for >3 weeks, and thus often requires slow tapering to allow recovery of a suppressed hypothalamic–pituitary axis.

▶ You may not need to taper steroids if used for <6 weeks.
  A potential regimen from 20 mg/daily prednisone might be:
  - Reduce by 5 mg every 2 weeks until on 5 mg/day.
  - Reduce to 5 mg alternating with 2.5 mg daily for 2 weeks.
  - Reduce to 2.5 mg daily for 2 weeks.
  - Reduce to 2.5 mg alternate days for 2 weeks.
  - Stop drug.

Advise patient of Addisonian symptoms, and warn patient to seek medical help if they become ill.

IgA nephropathy

IgA nephropathy (IgAN) is the most common primary glomerulonephritis in the world, often presenting with hematuria in the second and third decades. Although usually idiopathic, IgAN may be found in association with Henoch–Schönlein purpura, GI disorders (alcoholic cirrhosis, celiac disease, inflammatory bowel disease), and skin and joint disorders (spondyloarthropathies, dermatitis herpetiformis, psoriasis). Generally, IgAN is an indolent glomerulopathy, but long-term renal damage is common—renal survival is 50%–80% at 20 years.

Pathogenesis

Abnormally galactosylated IgA1 is deposited in the mesangium of the glomerulus (Fig. 6.4). Autoantibodies are formed against abnormal galactosylated IgA1. IgA activates complement and mesangial cells, which produce inflammatory mediators, growth factors, and cytokines. This results in mesangial cell proliferation and matrix synthesis, with inflammatory cell recruitment and subsequent local injury.

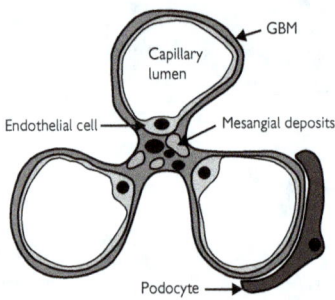

Fig. 6.4 Diagram of mesangial IgA deposits.

Symptoms and signs

IgAN often presents as asymptomatic urinary abnormalities, particularly microscopic hematuria (30%–40%). Hematuria may be macroscopic, classically timed 2–3 days after a viral pharyngitis (so-called synpharyngetic hematuria [30%–50%]) and, less commonly, gastroenteritis, or pneumonia. Associated proteinuria is common, although nephrotic-range proteinuria (>3 g/day) is unusual (<15%). IgAN may present as a rapidly progressive GN with acute renal failure (p. 60). Hypertension is common and often difficult to control.

Investigations

These include BUN, Cr, electrolytes, Ca, PO_4, albumin, lipid profile. Elevated serum IgA occurs in ±50%. Do urine microscopy for dysmorphic RBCs and RBC casts. Spot urine PCR or 24-hour urine protein and creatinine collection is required. If there is associated skin rash, a skin biopsy may show IgA deposition on immunofluorescence for Henoch-Schönlein purpura. In adults do a *renal biopsy*.

Histology

Mesangial cell proliferation and increased mesangial matrix may be focal or diffuse seen on light microscopy. Immunofluorescence (IF) confirms mesangial IgA deposits with C3. There may be co-deposited IgG. Electron microscopy shows mesangial deposits near the paramesangial GBM.

Henoch–Schönlein purpura (HSP)

HSP is a systemic vasculitis affecting predominantly children, presenting as a tetrad of abdominal pain, arthralgias, skin rash, and renal involvement. It is most prevalent in winter, often precipitated by an upper respiratory tract infection, with a 2:1 ♂:♀ ratio. There is recurrence in 1/3 of patients.

- Purpuric rash affecting legs, buttocks, and arms. Skin biopsy shows leukocytoclastic vasculitis with vascular IgA deposition on immunofluorescence.
- Abdominal colic and often GI bleeding related to bowel vasculitis
- Symmetrical polyarthralgias
- GN presenting as hematuria, proteinuria ± renal impairment, and hypertension secondary to IgAN. Usually after systemic symptoms.

In children the illness is usually self-limiting (<2 month duration), with skin manifestations predominating. In adults, HSP more commonly affects the kidneys. Complete resolution is the norm, but persistent urinary abnormalities (especially proteinuria) impart a worse outcome, and long-term follow-up is required. Crescentic IgAN in the context of HSP should be treated as 📖 p. 374.

Management of IgA nephropathy

There is no consensus on treatment because of the heterogeneity of patients and the disease itself. Few adequate trials have been performed, adding to the therapeutic dilemma. Prevention of progressive renal impairment is the goal.

Poor prognostic features at presentation include:
- Impaired renal function
- Proteinuria > 1 g/day (worst if >3 g/day)
- (Difficult to control) hypertension
- Tubulointerstitial fibrosis and glomerulosclerosis on biopsy
- Rapidly progressive crescentic IgAN

Low-risk patients (no poor prognostic features)
- Normal renal function
- <500 mg/day proteinuria
- No hypertension
- Episodic macroscopic hematuria is possibly a good prognostic sign.

▶ Treat BP and reduce proteinuria.

Aim for target BP of ≤125/75 mmHg, ideally with ACEI as the first agent. If patient is normotensive but proteinuric, treat with ACEI for proteinuria reduction. Dual blockade of AII using combined ACEI + ARB may offer additional benefit. Aim to increase ACEI/ARB dose so proteinuria <500–1000 mg/day.

⚫ *Fish oils* (ω-3 fatty acids) have been given to limit progression. They are presumed to act through modulating eicosanoid production and action. They are given as fish oil (OMACOR® or Maxepa®) 3 g qd–often limited by tolerability (GI upset). It is safe. Evidence supporting its use is debated, but it remains a reasonable adjunct to ACEI/ARB if proteinuria persists >1 g/day.

⚫ Use HmG-CoA reductase inhibitors for hypercholesterolemia.

High-risk patients
▶ High-risk patients are often difficult to treat, with frequent progression to ESRD despite therapy.

If treatment with ACEI ± ARB, ± fish oil does not stabilize renal function and reduce proteinuria to < 1 g/day, consider trial of methylprednisolone 1 g for 3 days on months 1, 3, and 5 with prednisone 0.5 mg/kg on alternate days for 6 months (⚫) or perhaps 1 mg/kg/day for 2–3 months followed by taper to 0.5 mg/kg/day for a total of 6 months. Clearly, this is a high-dose corticosteroid regimen with risks.

If there is crescentic IgAN, treat aggressively to spare renal function: prednisone 0.5–1 mg/kg/day + cyclophosphamide 2 mg/kg/day for 8–12 weeks of induction, followed by tapering prednisone and azathioprine 2 mg/kg/day for maintenance.

There is no robust evidence to support treatment of IgAN by removing the nephritogenic IgA1 through diet, tonsillectomy, or drug therapy. Tonsillectomy may help if the IgA does not have poor prognostic signs (↑BP, >1 g/d proteinuria). Whether anti-platelet agents and anticoagulants (as warfarin + dipyramidole) or HMG CoA reductase inhibitors add benefit is also uncertain, but the latter is recommended for hypercholesterolemia and possible further reduction of proteinuria when added to AII inhibition.

Recurrence after transplantation

Mesangial IgA deposition occurs in ± 50% of patients receiving a renal transplant for the treatment of ESRD secondary to primary IgAN, but it does not usually cause accelerated graft loss. It is not a contraindication to transplantation. The same is true for HSP.

Postinfectious glomerulonephritis

This is classically post-streptococcal GN, but infection of almost any cause may be associated with an acute GN and similar findings on kidney biopsy (a diffuse proliferative GN) or MPGN pattern. These include:

- Staphylococcal, pneumococcal, gram-negative infection
- Syphilis
- Influenza B, mumps, Coxsackie, hepatitis B, and Epstein–Barr virus
- Malaria, toxoplasmosis, or schistosomiasis

▶ Endocarditis, (□ p. 486), foreign bodies (shunt nephritis, opposite page), or abscess formation (deep-seated sepsis) often provides the source of chronic infection.

Acute post-streptococcal GN

An immune complex–mediated GN usually occurring in childhood (<7 years old), this form is now rare in developed countries. Classically, the trigger is a streptococcal throat infection some 10–21 days prior to the nephritis, although streptococcal infection elsewhere (or other organisms) may be implicated. Tonsillitis or pharyngitis (commonly), impetigo, otitis media, and cellulitis are common sites of associated infection.

Infection with nephritogenic Lancefield group A [β]-hemolytic streptococcus (especially types 12 and 49) is followed by a latent interval in which immune complex formation and glomerular deposition occurs, before symptoms manifest.

Symptoms and signs
Often gross hematuria (Coca-cola, tea colored), oliguria, edema (peri-orbital and ankle), ↑BP, and pulmonary edema occur. Bilateral loin pain or costovertebral angle (CVA) tenderness is secondary to renal engorgement.

Investigations
Urine microscopy for RBC casts ± pyuria. BUN, Cr, electrolytes, Ca^{2+}, LFTs. Spot urine PCR or 24-hour protein and creatinine. Anti-streptolysin-O titer (ASO) or anti-DNase B (for group A streptococci) may be positive. ↓C3 with normal C4, rheumatoid factor/cryoglobulins may be positive.

Histology
Diffuse and proliferative changes with marked hypercellularity can occur. Cellular crescents and frank necrosis are not common. Extensive neutrophilic infiltration is seen. Subepithelial IgG and complement deposition is seen on immunofluorescence ("starry sky pattern"). Electron microscopy shows large electron-dense deposits ("humps") in the subepithelial aspects of the capillary walls, with endothelial cell swelling. There may be smaller subendothelial deposits. Biopsy changes seen with postinfectious GN are very similar to those of MPGN.

Clinical course
Generally, postinfectious GN is self-limiting if the underlying infection resolves; it is associated with a full renal recovery (even after ARF) in children. In adults, prognosis is more guarded, with only ~50% having full renal recovery. Diuresis usually begins after 7–10 days and heralds resolution. Urinary abnormalities may persist for years after recovery. Patients should be offered long-term follow-up, as HTN and CKD are more common in this group (reflecting post-GN scarring).

Treatment
▶ *Ensure the predisposing infection has resolved, or treat vigorously.*
- Restrict Na^+ (<2 g/day) and fluid. Assess volume status and weight daily. Monitor UO to tailor fluid restriction (1000 mL/day).
- Treat HTN: as Na^+ and water overloaded, start with loop diuretics (e.g., furosemide 40–400 mg po/IV). Add CCB such as amlodipine 5–10 mg qd. or ACEI/ARB after renal function has stabilized (ramipril 2.5–10 mg qd).
- Hemodialysis for standard indications (📖 p. 126).
- Penicillins or other antibiotics only have a role in *ongoing* infection.
- Immunosuppression has not been shown to improve outcome, even with crescents on biopsy, although it is not studied in well-controlled trials. It is used by some with these findings.

Shunt nephritis

This term was originally coined to describe a GN associated with chronically infected ventriculoatrial (but *not* ventriculoperitoneal) shunts used to treat hydrocephalus. In the contemporary era, bacterial biofilms on in-dwelling central lines or pacing wires are more likely to → low-grade infection, immune complex formation, and deposition in the glomerulus. Clinical features in patients with implanted foreign bodies include
- Fever, HTN
- Hematuria, proteinuria, and ↑Cr.

Characteristic findings include positive blood cultures and ↓C3 and C4. Histology shows MPGN with diffuse deposits of IgG, IgM, and C3. Removing the foreign body is essential for resolution.

Endocarditis

Often there is *Staph. aureus* in acute bacterial endocarditis (BE), *Strep. viridans* in subacute BE. Clinical features include
- Fever
- Hematuria, proteinuria (30% have nephrotic syndrome) and ↑Cr.

Characteristic findings include positive blood cultures, ↑ESR, ↓C3 and C4. Histology shows diffuse proliferative, focal proliferative, or MPGN with diffuse deposits of IgG, IgM, and C3. Treatment of the infection.

Visceral abscess

Chronic suppurative infections: intrathoracic, intra-abdominal, dental abscesses, and osteomyelitis. Proliferative glomerulonephritis is seen. HTN, arthralgias, and purpura may be seen. C3 and C4 are normal.

Membranoproliferative glomerulonephritis (MPGN)

MPGN is also called *mesangiocapillary glomerulonephritis*. It is a descriptive histological term rather than a distinct GN with a single cause. MPGN is more commonly found at biopsy in the developing world. Chronic or repeated infection may predispose to the disease. As such, MPGN is frequently described in association with a variety of conditions. It tends to affect ♂ = ♀ aged 8–30 years, and is thought to carry a poor renal prognosis with 50% of patients reaching ESRD at 10 years.

Glomerular deposition of immune complexes localizing in the mesangium and subendothelial space reflects a common mechanism of injury (Fig. 6.5).

- *Type I MPGN* is described either in the *presence* of cryoglobulinemia (and usually hepatitis C) or less commonly in their *absence* as a true primary, or idiopathic MPGN.
- *Dense deposit disease (DDD)*, or type II MPGN, is related to deficiency in complement factor H (often with partial lipodystrophy and retinal abnormalities).
- *Type III MPGN* is similar to type I, but has added membranous change.

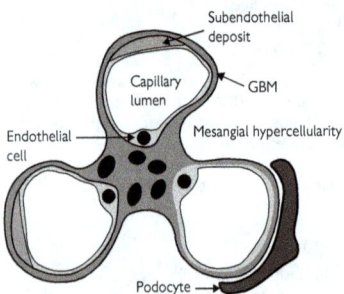

Fig. 6.5 Diagram of subendothelial deposits in MPGN.

Symptoms and signs

↑BP is common. All cases may present as asymptomatic urinary abnormalities, acute nephritis, nephrotic syndrome, or rapidly progressive renal failure.

Investigations

▶ Consider the underlying cause!

BUN, electrolytes (↑Cr), ↓ albumin, ↑ cholesterol, LFTs, immunoglobulins and serum protein electrophoresis (SPEP), spot urine PCR or 24-hour urine protein and creatinine, urine microscopy for RBC casts, hepatitis B+C, C3 nephritic factor, cryoglobulins, rheumatoid factor.

📖 p. 484 for hepatitis C and MPGN.

Complement in MPGN

Type I MPGN: The classical pathway is activated by immune complexes, leading to ↑C4 and normal/↑C3. In DDD (type II), the alternate pathway is activated: ↑C3, normal C4.

▶ An IgG that binds C3 convertase (C3Bb) is present in DDD → persistent cleavage of C3 (the so-called C3 nephritic factor). Findings are similar to those of DDD in type III, but without the C3NF.

Histology

All subtypes have a characteristic "double-contour" or "basement-membrane-splitting" appearance of GBM caused by mesangial cell cytoplasm intervening between endothelium and GBM.

- *Type I:* Diffuse mesangial hypercellularity ± mesangial immune complex deposition occurs. There is a lobular pattern to tufts that may show crescentic changes. Immunofluorescence shows granular IgG and C3 in the capillaries and mesangium.
- *DDD (type II):* May only see mesangial hypercellularity on light. There are widespread ribbon-like, intramembranous, electron-dense deposits containing C3 but no Ig, also in tubular basement membrane.
- *Type III* is similar to type I, but with prominent subepithelial deposits (membranous changes) as well.

Associations with MPGN

- Hepatitis C or B
- Cryoglobulinemia unrelated to HCV (primary, dysproteinemias)
- SLE, Sjogren syndrome
- Shunt nephritis and other chronic infections (📖 p. 377)
- Visceral abscesses, schistosomiasis, malaria, leprosy
- Complement deficiencies
- Thrombotic microangiopathy.

Treatment

❶ *Always exclude causes of secondary MPGN before planning treatment.*
For treatment of hepatitis C– or cryoglobulin-related MPGN, 📖 p. 378.

▶ Evidence-based treatment strategies are lacking for primary MPGN. General measures:
- Control BP and proteinuria with ACEI or ARB (aim for full dose).
- Treat dyslipidemia: HMG-CoA reductase inhibitor.

One option in the context of progressive renal failure or persistent nephrotic syndrome (limited evidence) includes:
- Aspirin 500 mg + dipyramidole 75 mg daily × 1 year

☛ Alternative strategies may offer benefit in nonresponders or as initial treatment, but no good evidence *in adults* exists to support their use:
- Corticosteroids (tapering prednisone started at 1 mg/kg/day) ± cyclophosphamide 2 mg/kg/day for 10 months (significant toxicity! 📖 p. 370)
- MMF ± corticosteroids
- For DDD, consider plasma infusion or plasmapheresis to provide factor H.
- Rituximab is being studied as a possible therapy.

Hereditary nephropathies

Include Alport syndrome and thin membrane disease (TMD) (or benign familial hematuria) in this category.

Alport syndrome
Classically it presents as a triad of
- Hereditary progressive nephropathy
- Sensorineural deafness
- Ocular abnormalities.

Defective basement membrane formation in the glomerulus, cochlea, and eye accounts for these findings. Although inheritance is varied, an X-linked-inherited mutation in the gene encoding α5 type IV collagen accounts for 80% of cases. (AR ~15%, AD ~5%). The X-lined disease leads to afflicted ♂, with ♀ carriers having thin GBMs and microscopic hematuria (but rarely renal impairment).

Thin membrane disease

TMD is an autosomal dominant (AD)-inherited familial condition presenting with urinary abnormalities (especially hematuria) almost always with normal renal function. The normal GBM is ±350 nm thick—in TMD it is often <200 nm.

A thin GBM may occur in 5% of people, but urinary abnormalities are less common. The underlying defect probably affects type IV collagen integration into the GBM, but results in a partial failure of basement membrane function.

Symptoms and signs
Both hereditary nephropathies present with asymptomatic hematuria early in life (in childhood with Alport syndrome) (see Table 6.1).

Alport syndrome Proteinuria (often nephrotic range) and ↑BP usually are present by adolescence. There is progressive CKD → ESRD by the fourth decade. High-tone sensorineural deafness and lenticonus (conical rather than spherical lens leading to distorted vision) are typical.

TMD is often a diagnosis of exclusion: proteinuria, ↑BP, or CKD is RARE, although stone formation and gross hematuria may occur.

Investigations
- Inheritance may differentiate TMD from Alport syndrome in early cases.
- BUN, Cr, electrolytes, LFTs, Ca, PO$_4$, lipid profile. Urine for microscopy (p. 12), spot urine PCR or 24-hour urinary protein and creatinine collection.
- ***Alport syndrome*** Audiometry and ophthalmic assessment. Skin biopsy using monoclonal antibody against α5 type IV collagen may assist if it is clearly negative in males and clearly mosaic in females. Molecular genetic testing will be used in the future. *Renal biopsy* may be required.

Histology

Alport syndrome Nonspecific glomerulosclerosis and tubulointerstitial scarring are present on light microscopy (especially if ↑Cr). A thin GBM on electron microscopy with a characteristic "basket weave" pattern is diagnostic, and negative staining with antibodies directed against type IV collagen in the GBM secures the diagnosis.

TMD Normal light microscopy. Electron microscopy demonstrates reduction in GBM diameter.

Treatment

- Patients with uncomplicated TMD can be reassured, but should be followed up at yearly intervals (for urinalysis, BP and creatinine check).
- No specific treatment for Alport syndrome exists. As with all progressive nephropathies, good control of BP and use of ACEI/ARB should be considered early (📖 p. 342). (Cyclosporine has been used for heavy proteinuria in a case series with success; however, its role is uncertain.)
- Family members should be screened for hematuria and ↑BP.

Transplantation and Alport syndrome

In <5% of cases, transplanted Alport patients may develop de novo anti-GBM antibodies and a rapidly progressive crescentic glomerulonephritis, as donor α5 type IV collagen is recognized as non-self. It is not a contraindication to transplantation.

Table 6.1 TMD or Alport syndrome?

	TMD	Alport syndrome
Hematuria	+ to +++	++
Proteinuria	±	+++ (>3 g/day)
↑BP	–	+++
Renal dysfunction	±	+++
Deafness/lenticonus	–	++
Family history of ESRD	–	++
Father-to-son transmission	+	–

Other forms of glomerulonephritis

Often referred to as "mesangial proliferative GN," C1q and IgM nephropathies remain ill-characterized and unusual lesions, thought by some to represent a spectrum between minimal change nephropathy (MCN) and focal and segmental glomerulosclerosis (FSGS). Patients present with proteinuria (often nephrotic range) and hematuria ± ↑Cr. Focal or diffuse mesangial proliferation, a relatively nonspecific glomerular response to a variety of injuries, is found at biopsy.

The differential diagnosis includes.
- Lupus nephritis
- IgA nephropathy
- Mild postinfectious GN.

C1q nephropathy

This is a mesangial proliferative GN that closely resembles lupus nephritis histologically, but without any serological or clinical criteria for the diagnosis of SLE. Histology shows a characteristic heavy deposition of C1q-containing deposits in the mesangium and elsewhere, with varying degrees of mesangial hypercellularity and "wire loop" capillary wall thickening. Secondary FSGS-like lesions occur as well.

IgM nephropathy

This is a similar lesion, presenting with the nephrotic syndrome, and characterized by prominent IgM and complement deposition in the mesangium.

Idiopathic mesangial proliferative GN

This is a diagnosis of exclusion, with mesangial proliferation on biopsy, but no immune complex deposition on immunofluorescence. There is considerable uncertainty over the efficacy of specific treatment.

Treatment

It seems reasonable to treat these GNs presenting with nephrotic syndrome with corticosteroids as one would for MCN or FSGS and perhaps those with progressive renal impairment with an additional agent as well (p. 368–370). As a group, they are not felt to be as steroid responsive as minimal change disease.

The nephrotic syndrome

This clinical syndrome is defined as having >3.5 g proteinuria/1.73 m^2 body surface area/day with hypoalbuminemia, edema, and hyperlipidemia. The syndrome arises from the failure of the glomerular filtration barrier to restrict the passage of protein into the urine, and reflects structural abnormalities within the glomerular filter, made up of a charged endothelial cell layer, and its fenestrations, the glomerular basement membrane (GBM), and interdigitating podocytes with slit diaphragms between podocyte foot processes.

Normally, the passage through the glomerular filter of albumin in particular, with its net negative charge, is prevented by size-specific factors (such as the slit diaphragm), and charge-specific factors (the anionic endothelial glycocalyx and GBM). Albumin escaping into the proximal tubule is efficiently absorbed by receptor-mediated endocytosis, degraded, and returned to the circulation as peptide fragments.

Many primary and secondary causes of the nephrotic syndrome are now thought to be due to abnormalities of or injury to the podocyte slit diaphragm or the GBM.

Causes of the nephrotic syndrome
- Diabetic glomerulosclerosis
- Membranous nephropathy
- Minimal change nephropathy
- Focal and segmental glomerulosclerosis
- Membranoproliferative glomerulonephritis
- Renal amyloidosis
- Light-chain deposition disease
- SLE.

Investigation of the nephrotic syndrome
- BUN, Cr, electrolytes, total protein and albumin, Ca, PO_4, LFTs
- Fasting lipid profile
- Urinalysis for microscopy for casts or lipid bodies
- Spot or 24-hour urinary protein and creatinine excretion, UPEP for selectivity. Selective proteinuria is the loss of albumin (minimal change disease), whereas nonselective proteinuria includes both albumin and small molecular-weight proteins <100 kDa such as immunoglobulins appearing in the urine.
- Creatinine clearance or estimated GFR
- Full nephrotic screen (📖 p. 48)
- Ultrasound of the kidneys
- Renal biopsy.

General principles of management

Salt and fluid restriction
↑ Primary Na^+ retention and ↑ blood volume → dependent edema. A fall in plasma oncotic pressure as a result of severe hypoalbuminemia (minimal change disease) may contribute further to fluid losses into the interstitium.
- Restrict sodium to 88 mEq/day (<2 g/day).
- Diuretics: a loop diuretic such as furosemide, at 40 mg/day po increasing to 200 mg daily. If grossly edematous, the patient may require IV diuretics to overcome impaired oral absorption of drugs secondary to gut edema.
- Furosemide with salt-poor albumin (as 50–100 mg in 100 mL 20% human albumin solution over 1 hour) may enhance diuresis; this has not been systematically studied.
- ▶ Monitor for volume overload.
- Addition of thiazide-type diuretics such as metolazone 2.5–5 mg on alternate days to daily may promote diuresis with high-dose loop diuretics.
- ▶ *Daily measurement of Na^+ and K^+ is required to prevent profound electrolyte imbalance—use cautiously in the outpatient setting.*

Fluid losses are best measured by regular weighing, aiming for 0.5–1 kg loss/day. Intake and output should be charted (in-dwelling urinary catheters are rarely needed).

Protein restriction and reducing proteinuria
Proteinuria itself leads to tubulointerstitial inflammation and fibrosis, accelerating declining renal function. Hypoalbuminemia leaves nephrotic patients susceptible to infection and malnutrition.
- Anti-proteinuric drugs (ACEI or ARB) titrated carefully toward full dose (administer at night if hypotension) may reduce proteinuria by up to 50% by 8 weeks and prevent or delay further progression.
- Treat hypertension aiming for 125/75 mmHg.
- Protein restriction is controversial. It is avoided with massive proteinuria. Some recommend 0.8 g/kg/day ±1 g for every gram urine protein loss, along with careful nutritional assessment.

Hypercoagulability
Increased hepatic synthesis of procoagulant factors, ↑platelet aggregation, and ↑ urinary losses of anticoagulant factors occur with nephrotic syndrome. Up to 20% of patients with membranous nephropathy (p. 390) as an underlying cause will develop a deep vein thrombosis (DVT) and up to 30% will develop renal vein thrombosis, both of which may be associated with pulmonary emboli. Membranous, membranoproliferative GN and minimal change disease are the most common causes of nephrotic syndrome associated with thromboemboli.
- Shortness of breath with pleuritic chest pain in a nephrotic patient should make you suspect pulmonary emboli. Many with PE are asymptomatic.
- New-onset hematuria and flank pain may imply renal vein thrombosis (p. 414). Usually this has an insidious presentation and is asymptomatic.

- Anticoagulate all patients with proven DVT with warfarin.
- Treat for the duration of the nephrotic syndrome for an INR 2–3.
- Consider prophylactic anticoagulation for high-risk patients with severe nephrotic syndrome such as those with membranous or membranoproliferative GN with serum albumin <2–2.5 g/dL.

Infection

Infections should be treated promptly, with coverage for encapsulated organisms (low IgG levels predispose to infection). Persistently nephrotic patients should be offered vaccination against pneumococcal disease.

Dyslipidemia

Increased hepatic synthesis (possibly as a response to reduced plasma oncotic pressure) and reduced catabolism of LDL cholesterol contribute as causes. Successful treatment of elevated LDL cholesterol may prevent cardiovascular morbidity and slow decline in renal function.
- Dietary restriction is usually insufficient.
- Use HMG-CoA-reductase inhibitors (statins).

Definition of response
- Complete remission is reduction of urine protein <300 mg/day.
- Partial remission in usually defined as >50% reduction in urine protein excretion with total urine protein <3.5 g/day. Some have used a definition of >50% reduction in urine protein excretion.

Minimal change nephropathy

This is the most common cause of the nephrotic syndrome in children; it is less common in adults (10%–25% of cases). In adults, 1♂:1♀. Generally, the prognosis is excellent.

The pathogenesis of minimal change nephropathy (MCN) is unknown, but a disorder of T lymphocytes is proposed. There is a postulated circulating T-lymphocyte factor that damages or alters podocytes. Subsequent albuminuria may be a result of loss of net membrane negative charge, leading to failure of the glomerular filtration barrier.

Symptoms and signs

Edema is often massive, with facial and periorbital swelling, and ascites. Nephrotic-range proteinuria is always present, with microscopic hematuria being uncommon. Urine may be described as foamy (protein has a detergent effect). There may be lipiduria, visible on microscopy as oval fat bodies. MCN may present with infections (especially skin and soft tissue) or hypotension (secondary to hypovolemia), more often in children. Abdominal pain may be due to spontaneous peritonitis.

Certain factors have been reported to trigger the nephrotic syndrome: allergens and immunizations, malignancies (especially lymphomas), viral infections, NSAIDs, and, rarely, lithium and tiopronin. The clinical course may be complicated by oliguric ARF secondary to ATN in up to 25% of patients. Patients are at increased risk for thromboemboli (renal vein thrombosis in 24%).

Investigations

BUN, Cr, electrolytes, ↓ albumin, LFTs, Ca, PO_4, ↑ cholesterol. Urinalysis may show hyaline, granular, fatty casts. Order spot or 24-hour urinary protein and creatinine collection (selective proteinuria, 📖 p. 384). There are no specific markers of MCN. Adults require *renal biopsy*.

Histology

Histological findings are normal on light microscopy (hence "minimal change"), and immunofluorescence is negative. Electron microscopy reveals diffuse effacement of podocyte foot processes. If there is concurrent acute renal failure, you may see ATN in elderly patients with hypertensive disease, or interstitial nephritis with NSAIDS.

Treatment

Follow symptomatic treatment as outlined (📖 p. 385).

In both adults and children, MCN remits to corticosteroids. Almost all children respond rapidly by 8 weeks; however, adults may take longer with 75%–80% achieving remission by 12–16 weeks of therapy.

- Prednisone 1 mg/kg daily (to maximum of 80 mg/day) until remission is achieved. Taper prednisone every 2 weeks, then weekly, until discontinued. Treat for not less than 12 weeks at first presentation (some advocate 2 mg/kg qod)
- Relapse can be expected in 30%–70% cases.

- Relapse should be treated as above, but taper steroids immediately on remission, aiming for short courses.
- 📖 p. 368 on initiating immunosuppression.

Certain subgroups will experience recurrent relapses off steroids after responding to treatment ("frequently relapsing," two relapses inside 6 months), or relapse during or within 2 weeks of steroid withdrawal ("steroid-dependent"), or not respond to steroids at all (no remission within 12 weeks of treatment, "steroid-resistant").

▶ Ensure that the histological diagnosis is MCN rather than FSGS (📖 p. 388)—you may need repeat kidney biopsy to get adequate sampling.

Consider
- Cyclophosphamide 2 mg/kg/day for 8–12 weeks then stop for frequent-relapsing or steroid-dependent patients. Usually start cyclophosphamide while in remission with steroids.
- Calcineurin inhibitor. Cyclosporine 4–5 mg/kg/day or tacrolimus in two divided doses for 12 months. Use especially if there are relapses on cyclophosphamide. May use if steroid resistant. Monitor GFR to prevent calcineurin inhibitor nephrotoxicity.
- If remission is not achieved with one regimen, consider the other.
- Mycophenolate mofetil and azathioprine have been used as alternative therapies in small case series and case reports.
- Steroid-resistant disease may be treated with calcineurin inhibitors. There is a poor overall response to cyclophosphamide in this population.
- 📖 p. 368 on initiating immunosuppression.

Membranous nephropathy (MN)

This is one of the most common worldwide causes of the nephrotic syndrome, with a peak incidence in the fourth to sixth decades, 2♂:1♀. It may be idiopathic (IMN) or secondary (📖 p. 392).

MN is characterized by IgG-rich immune deposit accumulation on the outer aspect of the GBM (Fig. 6.6), possibly due to antibodies being directed against an unknown antigen expressed either on or next to the podocyte foot processes. Antibody-mediated complement activation and formation of membrane attack complex lead to free-radical generation, podocyte injury, and abnormal GBM synthesis. Trapped circulating immune complexes derived from exogenous antigens may be responsible in secondary forms of the disease.

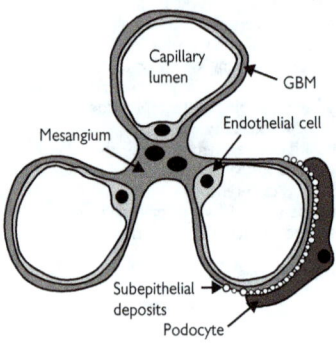

Fig. 6.6 Diagram of subepithelial deposits in MN.

Symptoms and signs

Most present with the nephrotic syndrome. There may be edema, microscopic hematuria, or hypertension. Consider underlying disease to rule out secondary membranous nephropathy.

If a patient has shortness of breath think of pulmonary embolus in the setting of ↓↓ serum albumin (<2–2.5 g/dL) and severe proteinuria (>10 g/day). A slow increase in serum creatinine, rarely flank pain or gross hematuria, may occur with renal vein thrombosis. It is usually asymptomatic.

Investigations

BUN, Cr, electrolytes, ↓↓ albumin, LFTs, Ca, PO_4, ↑LDL cholesterol, ↓immunoglobulins are common (IgG > IgA). Get 24-hour urine protein and creatinine collection or spot urine PCR (nonselective proteinuria, 📖 p. 384). Test for hepatitis B and C, ANA, anti-DNA, RPR, and age-appropriate cancer screening if clinically suspicious. Proceed to *renal biopsy*.

Histology

There may be normal light microscopy early, or in more advanced cases biopsy will show GBM thickening and "spikes" of GBM extending around subepithelial deposits; this is often best seen on silver stains. There may be a variable degree of ATN and tubulointerstitial fibrosis. Granular IgG ± C3 deposits are present on immunofluorescence. Presence of the IgG4 subclass points toward idiopathic MN. Subepithelial electron-dense deposits with foot process effacement are evident on electron microscopy. Secondary membranous nephropathy may show mesangial or subendothelial deposits with other IgG subclasses. Tubular staining on immunofluorescence or tululoreticular inclusions in endothelial cells on electron microscopy are suggestive of lupus membranous nephropathy rather than the idiopathic form.

Treatment

Symptomatic treatment 📖 p. 385.

Disease-modifying treatment

The natural history of MN is variable, with 20%–33% of patients having spontaneous remission, 20%–30% progressing to ESRD, and about 25%–40% with persistent proteinuria. The aim is to predict the course of the disease and treat those with high risk of progression.

Low risk
- Normal renal function
- Proteinuria <4 g/day or spontaneously decreasing proteinuria
- Women, <50 years old
- Nl Cr.

Symptomatic treatment. Expect remission (up to 4 years after diagnosis), but regularly reassess risk. Measure BUN, Cr, electrolytes, albumin, and proteinuria regularly.

High risk
- ♂ >50 years old
- Impaired renal function
- Proteinuria >10 g/day
- Persistent proteinuria >8 g/day for >6–12 months
- Interstitial scarring on renal biopsy.

▶ Disease-modifying therapy reduces proteinuria, spares renal function, and induces remission.
- Corticosteroids alone are not thought to be beneficial.
- Alternate monthly, steroids and alkylating agents for 6 months. Give steroids as methylprednisolone 1 g IV daily x3 days, then prednisone 0.4 mg/kg/day for the remainder of month on months 1, 3, and 5. Two alkylating agents have been used successfully with steroids: either chlorambucil at a dose of 0.1–0.2 mg/kg/day, or cyclophosphamide, 1.5–2.5 mg/kg/day given on months 2, 4, and 6.
- Another regimen is daily po prednisone 1 mg/kg/day + cyclophosphamide 1.5 mg/kg/day, tapering steroids against response.
- Treatment is often limited by toxicity (📖 p. 392).
- Alternatively, give cyclosporine 3.5–4 mg/kg/day (levels of 125–175 ng/mL) or tacrolimus (levels of 5–7 ng/mL) in two divided doses with steroids

for 12 months. Shorter courses often lead to relapses. Monitor GFR to exclude calcineurin inhibitor nephrotoxicity.
- MMF in combination with steroids may also induce remission in some case series.
- Rituximab, a monoclonal anti-CD20 antibody, has been used with success in one series.
- With declining renal function, you may need to continue treatment with steroids and alkylating agent.

Secondary MN

This is not uncommon in children and older adults. Presentation with nephrotic syndrome may not necessarily coincide with presentation of underlying disease. Malignancies in particular may rarely be preceded by MN by 1–2 years. Causes include the following:

Infections
- Hepatitis B and C
- Malaria
- Streptococcal infection
- Syphilis or leprosy
- Schistosomiasis.

Neoplasms
- Solid tumors (lung, colon, breast, kidney, stomach)
- Hodgkin's disease
- Non-Hodgkin's lymphoma.

Multisystem disease
- SLE
- Rheumatoid arthritis
- Autoimmune thyroiditis
- Dermatitis herpetiformis
- Sarcoidosis.

Drugs and toxins
- Captopril
- Gold
- D-penicillamine
- NSAIDs.

Approaching MN
Take a careful history focusing on the following:
- Medications
- Risk factors for hepatitis viruses or other infections (travel, sexual history, transfusions)
- Malignancy. If history and physical examination alone do not suggest an associated neoplasm, extensive investigation is unwarranted and unlikely to reveal any tumor. Some older patients (>50) may need further imaging or colonoscopy per age-appropriate screening.

Treatment of secondary MN
This involves treating the underlying condition and leads to remission of the nephrotic syndrome in many cases.

Focal and segmental glomerulosclerosis (FSGS)

FSGS is a histological description rather than a disease (see Fig. 6.7). *Secondary FSGS* occurs against a background of glomerular damage and dropout in an already abnormal kidney, causing hemodynamic stress on remaining nephrons, and a so-called hyperfiltration injury. *Idiopathic* or *primary FSGS* differs from secondary FSGS in being a *de novo* glomerulopathy rather than as a result of an associated disease.

FSGS occurs more often in ♂ than ♀ (2:1) and two thirds of the nephrotic syndrome in the African-American population is due to FSGS. It is the leading cause of ESRD due to primary glomerular disease in the U.S.

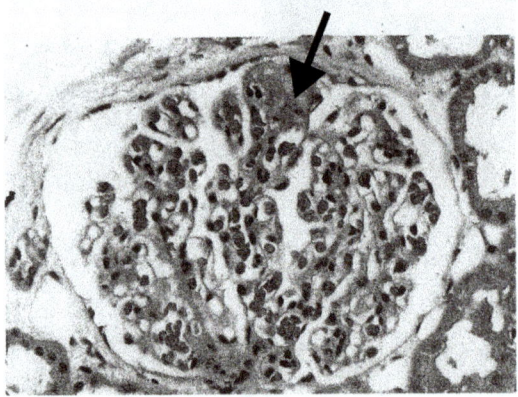

Fig. 6.7 A segmental sclerosis in an affected tuft.

Primary FSGS

The cause remains unknown. Because the disease may recur immediately after transplantation and may be improved after plasmapheresis, a circulating permeability factor(s) has been implicated, but not yet identified. Injury to the podocyte and a subsequent abnormal podocyte response to injury are features of the disease. Some familial and steroid-resistant forms are due to specific podocyte mutations.

Symptoms and signs

Proteinuria is often heavy, with microscopic hematuria and ↑BP. Impaired renal function is common. Young black males presenting with heavy proteinuria (>10 g/day), profound hypoalbuminemia (albumin <2 g/dL), and renal impairment tend to follow a more severe course, often ending in ESRD.

FOCAL AND SEGMENTAL GLOMERULOSCLEROSIS (FSGS)

Investigations
BUN, Cr, electrolytes, ↓ albumin, LFTs, Ca, PO_4, ↑LDL cholesterol. Get spot or 24-hour urine protein and creatinine collection (nonselective proteinuria, 📖 p. 384). Proceed to renal biopsy.

Histology
A focal (affecting some but not all glomeruli) and segmental (affecting part but not all of a glomerular tuft) process with mesangial matrix expansion, glomerular sclerosis, and hyalinosis is apparent. No abnormality may be seen if the sample size is small, reflecting the focal nature of the disease. Some IgM and C3 may be trapped in sclerotic lesions on immunofluorescence. Electron microscopy demonstrates diffuse podocyte foot process effacement. Tubulointerstitial fibrosis is not uncommon. Subclassification has five different variants (FGS NOS [not otherwise specified], collapsing, tip, perihilar, and cellular). The particular variant may have prognostic importance: the presence of "tip lesions" (segmental scleroses affecting the outer tip of the glomerulus alongside the proximal tubule) implies a better, more steroid-responsive course. The collapsing variant has a worse prognosis than that of other subtypes.

Secondary FSGS
This may be found with the following conditions:
- Reduced nephron number
- Glomerular disease and obsolescence with glomerular hyperfiltration
- Any cause of quiescent glomerulonephritis with scarring

Secondary FSGS tends to present with less proteinuria and hypoalbuminemia than the primary variant.

Collapsing glomerulopathy describes an FSGS-like lesion with glomerular tuft collapse, GBM wrinkling, and cystic tubular changes with interstitial fibrosis. It is usually due to HIVAN (📖 p. 480). It may be idiopathic, or associated with other viral diseases (parvovirus) and high-dose *pamidronate* (possibly other bisphosphonates as well). It presents with severe nephrotic syndrome and declining renal function, and generally carries a poor renal prognosis.

Secondary FSGS causes
- Reflux nephropathy
- Renal dysplasia
- Renovascular disease
- Diabetic nephropathy
- HIV-associated nephropathy
- Heroin-associated nephropathy
- Preeclampsia
- Sickle cell disease
- Membranous nephropathy
- Alport syndrome
- Morbid obesity.

Treatment of FSGS

In secondary FSGS, treat the underlying cause if possible. The general approach is as for any progressive proteinuric nephropathy (📖 p. 158). Even in biopsy-proven primary FSGS, in those with <2 g/day proteinuria, symptomatic treatment with ACEI and ARB with watchful waiting are advised.

For symptomatic treatment for the nephrotic syndrome, 📖 p. 385. Particular attention to anti-proteinuric agents should be given.

Disease-modifying treatment

- Prednisone 1 mg/kg/day (max 80 mg) for upto 12–16 weeks to determine responsiveness with total course in 6 months. FSGS is slow to respond and shorter courses of steroids are of little use. If there is a response (remission of nephrotic syndrome), taper steroids after a further 12 weeks. Unlike minimal change disease, a degree of proteinuria usually persists. (Presence of "tip lesions" (📖 p. 395) improves the likelihood of response.)
- Alternatively, use calcineurin inhibitor with low-dose or even no steroids if patient is felt to be a poor steroid candidate (see below).
- MMF is being used in an NIH-sponsored randomized controlled trial with oral dexamethasone and prednisone vs. cyclosporine and prednisone. Some success and failure with MMF has been reported in various case series.

After a 6-month course of steroids, 30%–65% of patients will achieve a meaningful reduction (>50%) in proteinuria. Those who relapse while on (tapering) steroids are defined as "steroid-dependent," and those in whom no reduction in proteinuria is achieved are deemed "steroid resistant." In these groups:

- Continue low-dose (10–15 mg/day) prednisone and add cyclosporine (3.5 mg/kg/day) or tacrolimus in two divided doses. Aim for trough cyclosporine levels 125–175 ng/mL or tacrolimus 5–7 ng/mL. Treat for 1 year, then taper dose and stop if response continues. In small trials, response rates of 70% have been reported. Many responders will be calcineurin inhibitor dependent, relapsing with drug withdrawal, especially if used for shorter time courses.
- Consider MMF in patients who are steroid resistant or dependent and calcineurin inhibitor dependent or intolerant.

🔑 Few data exist on how to treat the more aggressive form of the disease, presenting as severe nephrotic syndrome and progressive renal impairment in younger patients.
An alternative to cyclosporine in such patients is
- Cyclophosphamide 2 mg/kg/day for a minimum of 12 weeks.

The toxicity of all such treatment regimes needs to be considered on an individual basis.

Thrombotic microangiopathy (TMA)

TMA is caused by a disparate group of systemic disorders due to endothelial injury characterized by a triad of microangiopathic hemolytic anemia, thrombocytopenia, and organ dysfunction from platelet or platelet-fibrin aggregation and hyaline thrombotic occlusion of small vessels. Widespread thrombosis consumes platelets and causes nonimmune hemolysis.

Trying to distinguishing hemolytic-uremic syndrome (HUS) from thrombotic thrombocytopenic purpura (TTP) is often difficult and somewhat controversial. Some prefer the term *thrombotic microangiopathy (TMA)* or *HUS/TTP*. Generally, renal failure is considered a feature in HUS, whereas neurologic complications may be more prominent in TTP; however, there may be an overlap in symptoms. Patients may have multiorgan failure with pancreatitis, and cardiomyopathy.

Shiga toxin, *S. pneumoniae*, and genetic forms cause HUS. Inhibitors or deficiencies in ADAMTS13 activity result in TTP. Other causes are often lumped together as TMA.

Causes

Thrombotic thrombocytopenic purpura (TTP)
- Idiopathic, genetic forms

Hemolytic-uremic syndrome (HUS)
D+ form (typical shigatoxin)
- Associated with diarrhea *E. coli* O157:H7 (*Shigella dysenteriae* serotype 1, *Salmonella*, *Campylobacter*, or *Yersinia*)

D− form, atypical
- Complement deficiencies in factors H, I, or B, or membrane cofactor protein
- *S. pneumoniae*

Other thrombotic microangiopathies
- Pregnancy—near term or postpartum
- Systemic lupus erythematosus (SLE) (📖 p. 468), rheumatoid arthritis (RA) (📖 p. 476) and system vasculitis (📖 p. 456), scleroderma (📖 p. 474), others
- Anti-phospholipid syndrome (primary or as part of SLE, 📖 p. 472)
- Hematopoietic stem cell or solid-organ transplant
- Medications: cyclosporine A, tacrolimus, mitomycin C, quinine, sirolimus, ciprofloxacin, oral contraceptives, clopidogrel, and bevacizumab
- Malignancy
- HIV
- Malignant hypertension (📖 p. 350)
- Scleroderma renal crisis

General points
Take a careful history for diarrheal illness. Examine for petechiae and purpura. Check dipstick for hematuria, proteinuria, and bilirubinuria (hemolysis). Check BP and fundi. ?Skin signs of systemic sclerosis. ?Splenomegaly.

Investigations
- CBC (↓Hb, ↓↓Plt), smear for RBC hemolysis, INR, PTT, D-dimers/FDP, reticulocyte count, ↓haptoglobin, Coombs' test (negative)
- β-HCG. ↑LDH, BUN, Cr, electrolytes, LFTs (↑bilirubin), uric acid. Blood and stool cultures
- ANA, dsDNA, complements, anti-phospholipid antibodies
- Renal biopsy if platelet count allows.

Histology
TMAs share similar renal histology. Thrombi are present in the glomerular capillaries with resultant ischemia. Immunofluorescence for Ig and complement are negative. Electron microscopy shows capillary thrombi composed of either platelet-fibrin (HUS) or platelets (TTP), and endothelial injury and swelling with subendothelial deposits. Pathology may show renal limited disease without systemic effects (some cases with calcineurin inhibitors).

Thrombotic thrombocytopenic purpura (TTP)

Ultra-large von Willebrand factor (ulvWF) is released from endothelial cells as a large polymer and normally cleaved to form the mature polypeptide (vWF) that acts as a matrix for hemostasis. The protease responsible for this cleavage is the zinc metalloproteinase ADAMTS13. If the ulvWF cleaving protein activity is severely (5%) impaired (IgG autoantibody directed against the protease or inherited mutations encoding ADAMTS13), ultra-large vWF multimers enter the circulation and, under shear stress, bind and activate platelets. This leads to spontaneous platelet aggregation, platelet-rich (though fibrin-poor) thrombus formation, and a *systemic* microangiopathy.

Although ADAMTS13 activity and inhibition tests predict repalse, these bests results do not come back quickly enough to influence therapy if TTP is suspected clinicallly.

Symptoms and signs (in addition to general features, 📖 p. 398)

A pentad of microangiopathic hemolytic anemia, thrombocytopenic purpura, central nervous system involvement (confusion, seizures, or any other neurological abnormality), fever, and ARF (oliguria, anuria) occurs.

Investigations (📖 p. 399)

Monitor disease: ↓↓Plt, red cell hemolysis on smear, ↑↑LDH, ↓haptoglobin. Very low ADAMTS13 activity (<5% normal) in the correct clinical setting is diagnostic, but assays differ and may have higher values. In the acute setting, unless this test is performed on site, results from reference labs can take >1 week, so diagnosis is dependent on clinical judgment.

Hemolytic-uremic syndrome (HUS)

HUS may be associated with diarrhea due to Shiga-like toxin (D+, Shiga-toxin+), with peak incidence in summer. It usually affects children <5 years of age. HUS occurs after food poisoning (undercooked meat, unpastuerized milk, or contract with animal feces). Pathogenic bacteria produce a Shiga-like endotoxin that translocates across inflamed colonic mucosa, binding glomerular endothelial, mesangial, and tubular epithelial cells. An ↑ in prothrombotic factors, and ultra-large vWF multimers are released from damaged endothelial cells.

In the absence of diarrhea (D– or atypical HUS), hereditary mutations in factor H (a complement regulatory protein), complement factor I, complement factor B, and membrane cofactor protein are responsible in 50% of these cases. These genetic mutations result in decreased degradation of complement with resulting increase in renal endothelial injury during states of complement activation either directly or indirectly (endothelial injury). There is no reduction of ADAMTS13 in most cases of HUS (i.e., it has a different pathophysiology from TTP).

Infections associated with D+ HUS

- *E. coli* O157:H7
- *Shigella dysenteriae* serotype 1
- *Salmonella, Campylobacter,* or *Yersinia*

Associations with D– HUS

- Atypical HUS (mutations in factor H, membrane cofactor protein, complement factor I, complement factor B)
- *S. pneumoniae* or rickettsial infection

Symptoms and signs (in addition to general features, p. 398)

A triad of microangiopathic hemolytic anemia, and thrombocytopenia + renal involvement occurs. Diarrhea is bloody in most children and occasionally in adults. There is also fever, ↑BP, oliguria, and fluid overload.

Investigations (p. 399)

- ↑CBC common. Stool for culture and shigatoxin assay
- Monitor disease: ↓↓Plt, RBC fragments on film, ↑↑LDH.

Management of HUS, TTP, and TMA

Plasmapheresis (PP)
This is used for idiopathic TTP, drug-induced TTP, pregnancy HIV, Transplant Associated, autoimmune TMA, and Drug (quinine, clopidogel), and is considered in adults with D+ HUS. PP is not felt to be efficacious in childhood D+ HUS. The use of PP in cancer-associated disease and bone marrow transplant-associated disease is controversial.

PP allows for large-volume plasma infusion as well as removal of vWF cleaving protein inhibitor, especially if the patient is oligoanuric.

- Administer daily PP until plt count and LDH are normalized for 2 days (usually 7–16 days).
- Exchange 1–1.5 plasma volume/day. Use 1.0 volume/day for ARF to avoid volume overload (📖 p. 640).
- Patients are usually treated with steroids, prednisone 1–2 mg/kg or 1 g IV methylprednisolone for 3 days until there is improvement in idiopathic TTP, pregnancy, and autoimmune disorders. You may need to prevent allergic reactions to large volumes of plasma. Rituximab has been used with success in refractory or relapsing TTP.

Fresh frozen plasma is used as replacement fluid until there is improvement. Plasma infusion is inferior to plasma exchange, but *is* efficacious if PP is unavailable. Beware of fluid overload.

⚠ Avoid platelet transfusion unless there is life-threatening bleeding (it "fuels the fire"). There is no role for aspirin or anticoagulants. Resistant disease may be treated by increasing PP to twice daily, or using rituximab (anti-CD20 monoclonal antibody).

If prompt plasma infusion or exchange is instituted, patient survival should be up to 90%. Renal survival is good, with dialysis-requiring ARF being unusual. A third of patients may be expected to relapse.

⚠ If in doubt of diagnosis, use plasmapheresis.

For D+ HUS, management is supportive alone in children. PP has not been shown to consistently improve outcome in some TMA cases (malignancy, mitomycin C, gemcitabine, hematopoietic transplant).

Tubulointerstitial diseases

Acute interstitial nephritis (AIN)

AIN, or acute tubulointerstitial nephritis, is a common parenchymal cause of unexplained acute renal failure, usually in response to drugs. Incidence in ♂ = ♀, usually in their 50s and 60s, but can occur at all ages. Although the spectrum of causative drugs has changed, drug-induced AIN now accounts for 70%–90% of cases.

The provoking agent is associated with an inflammatory cell infiltrate in the renal interstitium, sometimes with delayed-type hypersensitivity reaction phenomena (fever, arthritis, rash) elsewhere. Rechallenging with drugs often leads to recurrent disease, confirming the immune-mediated nature of AIN.

Common causes of AIN

- Drugs
  - NSAIDs (including COX-2 inhibitors)
  - Penicillins, cephalosporins, rifampin, sulfonamides, quinolones
  - Diuretics
  - Allopurinol
  - Proton pump inhibitors
  - Cimetidine
  - Antiretrovirals
  - 5-amino salicylates
- Infections (streptococci, tuberculosis, legionella, leptospirosis, CMV)
- Autoimmune disease—TINU (see below), sarcoidosis, Sjogren syndrome.

Symptoms and signs

The classic triad of fever, arthralgias, and rash along with renal impairment is uncommon in the present antibiotic era and with most drugs, with the exception of penicillins and cephalosporins. Pyruria may be present. Nausea, vomiting, and oliguria may reflect renal failure. Flank pain may be present (renal swelling stretches the capsule). Causative drugs usually have been started 2 to several weeks previously, although AIN may occur up to 18 months after starting NSAID. On rechallenge with a previous offending drug, AIN may recur within 2–3 days.

Investigations

Urinalysis may be bland, or have modest hematuria and proteinuria (often <1 g/day), and may reveal pyuria, eosinophiluria and white cell casts or a bland urinalysis. BUN, Cr, electrolytes, Ca, PO_4, LFTs, CBC + diff (?eosinophilia), ↑ESR.

US shows normal-sized (or slightly enlarged) kidneys. CXR and serum ACE level if ?sarcoidosis. ANA, anti-Ro and La if ?Sjogren syndrome.

Renal biopsy: if clearly drug related, and the renal dysfunction is mild, withdraw drug and observe. If resolution does not occur in <10 days, biopsy. All dialysis-requiring patients should be biopsied to exclude other diagnoses and predict longer-term outcome.

Histology

Glomeruli are normal. An intense inflammatory cell infiltrate of lymphocytes and monocytes (± eosinophils) is present in the interstitium. Giant cells and granulomata may point to TB or sarcoidosis. The presence of interstitial fibrosis imparts a worse prognosis, as in all renal diseases.

Treatment

Treatment depends on the cause. Concentrating on drug-related AIN, the outcome is generally good, with most of those patients who required dialysis regaining independent renal function. However, there will invariably be some residual CKD. The mortality rate is reported at <5%.

▶▶ Stop the offending drug(s).

✦ Corticosteroids: have been widely used, if only to hasten renal recovery—there is no good evidence to support their use. Nevertheless, many treat those who are not improving or are worsening after drug withdrawal and if there are no contraindications to prednisone. Most patients, unless there are contraindications, should have a renal biopsy prior to steroid treatment. A reasonable algorithm is:
- Dialysis-requiring: treat with corticosteroids.
- Dialysis-independent: observe for 3–7 days.
  - If renal function improves, use expectant management.
  - If there is no improvement, treat with corticosteroids.

Treatment is prednisone 1 mg/kg/day po, with taper for a total 2- to 3-month course. If there is no response within 2 weeks, the patient may not respond. A small series showed success with MMF for steroid-resistant disease (NSAIDs). The treatment of tubulointerstitial nephritis with uveitis syndrome (TINU) is outlined in Box 6.1. Sarcoidosis may require a long course of steroid treatment (see Chapter 7).

Box 6.1 Tubulointerstitial nephritis and uveitis syndrome (TINU)

Unlike AIN, TINU affects predominantly young women and adolescents, presenting as anterior uveitis (eye pain and redness, often bilateral) and AIN (may be separated in time).

Additional features include weight loss, ↓Hb, ↑ESR, and deranged LFTs. You may see positive serologic workup (ANA, ANCA, RF). An ophthalmology opinion should be requested urgently. Patients treated with 1 mg/kg/day prednisone usually respond to treatment, with concurrent uveitis. They may require a longer course with treatment for 3–6 months. The differential diagnosis includes Sjogren syndrome and sarcoidosis, among others.

Chronic tubulointerstitial diseases

Chronic tubulointerstitial disease includes a wide range of disorders of varying causes linked by a common histological appearance on kidney biopsy. Glomeruli may be spared (although obsolescent glomeruli may be seen as a result of nephron dropout), and the tubulointerstitium is extensively fibrosed, often with a lymphocytic infiltrate in scarred areas. Many tubules are dilated and atrophic.

Although chronic tubulointerstitial nephritis exists as a distinct diagnosis (AIN of any cause may progress if exposure is not limited, or the underlying condition is not treated), *any* glomerular renal lesion associated with impaired renal function over time will develop the above histological changes (p. 154). Chronic tubulointerstitial nephritis secondary to glomerular disease will be apparent by the degree of proteinuria and primary glomerular changes on biopsy.

Specific causes include the following:
- Chronic analgesic use
- Reflux nephropathy
- Sarcoidosis
- Tuberculosis
- Autoimmune diseases (Sjogren syndrome)
- Metabolic causes, e.g., chronic ↓K^+
- Heavy metals
- Balkan endemic and Chinese herbal nephropathies.

Features include

- Impaired urinary concentration (nocturia, polyuria)
- Often normal BP (due to salt-losing state)
- Low molecular-weight (LMW) tubular proteinuria (β_2-microglobulin)
- Glycosuria (impaired tubular handling) ± renal tubular acidosis
- CKD
- Small, symmetrical kidneys on US (exception is reflux nephropathy, where polar scars may be seen)

Investigations

Urinalysis and urine culture, AFB. Spot urine PCR ratio or 24-hour protein and creatinine (often <1 g/day), BUN, Cr, electrolytes, Ca^{2+} (?↑Ca^{2+}), PO_4-, serum ACE level, ANA, anti-Ro/La, rheumatoid factor, US kidneys.

Lithium-induced nephropathy

Lithium therapy for bipolar disorder is associated with nephrogenic DI (p. 528), and may be associated with tubulointerstitial fibrosis and tubular dilatation with long-term use. Lithium dosing should aim for the lowest levels that control symptoms, with yearly labs obtained to monitor for ↑Cr. It is usually a mild and nonprogressive renal lesion, taking years to evolve. Some literature suggests that ACEI may adversely interact with lithium to cause progressive CKD.

Chinese herb nephropathy

Tubulointerstitial scarring with little acute inflammation and spared glomeruli are the principal histologic features. Although not conclusively proven, it appears to be due to aristolochic acid, an ingredient in many Chinese herbal preparations (notably used as a slimming agent). Patients are usually normotensive or have mild hypertension and mild proteinuria (<1.5 g/day). Cr on presentation may be varied. If herbs are stopped before severe CKD (Cr <2) the process may stabilize; however, more severe CKD progresses to ESRD. The incidence of urothelial malignancies is very high, and surveillance is mandatory. In those patients considered for transplantation after ESRD, bilateral native nephrectomies have been proposed to reduce the risk of malignant disease with immunosuppression.

Balkan endemic nephropathy (BEN)

BEN presents in men and women, usually farmers from the lands drained by the Danube who are >30 years old, with a tubulointerstitial atrophy and scarring. The cause remains unknown (? exposure to trace elements, aristolochic acid). Patients are usually normotensive with a urinary concentrating defect (polyuria), may have LMW tubular proteinuria (<1 g/day) and glycosuria. US shows small but symmetrical kidneys. There is an increased tendency for transitional cell carcinoma of the entire urinary tract: new hematuria should be investigated, and urine cytology should be performed for urothelial atypia regularly.

Lead nephropathy

Occupational (exposure to batteries, aerosols) or other exposure (moonshine or lead paint ingestion) cause chronic lead poisoning, with a chronic and progressive tubulointerstitial nephritis. Tubular injury results in decreased uric acid excretion, hyperuricemia, and gout. In at-risk individuals with unexplained CKD associated with high uric acid concentrations, the total lead burden should be established by bone X-ray fluorescence (not often available), or an EDTA lead chelation test (2 g IM 8–12 hours apart with 24-hour urine collection if Cr <1.5 mg/dL, 72-hour collection if > 1.5). Hypertension is invariably present. There may be neurologic symptoms (headache, tremors) as well. Treatment includes long-term lead-depletion with EDTA or oral succimer. Lead has also been shown to be an important determinant of progression of CKD of other causes. *Cadmium* exposure causes a similar nephropathy.

Analgesic nephropathy

Analgesic nephropathy (AN) was first described after chronic phenacetin (a pro-drug of acetaminophen, with toxicity independent of the latter) use, but is now recognized as a common cause of ESRD, accounting for up to 10% of cases. Incidence is 2♀:1♂ after the fifth decade.

Analgesics, in combination analgesic preparations or more than one taken separately, account for most AN (e.g., phenacetin + aspirin). Aspirin alone does not usually cause AN. Acetaminophen, if used in sufficient amounts (2 kg cumulatively, equivalent to about 8 years of daily full-dose ingestion) is strongly suggestive but not definitively proven to cause AN.

Injury begins in the medulla, with ischemic changes, and progresses to tubulointerstitial scarring, secondary focal and segmental glomerulosclerosis, and papillary necrosis (PN, see opposite page and Fig. 6.8).

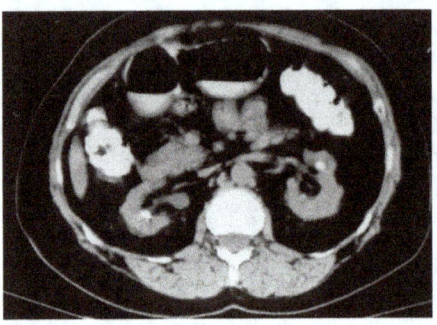

Fig. 6.8 Irregular, ragged renal outline characteristic of AN. Reproduced with permission from Davison AMA, Cameron JS, Grunfeld J-P, et al. (2005). *Oxford Textbook of Clinical Nephrology*. Oxford: Oxford University Press.

Symptoms and signs

A history of analgesic use may be difficult to elicit: direct questioning toward history of chronic headaches or backache. Dyspepsia is common. Nocturia and polyuria (loss of concentrating ability), episodic, colicky flank pain and frank hematuria due to papillary necrosis—sloughed papilla may be evident in the urine. ↑BP occurs as CKD develops.

Investigations

Urinalysis is often bland or shows modest proteinuria. You may see sterile pyuria on urinalysis. There is ↓Hb and ↑Cr. CT of kidneys may show calcified papillae and an irregular renal contour, and offers a contrast-free investigation to confirm AN. (IVU may show small kidneys ± clubbed calyces, but its use is limited because of the nephrotoxic dye.)

Management

Stop all analgesics. This is often difficult, but reducing the analgesic burden slows disease progression.

▶ Surveillance for urothelial malignancies is needed (transitional cell carcinoma occurs in up to 10% of confirmed AN). These may be multiple, in unusual sites, or even bilateral. New hematuria merits investigation (± cystoscopy), and yearly urine cytology provides a useful screening tool.

Analgesic nephropathy is also associated with accelerated atherosclerosis, though the mechanism is unclear.

Papillary necrosis

This is the end result of chronic medullary hypoxia: the vulnerable renal papilla (normal PaO_2 of 10–20 mmHg) suffers further (acute) ischemic injury, undergoes necrosis, and is shed into the renal pelvis. This may be associated with the following:
- Colicky flank pain (as the papilla traverses the ureter)
- Passage of a papilla (or part thereof)
- Gross hematuria
- Unilateral obstruction.
- Pyelonephritis of infected papilla
- No symptoms.

Non-contrast CT kidneys may show calcified papillae and an irregular renal contour as stated above. Alternatively, in patients without renal dysfunction, on IVU contrast tracking into eroded papilla, ring shadows around detached papilla ± calcification may be apparent. A CT urogram with contrast may be superior to IVU for papillary necrosis.

Diseases associated with papillary necrosis

- Analgesic nephropathy
- Diabetes mellitus
- Postobstructive uropathy
- Sickle cell nephropathy
- Tuberculosis
- Following severe acute pyelonephritis

Renovascular disease

Renovascular disease (RVD) remains an imprecise term for diseases of the large, medium-sized, and small renal vessels, excluding autoimmune vasculitis. Atherosclerotic renal artery stenosis (ARAS) and fibromuscular dysplasia (FMD) predominantly affect the larger vessels. We use the umbrella term *ischemic nephropathy* to describe the vasculopathy of vessels. The treatment of each differs, so careful diagnosis has real benefits.

ARAS and ischemic nephropathy

This combination is common with ↑ age (± 7% in people >65 years) and in those known to have atherosclerosis (± 50% if known PVD). However, anatomically proven ARAS may be hemodynamically unimportant and associated with ↑BP in only 50% of cases. Generally, stenoses >70% tend to be functionally significant, as is bilateral ARAS or disease in the artery to a single functioning kidney. Patients with ARAS or ischemic nephropathy have a substantial excess risk for cardiovascular death (MI and stroke).

Suspect ARAS in abrupt onset of hypertension in patients older than 65, and in older patients with onset of severe, accelerated or malignant hypertension, especially with known peripheral, coronary, or cerebrovascular atherosclerotic disease + risk factors (dyslipidemia, smoking, diabetes, ↑BP), or unexplained renal dysfunction.

Clinically
- Hypertension, often difficult to control (i.e., >140/90 on three drugs)
- Renal dysfunction
- ↑Cr (of >20% above baseline) with ACEI or ARB
- Sudden, unexplained pulmonary edema.

Pathophysiology
Atherosclerotic plaque involves the ostium or proximal 2 cm of the renal artery, often extending from the aorta. Disease is caused by a fall in renal perfusion, resulting in sympathetic overactivity and renin release. This leads to overproduction of the vasoconstrictor angiotensin II (AII), and aldosterone release with salt and water retention. The profibrotic actions of these factors in time cause renal scarring and CKD.

Symptoms and signs
Evidence of central or peripheral vascular disease is perhaps the most important clinical finding. ↑BP, edema, and flash pulmonary edema (see below), abdominal bruits (low predictive value in isolation), palpable abdominal aortic aneurysm (AAA), and bland urine on urinalysis are other findings. Flash pulmonary edema refers to sudden and episodic pulmonary edema with hypertension without a precipitating cardiac event, caused by exaggerated activation of the renin–angiotensin system and salt and water retention.

Investigations
These include BUN, Cr, electrolytes, ?↓K$^+$ and metabolic alkalosis due to ↑aldosterone), cholesterol, and urinalysis (bland or modest proteinuria). Screen for evidence of hypertensive end-organ damage (ECG or echo for LVH, dilated fundoscopy). Potential imaging includes the following:
- US kidneys for renal size and symmetry. A difference of >1.5 cm in renal length is suspicious.
- Duplex US with Doppler examination for resistive index (RI) as a surrogate for impeded flow. *Only* in experienced hands is this a useful dynamic test. It may predict responders to angioplasty and stenting, and follow-up if a procedure is performed.
- Gadolinium-enhanced magnetic resonance angiography (MRA) or multislice CT angiography is increasingly good at visualizing ostial lesions. Either one is more accurate than duplex US; however, gadolinium may cause nephrogenic systemic fibrosis if eGFR<30 mL/min and CT angiogram usually requires a large amount of contrast dye, which is suboptimal for patients with renal dysfunction.
- (Captopril renogram. With captopril, affected kidneys may show a 30% decline in GFR using DTPA or MAG-3 [p. 43]. It is the least accurate of these screening tests in a setting of CKD, bilateral RAS. It is **NOT** recommended for screening by 2005 ACC/AHA guidelines.)
- Angiography secures diagnosis and allows intervention. Perform this test if the screening tests above are equivocal and there is strong clinical suspicion.

Management of ARAS

General management
Modify risk factors—advise patient to stop smoking, use HMG-CoA reductase inhibitors, exercise, maintain glucose control if diabetic, and go on a low-salt diet. Consider giving aspirin 81 mg qd.

Control BP
Ideally aim for <130/80, but this is difficult to achieve. Be concerned about underperfusing the kidneys, which are accustomed to a higher blood pressure.
- ACEI/ARB (± diuretic). These may increase Cr, especially in bilateral disease. However, one can use these meds if Cr is monitored carefully. You may need to stop diuretic.
- β-blocker
- Calcium channel blocker.

Prevent renal complications
The prime aim is to prevent loss of renal function. Two treatment options exist, conservative or interventional. Selection can be very difficult.

Intervention is reasonable in progressive CKD with bilateral RAS or unilateral RAS with solitary functioning kidney, resistant or malignant hypertension, inability to tolerate antihypertension meds, unilateral small kidney, recurrent episodes of flash pulmonary edema, or unstable angina. It is unclear if revascularization is warranted in the absence of end-organ dysfunction or unilateral RAS and CKD.

Interventional management
This includes percutaneous transluminal renal angioplasty (PTRA) ± stenting, or surgical revascularization. PTRA alone is associated with a high incidence of restenosis—stenting is thus recommended. However, with PTRA and stenting:
- ~30% will see an improvement in Cr
- ~50% will experience no change
- ~20% will *deteriorate*.

Selected candidates who are more likely to benefit from PTRA and Stenting (or surgery):
- Known recent onset, Cr <3–4 mg/dL
- Low resistive index by Doppler US (<0.8)
- Rapidly declining renal function.

The kidney(s) should be >8 cm in length, implying there is meaningful nephron mass capable of recovering renal function, and the stenosis is high grade (>70%). The presence of heavy proteinuria may imply hyperfiltration injury in a scarred kidney with poorer prognosis (p. 154).

The risk of cholesterol emboli, arterial dissection, and contrast nephrotoxicity should be weighed against the potential benefits. Drug-eluting stents may alter the indications for PTRA + stenting.

Surgical revascularization is usually reserved for those undergoing simultaneous aortic surgery or those with early primary artery branching.

Conservative management
- A trial of ACEI/ARB.
- Patients must be well hydrated (check for postural drop). Start with low-dose ACEI (e.g., ramipril 2.5 mg qd) and measure Cr frequently. Continue and increase therapy as long as it is *efficacious* (BP control) and there is *no deterioration of >10%–20%* in Cr.
- ACEI/ARB will reduce CV risk, as well as block AII-mediated vasoconstriction and fibrosis. As above, this *will* drop perfusion pressure, and *may* precipitate ARF.
- ACEI/ARB will not prevent progression of stenotic lesions.

Other renovascular diseases

Fibromuscular dysplasia (FMD)
This primarily affects otherwise asymptomatic young women (15–50 years old) often with severe hypertension. It is much less common than ARAS. FMD is caused by arterial fibroplasia of intima, media (most common), or adventitia that may affect many vascular beds. These include intracranial, carotid, visceral (celiac, superior and inferior mesenteric), iliac, and subclavian arteries. FMD may affect both renal arteries, and classically affects the mid-distal renal artery (rather than the ostium as in ARAS).

Do angiography if you strongly suspect FMD; angiography may show a "string-of-beads" appearance with otherwise normal-caliber vessels on either side in medial disease. Smaller beading, smooth stenosis, or dissection is seen in other forms. ↑BP of FMD may be *cured* (withdrawal of all drugs) or improved by angioplasty (without stent), particularly in women <50 years with recent hypertension, refractory or intolerant to antihypertension meds, and having ischemic loss of renal mass. Consider surgery if BP is not controlled by medications or angioplasty.

Renal vein thrombosis (RVT)
RVT is usually found in association with the nephrotic syndrome (particularly membranous nephropathy [MN], 📖 p. 390, and MPGN, p. 378), when it may be uni- or bilateral. It is very rare outside of the hypercoagulable state found with severe hypoalbuminemia (usually <2–2.5 g/dL) and severe nephrotic-range proteinuria (often >10 g/day); it may be seen with tumors (especially renal cell carcinoma) invading and distorting the renal vein.

RVT may present as
- ↑Cr, loin pain, hematuria, renal infarction and ↑LDH (rare)
- Shortness of breath with pulmonary emboli or unilateral edema with DVT (general hypercoagulable state with NS).

Spiral CT, magnetic resonance venography, or Doppler US of the renal veins should be diagnostic. The gold standard is renal venography. Proven RVT should be treated with anticoagulation until non-nephrotic. Some patients have been treated with thrombolytic therapy or catheter thrombectomy. Prophylactic anticoagulation is controversial: no benefit has been proven in routine anticoagulation of either nephrotic patients in general or those with MN. Consider this treatment in severely nephrotic patients (albumin <2) with MN, but this is not agreed upon.

Cholesterol emboli
These may cause partial occlusion of the renal small vessels, with resultant luminal changes leading to downstream ischemia. Showers of emboli may present suddenly as ARF, or more commonly as a more gradual decline in renal function. This condition usually occurs in elderly patients known to have extensive atherosclerosis with recent
- Instrumentation of or surgery to the aorta (usually angiography)
- Thrombolysis or anticoagulation.

ARF in this setting may suggest the diagnosis. Patients may have embolic infarcts in end-arterial territories (digits, retina [Hollenhorst plaques]), pancreatitis (gut emboli), or livedo reticularis. The urine is usually bland (though heavy proteinuria may be a feature due to ischemic focal segmental glomerulosclerosis). Eosinophilia, eosinophiluria, and ↓C3/C4 may be seen early in the disease course. Renal biopsy shows characteristic intravascular clefts left by cholesterol. No specific therapy works, though aggressive BP and cholesterol lowering may improve longer-term patient survival.

Adult dominant polycystic kidney disease (ADPKD)

ADPKD is the most common inherited disease, affecting ± 1:800 live births, and responsible for 5%–10% of ESRD.

Autosomal dominant mutations in the genes *PKD1* (located on chromosome 16) and *PKD2* (chromosome 4) result in defective synthesis of the proteins polycystin-1 and -2, respectively. *PKD1* mutations are seven times more common than *PKD2* mutations, and are associated with more aggressive disease.

Polycystin-1 is a signaling membrane receptor protein that colocalizes with polycystin-2 (a calcium channel) in the cilia of renal collecting duct epithelial cells. The polycystin complex acts as an extracellular mechanosensor (flow in the lumen disturbs cilia and triggers the complex) regulating cell proliferation, adhesion, differentiation, and maturation to maintain normal tubular caliber.

Failure of normal polycystin complex formation results in dysregulated cell turnover, with uncontrolled cell proliferation in response to normally occurring growth factors. Proliferating tubular cells form disorientated cysts that rapidly close off from the original nephron and expand in size over time (Fig. 6.9). These changes are accompanied by the release of mitogenic and profibrotic cytokines that exacerbate local ischemia and scarring, leading to progressive renal failure.

Understanding the pathogenesis of ADPKD offers the best hope for meaningful therapies aimed at preventing the development of cysts. As cyst formation begins in utero, tailored therapy would require early diagnosis and treatment in childhood. In animal models, some experimental therapies seem promising:
- *Vasopressin receptor antagonists* inhibit cyst formation via ↓cAMP
- *Rapamycin or paclitaxel* to block disordered cell proliferation
- Therapies that block the actions of *epidermal growth factor*.

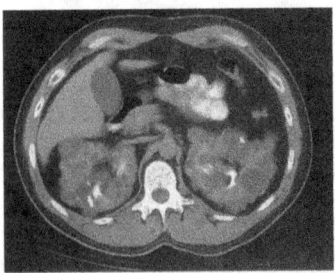

Fig. 6.9 Contrast-enhanced CT scan of a patient demonstrating the number, size, and location of cysts in the anterior portion of the left kidney and posterior aspect of the right kidney. Reproduced with permission from Watson ML, Torres VE (eds) (1996). *Polycystic Kidney Disease*, p. 214. Oxford: Oxford University Press.

Symptoms and signs

Most patients will present with a family history of ADPKD—a careful history for familial ↑BP, intracranial hemorrhage, or premature death may point to carriers of the gene mutations. Importantly, 25%–40% of new patients will have *no* family history. Inheritance is autosomal dominant, so 50% of offspring should be affected. Patients being investigated for ADPKD *should* be counseled before and after testing.

Clinical features include the following:
- Flank and abdominal pain arising from large cysts
- Nocturia and polyuria (loss of urinary concentrating ability)
- Microscopic or gross hematuria
- Microalbuminuria or less commonly, proteinuria (usually <1 g/day)
- ↑BP
- If presenting late, uremic symptoms
- Nephrolithiasis
- Severe headaches from cerebral aneurysms
- Abdominal hernias, colonic diverticuli
- Cardiac valve disease.

Investigations

Ultrasound remains the test of choice. As ADPKD is an evolving disease, the timing of the scan is important. For confirming a diagnosis, use the Ravine criteria (Table 6.2).

These criteria are valid for *PKD1* mutation alone. As *PKD2* mutations present with disease later, the criteria tend to give false negative results.
- Increased renal size is common (often 20 cm in length). Cysts in other organs (liver, pancreas, spleen) are suggestive of ADPKD.
- Genetic testing is available, though not widely used yet.

Table 6.2 Ravine criteria

Age	+ Family history	− Family history
<30 years	2 cysts in either kidney	5 cysts in either kidney
30–60 years	4 cysts in either kidney	5 cysts in either kidney
>60 years	8 cysts in either kidney	8 cysts in either kidney

Complications of ADPKD

Hypertension

↑BP is often the first sign of ADPKD, affecting ±60% with normal renal function. It is thought to be due to ↑ renin generation from ischemic renal tissue compressed by expanding cysts. Tight BP control (aiming for target BP ≤120/80) protects this often young cohort from end-organ damage. Choice of agent:
- ACEI/ARB as first-line therapy
- Add in calcium channel blocker, β-blocker, or diuretic.

Chronic kidney disease

Many patients with ADPKD will never reach ESRD; however, once renal impairment is established, some progression is the rule. Diagnosis in men at a younger age, with early hypertension, and large kidneys are risk factors for a worse renal prognosis. Those with *PKD2* mutations tend to develop symptoms and CKD later than those with *PKD1* mutations.

On dialysis and after transplantation, ADPKD patients have a better survival rate than that of the general ESRD population.

Cyst hemorrhage

This presents as abrupt-onset unilateral flank pain ± hematuria (Table 6.3) (cysts may rupture without communication into the collecting system). Conservative management is bed rest, hydration, and analgesics.

Cyst infection

Suspect this in the febrile and systemically ill ADPKD patient with flank pain. Culture blood and urine, and give a prolonged course of ciprofloxacin or trimethoprim/sulfamethoxazole (these have good penetration into cysts). Urine culture may be negative because the cyst may not connect with the collecting system. Consider pyelonephritis as a differential diagnosis—this may require IV antibiotics. A CT scan may demonstrate infected cysts in cases of doubt.

Nephrolithiasis

Twenty percent of these patients have associated renal stones, ~50% uric acid and 50% calcium oxalate in origin. Diagnosis is best made with CT scanning, and preventative measures are outlined on p. 430.

Table 6.3 Hemorrhage, infection, or stone?

	Hemorrhage	Infection	Stone
Fever	±	++	±
Leukocytosis	±	++	−
Frank hematuria	++	−	+
Renal colic	−	−	+
+ blood cultures	−	+	−

Extrarenal cysts

Hepatic cysts are particularly common, occurring in 10%–40% of ADPKD patients (most commonly in multiparous women). They do not interfere with synthetic liver function. Pancreatic and splenic cysts also occur, usually without symptoms.

Intracranial aneurysms (ICAs)

In ADPKD 4%–10% of patients have ICAs: specific mutations appear to predispose to aneurysm formation, so certain families have a history of intracranial bleeds. These families merit screening with MRA.

Symptomatic ICAs or those >10 mm in diameter need surgery. It is less certain what to do with asymptomatic ICAs <10 mm in size.

Rupture presents as subarachnoid hemorrhage, most commonly in patients <50 years old with poor BP control, and results in 50% mortality or severe disability.

Other manifestations

Mitral valve prolapse and aortic regurgitation, diverticular disease, and abdominal and inguinal hernias are more common in ADPKD patients.

Other cystic kidney diseases

Simple cysts
Solitary or multiple renal cysts are common in the elderly: 50% of those aged 50 years or more have one or more such cysts. So-called simple cysts are usually asymptomatic and are found on imaging the urinary tract for other reasons. Simple cysts have no further significance—complex (echoic) cysts need detailed evaluation by CT scanning to exclude renal malignancies.

Acquired cystic disease
Acquired cystic disease refers to cysts arising in the context of CKD with tubulo-interstitial scarring. These can be multiple and bilateral, and may be confused for ADPKD. Unlike ADPKD, acquired cysts occur in scarred and thus small kidneys, and are rarely >2–3 cm in size (most are ±5 mm). Complications include renal cell carcinoma and hemorrhage.

The age of presentation, family history, presence of hypertension, and cyst site may differentiate the various cystic renal diseases (Table 6.4).

Autosomal recessive polycystic kidney disease (ARPKD)
ARPKD is caused by a rare mutation on the *PKHD1* gene (located on chromosome 6) encoding for polyductin. It is a disease of infancy and childhood, presenting with polycystic kidneys progressing to ESRD, congenital hepatic fibrosis, and portal hypertension.

Nephronophthisis
This autosomal recessively inherited condition (6 mutations identified) is characterized by cystic change and tubulointerstitial fibrosis and usually presents in early childhood (>1 year) with impaired urinary concentration, leading to ESRD in adolescence. Unlike medullary cystic kidney disease, extrarenal manifestations (cerebral degeneration, bone abnormalities, and hepatic and portal fibrosis) occur.

Table 6.4 Classification of cystic kidney diseases

	Age	Family history	↑Cr	↑BP	Site
ADPKD	Any	++	±	+	Cortex
Juvenile PKD	<10	±	+	+	Cortex
Simple cysts	>65	–	–	±	Cortex
Medullary sponge kidneys	Any	–	–	–	Medulla
Medullary cystic kidneys	20–30	++	++	–	Medulla + cortex or netiher
Nephronophthisis	<15	+	++	–	Medulla

Medullary cystic kidney disease

This disease has autosomal dominant inheritance, presenting in early adulthood with progressive CKD and possibly gout. The affected genes, *MCKD1* and *MCKD2*, encode key signaling proteins located in the renal cilia. This manifests as small cysts (1–10 mm) forming at the corticomedullary junctions with associated tubulointerstitial inflammation and scarring, with unaffected glomeruli.

Clinically, affected individuals have a positive family history, and may present with nocturia, polydipsia, and polyuria (impaired concentrating ability). Urinalysis is usually bland, and BP is often normal (due to salt losses). Investigation shows small to normal-sized kidneys on US. CT of kidneys may demonstrate cystic changes. Hyperuricemia (± gout) may occur (*MCKD2* > *MCKD1*). Renal function declines to ESRD usually by 60 years of age. Treatment includes correcting salt and water depletion; there is no specific therapy.

Medullary sponge kidney

This is a benign, common condition characterized by malformations in terminal collecting ducts which result in diffuse microscopic medullary cyst formation. It is a developmental rather than genetic anomaly.

Clinically, there is no family history, and patients are identified incidentally or when investigated for UTIs, hematuria, or calcium oxalate or phosphate stones (Table 6.5). Hypercalciuria, hyperuricosuria, and hypocitraturia and urinary stasis in the collecting ducts predispose to formation of calcium-containing stones (often in microscopic cysts). Medullary sponge kidney should be considered particularly in young women presenting with calcium stones. Hematuria (microscopic or gross) and recurrent UTI also complicate the disorder.

Diagnosis is made on IVU, with a typical "calyceal brush" seen with adequate studies. A CT urogram may show this as well. CKD is very rare, and management should be directed toward treating infection and preventing stone formation.

Table 6.5 Sponge or cystic kidney disease?

	Medullary sponge kidney	Medullary cystic kidney disease
Age	Any	20–30 years
↑ Creatinine (ESRD)	–	++ (ESRD <60)
Salt-losing state	–	++
Calcium stones	++	–
UTI	+	–
+ Family history	–	+
Gout	-	+

Urinary tract infections (UTIs)

Approximately 50%–60% of women will experience a UTI in their lifetime.

A second infection is common in women who have had one UTI, but only 3%–5% will have recurrent UTIs (p. 425). In men and children, UTI is rarer and usually has associated abnormalities in the urinary tract needing further investigation (p. 423). Men may have uncomplicated UTIs associated with homosexual intercourse, intercourse with a partner with UTI, or lack of circumcision. Although serious morbidity from UTI is usually low, gram-negative septicemia and renal scarring do result from sporadic or recurrent infections. UTI in pregnancy is discussed on p. 570.

Pathogenesis

In women, the pathogens responsible for UTI are found in the colonic flora. Subsequent UTI is usually ascending, i.e., after perivaginal, perineal and transurethral colonization, often triggered by intercourse. *Lactobacilli*, vaginal bacterial flora, prevent urinary pathogens from colonizing the perineum. Spermicides may alter vaginal flora, predisposing patients to UTIs.

Bacteriology

- *Escherichia coli* 70%–90%
- *Staphylococcus saprophyticus* 5%–20%
- *Klebsiella* spp.
- *Enterococcus faecalis*
- *Proteus mirabilis*

Some women express an inherited and unique receptor on urothelium that aids *E. coli* binding. Also, *E. coli* expressing type *P. fimbriae* (pili) is an adhesin that promotes bacterial attachment to urothelium.

Host factors predisposing to UTI

- Recent or frequent intercourse
- Highly concentrated urine (>800 mOsm/kg) or failed urinary acidification (pH >5)
- Urinary stasis or incomplete bladder emptying
- ↑ Age (estrogen vaginal pH) ↓
- Eradication of vaginal colonizing organisms (use of spermicides)
- Renal or bladder stones

Diagnosis of UTI

Symptoms and signs

Cystitis or lower UTI

Dysuria, frequency, urgency, and nocturia. Suprapubic pain or tenderness. Foul-smelling urine or frank hematuria. Ask about sexual intercourse, new partners, and spermicidal or condom use, as well as recent antibiotic use or previous episodes of UTI.

▶ In the *elderly*, this may present as confusion ± incontinence. Vaginal irritation ± discharge makes UTI *less* likely (vaginitis more so).

Pyelonephritis or upper UTI

Fever, chills, night sweats, ± rigors, nausea ± vomiting, loin pain, and costovertebral angle (CVA) tenderness. The patient may be systemically ill or even in septic shock.

▶ In the immunocompromised and children, all of the above may be absent—maintain a high index of suspicion if they are ill appearing.

Investigations

- Dipstick urine: positive leukocyte esterase ± nitrite reductase. May be modest hematuria or proteinuria. *In low-risk cases, no further investigation is needed for positive dipstick with characteristic symptoms.*
- Clean-catch mid-steam urine for analysis with microscopy at ×40 magnification (i.e., high powered field [hpf]): pyuria (≥10 WBC/hpf on unspun specimen), WBC casts strongly suggest pyelonephritis.
- Culture: sample should be cultured within 2 hours of sampling. If this is not possible, store at 4°C for <48 hours.

Positive diagnosis of UTI

A pure growth of a urinary pathogen:
- $\geq 10^5$ colony-forming units (cfu)/mL of urine remains the standard.

However, at this cutoff, 30%–50% of UTI will escape diagnosis. In addition, then:
- $\geq 10^{2\text{-}3}$ cfu/mL in young women with suspected uncomplicated cystitis, or in *men*
- $\geq 10^4$ cfu/mL if pyelonephritis is suspected, or childhood UTI

If there is suspected pyelonephritis: ↑WCC, BUN, Cr, electrolytes. Imaging is only required in failure to defervesce >72 hours, or with renal colic, unusual pathogen, rapid relapse, or incomplete response. Non-contrast CT is the initial investigation of choice.

Persisting or repeated symptoms

Exclude urethritis or vaginitis if symptoms persist despite treatment. Re-infection is common, often <1 year after the first episode. Approach as a new infection. Repeated symptoms are usually due to persistent predisposing factors (colonization). *Complicated UTIs* refers to those occuring in patients who are pregnant, immunosuppressed, or very young or very old, or who have an anatomically abnormal urinary tract.

Who needs closer attention?
- Patients with symptoms >14 days
- Patients with recurrent UTI
- Men
- Children
- Pregnant women
- Diabetics
- Immunocompromised patients
- Those with *Proteus* UTI—? associated struvite stones
- Patients with a known abnormal urinary tract
- Patients with an in-dwelling catheter

Possible investigations
- *CT scanning* supercedes the above investigations. It is best for stones, hemorrhage, obstruction, and inflammatory masses.
- *Plain abdominal X-ray* for suspected stones (radio-opaque)
- *US kidneys* with pre- and post-micturition imaging of bladder will identify parenchymal pathology, hydronephrosis, and incomplete bladder emptying (but *not* many pelvic and ureteric abnormalities).
- ^{99M}Tc-*DMSA* scanning detects scars (reflux nephropathy).
- In men, assess the prostate (including PSA) and bladder emptying with *urodynamic flow studies* of lower urinary tract function.
- *Cystoscopy* is indicated in those at risk for bladder or prostate cancer, or those with evidence of impaired bladder emptying who may benefit from urethral dilatation.

Treatment of UTI

Duration of therapy varies widely, as does antibiotic prescribing. The choice of antibiotic should always be informed by local resistance patterns among common causative organisms.

Uncomplicated lower UTI (cystitis)
Either short-course (3 days) therapy:
- Trimethroprim/sulfamethoxazole 160/800 bid
- Fluoroquinolones such as ciprofloxacin 250 mg bid—offer a useful alternative

Or long-course (7–10 days) therapy:
- Nitrofurantoin (as monohydrate macrocrystals) 100 mg bid (not used with renal impairment)

▶ If symptoms persist, (re-)culture the urine.

Encourage high fluid intake of >2 L/day. Ampicillin/amoxicillin is less effective at eradicating vaginal and periurethral colonization.

Complicated lower UTI
See "at-risk patients" for criteria, 🕮 p. 422. Antibiotic therapy should *always* be tailored against urine culture results. Empirical therapy should be started immediately, and modified once sensitivities are known.
- Fluoroquinolones for 7–14 days (ciprofloxacin 500 mg bid).

For pregnant women, 📖 p. 570. In the immunocompromised, consider additional single-dose aminoglycoside (e.g., gentamicin 3–5 mg/kg IV). For renal transplant recipients, 📖 p. 274.

Acute pyelonephritis

After full assessment, if the patient is well, treatment can be as an outpatient. If nausea and vomiting predominate, or if the patient is systemically ill, admit the patient. ▶ Antibiotic therapy should *always* be tailored against urine culture results.

- Fluoroquinolones (e.g., ciprofloxacin 250–500 mg po bid) or levofloxacin (250–500 mg qd) for 14 days
- Alternatives include amoxicillin/clavulinic acid (especially for enterococcus), or a third-generation cephalosporin po for 14 days.
- If patient is systemically ill and unable to take meds po, IV therapy ± single-dose gentamicin 3–5 mg/kg IV qd or ceftriaxone 1 g IV qd
- Volume repletion with NS
- Antiemetics for nausea and analgesia

Catheter-related UTI

This is a common problem in hospitalized patients. Treatment is only effective after removal of the catheter (if possible). Diagnose if cultures are positive for >10^5 cfu/mL *and* heavy pyuria (colonization in the absence of pyuria does not merit treatment in most cases). Generally, only treat if there are significant local symptoms or patient is systemically ill. Use ceftrixone 1 g IV qd, ciprofloxacin 500 mg po bid, and remove catheter.

Recurrent UTIs

Establish whether the UTI is related to intercourse. Investigate and manage for abnormal urinary tract.

- Spermicides or spermicide-coated condoms should be discouraged.
- You may advise to increase fluid intake >2 L/day and perform postcoital voiding, but these measures have no proven efficacy.

The following *do not* predispose to UTI: wiping patterns, voiding after intercourse, personal hygiene, showering, hot baths or saunas, pantyhose, tights, or synthetic fabrics.

Prophylactic antibiotics should be offered if no underlying cause is identified. Ensure that any current infection is successfully eradicated.

- If UTI is related to sexual activity: trimethroprim/sulfamethoxazole 40/200–80/400 mg, or nitrofurantoin 50 mg after intercourse.
- If UTI has no relation to sexual activity, you may offer nightly low-dose prophylaxis for 6 months to 3 years: trimethoprim/sulfamethoxazole 40/200, nitrofurantoin 50 mg, then cephalexin 125–250 mg.

A *recurrence* is not the same as a *relapse* (defined as return of symptoms with culture of the same organism following UTI). Relapse should be treated with a prolonged (4- to 6-week) course of antibiotics.

Interstitial cystitis
This difficult-to-treat, sterile, inflammatory cystitis presents in women ~40 years old (often with a history of recurrent UTI). Symptoms include frequency, dysuria, and disabling suprapubic or pelvic pain. It may be sterile pyuria. Cystoscopy and biopsy may show characteristic inflammation and ulceration. Amytriptylline treats neuropathic pain. Oral pentosan polysulfate sodium 100 mg tid treatment has conflicting results in terms of efficacy.

Xanthogranulomatous pyelonephritis
This chronic, unilateral pyelonephritis is associated with calculi with obstruction causing widespread parenchymal destruction. It usually affects women >40 years old, often with a history of recurrent UTI. It presents as fever, nausea, anorexia, and weight loss along with a palpable kidney. Urinalysis confirms the UTI, usually with *Proteus* spp. or other gram-negative organisms. Diagnosis is on CT of kidneys and requires nephrectomy. This condition may be confused with renal cell carcinoma.

Reflux nephropathy

Reflux nephropathy (RN) describes a progressive lesion caused by repeated infections in either or both kidneys, almost always developing in childhood in the setting of an abnormal renal tract. The long-term renal scarring and CKD resulting from early injury is called RN, or *chronic pyelonephritis*. RN causes 5%–12% of ESRD in the developed world.

The anatomical abnormality is usually vesicoureteric reflux, but RN can occur with incomplete bladder emptying or outflow obstruction as well (see Box 6.2). By adulthood, the ureter usually inserts obliquely through the bladder wall, forming a compressible tunnel that acts as a one-way valve to prevent further reflux.

Lack of valves on the intravesicular ureter may allow reflux of urine into the ureters with bladder contraction and micturition. As the bladder is rarely empty, superinfection is the norm. The renal papillae do not restrict refluxing infected urine, so the tubulointerstitium becomes chronically infected and inflamed, leading to localized scarring in affected areas.

Symptoms and signs

In children, all males with UTI, females <3 years old with UTI, either gender <5 years old with febrile UTI, or children who had a prenatal renal anomaly should be referred and evaluated for RN. In adulthood, the presentation usually reflects progressive CKD. Consider screening siblings and parents of children with RN.

In adults, a history of renal colic, hematuria, or the passage of a stone may be offered. Findings include ↑BP (±50% of adults), sterile pyuria, and WBC casts on microscopy. Little proteinuria (<1 g/day) is present unless there is progressive CKD (often secondary FSGS at biopsy), when it may be heavy.

Investigations

A single infection with complete recovery and a normal US of the urinary tract requires no further assessment.

^{99M}Tc-DMSA scintigraphy (which is taken up in functioning renal tubules) will demonstrate renal scars at poles in areas of reduced uptake. IVU will show renal scarring (as parenchymal loss) and "clubbed calyces" (Fig. 6.10). Localized papillary scars do not take up contrast well, blunting the normal appearance of the renal calyx. Voiding cystourethrogram (VCUG) may show active reflux of contrast back into calyces while patients void.

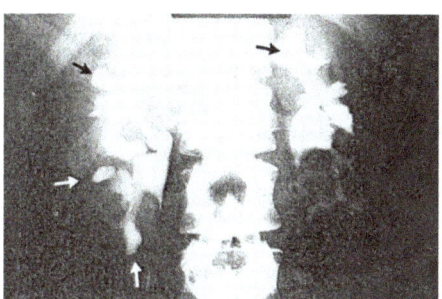

Fig. 6.10 Clubbed calyces (arrows) on IVU. Reproduced with permission from Warrell D, Cox T, Firth J, and Benz EJ (eds) (2004). *Oxford Textbook of Medicine*, fourth ed., p. 326. Oxford: Oxford University Press.

Histology

Histology shows typical features of chronic tubulointerstitial scarring, with dilated and atrophied tubules and an infiltrate of inflammatory cells. Secondary hyperfiltration injury develops over time, with compensatory hypertrophy of nondiseased segments, causing secondary FSGS.

Box 6.2 Vesicoureteric reflux (VUR)

This condition is genetically heterogeneous, but
- affects 0.1%–1% of newborns;
- underlies 12%–50% of children with a proven UTI;
- is almost always present in children with proven renal scars;
- is a leading cause of childhood ↑BP and ESRD.

Overt scar formation ceases at about 5–6 years, when the renal papilla no longer allows reflux into the renal parenchyma itself. VUR ceases around puberty, when the bladder base thickens and the ureteric tunnel elongates, and free reflux no longer occurs. Surgical correction of incompetent valves is required for those who have poor compliance or fail medical therapy. Otherwise, treat with antibiotic prophylaxis.

Management

Given no new scar formation occurs in adulthood, treatment is aimed at preventing progression of CKD.
- Treat ↑BP and proteinuria.
- Use ACEI or ARB as first-line therapy.
- Add on antihypertensive meds aiming for target BP <130/80 mmHg.
- Treat new infections vigorously.
- Ureteric reimplantation is no longer widely practiced.

Pregnant women with RN frequently develop UTI, functional deterioration, or hypertension ± preeclampsia, and should be referred early for specialist care.

Nephrolithiasis

Kidney stones affect 8%–15% of people, with an incidence of 2♂:1♀, aged 20–60 years. After a single stone, the likelihood of a second episode within 7 years is ±50%. Prophylaxis is effective in most cases.

Stones form around a nidus when the solubility of a urinary salt is exceeded: high solute delivery, concentrated urine (low volume) or areas of stasis (anatomically abnormal urinary tract), and an excess of stone promoters over inhibitors predispose to their formation. The key to management is identifying the stone components and any metabolic predisposition to stone formation.

Calcium oxalate/phosphate stones

These occur with an associated metabolic abnormality in most cases, but they may be idiopathic. Family history may be positive. Risk factors (in addition to predisposing factors above) are as follows:
- *Idiopathic hypercalciuria*: increased Ca^{2+} in urine. This is common.
- *Secondary hypercalciuria* (e.g., hyperparathyroidism, sarcoidosis)
- *Hyperuricosuria*: uric acid crystals form a nidus for calcium oxalate stone formation.
- *Hyperoxaluria*: increased dietary oxalate, reduced calcium intake, enhanced oxalate uptake due to ileal disease (Crohn's disease) or resection (bariatric surgery) and is named enteric hyperoxaluria. Ileal disease with malabsorption leads to increased free fatty acid and bile acid delivery to the colon. This increases the oxalate permeability in the colon.
- *Hypocitraturia*: Calcium stone inhibitor—citrate forms a soluble complex with calcium. (Low urinary citrate leads to clacium stone formation).
- *Alkaline urine* from distal RTA predisposes to calcium phosphate stones.

Uric acid stones

Acidic urine (chronic diarrhea, metabolic syndrome) is the most common risk factor (70%) for uric acid stones, as acidic urine decreases uric acid solubility. ↓ urinary pH <5.5 → insoluble uric acid stones. ↑ urinary uric acid with hyperuricemia (10%–20% will have frank gout) is seen with excess dietary purine intake, gout, and myeloproliferative disease.

Cystine stones

Cystinuria may be suspected in childhood stone-formers. Mutations in the gene encoding an amino acid transporter lead to urinary overexcretion of the amino acids cystine, ornithine, lysine, and arginine.

Stone composition and incidence

Calcium oxalate/phosphate	70%–80%
Struvite	10%
Uric acid	5%–10%
Cystine	1%

▶ *Calcium-containing or struvite stones are radio-opaque. All stones will cast acoustic shadows on US. Uric acid stones will not be seen on plain radiographs.*

Bladder stones

These occur in abnormal bladders, often following surgical reconstruction. Predisposing factors include UTI, bladder diverticula, and neurogenic bladders, ± bladder outflow obstruction.

Staghorn calculi

Struvite or magnesium ammonium phosphate stones are caused by a *Proteus, Klebsiela,* or *Serratia* urinary tract infection where these bacteria split urea to ammonium and hydroxyl ions (thus ↑ urinary pH). The alkaline urine predisposes toward phosphate stone formation. Such stones act as a reservoir for infection and often expand to fill much of the collecting system. Treatment depends on stone removal. Infection should be treated vigorously.

Investigating recurrent stone-formers

In patients presenting with a first urinary stone, 24-hour urine investigation into an underlying cause with a view to prevention may *not* be cost-effective. Routine evaluation includes the following:
- Urinalysis, urine culture
- Biochemical analysis of passed stones
- BUN, Cr, electrolytes, calcium, phosphate, uric acid
- Parathyroid hormone level if hypercalcemic
- Imaging (see below).

Risk factors for recurrent stones include positive family history, gout, diarrhea, and procedure required to remove stones. For these you may wish to obtain a 24-hour urine stone risk profile after a first stone. Obtain this for all recurrent stone-formers.

Goal values for 24-hour urine stone risk profile

Ensure that the collection is adequate. Urine creatinine of ± 20–25 mg of creatinine/kg body weight/day in men and 15–20 mg/kg body weight/day in women implies an accurate collection (urine Cr decreased if there is low muscle mass, such as in the elderly). Goal ranges:
- Volume >2 L/day. Urine osmolality of 300–350 mOsm/kg
- Calcium <250 mg/day in women, <300 mg/day in men or 4 mg/kg/day
- Oxalate <40 mg/day
- Uric acid <750 mg/day in women, <800 mg/day in men
- Citrate >320 mg/day (Some use higher goal values.)
- Phosphate <1200 mg/day—diet dependent
- Sodium <90–130 mEq/day if hypercalciuric. This reflects dietary sodium intake.
- Sulfate <30 mmol/day if hypercalciuric. Reflects animal protein intake (Urine urea nitrogen is also measured in some stone profiles.)
- Cystine negligible
- pH >6–6.5 for uric acid stone-formers
- Relative supersaturations for each stone. These are computer-generated numbers accounting for concentrations of inhibitors and promoters of stone formation for specific types of stones.

You may do one or two 24-hour collections on the first test and monitor each therapy change with one 24-hour collection ~4 weeks after an intervention.

Imaging in nephrolithiasis
- Unenhanced CT of kidneys is the gold standard.
- Plain KUB allows monitoring of radio-opaque stones.
- IVU is an alternative to CT for medullary sponge kidney.
- US kidneys for an abnormal urinary tract or if obstruction is suspected.

Management of recurrent nephrolithiasis

General measures:
- Increase fluids for daily UO >2–3 L/day. Urine osmolality of 300–350 mOsm/kg if measured. Urine creatinine to ensure accurate collection.
- Monitor urinary stone risk profile after 1 month of dietary or medication changes to assess the efficacy of therapy.

Calcium oxalate stones

Hypercalciuria
- Reduce salt intake if urine Na >130 mEq/L, as urine sodium excretion is linked to calcium excretion in the proximal tubule and loop of Henle. In idiopathic hypercalciuria, sodium restriction leads to decreased urinary calcium excretion.
- Reduce animal protein intake if urine sulfate is elevated, reflecting high animal protein intake. Animal protein is an acid load buffered by bone calcium carbonate, which may lead to hypercalciuria. Animal protein restriction may reduce urine calcium excretion. Less than 1 g/kg/day animal protein is optimal.
- Do not advise severe calcium restriction as it may worsen stone disease (see hyperoxaluria below). Low calcium intake predisposes women with idiopathic hypercalciuria to osteopenia as well.
- Thiazide diuretics (indapamide 2.5–5 mg daily, hydrochlorothiazide 25–50 mg daily, or the potassium-sparing–thiazide diuretic amiloride 2.5–5 mg/hydrochlorothiazide 25–50 mg daily) decrease urine calcium excretion. Patients may need potassium chloride or potassium citrate with thiazides because hypokalemia can lead to hypocitraturia.

Hyperoxaluria
Advise *normal* calcium intake (~1000–1200 mg/day) with meals; low Ca^{2+} intake leads to less dietary oxalate binding to calcium and increasing free oxalate in the gut, which ↑ urinary oxalate excretion. Hyperoxaluria with low calcium intake predisposes women with idiopathic hypercalciuria to osteopenia as well (may see this with lactose intolerance, Kosher meals). Also reduce dietary oxalate: spinach, tea, nuts, brewed tea, chocolate.

If there is enteric hyperoxaluria due to small bowel disease or resection you may want to give supplemental calcium with meals to bind up excess oxalate (calcium citrate or carbonate); the patient will usually have low urine calcium at baseline.

Hyperuricosuria
Try purine restriction (shellfish, meat gravies, organ meats, animal protein), and patient may need allopurinol 100–300 mg/day.

Hypocitraturia
Causes include diarrhea, distal RTA, hypokalemia, and high animal protein diet. Each of these causes increased proximal tubular reabsorption. Treat with potassium citrate 30–90 meq/day, usually as Urocit K 5–10 mEq pills tid.

Calcium phosphate stones

If the patient has pure calcium phosphate stones, rule out distal RTA and hyperparathyroidism. Elevated urine pH (>6.5) is favorable for phosphate stone precipitation. If there is distal RTA and hypocitraturia, treat with potassium citrate. Treat hypercalciuria as above.

Uric acid stones

Uric acid stones precipitate in acidic urine. They may be seen with diarrhea, gout, and metabolic syndrome where urine pH is often acidic. Alkalinize urine by testing with pH paper using potassium citrate (Urocit K 30–60 meq/day) to urine pH of 6–6.5.

Struvite stones

These stones require eradication therapy for associated UTI. Use urologic intervention for removal of stones and directed antibiotic therapy against cultures and sensitivities.

Cystine stones

These stones are treated with D-penicillamine 250–500 mg bid, or α-mercaptopropionylglycine 1000–2000 mg/day (considered less toxic than D-penicillamine with less severe GI side effects). Captopril may also be considered if the patient is hypertensive.

Cystine is a disulfide of two cysteine amino acids. The aim is to make a sulfhydryl group drug–cysteine disulfide bond instead of cysteine–cysteine disulfide found in cystine stones. Increased fluid intake is required, including at nighttime, to reduce urine cystine concentration <250–300 mg/L. Alkalinize urine to pH >7–7.5 (this is often impractical).

Acute renal colic

This syndrome is caused by stone(s) passage down the urinary tract. Patients, usually ♂ in their fourth decade, are often in severe pain. Predisposing factors include volume depletion (↓urine volume), exercise, or protein load.

Symptoms and signs

Colicky abdominal pain, often severe, radiates from loin to groin. There is nausea and vomiting along with CVA tenderness. Hematuria is often gross. Dysuria and frequency ± symptoms of UTI are present.

Investigations

Dipstick urine for hematuria, leukocyte esterase, and nitrate reductase. Get urine microscopy for crystals. Check BUN, Cr, electrolytes, and CBC. If there are signs of infection, culture blood and urine. Obtain an unenhanced stone protocol CT of the kidneys to confirm diagnosis and site of stone, and to exclude obstruction. A plain abdominal X-ray may reveal radio-opaque stones (±80%).

▶▶ Infection or obstruction is an indication for urgent intervention.

Treatment

- NSAIDs are effective analgesics and can be used as add-on therapy with *caution* (i.e., good renal function and volume repletion are required).
- Antiemetic: metaclopramide 10 mg IM/IV
- Oral fluids, or if vomiting, IV NS for UO >2 L/day
- If stone is ≤5 mm, 90% will pass spontaneously.
- If stone is 5–10 mm, ~50% will pass spontaneously.
- Flomax (or a calcium channel blocker) may prompt stone passage.

Some 10%–20% of stones will fail to pass. High-ureteric (proximal) stones may be treated with shock wave lithotripsy if <10 mm in size. Ureteroscopy is an alternative if the stone is >10 mm. Low (distal) stones can be successfully treated by endoscopic removal, although some clinicians perform lithotripsy. Percutaneous nephrolithotomy has excellent results for stones >20 mm or for complicated stones.

If there is associated infection, start IV antibiotic with good gram-negative coverage.

⚠ *An infected, obstructed system caused by stones (pyonephrosis) is an emergency.* Septicemia ± shock supervenes rapidly. Start IV antibiotics and arrange urgent referral for percutaneous nephrostomy to allow immediate drainage.

Chapter 7

The kidney in systemic disease

Diabetic nephropathy (DN) 438
Management of diabetic nephropathy 442
Management of ESRD in diabetes 444
The kidney in multiple myeloma 446
Managing myeloma kidney 448
Renal amyloidosis 450
Other non-amyloid dysproteinemias 453
Sickle cell nephropathy 454
Vasculitis and renal disease 456
ANCA-positive vasculitis 458
Treatment of ANCA-positive vasculitis 460
Churg–Strauss syndrome 462
Polyarteritis nodosa 464
Goodpasture's or anti-GBM disease 466
Lupus nephritis 468
Management of lupus nephritis 470
Anti-phospholipid syndrome 472
Scleroderma renal crisis 474
Rheumatoid arthritis (RA) 476
Sarcoidosis 478
HIV and renal disease 480
Hepatitis B–related renal disease 482
Hepatitis C–related renal disease 484
The kidney in infective endocarditis 486
Renal tuberculosis 488
Schistosomiasis 490
Malaria 492

Diabetic nephropathy (DN)

Diabetes mellitus (DM) is a state of chronic hyperglycemia leading to long-term organ damage, presenting as two types:
- Type 1 DM is due to autoimmune mediated islet B-cell destruction, presenting acutely, often in childhood (median age 12). it accounts for 5%–15% all DM.
- Type 2 DM is a heterogeneous condition, characterized by insulin resistance and islet failure.
  - It presents >40 years of age.
  - Peak incidence is 60–65 years.
  - ♂ predominance.
  - Incidence is 2% in Caucasian population, and higher in African Americans and Mexican Americans.

Definition and epidemiology

Diabetic nephropathy is now the most common underlying cause of ESRD in Europe and the United States, with an annual incidence of 140 cases per million population (pmp) (nondiabetic renal disease has an incidence of 15–42 pmp). The incidence depends on the ethnicity of the population: Pima Indians have a 40% incidence of ESRD after 10 years of DM and microalbuminuria. There is a higher incidence of DN in men. In type 1 DM, age at diagnosis is predictive of outcome:
- Diagnosis at <12 years: time to overt nephropathy = 14 years
- Diagnosis at 12–20 years: time to overt nephropathy = 8 years
- DN affects 30%–40% of type 1 DM after 20 years.

There is improvement in renal prognosis more recently in type 1 diabetes, perhaps due to better glycemic and BP control and use of ACEI/ARB.

Pathogenesis of DN

Renal hypertrophy, hyperfiltration (initially with ↑GFR to above normal), and intrarenal hypertension lead to glomerulosclerosis and tubulointerstitial fibrosis. ↑ glucose mediates this through the following:
- ↑shear stress and changes in glomerular hemodynamics
- Local ↑ angiotensin II release → hemodynamic and fibrotic changes.
- Modification of proteins by glucose-degradation products
- Activation of cytokines and TGF-β → excess matrix deposition.

In addition, a poorly understood genetic predisposition exists in both type 1 and type 2 DM that is associated with progressive renal failure.

Mean $HgbA_{1C}$ over time correlates with loss of renal function. In long-term studies in type 1 (Diabetes Control and Complications Trial [DCCT]) and type 2 (UK Prospective Diabetes Trial [UKPDS]) DM, blood glucose concentration is related to the development of microalbuminuria and progression to overt proteinuria.

Natural history

For type 1 DM, the evolving renal lesion develops serially:

Stage

1	Renal hypertrophy with ↑GFR
2	Early histological changes, though still clinically silent
3	Microalbuminuria—BP now starts to rise
4	Overt diabetic nephropathy with declining GFR
5	ESRD

One-third of type 1 diabetics develop diabetic renal disease, reaching stage 3 about 10 years after diagnosis—after 20 years, this subgroup will have progressed to overt DN.

Type 2 diabetics follow a similar pattern; but as they present in middle age, many will not progress to ESRD. However, enough do progress to make type 2 DM the most common cause of ESRD in the Western world. Type 2 diabetics also present *with* ↑BP, and often microalbuminuria. The long-term UKPDS studies demonstrated the following:
- 2% prevalence microalbuminuria/year (incidence 25% over 10 years)
- 2.8% microalbuminuria to overt proteinuria/year (5% over 10 years)
- 2.3% proteinuria with decreasing GFR (progression to CKD stage IV–V is 1% at 10 years)—this equates to 12 times the risk of CKD compared to that of the nondiabetic population.

Indications for renal biopsy

Renal biopsy is rarely required for diagnosis of DN. Consider biopsy if the following occur:
- Absence of retinopathy/neuropathy in type 1 (retinopathy is observed in 85%–99% of type 1 patients with nephropathy, this is less reliable in type 2; lack of retinopathy does not entirely rule out disease, neuropathy may be present)
- Dysmorphic red cells, red cell casts or frank hematuria (microscopic hematuria was seen in up to 66% in one series)
- ARF or rapidly worsening CKD months after ACEI/ARB
- Rapidly increasing proteinuria, or the nephrotic syndrome (<5 years from diagnosis in type 1; it is harder to know the exact onset of disease in type 2).
- Symptoms suggestive of multisystem disorder

▶ 23%–37% of diabetics with various indications for biopsy will not have DN at kidney biopsy (membranous GN, IgA, etc.).

Pathology

Mesangial expansion, GBM thickening, and glomerulosclerosis (possible nodule formation: Kimmelstiel–Wilson lesions) are present, with capillary lumen encroachment. There may be variable degrees of interstitial fibrosis or vascular arteriosclerosis and occlusion.

Other renal disease in diabetic patients

Papillary necrosis (📖 p. 409)
This disease occurs in up to 1:20 patients with diabetic nephropathy. It may be asymptomatic. It can present as pain (recurrent renal colic) or infection. Hematuria and modest proteinuria (<2 g/24 h) are common, and there may be sterile pyuria.

Renovascular disease (📖 p. 410)
This disease results from associated atherosclerotic renal artery stenosis. Suspect it if there is difficult to control BP, fluid retention, or a >20% rise in creatinine with ACEI.

Autonomic neuropathy of the bladder
Some 40% of long-standing diabetics have bladder dysfunction, with loss of sensation of fullness and incomplete emptying leading to large-volume bladders with significant post-void residual urine volume and stasis.

The patient often presents with UTI or incontinence. Assessment should include a measure of post-void volume and urodynamic studies. Interventions include regular voiding in the absence of urge, or intermittent self-catheterization. This may lead to ↓ bladder volume or partial recovery of detrusor function.

Urinary tract infection (📖 p. 422)
Women with diabetes have twice the incidence of UTI compared to that of nondiabetic ♀, and a higher incidence of pyelonephritis or renal abcess formation. Ninety percent of cases of emphysematous pyelonephritis (📖 p. 426) occur in diabetics.

Contrast nephropathy (📖 p. 142)
Diabetics with an elevated Cr, perhaps as a result of intrarenal microvascular disease, are more susceptible. There is ↑Cr following the use of contrast media.

⚠ Stop metformin for 2 days pre- and post-contrast procedure. (There is an increased risk of lactic acidosis due to metformin in the setting of ARF from contrast nephropathy. Metformin itself does not cause ARF.)

Management of diabetic nephropathy

Screening patients for proteinuria/microalbuminuria
Early detection of diabetic nephropathy delays and may prevent progression to ESRD. Annual screening by urinary albumin/creatinine ratio (ACR, expressed in mg albumin/g creatinine) should be performed
- In the absence of overt urinary tract infection
- In patients with stable glucose control.

ACR in a random urine specimen accurately reflects microalbuminuria:

ACR	24-hour albuminuria
<30 mg/g	<30 mg/day
30–300 mg/g	30–300 mg/day
>300 mg/g	Overt proteinuria

Investigations in DN
- Measure BP and examine peripheral pulses.
- Urinalysis (?hematuria → if so, microscopic for ?RBC casts)
- Quantify proteinuria (as above).
- Check visual acuity and perform fundoscopy.
- Test for peripheral neuropathy (other microvascular disease).
- BUN, Cr, electrolytes, albumin.
- HgbA$_{1C}$, cholesterol.
- US (kidneys are often of normal to large size despite ↓GFR).

Primary prevention of nephropathy (Table 7.1)
- Improve glycemic control:
  - HgbA$_{1C}$ <7% in insulin-requiring patients; watch for hypoglycemia
  - HgbA$_{1C}$ <6%–7% not on insulin
- Control BP, aiming for target <130/80 or lower if tolerated.
- Stop smoking, lose weight, and exercise.

Management of microalbuminuria and proteinuria
- Glycemic control
  - HgbAIC <7%
  - Stop metformin when creatinine >1.5 mg/dL eGFR <60 mL/min (☛risk of lactic acidosis).
- BP control (see next page).
- Other interventions:
  - Treat dyslipidemia: HMG-CoA reductase inhibitors significantly reduce cardiac events in diabetics. They may also ↓proteinuria and preserve GFR in overt nephropathy.
  - Dietary protein restriction of 0.8 g/kg/day is recommended per KDOQI guidelines, 📖 p. 161) to possibly slow decline in GFR. (With carbohydrate and fat restriction, this may be difficult to

achieve.) Evidence of benefit (Cochrane Database analysis) shows a small, statically insignificant slowing of renal progression with protein restriction in type 1 and type 2 diabetics.

BP control in DN

- Good blood pressure drastically alters renal prognosis.
  - 30% have ↑BP at diagnosis of type 2 diabetes.
  - 70% have ↑BP at diagnosis of DN.
  - ↑BP is proportional to ↑albumin excretion.
  - Good BP control reduces the decline in GFR associated with DN from ±12 mL/min/year to <5 mL/min/year.
  - ACEI/ARB may restrict progression to as little as −0.3 mL/min/year.
- Emphasize importance of a low-sodium diet 2–3 g/day (📖 p. 198–199).
- Use drug therapy.

✦ *Start inhibitors of the renin–angiotensin system (ACEI, ARB).* We recommend (▶ usually need multidrug therapy) the following:
  - Start with low-dose, long-acting ACEI (e.g., ramipril) or ARB (e.g., irbesartan) and titrate to maximum dose.
  - Step-wise, add on therapy aiming for BP <130/80 and consider <125/75 with >0.5–1 g/day proteinuria (avoid diastolic BP <75 if there is active coronary artery disease and keep systolic BP >110).
    —Diuretic
    —Non-dihydropyridine calcium channel blockers (e.g., diltiazem)
    —β-blocker (caution with hypoglycemia)
  - Combination therapy with both ACEI and ARB may have additive effects in ↓proteinuria and slowing progression, and we recommend this if proteinuria > 1 g persists despite measures used above. This therapy may require low K^+ diet ± diuretic.
- 📖 p. 348 for difficult ↑BP.

Table 7.1 Summary of recommended interventions to slow progression of renal disease in patients with DM

	Target
BP control	<130/80 (if > 0.5–1 g/day proteinuria, consider <125/75 as above)
Inhibition of RAS	Urinary protein <0.3 g/day
Glycemic control	$HgbA_{1C}$ <7%
Correction of dyslipidemia	LDL cholesterol <100 mg/dL

Management of ESRD in diabetes

It is generally felt that diabetic patients should initiate dialysis at an earlier stage than patients with another cause of end-stage renal failure, i.e., GFR 10–15 mL/min, or creatinine >500 μmol/L, as diabetics are more susceptible to uremic symptoms, fluid retention, and hyperkalemia.

Survival and causes of death in diabetics on dialysis

Diabetics with ESRD have a 5-year survival rate of 25.5%. This difference is due to greater comorbidity, particularly macrovascular disease. There is also a higher incidence of withdrawal from dialysis reported among diabetics.

Outcome of dialysis: peritoneal dialysis (PD) versus hemodialysis (HD)

A clear difference in outcome between PD and HD has not been observed. Early data showed better survival on PD while the USRDS showed worse survival on PD, especially for elderly diabetics. Another study showed better survival on PD for younger diabetics but worse survival on PD for older diabetics.

Renal transplantation in diabetics

Renal transplantation is both safe and effective, offering improved survival and rehabilitation over that with dialysis (5-year survival rates of 75%–83% vs. 25.5% on dialysis). This difference is in part due to selection criteria. Recent studies have shown similar 1- and 5-year graft survival for diabetics and nondiabetic patients, when data are censored for patients dying with a functioning graft. Living-donor graft survival is superior to cadaveric-donor grafts (80% vs. 64% graft 5-year survival).

Type 1 diabetics should be considered for combined kidney–pancreas transplantation.

The kidney in multiple myeloma

Multiple myeloma (MM) is characterized by an aberrant clone of plasma cells producing an immunoglobulin (IgG or IgA) or immunoglobulin light chain, generally presenting >60 years of age, in ♂ > ♀. Median survival after diagnosis is 3 years. The annual incidence is about 4–5 per 100,000. Proliferation of these plasma cells leads to bone marrow failure, skeletal destruction, and ↑Ca^{2+}. Paraproteinemia (or monoclonal Ig produced by plasma cells) may cause renal failure, recurrent bacterial infections, or hyperviscosity.

Diagnosing MM

- Monoclonal immunoglobulin band (M-band) in serum or urine.
- >10% plasma cells on bone marrow
- Evidence of end-organ damage: ↑Ca^{2+}, ARF/ CKD, anemia or bone lesions

Renal impairment is a major complication of MM, found at or preceding diagnosis in 20%–30% of patients, and occurring in 50% of patients during the course of the disease. Causes, often multifactorial, are as follows:
- Hypercalcemia and dehydration
- Cast nephropathy (myeloma kidney, 30%–65%)
- AL amyloidosis (usually lambda-subtype light chain, 20%)
- Light-chain deposition disease (usually kappa light chains, 10%).

Symptoms and signs

Think of MM in any patient (especially if elderly) with unexplained renal impairment, normal-sized kidneys, and a bland urinalysis.
Bone pain (especially backache), weakness, fatigue, symptoms of ↑Ca^{2+} (📖 p. 447), easy bruising, pallor, and hepatomegaly (20%) are possible symptoms.

▶ Urinalysis may be negative for protein (dipstick detects albumin, does NOT detect light chains).

Investigations

Check CBC (↓Hb), ↑ESR, electrolytes (↑BUN and Cr), total protein, albumin, ↑Ca^{2+}, ↑ uric acid (rarely have tumor lysis) (↑cell turnover). Do serum protein electrophoresis (SPEP) and check quantitative immunoglobulins (may see decrease in uninvolved Igs), M-band, and β_2-microglobulin (activity monitoring). Assess 24-hour urine protein electrophoresis (UPEP), urinary free light chains. Run serum light-chain assay.
Do a skeletal survey (?osteolytic lesions, osteoporosis, pathological fractures). Bone marrow aspirate or biopsy is diagnostic (>10% plasma cells). If there is renal impairment, proceed to *renal biopsy*.

What is in an Ig?

Immunoglobulin is made up of two heavy chains (with a complement fixing site) and two light chains (with an antigen binding site). Plasma cell dyscrasias may produce whole Ig (monoclonal), whole light chains or heavy chains, or parts of either.

Pathogenesis and histology

Cast nephropathy is characterized by freely filtered light chains that bind tubular Tamm–Horsfall protein (📖 p. 23), forming proteinaceous casts that obstruct the tubular lumen. Light chains are toxic to tubules as well. Multiple large casts are apparent on light microscopy, particularly in the distal tubule and collecting duct, with a fractured appearance (Fig. 7.1). Casts may be surrounded by multinucleated giant cells, with tubulitis and interstitial inflammation being common. Casts are polychromatic with Masson's trichrome, and may stain with Congo red, but are not birefringent under polarized light (see amyloid). The risk of developing renal failure is 5- to 6-fold greater if Bence Jones proteinuria >2.0 g/day compared to those with proteinuria <0.05 g/day.

AL amyloidosis (📖 p. 450) and *light-chain deposition disease* (📖 p. 453).

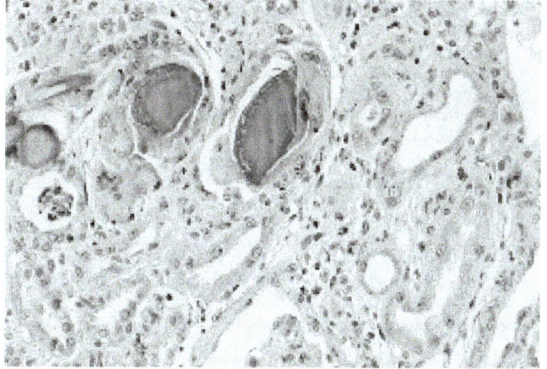

Fig. 7.1 Fractured tubular casts characteristic of myeloma kidney. Reproduced with permission from Davison AMA, Cameron JS, Grunfeld J-P, *et al.* (eds) (2005). *Oxford Textbook of Clinical Nephrology*, 3rd ed. Oxford: Oxford University Press.

Managing myeloma kidney

▶ Correct associated reversible causes of acute renal failure: volume depletion, and hypercalcemia.
- Replete volume:
  - NS IV—may require large volumes (>5 L) if ↑Ca^{2+}
  - Monitor orthostatic BPs, daily weights, input and output.
  - Hb may fall—consider need for transfusion.
- Correct hypercalcemia (📖 p. 544).
  - *Once euvolemic*, if still ↑Ca^{2+}, consider IV bisphosphonates (📖 p. 545).
- Tumor lysis is rare with multiple myeloma.
  - May use allopurinol or rasburicase (📖 p. 145)
- Encourage all patients with CKD and MM to maintain a high fluid intake.

Specific treatment for cast nephropathy

Treatment involves reducing Ig or light-chain deposition:
- ↓ synthesis: Most treatment regimes include corticosteroids (either dexamethasone or prednisolone) with alkylating agents. Newer treatments include thalidomide or proteasomal inhibitors. Autologous stem cell transplantation offers hope of complete remission.
- ↑ clearance: Plasmapheresis by removing circulating light chains is controversial for ARF. The MERIT trial did not show a statistically significant benefit. It is NOT considered routine, but consider it in those patients with high levels of circulating light chains and severe ARF.

When myeloma isn't myeloma

Finding a paraprotein in serum or urine is not always due to MM!
- *Monoclonal gammopathy of uncertain significance (MGUS)* is characterized by
  - M-band (monoclonal IgA, IgG, or IgM) <3 g/dL
  - <10% plasma cells in the bone marrow
  - Minimal Bence–Jones proteinuria
  - No end-organ damage

The paraproteinemia tends to remain stable over time—but MGUS may evolve into MM (1% year). Follow-up should include 6-monthly testing of SPEP and urine light chains.
- *Smoldering MM* refers to asymptomatic patients with M-band >3 g/dL and a plasma cell infiltrate, but no end-organ damage. Evolves into MM in 3% patients/year
- *Plasmacytomas* are solid tumors made up of plasma cells in bone or elsewhere that do not (usually) produce an M-band.

ESRD in MM

Patients who require renal replacement therapy can start either HD or CAPD. Of patients surviving beyond 2 months after diagnosis, actuarial survival is approximately 45% at 1 year, and 25%–30% at 3 years. Patients who respond to chemotherapy with a reduction in light-chain burden do much better, with a mean survival rate in one study being as high as 47 months versus only 17 months in nonresponders.

Renal amyloidosis

Amyloidosis is a group of conditions characterized by tissue deposition of degradation-resistant fibrillary proteins as a β-pleated sheet leading to disease. Classically, amyloidosis appears as an apple-green color on Congo red staining when viewed under birefringent light. Amyloid is deposited within the kidney in the mesangium and capillary walls: evolving glomerular involvement presents as worsening proteinuria and renal dysfunction.

Types of amyloidosis

Primary (AL) amyloidosis Monoclonal light chains (usually lambda) or light-chain fragments found alone or with myeloma form amyloid sheets. It is more common in ♂ than ♀ (2:1) >50 years old. Prognosis is poor.

Secondary (AA) amyloidosis Reactive amyloidosis results from deposition of fragments of serum amyloid A (SAA) proteins (an acute-phase reactant) in patients with underlying inflammatory conditions (see below). Prognosis depends on the cause of inflammation.

Familial amyloidosis Inherited defects of (usually) transthyretin lead to amyloid formation in middle age. This type has a better prognosis.

Symptoms and signs

Asymptomatic or nephrotic syndrome ± CKD. Fatigue, weight loss, bruising, and easy bleeding (including GI tract) occur. Cardiomyopathy and cardiac failure (AL alone) autonomic and peripheral neuropathy, hepatomegaly, splenomegaly, and macroglossia (AL alone) ± lymphadenopathy also occur.

Causes of secondary (AA) amyloid

- Rheumatoid arthritis (40% of AA amyloid)
- Other arthropathies: ankylosing spondylitis, psoriatic arthritis
- Inflammatory bowel disease
- Chronic suppurative infections (osteomyelitis, bronchiectasis, leg ulcers)
- TB or leprosy
- Malignancies (renal cell carcinoma, lymphoma)
- Familial Mediterranean fever (FMF).

FMF affects Sephardic Jews, Armenians, and Turks, and is inherited by autosomal recessive transmission. Periodic acute attacks present before the age of 20, with fever, severe abdominal pain, arthritis, and pleurisy (though 25% will have fever alone), lasting 48–72 hours and resolving spontaneously. During the attack, there is ↑WBC and ↑CRP.

Investigations

Dipstick urine (no or little hematuria). BUN, Cr, electrolytes, ↓ albumin, ↑CRP, cholesterol. Spot urine protein/creatinine ratio (PCR) or 24-hour urine protein and creatinine. Consider diagnostic fat pad aspirate for amyloid staining US kidneys (may be ↑size). Renal biopsy. Radiolabeled serum amyloid protein P component (SAP scan) binds to all types of amyloid fibrils and allows quantitation of disease load and response to treatment.

▶ Cardiomyopathy (echocardiogram).

AL suspected: SPEP, M-band (positive in 90%), immunoglobulins and serum free llight chains. Get 24-hour urine for Bence–Jones proteinuria (73% will have urinary free light chains, usually lambda). Do bone marrow aspirate or biopsy (56% will have ↑ plasma cells, 15% will have true myeloma).

AA suspected: SAA protein (useful to monitor response). Search for an underlying cause.

Familial amyloid suspected: Can check for mutant transthyretin gene mutations.

Histology

Amyloid fibrils have characteristic appearance on electron microscopy (Fig. 7.2) and bind Congo red (→ apple-green birefringence under polarized light) or thioflavine-T (→ yellow-green fluorescence). Amorphous deposits of pale hyaline material are demonstrated in the mesangium and capillary loops, staining positive with Congo red. Immunofluorescence may be positive (for light chains) in AL, but is negative in AA amyloid. Electron microscopy will show small (8–10 nm) fibrils.

Management

AL amyloidoisis

Consider chemotherapy as melphan + prednisolone (± autologous stem cell transplant). In responders (~30%) there is ↑ patient survival, ↓proteinuria, and ↓ progression to ESRD. All patients considered candidates for therapy are thus treated. In elderly or frail patients with much comorbid disease, an alternative is pulse dexamethasone + alkylating agents and interferon.

AA amyloidosis

Treat the underlying cause. Consider immunosuppression (cytotoxic therapy or monoclonal antibodies) in autoimmune diseases. Give antibiotics ± surgery for chronic infectious causes. FMF treated with colchicine 1.2 mg/day reduces acute attacks and improves renal outcome. Eprosidate, an anionic sulfonate, interferes with AA fibril formation. It reduced risk of worsening renal function in a placebo-controlled trial, but is not yet available.

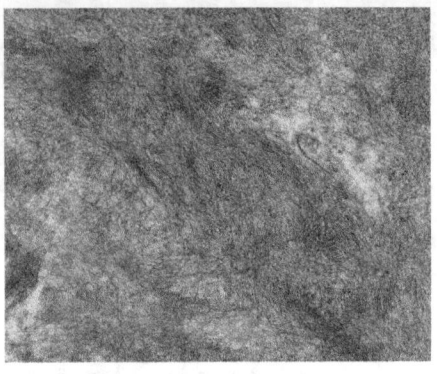

Fig. 7.2 Amyloid fibrils on renal biopsy. Reproduced with permission from Davison AMA, Cameron JS, Grunfeld J-P, et al. (eds) (2005). *Oxford Textbook of Clinical Nephrology*, 3rd ed. Oxford: Oxford University Press.

Other non-amyloid dysproteinemias

Light-chain deposition disease (LCDD)

LCDD is caused by a plasma cell dyscrasia leading to tissue deposition of monoclonal Ig light chains (kappa [κ] chains in 65%). It differs from amyloid in that the light chain lacks hydrophilic residues and cannot organize into fibrils *or stain positive for Congo red*. It may be associated with overt myeloma in 50% (or MM may subsequently develop). Absence of a monoclonal band on SPEP (up to 30% patients) or plasma cell expansion in the bone marrow is still consistent with LCDD. Free light chains may be detected in serum (usually kappa vs. lambda present in AL amyloid).

Patients usually present with nephrotic syndrome ± progressive renal failure with eventual ESRD. There may be features of AL amyloid (rarely diastolic dysfunction on echocardiography).

On renal biopsy, a nodular glomerulosclerosis is present that is Congo red *negative*. Immunofluorescence is positive for monoclonal light chains in capillary walls and the mesangium. Electron microscopy demonstrates widespread amorphous, granular deposits without fibril formation.

Heavy-chain deposition disease

This is a rare disorder in which abnormal heavy chains deposited in the glomerulus cause similar disease.

Immunotactoid and fibrillary glomerulonephritis

These are poorly understood disorders characterized by the deposition of non-amyloid (i.e., Congo red *negative*) proteinaceous fibrils derived from Ig. Although two forms are described, they may represent a spectrum of a single process.

Fibrillary GN (FGN)

FGN involves deposition of polyclonal Ig (and C3) fibrils (18–22 nm) in mesangium and glomerulus. There may be focal and diffuse GN with or without crescents.

Immunotactoid GN (ITGN)

Monoclonal Ig deposits form rod-like microtubular structures. Fibrils are larger (30–40 nm diameter) than FGN. There may be an underlying M-band, 📖 p. 87, chronic lymphocytic leukemia (CLL), B-cell non-Hodgkin's lymphoma (NHL), hepatitis C virus (HCV) infection, or other autoimmune disease.

▶ There are no extrarenal features of the disease. It presents with proteinuria (nephrotic range in 60%), hematuria, ↑BP, and progressive CKD. There is no specific diagnostic test, so proceed to renal biopsy, where larger fibrils are seen infiltrating the glomerulus. Always exclude M-band or HCV.

There is no proven effective treatment to slow progression in either fibrillary or immunotactoid GN. Although there are anecdotal reports of success, small trials of immunosuppressive therapy have been disappointing, except in patients with crescentic changes on renal biopsy (prednisone 60 mg qd after pulse methylprednisolone + cyclophosphamide 1.5–2 mg/kg/qd).

Sickle cell nephropathy

Renal involvement affects 4%–8% of patients with sickle cell disease, in patients with homozygous sickle cell anemia (HgbSS) or combined HgbSC disease. HgbS carriers (sickle cell trait) can develop milder tubular defects.

Erythrocyte sickling in the low oxygen environment of the medullary capillaries (vasa recta) → obstruction and occlusion of capillaries, ischemia, interstitial fibrosis, and papillary necrosis. The medullary counter-current mechanism is also impaired, resulting in impaired urinary concentration. Glomerular hypertrophy, hyperfiltration, and secondary FSGS (≈FSGS, 📖 p. 394) may evolve, leading to ESRD.

Symptoms and signs

Impaired concentrating ability presents as nocturia or polyuria (occurs early). Asymptomatic hematuria is common. Sloughed necrotic papillae may present with frank hematuria and either painless or painful colic (and ureteric obstruction, usually left-sided). Proteinuria and CKD may occur over time. Hypertension occurs less frequently than in the general African-American population due to increased sodium and water loss.

Renal medullary carcinoma

This is a rare, aggressive malignancy found in patients with sickle cell trait, occurring at a young age. It presents as abdominal or flank pain, hematuria, and weight loss ± an abdominal mass. Treatment is surgical, but metastasis is common at diagnosis—median survival is usually less than 4 months.

Investigations

Electrolytes, BUN, Cr, albumin, CBC. 24-hour urinary volume (↑), urine osmolality or specific gravity (SG)—↓ concentrating capacity. There may be an incomplete distal RTA (UpH ↑ with normal serum bicarbonate, 📖 p. 556).

Get US if there is gross hematuria (papillary necrosis [PN] ± obstruction, 📖 p. 500). IVU may show clubbed calyces from PN. New gross hematuria should not be assumed to be PN, and therefore a workup is recommended.

Management

No specific therapy prevents the disease—aim to limit sickle crises, and prevent infection. Encourage fluids for target UO >2 L/day.
- Massive hematuria (?PN)
  - Bed rest
  - Start vigorous IV hydration with 0.45% NaCl with urine alkalinization.
  - In resistant cases, consider transfusion ± DDAVP, Epsilon-amino caproic acid, ureteroscopy with electrocautery or laser treatment. Consider renal angiography and embolization.

- Progression
  - ACEI (♦ unproven) to maximum tolerated dose to decrease proteinuria (📖 p. 342).

ESRD in sickle cell disease

Anemia may be resistant to EPO, and patients may continue to be transfusion dependent. Patients may become iron overloaded—deferoxamine chelation may be useful.

It is estimated that 4.2% of patients with sickle cell disease progress to ESRD. Renal replacement therapy by either HD or PD is well tolerated.

Renal transplantation is successful, with graft survival being comparable at 1 year with that of the general transplant population, although patient survival is lower. Recurrent disease is likely, but graft loss is rare.

Vasculitis and renal disease

The systemic vasculitides are a group of inflammatory diseases of unknown cause, which are often fatal if untreated. The term *vasculitis* simply reflects the underlying process: inflammation and leukocyte infiltration of the walls of blood vessels (Fig. 7.3). This may lead to local inflammation (e.g., purpura), vessel wall damage (aneurysm formation or hemorrhage), or vessel occlusion (ischemia or infarction).

Some vasculitides do not present with renal impairment—however, most of the potentially fatal diseases do. This may present as gradually progressive CKD or oligoanuric ARF with life-threatening multisystem involvement.

⚠ When considering a diagnosis of vasculitis, three important differential diagnoses ALWAYS need to be considered:
- ▶ Infective endocarditis
- Systemic or occult infection
- Paraneoplastic states.

A brief primer on vasculitides

- Takayasu's arteritis affects the thoracic aorta and its branches in ♀, presenting with ↑BP, pulse deficits, and ischemic limbs or viscera (brain, heart, lungs, and GI tract).
- Giant cell arteritis (temporal arteritis) presents in older patients with headache, jaw claudication, visual symptoms, and myalgias.
- Kawasaki's disease affects children, presenting as a febrile illness with lymphadenopathy, skin rash, conjunctivitis, and mucositis (lips, tongue).
- Classic polyarteritis nodosa (📖 p. 464)
- Churg–Strauss syndrome (📖 p. 462)
- ANCA-positive small-vessel vasculitis (📖 p. 458)
- Henoch–Schönlein purpura (📖 p. 373)
- Cryoglobulinemia (📖 p. 484)
- Other vasculitides include
  - Those associated with other autoimmune diseases (SLE, RA, Sjogren's, Behçet's)
  - Hypersensitivity vasculitis (related to drug reactions)
  - Those associated with viral infection (hepatitis B+C, CMV, EBV, and others)

All vasculitides tend to present with constitutional symptoms (fever, weight loss, malaise)—there is often myalgias ± arthralgias, and may be a skin rash (described as a leukocytoclastic vasculitis on skin biopsy). Acute-phase markers (ESR, CRP, ferritin) are usually elevated. The size of vessel and organ affected will then dictate how the disease presents and evolves.

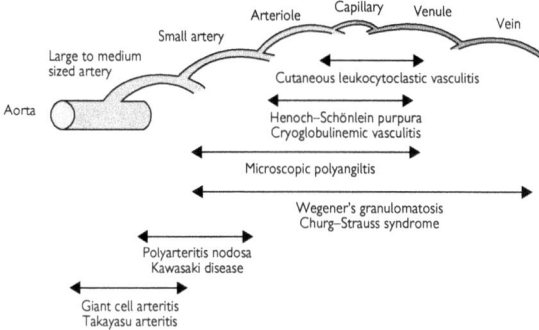

Fig. 7.3 Chapel Hill classification of vasculitis based on the size of vessel. Modified with permission from Jeanette JC, Falk RJ, Andrassy K, et al. (1994). Nomenclature of systemetic vasculitides. Proposal of an international consensus conference. *Arthritis Rheum* **37**: 187–92.

ANCA-positive vasculitis

Small-vessel vasculitides are characterized by the presence of anti-neutrophil cytoplasmic antibodies (ANCA), a group including Wegener's granulomatosis (WG), microscopic polyangiitis (MPA), and renal-limited vasculitis (see below). Churg–Strauss syndrome, often ANCA+, is dealt with elsewhere (p. 462). ANCA-positive vasculitis affects ± 20 pmp (in Europe), ♂ = ♀, with an increasing incidence with age (peak 55–70 years). Wide geographic, ethnic, and seasonal differences are described. Untreated, prognosis is poor (90% mortality at 2 years), but with immunosuppression the outlook is much better (70%–80% 1-year patient survival). However, aggressive disease remains difficult to treat, and treatment-related morbidity is substantial.

Symptoms and signs

These include fever, weight loss, malaise, myalgias, and polyarthralgias. Other features depend on the affected organ system(s):
- Upper respiratory tract (▶ usually WG): nasal discharge, epistaxis, sinusitis, oral or nasal ulcers, otitis media (deafness), cartilaginous involvement (collapse of nasal bridge and tracheal stenosis)
- Lungs: cough, dyspnea, hemoptysis → pulmonary hemorrhage
- Kidney: asymptomatic urinary abnormalities to a rapidly progressive GN and ARF
- Skin: palpable purpura or diffuse, fine vasculitic rash
- Mononeuritis multiplex presenting as peripheral neuropathy
- Eyes: conjunctivitis, episcleritis, uveitis. Optic tract granulomata and proptosis (WG)
- GI: abdominal pain and bloody diarrhea
- Deep vein thrombosis or arterial thrombosis.

Investigations

Urinalysis shows dysmorphic RBCs, RBC casts; get 24-hour urine protein and creatinine or spot urine PCR. Check ANCA, anti-GBM (double-positive ANCA+ and anti-GBM+ disease occurs, and behaves more like Goodpasture's disease). Get full RPGN screen, p. 86. Complement levels are normal. CBC (↓Hb, ↑Plt). Electrolytes, BUN, Cr (ARF), albumin, LFTs. ↑ESR, ↑CRP.

Chest X-ray may show patchy or diffuse alveolar infiltrates—cavitating nodules may be seen with WG. If ↓O_2 saturation, get ABG.

Skin biopsy will suggest leukocytoclastic vasculitis without immune deposits. Renal biopsy is important for diagnosis, prognosis, and treatment.

Histology

A focal and segmental necrotizing, crescentic glomerulonephritis is apparent ± granulomatous small-vessel vasculitis. On immunofluorescence, there is no significant immune complex or complement deposition seen, i.e., *pauci-immune*. The presence of renal (or other tissue) granuloma formation is characteristic of WG.

Renal-limited vasculitis refers to a pauci-immune GN (as above) in patients who are often ANCA positive but have no systemic disease.

WG and MPA

Treatment of these two diseases is similar and clinical presentations and serologic markers may overlap, compared to the usual characteristics shown in Table 7.2.

A–Z of ANCA

Anti-neutrophil cytoplasmic antibodies are antibodies directed against intracellular antigens, most commonly proteinase-3 (PR3) or myeloperoxidase (MPO) detected by ELISA assays. On indirect immunofluorescence, the cytoplasmic or c-ANCA is now known to be PR3-ANCA on ELISA, and the perinuclear or p-ANCA is MPO. Antigen-specific ELISA testing has improved assay reliability, and a positive ANCA is 99% specific and 70% sensitive in the right clinical context. Many labs will screen for ANCA with the indirect immunofluorescence test and will confirm positive results with ELISA tests.

▶ Low-titer P-ANCA–positivity is recognized with other connective tissue disorders or systemic infection. Higher-titer MPO ANCA-positivity is also recognized with drug-induced vasculitis (especially anti-thyroid drugs).

Table 7.2 Characteristics of WG and MPA

	WG	MPA
ENT involvement	Yes	No
ANCA specificity	c-ANCA (PR3)	p-ANCA (MPO)
Granulomata	Yes	No
Pulmonary hemorrhage	Yes	Yes
Necrotizing GN	Yes	Yes
Peripheral nerve	Uncommon	More common

Does ANCA cause disease?

In mice, evoking ANCA causes a systemic small-vessel vasculitis. In humans, we do not yet know if ANCA is pathogenic or an epiphenomenon. More is known about how ANCA may contribute to disease.

It is thought that ANCA+ vasculitis is a "two-hit" disease: the release of local or systemic proinflammatory cytokines (especially TNF) in response to infection (nasal *S. aureus* carriage, viral infection) or non-infectious toxins primes neutrophils (→ surface expression of MPO and PR-3) and activates endothelial cells. ANCA binds primed neutrophils, increasing

- Neutrophil tethering and migration on and across endothelium.
- Neutrophil degranulation → secondary recruitment of monocytes.
- Augmentation of inflammation and endothelial cell injury through free-radical generation.

Treatment of ANCA-positive vasculitis

Both the disease and the toxic therapy may cause morbidity or death. Balance the risk and benefit in pursuing treatment. For a full discussion on starting immunosuppression, 📖 p. 369. (▶ Preventative and protective measures should be taken when using immunosuppressants.)

Induction therapy (to achieve remission)

Prednisone
- If rapidly ↑Cr, or pulmonary hemorrhage, "pulse methylprednisolone" as 500 mg—1 g IV x 3days, then po steroids as below
- Prednisone at 1 mg/kg/day, aiming to taper ↓10–15 mg/month (but not less than 7.5 mg/day at 6 months)

Cyclophosphamide
- Oral 1–2 mg/kg/day (to a maximum of 150 mg) for 3–6 months
- An alternative is monthly IV cyclophosphamide, as IV may be less toxic, but associated with higher rate of relapse.
- Toxicity is less usual if total dose is <10 g (📖 p. 370).

Using this regimen, expect 90% clinical improvement and complete remission in 75%—it often takes 12 months or longer of therapy. In those who achieve remission earlier (i.e., at 12 weeks), cyclophosphamide may be discontinued, and maintenance therapy commenced.

Plasma exchange

☞ The MEPEX trial recommends plasma exchange (PEX) instead of pulse methylprednisolone in ANCA + vasculitis if there is:
- Cr >5.7 mg/dL
- Coexisting anti-GBM antibodies

If used, treat with 7 plasma exchanges (combination of human albumin ± fresh frozen plasma [FFP]) within 2 weeks and reassess for benefit.

Maintenance therapy (to maintain in remission)
- Continue prednisone at 7.5–15 mg/day po.
- Convert cyclophosphamide to azathioprine 1.5–2 mg/kg/day po based on EUVAS data (or perhaps mycophenolate mofetil [MMF] 0.5–1.5 g po bid). Methotrexate is reserved for patients with mild renal disease.

The risk of relapse is ± 25%–50% within 3–5 years, and is more likely with:
- WG
- Persistently positive high-titer ANCA (especially anti-PR3).

☞ It is not known how long to continue therapy; most would treat for at least 12 months after remission is induced.

Monitoring response and predicting relapse

Disease remission may be judged by the following:
- Clinical assessment (absence of symptoms)
- Urinary abnormalities (↓ hematuria, ↓ proteinuria)
- ↓CRP
- Improving renal function.

The Birmingham Vasculitis Activity Score (BVAS) provides a good tool for monitoring Wegener's.

A rising ANCA titer may predict relapse, but there appears to be no role for presumptively increasing immunosuppression in the absence of other (clinical) features of ↑ disease activity.

Relapse should be treated as for first presentation. Novel therapies are being investigated for resistant or frequently relapsing disease, including rituximab (anti-CD20 antibody) and deoxyspergualin. Etanercept (anti-TNF-α antibody) has not proved useful in maintaining remission, but such therapies may yet have a role in inducing remission in difficult disease.

Churg–Strauss syndrome

This syndrome is a rare multisystem disorder presenting as allergic rhinitis, asthma, and eosinophilia, with a small- and medium-vessel vasculitis affecting predominantly the lungs and skin. Occurrence in ♂ = ♀, at age 30–50 (unlike WG or MPA, 📖 p. 459). The cause remains unknown.

Symptoms and signs

Disease evolves from an atopic prodrome to a life-threatening systemic vasculitis. Allergic rhinitis or other atopic conditions ± late-onset asthma precede vasculitis by weeks to years. Vasculitis is often steroid requiring and severe.

Vasculitis presents as fever, malaise, weight loss, and myalgias ± polyarthralgias. Skin rash (urticarial or vasculitic) ± mononeuritis multiplex is common.

Visceral involvement includes the following:
- Lungs: dyspnea, hemoptysis
- Kidneys: urinary abnormalities are common. Although renal impairment is usually mild, it may cause RPGN or interstitial nephritis. ↑BP is common (presumably renal ischemia).
- GI: abdominal pain and bloody diarrhea ± ischemic bowel
- Heart: coronary vasculitis (angina), myocarditis (LVF) or pericarditis (⚠ even tamponade).

Investigations

- Urinalysis for dysmorphic RBCs and RBC casts, 24-hour urine for protein and creatinine or spot urine PCR.
- CBC (↓Hb) with prominent eosinophilia (>10% total WBC, or absolute count >1.5 x 10^9/L) or eosinophilic-rich infiltrates on biopsy of affected tissues.

▶ Eosinophilia is exquisitely steroid-sensitive and may resolve rapidly on treatment. Check ↑ESR, ↑CRP, immunoglobulins (?↑IgE). Send electrolytes, BUN, Cr, albumin, LFT, CK. Order chest X-ray (patchy infiltration) ± ABG, ECG, echocardiogram. Patients are ANCA positive in only 38%–50% by indirect immunofluorescence (P or C ANCA), but higher using PR3 or MPO ELISA with slightly more MPO, 📖 p. 459.

Tissue biopsy may be required: classically this shows an eosinophil-rich granulomatous inflammation, and if vessels are sampled, a small- to medium-vessel necrotizing vasculitis. Renal biopsy may show vasculitis ± focal and segmental necrotizing GN, though with an eosinophilic infiltrate and granuloma formation in the interstitium.

Treatment

For crescentic GN, start with cyclophosphamide and methylprednisolone IV pulse therapy followed by po steroids.

Milder renal disease such as interstitial nephritis can be treated with prednisone po 1 mg/kg/day for 6–12 weeks or until remission. If full remission is achieved, discontinue steroids, and monitor for relapse using
- Eosinophil count
- Acute-phase reactants (ESR, CRP)
- ▶ ANCA positivity does not predict disease activity.

Relapse can be expected in ± 25% of cases. Difficult to control disease may be treated by adding cyclophosphamide (📖 p. 369), interferon-∞.

Polyarteritis nodosa

This disease is a rare, medium-vessel necrotizing arteritis involving principally the skin, nerves, gut, and kidney. It is *not* synonymous with microscopic polyangiitis, one of the ANCA-positive *small*-vessel vasculitides (📖 p. 458). It may be associated with hepatitis B infection. Onset is at age 40–60 years, with incidence of 1.5:1 males to females.

Symptoms and signs

These include fever, weight loss (>4 kg), arthralgias, and myalgias. Mononeuritis multiplex (peripheral neuropathy) occurs, rarely CNS disease. Livedo reticularis, skin ulcers, or erythematous nodules are also found. Medium-vessel involvement in the GI tract presents as abdominal pain or bloody stools. There may be testicular pain (orchitis).

Renal ischemia → ↑BP and renal impairment. Presentations include hematuria or loin pain with segmental renal infarcts. There may be rupture of renal aneurysms.

Investigations

Electrolytes, BUN, Cr, albumin, LFTs, ↑CK (muscle injury), CBC, ↑ESR, ANCA negative, hepatitis B (positive in a minority), and cryoglobulins. Diagnosis is made on angiography: arterial aneurysms are in the renal or mesenteric tree (Fig. 7.4). Renal biopsy may show segmental transmural fibrinoid necrosis in medium-sized arteries, but may sample downstream ischemic changes or frank infarction alone. Glomerulonephritis is not seen. Because small aneurysms may increase bleeding from renal biopsy, some advocate biopsy only after negative angiography.

Management and natural history

Untreated, the prognosis is poor. With therapy, 10-year patient survival is approximately 80%. Risk factors associated with poor outcome include
- Age >50 years
- Renal impairment
- GI or coronary involvement.

Treatment

- Low risk: prednisone 1 mg/kg/day against clinical and biochemical response
- High risk: (ARF, mesenteric ischemia, mononeuritis multiplex) prednisone as above (or IV methylprednisolone if life threatening or with nerve involvement), + oral cyclophosphamide 1–2 mg/kg/day (limit to 150 mg daily). See 📖 p. 264 for starting immunosuppression.
- If HBsAg positive, give short-term prednisone followed by interferon-α and plasma exchange.

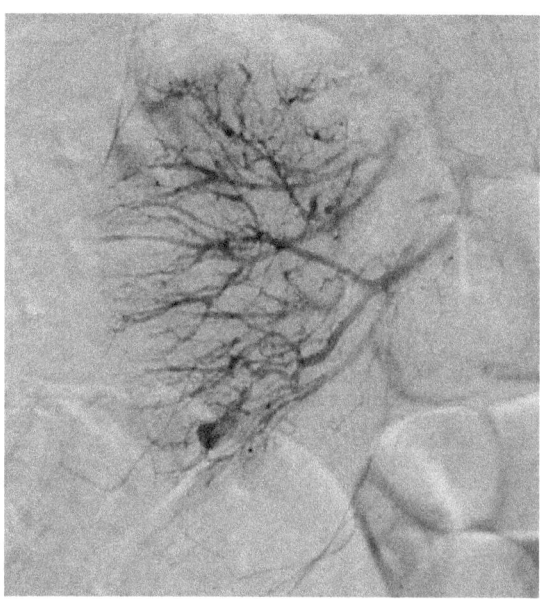

Fig. 7.4 Medium-vessel aneurysms in the kidneys at ateriography. Reproduced with permission from Wu K and Throssell D (2006). *Nephrol Dial Transplant* **21**:1710–12.

Goodpasture's or anti-GBM disease

Anti-GBM disease causes a rapidly progressive GN and is known as Goodpasture's disease or syndrome if there is pulmonary–renal syndrome with pulmonary hemorrhage. It has an incidence of <1 pmp, and affects two age groups: ♂ > ♀ aged 20–30 years, or ♂ and ♀ >60 years.

Pathogenesis
Pathogenic, predominantly IgG anti-GBM antibodies are directed against the α3 chain of type IV collagen (found in the basement membranes of glomeruli and alveoli) and cause disease. A trigger (?cigarette smoking, infections, ?other environmental) exposes antigenic epitopes on the normally "hidden" α3 chain. On binding, anti-GBM antibodies fix complement and cause local injury.

Symptoms and signs
Anti-GBM disease may present gradually (over months to years), or abruptly over days with fulminant lung hemorrhage and renal failure. Lung and kidney involvement can present separately or together. Severe pulmonary hemorrhage may present with profuse hemoptysis and respiratory failure requiring intubation and ventilation—usually in smokers.

Fever and weight loss may be present, but often there are few other constitutional symptoms. There may be dyspnea and cough (nonproductive → flecking or frank hemoptysis). Hematuria and proteinuria are found on urinalysis.

Investigations
Urinalysis (RBCs, RBC casts), 24-hour urine protein and creatinine or spot urine protein and creatinine. Electrolytes, BUN, Cr, albumin, LFTs, CBC (↓Hb), normal complement levels. ANCA (25% "double positive"—treat as for anti-GBM, but expect better outcome). Anti-GBM: by immunofluorescence or ELISA (note occasional false positive). Get chest X-ray (diffuse alveolar infiltrates), ABG (↓pO$_2$). Proceed to renal biopsy.

Pathology
A focal and segmental necrotizing, crescentic GN is evident. Bowman's capsule may be ruptured. Immunofluorescence shows *linear* capillary wall staining for anti-GBM (IgG) and C3 deposition in a similar pattern.

Treatment of renal disease
⚠ Oligoanuria (<200 mL/day) or Cr >5.7 mg/dL implies severe crescentic glomerular damage. If the patient requires dialysis within 72 hours of presentation or has evidence on biopsy of chronic disease (fibrous crescents or tubulointerstitial fibrosis), renal recovery is very unusual.

For those with Cr <5.7 mg/dL or not requiring dialysis within 72 hours and having no chronic changes on renal biopsy, therapy should include:
- Pulse methylprednisolone 0.5–1 g IV daily x 3 days, then prednisone 1 mg/kg/day (to a maximum 60 mg)
- Cyclophosphamide 1–2 mg/kg/day (to a maximum of 150 mg).

And unless patient requires dialysis with severe chronic damage on biopsy (when it offers little renal benefit):
- Plasma exchange as 8–10 treatments in <2 weeks of 4 L (by volume, usually albumin solution unless recent biopsy or pulmonary hemorrhage, then 1–2 L FFP). Daily pheresis is preferable if possible. Check anti-GBM titer weekly to confirm efficacy of therapy.

Continue prednisone + cyclophosphamide 3–6 months; consider discontinuing cyclophosphamide and keep low-dose prednisone ± azathioprine for total duration of therapy for 6–9 months.

Treating pulmonary hemorrhage

▶ Differentiating pulmonary edema from pulmonary hemorrhage can be difficult. Transfer to ICU for invasive monitoring.
- Such patients may (often do) require mechanical ventilation.
- Institute early plasma exchange as above in *all* cases of pulmonary hemorrhage with daily pheresis if possible.

Treatment continues until anti-GBM titer becomes negative; this usually is within 2–3 weeks but may take longer. The disease does not usually recur, and immunosuppression can be discontinued as above. Cigarette smoking should be discouraged, as it may be related to rare relapse.

Renal transplantation is successful for ESRD secondary to Goodpasture's—it should be deferred until 6 months after anti-GBM is negative in suitable recipient candidates. De novo anti-GBM disease can cause graft loss in ESRD patients transplanted for Alport syndrome (p. 381).

Lupus nephritis

Systemic lupus erythematosus (SLE) is a heterogenous multisystem disease characterized by autoantibody production and impaired immune complex clearance. SLE is more common among African Americans, Hispanics, or Asians ♀ (10♀:1♂), presenting in youth or young adulthood (although autoantibodies predate disease). Approximately 50% of patients will develop renal involvement within 3 years of diagnosis, and ~10% progress to ESRD by 10 years.

How do autoantibodies arise in SLE?

Genetic and environmental factors influence risk for developing lupus. Loss of tolerance to self-antigens is of prime importance in the etiology of SLE—a wide range of interacting immune defects has been described as a result of this self-tolerance.

Part of the explanation is as follows: apoptosis (programmed cell death) is part of normal cell replacement. Faulty phagocytosis and clearance of apoptotic waste → nucleosomal (and other) proteins being engulfed by circulating B cells. Processed peptides are presented to histone-specific CD4+ T cells, which in conjunction with appropriate co-stimulation → cytokine-dependent autoreactive B-cell activation with autoantibody production. Usually, IL-2-mediated pathways are responsible for the elimination of these autoreactive lymphocytes; patients with SLE have low T-cell IL-2 production.

Diagnosing SLE

The American College of Rheumatology offers clinically useful criteria:

▶ >3 criteria is diagnostic, but many patients with 2–3 criteria will evolve over time to develop full-blown SLE.

Malar rash	Fixed erythematous ("butterfly") rash
Discoid rash	Raised erythematous patches that may scar
Photosensitivity	
Oral ulcers	Painless (may be nasopharyngeal)
Arthritis	Nonerosive, x2 more peripheral joints
Serositis	Pleural or pericardial (pain), rub or effusion
Renal disease	Urinary RBC casts or proteinuria >0.5 g/day
CNS disease	Psychosis or seizures
Blood disorder	Hemolysis, ↓WBC, ↓Plt or lymphopenia
Immunology	Positive anticardiolipin, anti-dsDNS or anti-Sm antibodies, or false positive syphilis serology (RPR)
Anti-nuclear factor	

Other clinical features include constitutional symptoms (fever, weight loss, fatigue), lymphadenopathy, Raynaud's phenomenon, scleritis or sicca symptoms, polyarthralgias, myalgias, pneumonitis, interstitial lung disease (or pulmonary hypertension), sterile (Libman–Sacks) endocarditis, or vascular thrombosis (▶ anti-phospholipid syndrome).

Investigations

CBC (Hb↓, ↓Plt, lymphopenia), ↑↑ESR. Screen for hemolysis (including Coombs' test). Electrolytes, BUN, Cr, Ca^{2+}, LFTs, CK. ANA, dsDNA (may be useful to monitor response to treatment), anti-RNP, anti-Smith, anticardiolipin antibodies. Check complement levels (active disease → ↓C3/C4).

Get urinalysis for dysmorphic RBCs or RBC casts (📖 p. 23), 24-hour urine for protein and creatinine or spot urine PCR. US kidneys ± renal biopsy is indicated if there is hematuria (especially if RBC casts or >300–500 mg proteinuria/day ± ↓ GFR).

Pathogenesis and histology of lupus nephritis

Circulating (or locally derived) immune complexes deposit within the glomerulus, activating (and consuming) complement. Recruited monocytes and leukocytes → proinflammatory cytokines, neutrophil-induced oxidant injury, and activation of the coagulation cascade. The histology that results is often varied. Characteristic deposition of IgG- and complement-rich (C3 and C1q) immune deposits are seen in the mesangium or subendothelial space. A lupus membranous-like lesion is characterized by deposits in the subepithelium and mesangium. The histological lesion has important therapeutic and prognostic implications.

ISN/RPS classification of lupus nephritis

I	Normal light microscopy (but mesangial deposits → electron microscopy)
II	Mesangial proliferation (hypercellularity)
III	Focal proliferative: affecting <50% of glomeruli
IV	Diffuse proliferative: affecting >50% of glomeruli, either segmentally (IV-S) or globally (IV-G)
V	Membranous (subepithelial deposits)
VI	Advanced sclerosing with >90% glomeruli obsolescent

Class III or IV is further subclassified as active or chronic as well as segmental or global (e.g., Type IV-GA is an active global diffuse proliferative lesion).

Management of lupus nephritis

🔑 How to treat LN is controversial. Attempt to do the following:
- Identify those most at (renal) risk.
- Induce (renal) disease remission (only 80% will achieve remission).
- Maintain (renal) disease remission (relapse can be expected in 30%).
- Prevent CKD → ESRD.
- Minimize drug toxicity (in the short and longer term).

Those at risk

▶ Type I and II LN patients rarely require treatment for renal disease (it may be required for other involved organs). Types III–V require treatment. Predictors of ↑ renal risk include the following:
- African American or Hispanic (especially if male)
- Poor socioeconomic status
- Renal impairment, neuropsychiatric, or other severe extrarenal disease
- High activity or chronicity index on biopsy
- Poor response to therapy or frequent relapse.

Induction therapy to induce remission (⚠ p. 369 for using IV cyclophosphamide)

- Type III or IV (or mixed-type III or IV with V)
  - *Either* pulse methylprednisolone 0.5–1 g IV for 3 days followed by prednisone as below if ARF, crescentic GN, and/or severe extrarenal manifestations
  - *Or* prednisone 1 mg/kg/day qd for 4–8 weeks tapering slowly to 7.5 mg qd over months against disease activity
  - Plus:
    1. IV cyclophosphamide $0.5–1 g/m^2$ over 30–50 min monthly for 6 months (check WBC at day 10–14). (↑dose to $1 g/m^2$ if possible). If GFR <60 mL/min, ↓ dose to $500 mg/m^2$.
    2. ▶ Mycophenolate mofetil 0.5–1.5 g bid is an alternative for induction with cyclophosphamide. Its efficacy is unclear if Cr is elevated with severe crescentic changes on biopsy (mean Cr 1.1–1.2 in MMF clinical trials).
- Type V
  - Prednisone 1 mg/kg/day for 4–8 weeks, ↓ to 7.5 mg by 6 months
  - Depending on severity, or lack of response, *add on either* azathioprine 1.5–2 mg/kg/day, cyclosporine 5 mg/kg in two divided doses, MMF or cyclophosphamide as above.

Maintenance therapy for remission

If remission is attained, consider switching from intermittent cyclophosphamide to *either*
- Mycophenolate mofetil 0.5–1.5 bid
- *or* azathioprine 1.5–3 mg/kg/day.
- (More effective and less toxic than older regimen of continued IV cyclophosphamide every 3 months for total of 2 years)
- *Continue* lower-dose (± 0.15 mg/kg/day) prednisone.

Prevent CKD → ESRD
- Stop smoking, limit salt, and do exercise.
- Control BP <125–130/75–80.
- If proteinuric >1 g/day, use ACEI ± ARB.
- Treat dyslipidemia with statins.

Minimize toxicity see 📖 p. 370

Monitoring disease activity
- Symptoms
- Urinary sediment (↓proteinuria <0.5 g/day, ↓RBC/hpf <10)
- Cr
- Anti-dsDNA antibody titer
- Complement levels.

Experimental therapies
- ▶ Rituximab is increasingly used for resistant disease and even as initiation therapy in case series. There are rare case reports of progressive multifocal leukoencephopathy with rituximab, but its relative role in this is unclear because of prior immunosuppression in these cases.
- Watch the relevant literature, as much is expected of clinical trials using new agents.

Anti-phospholipid syndrome

Antibodies directed against the phospholipid components of coagulation factors → recurrent arterial and venous thrombosis. This may be either 1° or 2° (usually SLE). Diagnosis requires either venous, arterial or small vessel thrombosis, or unexplained pregnancy morbidity in addition to laboratory tests identifying an anti-phosholipid Ab (see below).

Described antibodies may be directed against:
- Cardiolipin (a phospholipid)
- β2 glycoprotein I (binds to cardiolipin)
- Prothrombin.
- Phosphatidyl choline

These are often found in conjunction with the lupus anticoagulant.

Symptoms and signs
- DVT, spontaneous superficial thrombophlebitis ± pulmonary emboli
- Arterial thrombosis: TIA, RIND, or stroke
- Livedo reticularis (~ 20%)
- Recurrent miscarriges, premature births due to preeclampsia
- ↑BP (~ 30%)
- Features of SLE (📖 p. 469) or other connective tissue disorder
- Sterile (Libman–Sacks) endocarditis
- Hemolytic anemia, thrombocytopenia.
- Renal disease

The renal lesion tends to reflect occlusion of a range of possible vessels (main renal artery and vein to glomerular capillaries, 📖 p. 412, with ↓GFR and bland urine). Patients may have non-nephrotic proteinuria to ARF with active urinary sediment. The APS may present acutely with a thrombotic microangiopathy (📖 p. 398). Secondary FSGS may be seen late. May present with CKD.

Investigations
- CBC (↓Hb, ▶ ↓Plt), evidence of hemolysis (↑LDH, ↑Bili). Clotting (↑APTT). Electrolytes, BUN, Cr
- ANA, dsDNA, complement levels, RF. False positive syphilis serology
- Testing for antibodies:
  - Positive IgG/IgM anticardiolipin antibodies at (.40 unit GPL or >99th percentlie)
  - Positive lupus anticoagulant (failure to correct prolonged APTT after mixing with normal plasma)
  - Positive anti-β2 glycoprotein I IgG/IgM antibodies (>99th percentile).

A single positive test is insufficient to make the diagnosis—it needs repeating after 12 weeks (and can be done on warfarin).

Treatment
Some 20%–30% of untreated APS patients will have a further thrombotic event. Evidence is modest, but consensus suggests the following:
- Lifelong warfarin for INR 2–3
- If there is a new event on warfarin, aim for target INR 3–4.
- Catastrophic anti-phospholipid syndrome with ARF may respond to plasmapheresis to remove anti-phospholipid antibody and is also treated with steroids, anticoagulation ± IVIg.

Anti-phospholipid antibodies in ESRD
- May be found at a high prevalence in hemodialysis patients
- Appear to predict increased AVF stenosis and failure
- Increase the risk of early transplant failure due to graft renal artery or vein thrombosis, a risk only partly ↓ by anticoagulation

Scleroderma renal crisis

Systemic sclerosis (SS), or scleroderma, frequently involves the kidneys; scleroderma renal crisis, however, affects far fewer cases (5%–10%). SS characteristically causes sclerosis of the skin and subcutaneous tissue and an obliterative vasculopathy. It may be diffuse (traditional scleroderma), or limited (used to be called "CREST" syndrome). Other skin-limited varieties are also described.
- Diffuse: ↑ skin fibrosis score (sclerosis beyond the hands and face), frequent solid-organ involvement, positive anti-scl-70 antibodies, anti-RNP)
- Limited: ↓ skin fibrosis score (hands and face affected), unusual solid organ involvement, positive anti-centromere antibodies.

Symptoms and signs of SS

Patchy skin edema → fibrosis and calcinosis ± digital ulceration. Peri-orbital tethering and microstomia, nasal beaking, and tapering of the fingers (sclerodactyly) occur. Raynaud's phenomenon, facial and limb telangiectasias, nonerosive arthritis, and myalgias may be present. There is esophageal (and intestinal) dysmotility, as well as pulmonary fibrosis and pulmonary hypertension.

Scleroderma renal crisis

Severe and life-threatening renal disease develops in 12% of patients with diffuse disease, but only 1% of those with limited SS. Scleroderma renal crisis usually presents early in those with diffuse scleroderma and may be precipitated by high-dose steroids. It is characterized by the following:
- Acute renal failure
- ↑BP (10% can be *normotensive*, though these patients have higher BP than at baseline with marked vessel changes)
- Bland urine.

There may be accelerated ↑BP (📖 p. 350) with hypertensive encephalopathy or acute LV failure ± thrombotic microangiopathy (📖 p. 398).

Investigations
- Immediate
  - CBC (↓Hb, ↓Plts), RBC smear (?fragments), ↑LDH, ↓haptoglobin
  - Electrolytes, BUN, Cr, albumin, LFTs. Urinalysis, 24-hour urine protein and creatinine or spot urine PCR
  - US kidneys (proceed to renal biopsy once BP is controlled)
- Evaluate end-organ hypertensive damage
  - Fundoscopy for hypertensive retinopathy
  - ECG (LVH ± strain), echocardiogram
- To confirm systemic sclerosis if there are no obvious signs:
  - Nail-fold capillaroscopy (dilated capillaries)
  - ANA, anti-topoisomerase I (also called anti-Scl70), anti-RNA polymerase antibodies (rarely have positive anti-centromere antibody).

Renal histology

Within vessels, fibrinoid necrosis and fibrin thrombi are found, with "onion-skin" intimal thickening of interlobar arteries. There are varying degrees of collapsed and ischemic glomeruli or ATN.

Management

For severe hypertension, admit patient to ICU or higher-acuity care unit.
- Cardiac monitor
- Strict input and output (in-dwelling catheter)
- Arterial line for invasive BP monitoring if severe ↑BP.

▶ BP control with ACEI is the mainstay of therapy. ACEIs have reduced mortality in renal crises from 80% to 15%. Good BP control can prevent further renal deterioration, or even aid renal recovery and dialysis independence. Progression to ESRD occurs in 20%–50%.
- Start captopril (short-acting) 12.5–50 mg po tid.
- Add in calcium channel blockers.
- Aim for BP reduction 10–15 mmHg/day.
- Target diastolic BP 85–90 mmHg.
- Avoid β-blockers.

Unproven interventions include IV prostacyclin infusion for 24–48 hours, done in the United Kingdom, or fish oils (as for IgAN, 📖 p. 372).

⚠ If ACEI does not provide adequate BP control, or if there is a complicated hypertensive emergency (seizures, acute LVF), use calcium channel blockers (nifedipine). (ARB use is controversial.)

All SS patients should have urinalysis and BP measured every 3 months. ↑BP should be treated with ACEI as a first-line agent.

Rheumatoid arthritis (RA)

Renal conditions complicating RA
- Secondary membranous nephropathy (MN)
- Secondary amyloidosis (AA amyloid)
- Analgesic nephropathy (NSAIDs)
- Rheumatoid vasculitis
- Other glomerular lesions.

Secondary MN (p. 392)
Patients present with proteinuria (less commonly nephrotic syndrome), usually due to disease-modifying drugs (gold, penicillamine), timed with starting therapy (6–12 months). Stopping the drugs → remission (but the course of proteinuria may be prolonged, up to 1 year).

Secondary amyloidosis (p. 450)
Patients present with nephrotic-range proteinuria, and are often normotensive. There is a long history of poorly controlled active RA, often seropositive RF+) Control of RA can lead to improvement.

Analgesic nephropathy (p. 408)
This may present as papillary necrosis, or insidious renal impairment with bland urinalysis.

Rheumatoid vasculitis

This small- and medium-vessel vasculitis affects seropositive patients, often with rheumatoid nodules. It presents as a skin leukocytoclastic vasculitis and mononeuritis multiplex (peripheral neuropathy). The renal lesion is a pauci-immune necrotizing glomerulonephritis. There is ↑ESR, ↑↑RhF. ↓C_3, ↓C_4. ANCA testing may be positive.

⚠ This is an aggressive and life-threatening complication—treat as for ANCA-positive small-vessel vasculitis, with corticosteroids and cyclophosphamide (p. 460).

Glomerular lesions
A mesangioproliferative GN may also occur, presenting with an active urinary sediment, and less commonly, renal impairment. Crescentic GN has been reported with anti-TNF-α therapy.

Other connective tissue disorders associated with renal disease

- Sjogren syndrome may present with
  - Type 1 renal tubular acidosis (📖 p. 556)
  - Impaired concentrating ability (nephrogenic DI, 📖 p. 530)
  - Interstitial nephritis (📖 p. 404)
- Mixed connective tissue disorder is associated with
  - Membranous nephropathy (📖 p. 390)
  - MPGN (📖 p. 482)
- Polymyositis and dermatomyositis

Myositis and myoglobinuria may lead to false-positive hematuria (📖 p. 13), or less commonly, ARF secondary to rhabdomyolysis.

Almost all connective tissue disorders may have a degree of overlap or present atypically—renal disease is not uncommon, and kidney biopsy is often indicated in patients with urinary abnormalities, ↑BP, or renal impairment.

Sarcoidosis

Sarcoidosis is a multisystem granulomatous disease of unknown cause, usually affecting the lungs. It is more common in African Americans and usually diagnosed by age 40. It is characterized by noncaseating granulomata. Renal disease complicates sarcoidosis in up to 40% of cases (although often subclinically).

Symptoms and signs

Sarcoidosis is the great mimicker of the post-syphilis era, involving anything and everything.
- Lymphadenopathy, fevers, loss of weight, malaise
- Chest: bilateral hilar lymphadenopathy, infiltrates, pulmonary fibrosis
- Eyes: uveitis, keratoconjunctivitis sicca
- Skin: pigmentary changes, erythema nodosum
- Cardiac: conduction defects, arrythmias (▶ VT), cardiomyopathy
- CNS: mononeuritis multiplex, aseptic meningitis, pituitary infiltration (central DI, 📖 p. 530), or neurosarcoidosis presenting like multiple sclerosis
- Liver: granulomatous hepatitis
- Kidney: granulomatous tubulointerstitial nephritis, ↑Ca^{2+}, hypercalciuria, renal tubular dysfunction, rarely GN or obstruction.

Investigations

- Urinalysis (often bland) and 24-hour or spot urine PCR (≤1 g/day)
- Electrolytes, BUN, Cr, albumin, LFTs. ↑Ca^{2+}, ↑urinary Ca^{2+}
- If hypercalcemic, 1,25-$(OH)_2$ vitamin D, intact PTH (↓)
- CBC (↓Plt, lymphopenia), ↑ESR
- Polyclonal ↑Ig, ↑serum ACE level—produced by granulomata
- Chest X-ray (?bilateral hilar lymphadenopathy, diffuse nodular infiltrates), pulmonary function tests ±high-resolution chest CT
- Lymph node, salivary gland, skin or kidney biopsy.

Calcium homeostasis in sarcoidosis

Activated macrophages within granulomata convert 25-(OH) vitamin D_3 to its active metabolite, 1,25-$(OH)_2$ vitamin D, particularly during sunny months. This leads to increased GI calcium uptake, resulting in:
- Hypercalciuria (50%)
- Hypercalcemia (10%–20%)
- Calcium-containing renal calculi or nephrocalcinosis (📖 p. 430).

Sarcoidosis may also be associated with
- Diffuse nephrocalcinosis (▶ cause of ESRD)
- Retroperitoneal lymphadenopathy and obstruction
- Glomerulonephritis.

Granulomatous tubulointerstitial nephritis

This disorder presents as → progressive renal impairment (mean Cr 4.8 mg/dL) with mild proteinuria or bland urinalysis. Other features of sarcoidosis might suggest it as a cause, but biopsy often provides the diagnosis—histology shows a lymphocytic tubulointerstitial infiltrate with noncaseating epithelioid granulomata. The differential diagnosis may include
- TB (caseating granulomata!) or other infections
- Drug hypersensitivity (especially NSAIDs)

↑Ca^{2+} may contribute to renal impairment and replete volume prior to therapy.

Management
- Replete volume if ↑Ca^{2+} with NS.
- Prednisone 1 mg/kg qd: renal function and hypercalcemia often improve rapidly (If hypercalcemia is present alone, this responds to prednisone 20–40 mg/day.)
- Taper prednisone slowly once Cr is stabilized, which may lead to a prolonged course; usually there is residual CKD. There are few accurate predictors of remission or relapse, so maintain a high index of suspicion and regular follow-up.

HIV and renal disease

Almost 40 million people worldwide are infected with the human immunodeficiency virus-1 (HIV). HIV is associated with almost every described renal lesion, but HIV-associated nephropathy (HIVAN) has been the most common renal lesion identified in such patients in the developed world. The renal complications of HIV elsewhere (and especially in Africa) remain poorly described.

HIVAN

HIVAN results from direct HIV infection of renal proximal tubular cells and podocytes, causing the so-called collapsing variant of focal and segmental glomerulosclerosis (📖 p. 394) with cystic tubular dilatation. HIVAN has become a significant cause of ESRD, particularly in African-American adults. It usually occurs with advanced HIV infection (↓CD4 <200).

Symptoms and signs

Edema, nephrotic-range proteinuria, and usually significant renal impairment (often due to superimposed ATN) are common. BP is often normal.

Investigations

Urinalysis may be bland, get 24-hour urine protein and creatinine or spot urine PCR. Check electrolytes, BUN, Cr, ↓↓albumin, LFTs. ↓CD4 count. Check for hepatitis B and C. US kidneys (you may see large echogenic kidneys, but insensitive). Renal biopsy shows collapsing FSGS (📖 p. 394). Characteristically, the glomerular tuft is collapsed with a wrinkled basement membrane and microcystic tubular dilatation. Tubular atrophy, interstitial infiltrates, fibrosis, and edema are common. Tubuloreticular inclusions in glomerular endothelial cells may be seen on electron microscopy.

Management of HIVAN

Highly active antiretroviral therapy (HAART), a three-drug regimen of two reverse transcriptase inhibitors and a protease inhibitor, has transformed the outlook in HIV-infected individuals. HAART appears to have similar effects on HIVAN:
- ↓proteinuria ± induce full or partial remission of nephrotic syndrome
- Delays progression of CKD
- It may promote renal recovery and dialysis independence.

ACEI may reduce proteinuria and delay progression.

☙ Prednisone has been used in older case series prior to the development of HAART; consider if patient is intolerant to HAART or in combination with HAART for short course if there is severe renal failure, but weigh infection risk. Long-term efficacy with steroids alone is questionable.

Other renal lesions found with HIV infection

In HIV+ patients with renal disease, 40%–50% of lesions are *not* due to HIVAN, with wide ethnic and geographical variations.
- Diffuse proliferative GN
- Lupus-like immune complex GN
- IgA
- Thrombotic microangiopathy (📖 p. 398)
- Other GNs due to concomitant hepatitis B, C, or cryoglobulinemia
- Acute interstitial nephritis (📖 p. 404).

HAART-related renal side effects

Common problems include the following:
- Indinavir (and acyclovir): crystalluria, stones, interstitial nephritis—consider change to another protease inhibitor?
- Cidofovir, adefovir, tenofovir: proximal tubular cell injury causing a Fanconi-like syndrome and ATN
- *All* reverse transcriptase inhibitors may cause lactic acidosis, often severe, thought to occur through mitochondrial DNA damage.

HIV-infected patients with ESRD

Use standard universal precautions—patients do not require isolation on hemodialysis. Survival on either HD or PD seems comparable. Renal transplantation is possible, but patient selection is important. Those with stable disease, who are compliant with medications, and have low viral load and preserved CD4 counts can be referred for consideration—drug interactions and toxicities are a major challenge.

Hepatitis B–related renal disease

Hepatitis B (HBV) affects 350 million people worldwide, especially in Africa and Southeast Asia. It is a DNA virus transmitted from mothers to children, between close (family) or sexual contacts.

In adults, an acute seroconversion illness (with appearance of hepatitis B surface antigen, HBsAg) occurs 1–6 months after exposure. Ninety percent of adults clear the virus (and develop immunity)—chronic carriers then remain at risk for hepatic and extrahepatic complications.

▶ If acquired in childhood, chronic carriage is usual.

Chronic HBV (i.e., HBsAg positive) carriage is associated with renal disease—viral antigen (usually HBe antigen, HBeAg) and host antibody form immune complexes that deposit in the kidney, causing injury. Three common nephropathies are described.

Membranous glomerulonephritis (MN)

MN is common in children between 2 and 12 years of age ($\sigma > \varphi$). It presents with proteinuria. Usually patients are HBeAg positive. It tends to remit spontaneously with clearance of HBeAg and development of anti-HBe antibodies.

Adults present with a chronic nephrotic syndrome, viral liver disease, and progressive CKD (📖 p. 392).

Membranoproliferative glomerulonephritis (MPGN)

MPGN is seen in adults. It presents with ↑BP, heavy proteinuria, hematuria and progressive ↑Cr. Patients are HBsAg and anti-HB core antibody positive. Renal histology is similar to type 1 MPGN (📖 p. 378). Unlike hepatitis C–associated MPGN, usually cryoglobulins are not detected.

Classic polyarteritis nodosa (PAN)

PAN occurs within 4 months of infection in adults. This presents as a medium-vessel vasculitis (📖 p. 464).

Investigations

Order full hepatitis B serologies (sAg, e and core Ag and antibody) and, if indicated, HBV DNA load. Check for hepatitis C ± HIV. Send electrolytes, BUN, Cr, albumin, LFTs. Get 24-hour urine protein and creatinine or spot urine PCR, and other labs for nephrotic syndrome. Check CBC, INR, cholesterol. US liver and kidneys. Proceed to renal biopsy.

A brief primer: treatment of HBV-related liver disease

- Chronic HBeAg-negative, anti-HBe antibody-positive carriers with normal ALT should be monitored every 6 months for reactivation.
- HBeAg+ patients with >105 copies/mL HBV DNA and ↑ALT should have a liver biopsy.
- Treatments include oral lamivudine, interferon-α, or newer agents such as adefovir if patient is lamivudine resistant; combination therapy may provide the best option.

Treatment of HBV-associated GN in adults

Aim to clear the virus (HBsAg negative, undetectable viral DNA) and promote seroconversion to immune status (anti-HBs antibody positive). Significant renal disease tends not to remit without treatment (and may progress)—liver disease may require treatment on its own merits. Response rates are higher in MN (than in MPGN). Remission tends to follow clearance of HBeAg and the appearance of anti-HBe antibodies.

- Interferon-α_{2b} 5 million U SC 3x/week for 4–12 months (or longer) results in ± 50% response.
- Lamivudine 100 mg qd (lamivudine resistance develops in ~15% per year) may offer benefit with long treatment time, but trials are awaited (?Entecavir for future therapy).

⚠ Avoid corticosteroids: ↑ viral replication, and at withdrawal, may be associated with hepatic failure. However, in PAN a short course of steroids ± plasma exchange is required for severe vasculitis (📖 p. 464) + antiviral treatment.

The best means of controlling HBV-related renal disease is to prevent it. Offer vaccination against HBV to high-risk individuals.

▶ Household contacts and family members of HbsAg-positive patients should be vaccinated. Patients should avoid alcohol and sharing blood-contaminated items (toothbrushes, etc), and use condoms.

Hepatitis B-infected patients with ESRD

These patients require isolation in HD units in addition to standard universal precautions. Dedicated machines should be used, and dialyser reuse avoided. There is no contraindication to PD in otherwise healthy patients. Transplantation is thought to offer a survival benefit compared to remaining on dialysis, but selecting appropriate patients requires full HBV serology testing, viral load measurement, and may require liver biopsy to predict risk.

Yearly screening for hepatocellular carcinoma, with serum α-fetoprotein and US of liver, should be performed in high-risk patients (▶ ♂ >45 years).

Hepatitis C–related renal disease

HCV is a RNA virus with six different genotypes, causing hepatitis, cirrhosis, and hepatocellular carcinoma. It is transmitted parentally, affecting IV drug users and those accidentally infected through needle-sharing or blood products (prior to screening). Infection is mild and often subclinical after a long incubation period (6–9 weeks). Some 70%–85% of patients fail to clear the acute infection and become chronic carriers. Chronic HCV, and its associated mixed cryoglobulinemia, is now known to be the principal cause of type 1 MPGN (previously thought to be idiopathic). Hepatitis C can also cause membranous GN.

HCV-related type 1 MPGN (📖 p. 378) ± cryoglobulins

Membranoproliferative GN can occur with or without cryoglobulinemia. Cryoglobulins may deposit in medium and small vessels in skin, joints, and glomeruli, fixing complement and causing local inflammation and injury leading to GN.

Symptoms and signs with cryoglobulinemia

Fatigue, weakness, and weight loss occur. There may be an episodic palpable purpuric rash on legs (leukocytoclastic vasculitis on biopsy), arthralgias, myalgias, mononeuritis multiplex, hepatosplenomegaly, and Raynaud's phenomenon. This may present as acute and disseminated vasculitis. Renal manifestations include hematuria, proteinuria (often nephrotic range), ↑BP, and renal impairment (progressive or presenting as ARF).

Investigations

Urinalysis for RBCs, RBC casts, 24-hour urine protein and creatinine or spot urine PCR. Electrolytes, BUN, Cr, albumin, LFTs (↑ALT). CBC, ↑ESR. Rheumatoid factor (often positive, see below), cryoglobulins, serum immunoglobulins (polyclonal ↑), complements (normal C3, ↓C4), ANA, anti-smooth muscle antibodies (?autoimmune disease). US liver and kidneys. Anti-HCV antibody ± PCR for HCV RNA. HCV genotyping. Hepatitis B and HIV. Renal biopsy (📖 p. 634).

Cryoglobulins

These are immunoglobulins that precipitate at <37°C and dissolve once again on warming.
- Type I cryoglobulinemia is a monoclonal immunoglobulin (IgG or IgM), associated with lymphoproliferative disease (myeloma, lymphoma, CLL, Waldenstrom's macroglobulinemia).
- Type II or mixed essential cryoglobulinemia is monoclonal IgM with polyclonal IgG, associated with hepatitis C infection or autoimmune disease. Hepatitis C enters host cells (hepatocytes and CD5+ B cells) via the LDL receptor—infected B cells which are resistant to apoptosis and increase production of autoantibodies. This monoclonal IgM autoantibody is a *rheumatoid factor*, i.e., directed against the Fc portion of other immunoglobulins.
- Type III cryoglobulinemia is polyclonal IgM directed against IgG (as above), found in low concentration and associated with viral infection and autoimmune disease.

Management

Most HCV-infected patients have evidence of liver disease, and seemingly normal hepatic function does not exclude the presence of HCV. Patients with HCV infection are generally treated with pegylated interferon-α and the oral antiviral agent ribavirin (if CrCl >50 mL/min) for 24–48 weeks. Of the six known HCV genotypes, types 2 and 3 are more responsive to therapy than types 1 or 4, with sustained virologic response rates of 80% vs. 45%. Side effects are common, with hemolysis, depression, and others.

If severe vasculitis with cryoglobulinemia is present, treat with steroids and cyclophosphamide.

▶ Although interferon-α and ribavirin may clear HCV, most clinicians hold use of ribavirin with CKD. The treatment has modest effects on proteinuria and renal function; however, on cessation of treatment, HCV RNA and cryoglobulins may return. In addition, consider the following:
- EPO to maintain Hb >11 g/dL (ribavirin induces red cell fragility)
- ACEI to limit proteinuria
- HMG-coA-reductase inhibitors if LFTs are normal.

Also recommend to patients that they avoid alcohol, avoid sharing blood-contaminated items (toothbrushes, etc.), and use condoms.

Hepatitis C-infected patients with ESRD
- Standard universal precautions: patients do *not* require isolation on hemodialysis (unlike those with hepatitis B). Check ALT level every 6 months.
- Yearly screening for hepatocellular carcinoma ± cirrhosis by US liver and serum α-fetoprotein should be performed.
- Renal transplantation offers superior survival to maintenance HD or CAPD, but HCV-positive transplant recipients do less well over the long term compared to HCV-negative patients. A group of HCV-positive ESRD patients may benefit from anti-HCV treatment with interferon prior to transplantation.

The kidney in infective endocarditis

Bacterial infection of any valve on either side of the heart may be complicated by renal disease, including the following:
- Postinfectious immune complex–mediated GN
- Aminoglycoside-induced ATN
- Renal emboli (off infected valves)
- Drug-induced AIN.

Infective endocarditis (IE) should be suspected in a patient with a fever, new murmur, splenomegaly, and hematuria, especially if they are known to have a valvular abnormality or prosthesis. Careful examination may reveal splinter hemorrhages, although classical stigmata of IE are often absent.

Common causes include S. aureus in acute IE, or viridans streptococci or coagulase-negative staphylococci in more chronic IE.

▶ Repeated cultures and sensitivity testing are the key to management.

The severity of the glomerulonephritis is related to the duration of infection prior to the institution of antibiotics. Control of infection usually leads to rapid resolution, with return of renal function to or near the previous baseline. However, irreversible renal failure can occur if appropriate therapy is delayed.

Symptoms and signs
- Urinary abnormalities and ↑Cr *at presentation* suggest GN, especially if improving with antibiotics. ↑Cr over time on antibiotics with bland urine except granular casts → aminoglycoside toxicity. A new and persisting fever ± 10–14 days after starting antibiotics, especially if timed with a rash ± eosinophilia, → AIN from pencillins or cephosporins (📖 p. 404). Other medications causing interstitial nephritis may not be associated with rash, eosinophilia or pyuria. Check for prior aminoglycoside levels (?toxic).
- Renal emboli may present as acute (unilateral) flank pain ± frank hematuria.
- There may be peripheral emboli in other beds (▶ feet) that may occur months after bacteriologic cure.

Investigations
- Repeated blood cultures, urgent echocardiography (?TEE).
- Urinalysis (if sterile pyuria or eosinophiluria, ?AIN [absence of pyuria does not rule this out]), 24-hour urine protein and creatinine (>1 g/day → GN) or spot urine PCR.
- CBC (eosinophilia → AIN), ESR↑, electrolytes, BUN, Cr, albumin, CRP↑. Check aminoglycoside levels.
- ↓C_3, cryoglobulins if there is GN
- US kidneys ± DMSA for focal perfusion defects (if emboli are suspected).
- Patient may require kidney biopsy if diagnosis is unclear.

Histology

The histologic findings are similar to those for post-streptococcal glomerulonephritis (p. 376), AIN (p. 404), or ATN (p. 100).

Treatment

- If GN is present, treat IE using appropriate antibiotics against sensitivities ± valve surgery if indicated. There is no proven benefit for adjunctive treatments, even if there are crescentic changes on biopsy, especially in light of severe infection. However, some treat with immunosuppression for crescentic changes once infection is under control.
- If there is ATN, tailor aminoglycoside doses to levels, or change antibiotic.
- If there is AIN, change antibiotic. Steroids are not of proven benefit, and may be detrimental with severe infection.

Renal tuberculosis

Tuberculosis is caused by *Mycobacterium tuberculosis*, affecting 8–10 million people every year, usually presenting as pulmonary disease. The global burden of TB has risen sharply as a result of HIV infection. Extrapulmonary disease (in HIV-negative patients) presents in 15% of active cases (of which 27% is due to renal tract TB).

Genitourinary TB

This type is due to direct infection of the GU tract, either as a sole site of infection or with disseminated (miliary) disease. Both kidneys are usually infected, and disease tends to spread along the entire urinary tract (▶ ureteric strictures). The renal medulla is preferentially affected, but subsequent papillary and pelvic involvement can cause calcification and cortical scarring over time. Other sites infected by TB include the epididymus and prostate.

Symptoms and signs

⚠ Patients may be asymptomatic (25%): maintain a high index of suspicion in those at risk. Lower abdominal pain, dysuria and frequency, and back and flank pain often present as recurrent UTI unresponsive to antibiotics. Gross hematuria may be seen. Longer-term bladder fibrosis may present with urgency or incontinence. Secondary bacterial infection is common.

▶ Fever, weight loss, and night sweats are rare. Pulmonary symptoms may be absent (30% will have an abnormal chest X-ray). Foci in the urinary tract may remain dormant indefinitely, or activate with immunosuppression.

Chronic TB may cause AA amyloid, with renal involvement (📖 p. 450).

Investigations

- Sterile pyuria on microscopy and negative culture is characteristic.
- Three consecutive early-morning urine samples are needed: conduct microscopy on centrifuged urine for acid-fast bacilli (Ziehl–Nielson stain) and mycobacterial culture (takes 2–4 weeks).
- Polymerase chain reaction (PCR) for mycobacterial DNA may be helpful (but there are false positives). Check electrolytes, BUN, Cr, CRP, CBC, ESR, chest X-ray, and plain KUB (?renal tract calcification).

▶ Consider HIV testing.
   Skin tuberculin testing is of limited use (false positive results).
- IVU is abnormal (70%–90%), with calyceal tip erosions, filling defects and distortion. There are ureteric strictures ± obstruction. It may demonstrate absent kidney. Get US if obstruction is suspected.

Tuberculous interstitial nephritis (TIN)

TIN may be an underestimated worldwide cause of renal failure. TB causes a parenchymal reaction with (caseating) granuloma formation containing giant cells and chronic tubulointerstitial inflammation. It usually presents with ↑Cr in at-risk populations (South Asians). Urinalysis is bland, and US confirms ↓ renal size. Chest X-ray may demonstrate prior or active pulmonary TB, and skin tuberculin testing may often be strongly positive. Diagnosis is made at renal biopsy (M tuberculosis may be identified on tissue stains).

Anti-tuberculous treatment → ↑ improved renal function (and even recovery from advanced CKD).

Management
- Anti-TB therapy. Rifampin can cause ATN and AIN.

Schistosomiasis

Infestation with schistosomes (a water-borne trematode) affects as many as 200 million people worldwide and may lead to urinary tract disease or glomerulonephritis. S. haematobium is endemic in most of Africa and the Middle East, and preferentially migrates to the venous plexus surrounding the bladder. S. mansoni (additionally found in Latin America) and S. japonicum (found in Asia alone) establish in the mesenteric vessels or portal tree.

Acute infestation tends to occur in childhood in residents in endemic areas, but afflicts travelers of any age. This is characterized by dermal invasion ("swimmer's itch"), a later systemic serum-sickness-like syndrome (Katayama fever) and eventual maturation of a worm in blood vessels. Lodged eggs released from mature worms evoke granulomatous inflammation in local tissues.

Although worms have strategies to evade immune recognition, if incomplete, an antibody response may result in circulating immune complexes. These may become trapped in glomeruli (especially if liver fibrosis → poor immune complex clearance), leading to schistosomal glomerulonephritis.

Urinary schistosomiasis

This is caused by S. haemotobium infestation. Chronically, urinary tract infestation presents with terminal hematuria (frank blood at the end of voiding), dysuria, and frequency as a result of an inflammatory cystitis. Bladder fibrosis may be asymptomatic or lead to detrusor failure. Ureteric strictures and obstruction are common (10%). Recurrent bacterial infection, bladder calculi, and increased risk of bladder cancer may complicate chronic disease.

Diagnosis
- Typical ova on urine microscopy (centrifuge sample to improve yield)
- CBC (eosinophilia), electrolytes, BUN, Cr
- Anti-schistosomal antibodies (serological testing) may be helpful in excluding infestation (positive 1 month after exposure).
- Plain KUB may demonstrate calcification.
- US to exclude obstruction
- Cystoscopy may show a nodular, polypoid, and ulcerating hemorrhagic cystitis.

Treatment

Praziquantel 40 mg/kg po (80%–90% cure rate). If there is S. japonicum, ↑dose to 60 mg/kg in two divided doses 3 hours apart. Treatment can be repeated if needed.
- There may be some resolution of urinary tract lesions (especially if there is little fibrosis).
- Strictures may require surgical intervention.

Schistosomal glomerulonephritis

This occurs in 10% patients with *S. mansoni* (less commonly *S. haemotobium*). Most commonly, an MPGN-like lesion on kidney biopsy presents as nephrotic-range proteinuria, hematuria, and impaired renal function. Other investigations show ↑Igs, ↓C3, false positive syphilis serology, ± ova on fecal microscopy. This GN tends to carry a poor renal prognosis, progressing to ESRD. No treatment is of proven benefit (including praziquantel).

Other GNs include mesangial proliferative GN, and secondary amyloidosis.

Malaria

Malaria is caused by *Plasmodium* parasites transmitted via *Anopheles* mosquitoes. It is endemic to large parts of the globe and is responsible for 1–3 million deaths/year. Species causing disease:
- *P. falciparum*—sub-Saharan Africa, Indian subcontinent
- *P. vivax*—central America
- *P. malariae* and *P. ovale*—rare outside Africa.

▶ Only *P. falciparum* and *P. malariae* cause renal disease.

Transient glomerular abnormalities (≈ postinfectious GN, 📖 p. 376) occur in up to 18% of infected individuals, presenting with hematuria and proteinuria (may be heavy). Renal dysfunction is unusual. Biopsy shows mesangial matrix expansion with hypercellularity, with IgM and C3 in granular deposits in capillary walls. Prognosis is good, with complete recovery after treatment of malaria.

Acute malarial nephropathy

ARF complicates severe *P. falciparum* malaria in 1%–4% cases in endemic areas, but is more common in nonimmune travelers. The renal lesion is always due to ATN associated with circulatory collapse (as a result of "malignant" parasitemia, hemolysis, and a cytokine and oxidant "storm"). If severe >50% will require dialysis—mortality can be as high as 10%.

Symptoms and signs
Malaise, headache and confusion, fevers and chills, and often severe myalgias (→ rhabdomyolysis) occur. (Profound) ↓BP, peripheral vasodilatation, and oliguria (hemoglobinuria = Blackwater fever) are other signs. There can be nausea, vomiting, diarrhea, and jaundice (75%), as well as hepatosplenomegaly and anemia.

Investigations
CBC (hemolytic anemia), ↓Plt (70%). RBC smear for parasitemia (usually >5%). ↓Haptoglobin. DIC (↑APTT, ↑PT,↑D-dimers↑). BUN, Cr, electrolytes (severe ↑K^+, ↓Na^+, ↑Cr), ↑LFTs (↑ALP) and ↑lactic acidosis. Mild proteinuria (<1 g/24 h).

Management
- Manage in ICU setting and initiate continuous renal replacement therapy or HD early.
- Give supportive blood products as required.
- Culture blood and empirical broad-spectrum antibiotics (bacterial superinfection is not uncommon).
- Give IV quinine loading dose as 20 mg/kg (no more than 1.4 g) over 4 hours
  - 10 mg/kg IV q8h for 7 days and convert to po therapy once appropriate.
  - ⚠ If patient is G6PD deficient, consult local pharmacy.

Chronic malarial nephropathy

This disease is caused by *P. malariae*, affecting African children (~5 years old). It presents as proteinuria (may be nephrotic range) ± hematuria. Edema (coexistent malnutrition), ↓Hb, and hepatosplenomegaly may be present. Renal biopsy shows an MPGN with subendothelial deposits (📖 p. 378). The disease runs a progressive course to ESRD despite eradication of the infection.

Chapter 8

Urinary tract obstruction

Approaching obstruction 496
Imaging urinary tract obstruction 498
Acute obstruction 500
Chronic obstruction 502
UPJ and UVJ obstruction 504
Retroperitoneal fibrosis (RPF) 506
Investigation of a renal mass 508
Renal cell carcinoma (RCC) 510
Urothelial tumors 512
Benign prostatic hypertrophy (BPH) 514
Prostate cancer 516
Management of prostate cancer 518

Approaching obstruction

Obstruction of the urinary tract is a not uncommon and often silent cause of renal impairment or disease. It leads to delayed urinary transit and, over time, increased intratract pressures → renal impairment. Obstruction tends to present in infants and young children (as a result of anatomical abnormalities) or in older people, particularly men (tumors, stones and prostatic disease). The key to diagnosis rests on identifying the level of obstruction correctly (Table 8.1).

Normal physiology

Urine reaches the bladder as a result of three interrelated mechanisms:
- Glomerular filtration pressure
- Renal tract peristalsis
- Gravity

Coordinated smooth muscle contraction in the ureters directs urine toward the bladder, with maximum intraluminal pressures of ~25 mmHg.

Classification
- *Upper or lower*
  - Upper tract ≈ obstruction at the level of the ureter or higher.
  - Lower tract ≈ bladder or lower.
- *Unilateral or bilateral*
  - Lower tract obstruction affects both kidneys.
  - Upper tract obstruction may affect one or both kidneys.
  - Bilateral obstruction will cause renal impairment, as will unilateral obstruction of a single functioning kidney.
- *Complete or partial*
  - Complete obstruction is the most common cause of anuria. It may be easy to diagnose and imaging is often clear-cut in confirming this.
  - Partial obstruction may be more difficult to diagnose, as the patient's urine output may vary.

Table 8.1 Causes of urinary tract obstruction

Level of obstruction	Obstruction within the lumen	Obstruction within the wall	Extrinsic compression
Kidney	Stones Sloughed papillae	Cysts Tumors Anatomical abnormalities, e.g., UPJ obstruction	Lower polar renal vessels crossing at UPJ
Ureter	Stones	Tumors Stricture (malignant, post-surgery, or post-radiotherapy, tuberculous, schistosomiasis) Anatomical abnormalities, e.g., UVJ obstruction	Tumors Retroperitoneal fibrosis Retrocaval right ureter (congenital) Pancreatitis, inflammatory bowel disease (rare)
Bladder/bladder neck	Stones Clot retention	Tumors Functional obstruction (diabetes, neurological damage to bladder, drugs)	Pelvic tumors
Urethra	Stones Blood clots (after catheterization or surgery)	Stricture (post-infective, or post-surgical) Congenital urethral valves Tumors	Prostate enlargement

Imaging urinary tract obstruction

History and examination can often make a diagnosis in acute obstruction (📖 p. 500). ▶ A palpable bladder is an important finding → lower tract obstruction, but imaging is always required to diagnose upper tract obstruction.

Ultrasound (US)
- US is portable, noninvasive, and quick.
- It may demonstrate dilated ureters (Fig. 8.1).
- The upper (but not always the lower) ureter may be visualized.
- It is the imaging of choice in patients with renal impairment or who are pregnant.

However, US is operator dependent and (early) obstruction can occur without a dilated system in some circumstances. Moreover, a dilated system does *not* necessarily imply that obstruction is present (Box 8.1).

Box 8.1 How good is ultrasound at diagnosing obstruction?

▶ Do not rely on imaging alone to diagnose obstruction.

Obstruction without a dilated system
- Hydronephrosis may not be apparent in early (2–3 days) obstruction.
- Dilatation may not occur if tumor or fibrous tissue encases a kidney.
- Chronically obstructed kidneys fail → anuria ∴ no hydronephrosis.
- Partial obstruction may not show a hydronephrosis (but ↑Cr).

Dilated system without obstruction
- Anatomical variants include extrarenal pelvis, megaureter (possible secondary to vesicoureteral reflux).
- Pregnancy: hormonal changes cause dilated ureters and renal pelvis.
- Post-obstruction: a "baggy" system may remain long after relief of chronic obstruction. Review previous imaging and compare.
- If doubt exists, then consider (but not in pregnancy)
  - IVU
  - Diuretic renography

Computerized tomography (CT)
CT has superceded plain X-ray (which is still useful to identify radio-opaque stones).
- If clinical findings and US are unclear, CT is most likely to provide the most information on the site and cause of the obstruction.
- CT is useful in stone disease, especially renal colic (📖 p. 435).
- It is useful to diagnose the cause of extrinsic compression, staging of tumors, and retroperitoneal fibrosis.
- Beware of contrast nephropathy if renal impairment is present (📖 p. 142).

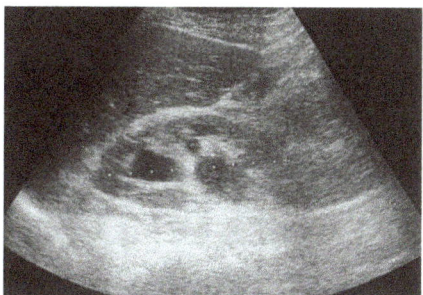

Fig. 8.1 Renal ultrasound appearances of acute obstruction with pelvicalyceal dilatation. Reproduced with permission from Warrell D, Cox T, Firth J, and Benz EJ (eds) (2004). *Oxford Textbook of Medicine*, 4th ed., p.451. Oxford University Press.

Intravenous urography (IVU)

IVU is more difficult to perform than CT and requires contrast. But it is useful if
- CT fails to demonstrate the level of obstruction.
- There are suspected obstruction and complicated staghorn calculi or multiple renal cysts (CT, US cannot differentiate hydronephrosis from cysts).

Obstructed nephrogram of unknown cause

Occasionally in the context of acute unilateral flank pain, IVU shows evidence of obstruction but no stone. Consider the following:
- Recent passage of radio-opaque stone
- Radiolucent uric acid stone (→ CT)
- Acute UPJ obstruction (distended pelvis may be seen)
- Sloughed papilla (📖 p. 408) (?clubbed calyces on IVU). Consider:
  - Diabetes
  - Analgesic abuse
  - Sickle cell disease and trait
- Blood clot (*always* with macroscopic hematuria)

Isotope renography

A DTPA or MAG-3 renogram (📖 p. 43) may show delayed excretion with obstruction. It is helpful in diagnosing unilateral obstruction (compare excretion with the normal side) or partial (with furosemide, increased urinary flow may reveal a partially obstructed system). It can be used to estimate split function. A t1/2 excretion of >20 min suggests at least partial obstruction.

Magnetic resonance imaging (MRI)

MRI has a growing role in tumor staging and detection of extrinsic compressive lesions.

Acute obstruction (see 📖 p. 3)

Clinical features
Complete bilateral obstruction presents with anuria and progressive ARF. Partial or unilateral obstruction may present with localized pain or signs of sepsis, or may be asymptomatic and diagnosed late with a nonfunctioning kidney.

Features resulting from the underlying cause include the following:
- *Prostatic disease* may present with symptoms of difficulty, dribbling, or poor stream (📖 p. 504). Examine for a palpable bladder and measure postvoid residual urine volume (PVR).
- *Retroperitoneal fibrosis* is suggested by backache ± AAA (📖 p. 506).
- *Stones* present with pain (acute obstruction secondary to stones is usually painful), hematuria (macro- or microscopic) (📖 p. 430).
- *Tumors* rarely present with acute obstruction. Intrinsic and extrinsic tumors compression → partial obstruction, hematuria or pain. (📖 p. 512). ♀ may require a vaginal examination if cancer is suspected.
- *Papillary necrosis* may present with pain ± hematuria (📖 p. 409).
- *Clot colic* is usually accompanied by frank hematuria.

⚠ Pain, fever, or systemic signs of sepsis are important features of an obstructed infected system(s). Proceed to *urgent* decompression.

Investigations
⚠ Always exclude obstruction in cases of unexplained renal impairment.
- If the bladder is palpable, then the diagnosis may be made at the bedside. If not, then US almost always leads to the diagnosis.
- Microscope urine for red cells, crystals. U+E, Ca^{2+}, CRP, CBC, ESR, culture blood, and urine if febrile. Run *PSA* in ♂.
- Further imaging may be and often is required (📖 p. 36). Once the nature and extent of obstruction are known, direct investigations appropriately.
- Cystoscopy ± ureteroscopy may eventually be required to make a definitive diagnosis when the cause is within the lumen.

Management of acute obstruction
The quicker obstruction is relieved, the better: chronic obstruction → irreversible decline in renal function.
- Do not delay: time = nephrons.
- *An obstructed urinary system is an emergency.*
- If there is bladder outflow obstruction, *catheterize*. If insertion is difficult, insert a suprapubic catheter—don't traumatize the urethra.
- If patient is ureteric, a *nephrostomy* or retrograde ureteric stenting is needed. If ARF with fluid and electrolyte abnormalities are present, then a nephrostomy to one kidney should be enough to secure the patient until definitive drainage is performed.

Further management depends on the cause:
- Before removing a nephrostomy, do a nephrostogram (injection of contrast via the nephrostomy to examine ureteric flow).
- Ureteric stents can be inserted from above (via nephrostomy) or from below (cystoscopically—can be technically difficult or impossible if the ureteric orifices are diseased and difficult to cannulate).
- Stones and tumors should be managed by the relevant experts.

Organizing a nephrostomy

Is it necessary?
- *Pros*: It relieves ureteric obstruction and corrects renal failure and its associated electrolyte abnormalities.
- *Cons*: It is invasive, has serious potential complications (bleeding, infection), and is temporary. If it is possible to relieve the obstruction from below, this may be preferable.

How urgent is it?
- Infection → emergency required nephrostomy. Often only clinical signs may suggest infection (pain, systemic signs of sepsis).
- If K^+ >6.0 or there is pulmonary edema or severe uremia (limiting patient cooperation), then it may be safer to dialyse the patient first. ▶ *Dialysis is not risk-free* (lines etc.).
- Otherwise, a delay of *hours* to ensure an expert operator may be justified.

What blood tests should I send?
Renal function profile, CBC, PT, PTT.

What about consent?
This must be obtained by the person doing the procedure, as always. Bleeding or trauma to the kidney is rare but does occur.

Which kidney?
In an emergency, relieve the one kidney most likely to work (i.e., the larger kidney with the thicker cortex). Otherwise relieve both.

Post-procedure care
- *Exact* fluid balance: there is likely to be a brisk post-obstructive diuresis, often >5–10 L UO/day.
- Patient may require IVI 0.9% NaCl replacement (as urine output + 50 ml/h initially).
- Watch for ↓K^+ or ↓Na^+ with diuresis.
- Make sure the nephrostomy is well strapped in or sutured!

Chronic obstruction

▶ The presentation may be insidious.
Importantly, unilateral obstruction may not present with renal failure (if the other kidney is functioning), but may cause ↑BP (renin–angiotensin activation). Symptoms and signs are similar to those described with acute obstruction (📖 p. 500), though pain is infrequent. More chronic features may include local feelings of fullness or pain, nocturia or urinary frequency, other prostatic symptoms (📖 p. 514), or symptomatic uremia. Always examine for a palpable bladder, enlarged prostate, or other pelvic masses.

Renal consequences of obstruction
- Acute obstruction causes an acute reduction in the GFR, which is *fully* reversible if relieved within a few days.
- In chronic obstruction, the renal parenchymal changes may never fully recover despite relief. The longer obstruction has been present, the longer renal function takes to recover. With severe renal failure (Cr >6.8 mg/L) recovery to <3.5 μmol/L is unusual.
- Chronic tubular damage may lead to
  - Salt-losing nephropathies (📖 p. 406)
  - Type 1 or 4 renal tubular acidosis (📖 p. 556)
  - A persistent "baggy" renal pelvis on imaging.

Management
Aim to relieve obstruction as for the patient with acute obstruction (📖 p. 500). Further management depends on the cause:
- Whenever possible, remove stones, treat tumors, treat prostatic enlargement, dilate strictures, and offer surgery if there are anatomical abnormalities.
- In some circumstances, a long-term catheter or ureteric stents may be the most practical and sensible option (e.g., for inoperable tumors or frail patients with advanced disease).
- Urethral catheters and ureteric (JJ) stents require long-term follow-up:
  - Change the catheter or stent at appropriate intervals (depending on the catheter or stent, this can be weeks–months if well tolerated).
  - Watch for infection (patient may require exchange or removal if antibiotics are ineffective) or blockage (▶ deterioration of renal function).

Mechanism of renal damage in chronic obstruction

This is not fully understood, but likely important mediators are the following:
- Back pressure: ↑proximal tubular pressure leads to ↓filtration pressure.
- Vasoconstriction in response to ↑ intratubular pressure. This is mediated locally by angiotensin II and thromboxanes (a physiological response redirecting blood away from nonfunctioning nephrons).
- Ischemic nephrons release mediators of inflammation, leading to local injury, interstitial fibrosis, and irreversible atrophy of the disused nephrons.

UPJ and UVJ obstruction

Both obstruction at the ureteropelvic junction (UPJ) and ureterovesicular junction (UVJ) are thought to be congenital in origin, perhaps arising from urinary tract adhesions or persisting fetal folds → mechanical and structural changes.
- UPJ obstruction: There is failure of normal urine flow from the renal pelvis into the ureter, resulting in a "baggy," high-pressure pelvis.
- UVJ obstruction: Urine cannot pass from the ureter into the bladder, with a resultant megaureter. Ureteric reflux may mimic it or coexist.

Symptoms and signs

UPJ obstruction is increasingly diagnosed antenatally, when it is often bilateral. Older children present with flank pain, a palpable mass, urinary tract infection, or hematuria after trauma. However, 20% of cases are diagnosed as adults, and presumably a large number are never diagnosed at all. Characteristic flank pain occurs after drinking alcohol or coffee or taking diuretics (i.e., anything that promotes diuresis). UVJ obstruction presents with a similar constellation of symptoms, but often later in childhood or as an adult.

Diagnosis

US is needed to confirm structural changes. IVU or isotope renography (with furosemide) will describe functional consequences. A micturating cystoureterogram (MCUG) may demonstrate reflux in ?VUJ obstruction.

Management
- Either obstruction is generally managed conservatively unless there is
  - Impaired renal function
  - Recurrent infection
  - Calculi
  - Persistent pain
- UPJ obstruction can be managed by open Anderson–Hynes pyeloplasty, laparoscopic pyeloplasty, or endopyelotomy (antegrade or retrograde). Balloon dilatation is usually unsuccessful.
- UVJ obstruction can be managed by reimplantation of the ureter. If there is positive reflux into the ureter (on MCUG), consider antibiotic prophylaxis against UTI. See 📖 p. 428 for full discussion on vesicoureteric reflux.

Posterior urethral valves

This is the most common form of lower tract obstruction in ♂ infants. Valves in the posterior urethra obstruct urinary flow with sequential dilatation of the proximal urethra, bladder wall hypertrophy, bilateral megaureters, and hydronephrosis → (if uncorrected) obstructive uropathy.
- It is often diagnosed during pregnancy.
- Reflux is often present as well.
- When diagnosed late, it tends to present with CKD or UTI.

Standard fetal US often makes the diagnosis. VCUG in infancy can be used to confirm features. Management includes immediate bladder catheterization followed by endoscopic resection of valves as early as possible. Bladder dysfunction may persist after correction.

Retroperitoneal fibrosis (RPF)

Obstruction at the mid to lower third of the ureter by an encasing inflammatory fibrous tissue → impaired ureteric contractility (Fig. 8.2). This leads to a chronic obstructive uropathy, often presenting with unexplained renal impairment. The etiology is not clear. Several mechanisms have been proposed and include (1) leakage of proinflammatory lipid-derived material across the wall of an atheromatous aorta. This in turn → a ureteric inflammatory response that over time heals as fibrosis. (2) A small-vessel vasculitis of the vasa vasorum of aorta can occur. RPF is one of the disease states classified under the broader term *periaortitis*. Other disease states in the category include inflammatory abdominal aortic aneurysms and perianeurysmal RPF. Idiopathic RPF usually occurs in patients over 50.

Causes
- Idiopathic: The underlying mechanism is as above.
- Drug induced: classically methysergide, but also some β-blockers
- Lymphoma and other lymphoproliferative disorders may mimic RPF on imaging studies.
- Prostatic and pelvic malignancies may have similar radiological features, but represent a different disease.

▶ Establish tissue diagnosis in all patients if possible. *Fine needle biopsy may miss this by sampling error, so open or multiple core biopsies are preferred.*

Clinical features
Patients typically present with unexplained back or abdominal pain, accompanied by weight loss, anemia, and elevated sedimentation rate.

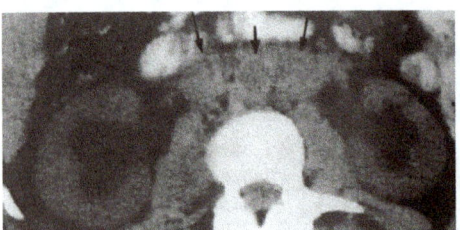

Fig. 8.2 Retroperitoneal fibrosis—CT appearances. Note the periaortic mass and aortic calcification. Reproduced with permission from Warrell D, Cox T, Firth, and Benz EJ (eds) (2004). *Oxford Textbook of Medicine*, fourth ed., p. 454. Oxford: Oxford University Press.

Investigations

Check renal function profile, TSH (iRPF associated with hypothyroidism), (↓Hb), ↑↑ESR (a consistent marker of inflammation, and useful for monitoring disease). CT and MRI are investigations of choice to
- Make or confirm the diagnosis.
- Image the aorta (and assess any aortic aneurysm).
- Characterize any lymphadenopathy.

CT-guided biopsy can be performed unless surgery and excision biopsy is planned (see above).

Management

The ideal management of these patients has not been determined.

Medical management
- Corticosteroids ↓ inflammatory tissue encasing the ureter(s) and may restore ureteric patency.
- Start prednisolone 30 mg/day for 12 weeks. Taper the dose, titrating down against ESR and serial imaging.
- Longer term, azathioprine, and mycophenolate have been used in patients unsuitable for surgery. ☞ Controlled trials are needed.

Surgery
- Insertion of bilateral retrograde JJ ureteric stents may obviate the need for nephrostomies to relieve obstruction.
- Definitive surgery is best if preceded by a course of steroids to shrink the mass.
- Ureterolysis and omental wrapping is the definitive surgical procedure. The ureters (with JJ stents in situ) are identified, freed and moved laterally, then wrapped in a protective layer of omentum.
- Aortic aneurysm repair may also be required.
- Steroids can be stopped after surgery, but relapse can occur.

Follow-up should be lifelong (renal function profile, ESR, CBC).

Investigation of a renal mass

Renal masses may be asymptomatic or symptomatic, single or multiple, cystic or solid (Table 8.2).

When is a cyst not a simple cyst?

Diagnosis is by US—criteria for a simple renal cyst are that it be:
- Round
- Smooth walled
- Anechoic
- With good transmission of ultrasound through the cyst.

If all these are present, then it is almost certainly benign. If not, then proceed to contrast-enhanced CT. On CT, simple cysts have
- Smooth, thin walls
- A density similar to that of water
- No enhancement with contrast.

Uncertain cases should be followed up every 6–12 months with repeat scanning. The differential diagnosis and investigation of cystic disease are discussed elsewhere (p. 420).

The solid renal mass

This type of mass may be benign (angiomyolipoma) or malignant. No imaging technique can completely reliably confirm that a solid lesion is benign, although MRI may detect small quantities of fat, highly suggestive of an angiomyolipoma. Worrying features of a solid lesion are as follows:
- Diameter >3 cm
- Enhancement with contrast
- Thick or irregular wall
- Necrotic areas (implying rapid growth).

Removal is usually advocated. Consider nephron-sparing surgery (i.e., partial nephrectomy), especially if there is reduced renal function or a problem with the other kidney. Borderline cases or indeterminate lesions should receive serial CT with or without ultrasound. MRI may be useful in evaluating the internal contents of the cyst. Even small lesions may progress.

Table 8.2 Types of renal masses

	Solid	Cystic
Single	Tumor Angiomyolipoma AV malformation	Simple cyst
Multiple	Congenital syndromes, e.g., von Hippel-Lindau syndrome, tuberous sclerosis	Polycystic kidney disease Acquired cystic disease (p. 420)

Renal cell carcinoma (RCC)

RCCs are adenocarcinomas accounting for 80% of primary malignant tumors of the kidney. They may be slow growing and hence commonly present as an incidental finding. Incidence is 4♂:1♀, with bilateral lesions occurring in up to 50% of cases. Smoking has been strongly implicated in development of RCC.

Clinical features

The classic presenting triad is pain, hematuria, and a palpable mass. In reality, other features are often as common. Flank or back pain (capsular stretch) radiating into the groin occurs with large tumors, as with cystic tumors complicated by hemorrhage or infection. ↑BP occurs. Hematuria is common and may be macroscopic. Tumor may obstruct a kidney. A quarter of patients present with distant metastases (lung, liver, bone, nodes, the other kidney) or extensive local disease. Some develop scrotal variceles due to occlusion of the testicular vein (these always arouse suspicion if found). Paraneoplastic symptoms also occur (see Box 8.2).

Differential diagnosis

⚠Most solid lesions in the kidney are renal cell carcinomas.
- Oncocytoma is benign and not reliably distinguishable on CT.
- Angiomyolipoma has a fat density less than that of water on CT. If bilateral, then it is likely a feature of tuberous sclerosis.
- Xanthogranulomatous pyelonephritis (📖 p. 426).

Box 8.2 Paraneoplastic syndrome with RCC

- Fever (up to 20%, often with night sweats)
- Cachexia
- Erythrocytosis (the tumor may make erythropoietin)
- Anemia (may be disproportionate)
- Hypercalcemia (due to bony metastases, or to production of PTH-related protein). This is a poor prognostic sign.
- Hepatic dysfunction without liver metastases
- Secondary amyloid deposition (AA amyloid)
- Polymyalgia
- Other hormonal effects (production of ACTH-like substance, gonadotrophins, renin, and insulin have all been reported)

Investigations

Perform urine cytology. Get UA, renal function profile, alkaline phosphatase, LFT. Check CBC, ↑↑ESR. Order CT of kidneys (or US + IVU). Use MRI if patient is unable to tolerate IV contrast. You may need a bone scan.

Preoperative work-up

Evaluate local spread of disease by CT. Invasion of the renal vein is best assessed by MRI (important if you are planning nephron-sparing surgery). Use MAG 3 renogram and estimation of GFR to assess differential renal function. Look for metastases with CT of the chest and a bone scan.

▶ Avoid needle biopsy of the renal mass as this has low reliability and a risk of seeding.

Staging

Using the TNM classification, prognosis is related to staging at diagnosis:
- If T1 lesion, 5-year survival >90%.
- If metastatic disease, 5-year survival <10%.

The grade of tumor or presence of paraneoplastic features also influences prognosis.

Treatment

Resection of the primary tumor is the treatment of choice (reports of metastases shrinking after removal of the primary tumor exist). Radical nephrectomy has been the standard, but nephron-sparing surgery is increasingly used to preserve renal function.

High-dose immunotherapy with interleukin-2 ± interferon in addition to debulking surgery has given promising results and, sometimes, cure.

Wilms' tumour (nephroblastoma)

This is the most common malignant tumor of the urinary tract in children, with a peak incidence at 3–4 years. Of mesodermal origin, it presents as a well-demarcated solid lesion in the kidney in the context of ↑BP. Some 15% of affected children have other congenital abnormalities.

Urothelial tumors

Bladder cancer

Over 90% of bladder cancers are transitional cell cancers (TCC), affecting 3♂:1♀ over the age of 60. Exposure to urothelial carcinogens → malignant transformation, with environmental factors playing a key role in tumor genesis. Squamous cell cancers are seen in areas of chronic schistosomiasis infection.

Risk factors
- ▶ Cigarette smoking
- Aniline dyes, aromatic amines, diesel fumes (truck drivers), and hair dyes (hairdressers) have all been linked to TCC.
- Significant levels of arsenic in drinking water
- Long-term exposure to laxatives or phenacetin (+ ?other analgesics)
- Previous radiotherapy to the pelvis
- Previous chemotherapy—especially with cyclophosphamide (📖 p. 369).

Pathogenesis
N-acetylation detoxifies potential carcinogens (such as arylamines)—an ↑ risk of bladder cancer is found in those with mutations → slower acetylation kinetics.

Clinical presentation
Occupational history is important. Hematuria (microscopic → frank) is the cardinal presenting feature. Pain is a feature of advanced disease. Urinary frequency, a feeling of incomplete emptying and urge incontinence may occur. Weight loss, fatigue, and anorexia occur late.

Investigations
Repeat urine cytology (×2) for cancerous cells. Get UA, renal function profile, alkaline phosphatase, FBC. Proceed to cystoscopy if patient is at risk: it allows visual inspection of the bladder ± ureters, collection of urine for cytology, and biopsy.

IVU allows examination of the upper tracts and detection of small lesions of the ureter or renal pelvis, and US may pick up renal parenchymal disease or hydronephrosis.

Staging
CT of the abdomen and pelvis (or MRI) is needed if locally invasive disease is suspected. Get a chest X-ray (if abnormal, then chest CT). Perform a bone scan if there is invasive disease, bone pain, ↑Ca^{2+}, or ↑alkaline phosphatase.

If tumor is superficial, the prognosis is good, though recurrence is common and surveillance with regular cystoscopy is necessary. Advanced tumors have a poor prognosis.

Management

Briefly, noninvasive superficial tumors are removed by transurethral resection of bladder tumor (TURBT). Because of recurrence, especially with high-grade tumors, adjuvant treatment with intravesical BCG may be recommended and reduce this risk by up to 40%. Invasive tumors require radical surgery ± radiotherapy and chemotherapy.

Tumors of the renal pelvis and ureter

- The urothelium of the renal pelvis and ureter may also develop transitional cell carcinomas (often multifocal). Such tumors are usually uncommon: <1% urinary tract neoplasms, ± 8% of renal tumors. They may occur in association with Balkan endemic nephropathy (p. 407).
- These tumors occur in 2♂:1♀ between 50 and 60 years of age. Investigate as for bladder TCC, though emphasis should be on IVU or CT, proceeding to flexible ureteroscopy ± brush biopsies. Careful evaluation for synchronous or multifocal urothelial tumors is required. Treatment is surgical (nephroureterectomy).

Benign prostatic hypertrophy (BPH)

BPH is a common and important condition in ♂, and a major cause of bladder outflow obstruction and renal impairment. The incidence rises steadily after the age of 50, affecting >50% of ♂ over 60. BPH is thought to be multifactorial in cause, with sex hormones and growth factors interacting with prostatic stromal epithelium → unbalanced cell proliferation and extracellular matrix production. Of the many implicated factors, age is clearly important, as are androgens (eunuchs do not get BPH). BPH is *not* an independent risk factor for prostatic carcinoma.

Clinical features

BPH classically presents with lower urinary tract symptoms (LUTS):
- Urinary frequency, hesitancy, and a poor stream
- Urgency, nocturia, and dribbling.

Chronic BPH may complicate as
- Long-term bladder outflow obstruction → bladder wall hypertrophy with ↑ post-void residual volumes and irreversible bladder dysfunction, UTIs, or bladder stones.
- Acute urinary retention ± obstructive uropathy.

On rectal examination, the prostate is characteristically enlarged, smooth, and symmetrical. Always exclude a palpable bladder (and obstruction).

Differential diagnosis

- Carcinoma of the prostate or bladder
- UTI or prostatitis
- Bladder stones
- Neurogenic bladder.

Investigations

Use urine dipstick (⚠ hematuria may occur with BPH—but *always* assess the bladder and upper tracts for other lesions). Get urine for UA, C+S. Get renal function profile, PSA.

Other tests that may be useful include the following:
- Frequency volume chart
- Urine flow rate measurement
- Post-micturition residual volume assessment
- Urodynamics if bladder dysfunction suspected.

Management

Symptom scoring systems exist to assess the severity of disease. Many ♂ benefit from conservative management ("watchful waiting") if symptoms are mild (the cost and side effects of drugs outweigh potential benefit).

If there is acute urinary retention use an in-dwelling catheter. After catheterization for acute retention, treat with α-blocker (e.g., tamsulosin 0.4 mg once daily) for 48 hours prior to trial without catheter to improve chance of success.

Active therapies for BPH
Indications for further intervention include the following:
- More severe symptoms
- Large prostate volume
- ↑PSA (reflecting ↑prostate volume rather than cancer)
- Low maximal flow rate
- High post-voiding residual volume.

α-blockers (e.g., tamsulosin, alfuzosin)
These agents cause bladder neck and prostatic smooth muscle relaxation. They provide effective symptomatic relief, ↑ quality of life, ↑ maximum flow rate, and ↓ risk of acute urinary retention, and may also ↓ need for surgery. Side effects (15%) are usually mild and include postural hypotension, headaches, and dizziness. Long-acting preparations are a significant advancement.

5-α reductase inhibitors (e.g., finasteride, dutasteride)
These inhibit conversion of testosterone to dihydrotestosterone (more active in the prostate). They have a slow onset of action (3–6 months) but long-lasting effects. Most effective in ♂ with large prostates, they improve symptoms, quality of life, flow rate, with ↓ prostate volume, ↓ risk of urinary retention and ↓ need for surgery. Side effects include impotence.

Combination of α-blocker with 5-α reductase inhibitor
This appears to be more effective than either class of drug alone. Stopping the α-blocker after several months may be possible.

Surgery
Surgery is recommended for severe symptoms or complications of bladder outlet obstruction:
- UTI
- Persistent retention of urine
- Renal failure.

Flow rates and urodynamic studies help with patient selection. Surgery is more successful in ♂ with proven BOO (flow rate <10 mL/s) and less successful in ♂ with symptomatic detrusor overactivity (frequency, urgency).
- *Transurethral resection of the prostate* (TURP) is usually the operation of choice.
- For small glands, a bladder neck incision may be all that is required.
- Very large glands may require a retropubic approach.

Acute complications of surgery include hemorrhage, sepsis, and the TUR syndrome (systemic absorption of glycine from the irrigated bladder leading to ↓Na^+). Longer-term complications may include impotence, retrograde ejaculation, urethral stricture, and urinary incontinence.

▶ Laser prostatectomy, thermotherapy, microwave therapy, transurethral needle ablation of the prostate (TUNA), and transurethral ethanol ablation of the prostate (TEAP) are rapidly evolving therapies for BPH.

Prostate cancer

Prostate cancer is the most common malignancy in ♂ after skin cancer, with an incidence of 50/100,000 ♂, rising with age (it is rare <45 years of age). Race (it is more common in the African-American population), genetics (it is more common in first-degree relatives of affected people), and diet (animal fats, dairy products) are implicated in the etiology.

Clinical features

These include LUTS (📖 p. 514), erectile dysfunction, hematuria, or hematospermia. Symptoms of bladder outlet obstruction or metastatic disease may lead to a digital rectal examination, with characteristic irregularity, nodules, or asymmetry. An abnormal-feeling prostate should always be investigated, even if the PSA is normal (20% of such patients have a normal PSA).

⚠ In early disease the prostate may feel normal!

Investigations

Get urine for UA and C&S, renal function profile, PSA, LFT. Order transrectal ultrasound (TRUS). Get US pre- and post-micturition + kidneys if there are symptoms of obstruction. Further investigations depend on stage and grade.

Staging and grading

Get TRUS-guided prostate biopsy of nodules or abnormal areas for tissue diagnosis. Other areas are also sampled ("sextant biopsy"). Up to 25% of cancers may be missed, and re-biopsy may be required.

- A Gleason score is calculated to grade the tumor: the degree of glandular differentiation and gland architecture are graded 1–5 (1 = well differentiated). These are combined to give a score out of 10.
- The TNM classification is used to stage the tumor (see below).
  - Patients with stage cT2 or less, PSA <10, and Gleason <6 do not need a bone scan as yield is low for these patients.
  - Similar criteria are used for CT of abdomen/pelvis, unless external beam radiotherapy is planned.
  - Endorectal-coil MRI has the best sensitivity at diagnosing extracapsular spread and seminal vesicle invasion (but is *not* routine).

TNM staging of prostate cancer

The *c* stage is based on clinical and ultrasound findings:
- cT1: clinically not apparent
- cT2: confined to the prostate
- cT3: extension through the capsule
- cT4: adjacent structures involved.

The *p* stage depends on the findings at the time of radical prostatectomy:
- pT2: organ-confined
- pT3: extraprostatic extension
- pT4: invasion of bladder/rectum

Nx: nodes not examined
N0: regional nodes not affected
N1: regional nodes affected

M0: no evidence of distant metastases
M1: distant metastases present.

Screening with prostate-specific antigen (PSA)

PSA is a glycoprotein produced by both normal and malignant prostate tissue. It rises with age after the age of 40. There is considerable overlap in PSA measurements between benign and malignant prostate disease. Causes of an elevated PSA:
- Carcinoma of the prostate
- BPH (📖 p. 514)
- Prostatitis
- Trauma (prostatic biopsy, TURP: avoid measuring PSA for 6 weeks)

Digital rectal examination causes a *clinically insignificant* rise in PSA. The normal range is *age-specific*, but as general rules:
- If PSA <4 ng/mL, cancer is possible, though diagnostic yield is lower, and disease is more likely to be confined to the gland.
- If PSA 4–10 ng/mL, there is ~20% chance of malignancy. Biopsy is usually recommended but depends on individual circumstances.
- If PSA >10 ng/mL, the probability of prostate cancer is >50%. Biopsy is usually recommended.

The rate of rise of PSA (>0.75 ng/mL/year may prompt biopsy), PSA density (PSA corrected for prostatic volume on US), and ratio of free to bound serum PSA (↓ fraction of free PSA in malignancy) may become useful tools in enhancing specificity. These are not yet useful in clinical practice.

Controversies
- Many older ♂ have asymptomatic prostate cancer and will go on to die of something else. They ∴ do not benefit from investigation, the associated anxiety, or the possible treatments offered.
- PSA is not sensitive or specific for cancer when normal or moderately raised (<10 ng/mL). More invasive tests (biopsy) and potentially needless anxiety may be generated.
- We do not yet know what the optimal treatment for early prostate cancer is: watchful waiting may be better management than radical prostatectomy and/or radiotherapy.
- Screening tests are only valuable if they allow earlier and more beneficial treatment to be instituted.

Management of prostate cancer

Early disease
The options are watchful waiting, radical prostatectomy, or radiotherapy; no good trial data separate these therapies. The general health of the patient, clinical stage, and grade are all important in the decision-making process, but it may boil down to the choice of the patient. Newer alternatives include brachytherapy, cryoablation, or androgen ablation.
- 5-year survival was 67% in the 1970s; it is 98% today. So earlier and aggressive treatment has ↑ survival (in early disease).
- ▶ Radical prostatectomy may → erectile dysfunction and incontinence.

Follow-up
Watchful waiting: Some individuals have disease that advances. Monitor as follows:
- Regular physical examination (? urinary retention or incontinence)
- PSA every 3–6 months
- Surveillance CT or bone scans are not justified.
- Repeat prostatic biopsy may be helpful with ↑PSA.

Post-radical prostatectomy/radiotherapy
- Regular PSA ± rectal examination, usually every 6 months.

Recurrence and late disease
Local recurrence after radical prostatectomy → radiotherapy. Local recurrence after initial radiotherapy treatment → salvage prostatectomy, with an increased risk of postoperative complications.

Metastatic disease is treated with palliative (*not* curative) androgen deprivation therapy. Measure PSA every 6 months. Patients who "escape" (↑PSA, usually after ~2 years) on anti-androgens have a poor prognosis (median survival = 12 months).

Androgen deprivation therapy
Prostate cells are androgen sensitive, and malignant cells respond to androgen manipulation. Androgen production can be ↓ by bilateral orchidectomy (produced in testes) + anti-androgen treatment (to block adrenal production), or estrogens (e.g., diethylstilboestrol) or LHRH agonists (e.g., goserelin). Competitive androgen-receptor blockers (bicalutamide, flutamide, cyproterone acetate) can contribute to combination therapy and are thought to improve survival marginally.

Chapter 9

Fluids and electrolytes

Sodium: salt and water balance 520
Hyponatremia 522
Management of hyponatremia 526
Hypernatremia 528
Edema and its treatment 531
Diuretics 532
Potassium 534
Hypokalemia 536
Bartter's, Gitelman's, and Liddle's syndromes 538
Calcium, magnesium, and phosphorus 540
Hypocalcemia 542
Hypercalcemia 544
Hypomagnesemia 546
Hypermagnesemia 548
Hypophosphatemia 549
Hyperphosphatemia 550
Acid–base 552
Metabolic acidosis 554
Renal tubular acidosis (RTA) 556
Lactic acidosis 559
Metabolic alkalosis 560
Mixed acidosis and alkalosis 564
Tubular rarities 566

Sodium: salt and water balance

The human body is made up of 50%–60% water by weight. More accurately, total body water (TBW) in liters can be estimated as weight (kg) × a correction factor as below:

	♂	♀
<65 years old	0.6	0.5
>65 years old	0.5	0.45

So, in a 70 kg ♂, TBW = 0.6 × 70 = 42 L. Water is contained in specific compartments:
- Intracellular space (~ $2/3$ TBW, or 28 L in a 70 kg ♂)
- Extracellular fluid (ECF) is then ~ $1/3$ TBW, or 14 L in a 70 kg ♂.
  This includes
  - Interstitial fluid (~ $2/3$ ECF water, or 9.4 L in a 70 kg ♂)
  - Plasma (~ $1/3$ ECF water, or 4.6 L in a 70 kg ♂)

The hydrophobic cell membrane acts as a barrier between intra- and extracellular fluid, and the capillary wall separates plasma from the interstitium. Every compartment maintains osmotic pressure through an actively retained, specific solute:
- Intracellular: K^+ (pumped inward by Na^+/K^+-ATPase).
- ECF: Na^+ (see below)
- Plasma: proteins (especially albumin, impermeable through the normal endothelial barrier).

Extracellular volume is controlled by Na^+ retention and excretion (water will passively follow sodium). The body does not sense the ECF volume as a whole, but senses the effective arterial blood volume (EABV).[1]
- This amounts to ~ 700 mL (blood in the arterial tree at any one time).
- EABV is a function of cardiac output (CO) and systemic vascular resistance (SVR).

Changes in EABV due to hypovolemia, ↓CO, or ↓SVR are sensed by
- Systemic baroreceptors (carotid sinus, aortic arch)
- Intrarenal volume sensors (juxtaglomerular apparatus).

With ↓EABV, these volume sensors activate the sympathetic nervous system, with Na+ retained by the kidney (often UNa < 10 mEq/L). Conversely, with ↑EABV, sodium-wasting (>100 mEq/L) takes place with appropriate changes in TBW. This requires intact renal sodium handling (and kidney function) for this homeostasis.

Low-pressure volume receptors in the atria and the great veins are also important: ↑ECF leads to increased atrial natriuretic peptide (ANP) release and renal sodium wasting, as well as suppressing sympathetic tone. These receptors may control nonosmotic ADH release if the ECF is underfilled.

---

1 Schrier RW (1988). *N Engl J Med* **319**: 1065.

Falling EABV increases sympathetic tone
- ↑ irculating catecholamines, leading to ↑CO and ↑ SVR
- Activated renin–angiotensin system (RAS), improving renal hemodynamics and sodium retention through secondary hyperaldosteronism.
- ↑ nonosmotic ADH (vasopressin) release.

Rising EABV (including low-pressure whole ECF sensing)
- ↑ ANP (atrial natriuretic peptide, a potent natriuretic)
- Suppressed renin production and, thus, decreased angiotensin and aldosterone.

Water handling

TBW is mainly regulated by hypothalamic osmoreceptors (*not* volume sensors) capable of sensing changes in ECF osmolality: ↑ osmolality triggers thirst and pituitary ADH (vasopressin) release. Relatively dilute urine arrives at the collecting duct, as Na^+ reabsorption in the ascending limb of the loop of Henle and distal convoluted tubule occurs without water (the loop allows the countercurrent mechanism, leading to a hypertonic medullary interstitium).

Without ADH, the final urine is dilute (which explains the polyuria of DI, 📖 p. 530). ADH binds V2 (vasopressin) receptors on the basolateral aspect of the principal cells in the collecting duct, leading to translocation of aquaporin 2 to the apical membrane, where these water channels allow free water absorption along an osmolar gradient into the hypertonic interstitium.

With water-loading, osmoreceptors sense a falling serum osmolality. Thirst and ADH release are suppressed → dilute urine formation, rapidly (within 6 hours) restoring normal serum osmolality (~285 mOsm/kg).

With water depletion, osmoreceptors sense ↑ osmolality and trigger ADH release, leading to water reabsorption by the collecting ducts with resulting highly concentrated urine. Increased thirst eventually corrects the absolute water deficit.

So, for normal water homeostasis, an individual needs
- An intact thirst sensation
- Access to water
- The ability to secrete and suppress ADH (vasopressin)
- A responsive collecting duct

Abnormalities in one or more of these components → abnormal water homeostasis.

Hyponatremia

As with many electrolyte disorders, ↓Na^+ is relatively common in hospitalized patients—symptomatic hyponatremia is associated with a mortality of 10%–50%. Hyponatremia usually occurs as a result of altered water balance, making clinical assessment of body water the key to management. The NR for Na^+ is 135–145 mEq/L. Causes include pseudo-hyponatremia (see below), dilutional hyponatremia with increased serum osmolality, iso-osmolal hyponatremia, and hyposomolal hyponatremia.

Hyperosmolal (dilutional) hyponatremia

Mannitol or hyperglycemia (▶ for every 100 mg/dL above the normal range for glucose, correct ↓ by 2.4 mEq/L). One can also see this with IV Ig (maltose) in renal failure.

Iso-osmolal hyponatremia

Non-Na^+ glycine or sorbitol containing bladder irrigants may also be absorbed, especially after prostatectomy, ↓Na^+. Neurological symptoms can occur. Glycine or sorbitol solutions can be metabolized to water.

Hypo-osmolal hyponatremia

With depleted ECF (Na^+ loss > water loss)
- Renal losses:
  - Diuretics
  - Osmotic diuresis (glucose, urea in recovering ATN)
  - Salt-wasting nephropathy (due to chronic tubular dysfunction)
  - Addison disease
- Nonrenal losses:
  - Diarrhea or vomiting
  - Sweating
  - "Third space" losses (burns, bowel obstruction, pancreatitis).

▶ Severe volume depletion causes a state of ADH secretion: although initially suppressed as Na^+↓, hypovolemia overrides osmoreceptor-induced inhibition, and is a potent stimulus for ADH release to maintain blood pressure through its vasopressor properties and through reabsorbtion of water from the collecting ducts, even though water will distribute predominantly in the intracellular fluid (ICF) rather than ECF. Sensed EABV depletion takes precedence over the low serum Na^+ concentration. ADH will increase thirst with intake of hypotonic fluids.

With excess ECF (water retention > Na^+ retention)
- CHF
- Nephrotic syndrome or CKD
- Cirrhosis.

If EABV is extremely low due to severely poor perfusion with CHF, severe splanchnic dilatation with cirrhosis, or severe loss of oncotic pressure in nephrotic syndrome (minimal change disease) will lead to stimulation of the renin–angiotensin system as well as ADH.

With normal ECF (water retention*)
- Syndrome of inappropriate antidiuretic hormone secretion (SIADH) (*In actuality, excess water retention leads to volume sensors excreting Na^+ to restore volume to normal.)
  - Pneumonia, COPD, TB, other lung diseases (usually with $\downarrow pO_2$)
  - Malignancy (usually small cell lung cancer, occasionally head and neck cancers)
  - Drugs (antipsychotics, SSRI antidepressants)
  - Neurological disease (e.g., CVA, trauma, acute psychosis, cancers)
  - Pain, opiates, stress (⚠ surgery)
- Cortisol deficiency
- Hypothyroidism (severe)
- MMDA (Ecstasy): both excess ADH and water intake are involved.
- Psychogenic polydipsia: Massive free water intake overwhelms the kidney's normal ability to dilute urine. These patients have psychiatric problems.
- Potomania: Ethanol consumption and/or moderately increased water intake in the absence of ethanol consumption with very low solute intake may cause hyponatremia.

Pseudohyponatremia

Pseudohyponatremia results when Na^+ is measured in plasma where the fraction of water is reduced by ↑lipids, ↑plasma proteins (▶ myeloma or hypergammaglobulinemia) compared to normal states. The measured sodium concentration is lower in the plasma, although the actual Na^+ is normal in plasma water. There are no neurological symptoms.

Symptoms and signs

Symptoms may be subtle or absent if chronic, or Na^+ >125 mEq/L. Common symptoms if acute, or Na^+ <110 mEq/L, include headache, apathy, confusion (especially in the elderly) → seizures and coma. Symptoms are due to cerebral swelling as serum osmolality falls; water will diffuse to relatively hypertonic brain intracellular space. (Defense vs. hyponatremia is loss of brain solutes; see "The brain and $\downarrow Na^+$"). Encephalopathy is exacerbated by $\downarrow pO_2$ of any cause.

If ↑ECF (overloaded) or↑ECF (volume depleted), the diagnosis is usually apparent.

Investigations
Recheck an abnormal result (⚠ blood drawn above IV in patients on 5% dextrose).
- Electrolytes, BUN, Cr, glucose, plasma osmolality (normal/↑ if pseudohyponatraemia)
- Urine osmolality (UOsm *should* be <100 mOsm/kg, and will be if ADH is suppressed [e.g., psychogenic polydipsia]).
- UNa (if <20 mEq/L = nonrenal Na^+ losses, if >40 mEq/L = SIADH [unless Na^+ intake is low or there is superimposed volume depletion with SIADH])—⚠ diuretics may confound interpretation of urinary electrolytes.
- Urinalysis for specific gravity and glucose
- TSH and morning cortisol level, if indicated
- Ca^{2+}, albumin, glucose, LFT. ↓ serum uric acid is common with SIADH.

▶ Consider Addison's if there is ↓Na^+, ↑K^+, and volume depletion—check AM cortisol and after ACTH stimulation, and if patient is ill, treat with vigorous NS replacement and hydrocortisone.

If patient has low cortisol and is euvolemic with normal K^+, consider isolated cortisol deficiency.

Diagnosing SIADH
- ↓Na^+ in patients not on diuretics
- Euvolemic (i.e., no edema)
- Normal renal, adrenal, and thyroid function
- Normal K^+ and HCO_3
- Urine osmolality >100 mOsm/kg, often >300 mOsm/kg
- UNa >20 mEq/L (unless salt-restricted, superimposed volume depletion)
- Low serum uric acid (<4 mg/dL)

▶ ADH may be released inappropriately from the pituitary, or from cells of neuroendocrine origin in the lungs.

Cerebral salt-wasting
Brain injury of any cause (SAH, trauma, tumor) → brain natriuretic peptide (BNP, ≈ ANP 📖 p. 626) release, resulting in Na^+ wasting and volume depletion. ↓ECF → appropriate ADH release and ↓Na^+.

Cerebral salt-wasting is probably overdiagnosed. Confirm the following:
- Is patient volume depleted?
- With volume resuscitation, UOsm rapidly rises (with ADH suppression).

Management of hyponatremia

In all cases
- Identify those at risk for neurological complications (osmotic demyelination syndrome):
    - Thiazide-induced ↓Na^+
    - Premenopausal ♀ (?estrogen, ↑ responsiveness to ADH)
    - Malnourished or alcoholic patients
    - Even if patient is well, ↑ surveillance as for symptomatic patients with repeated Na^+ checks (see below).
- *Assess the volume status correctly* (📖 p. 377). This is key to correct diagnosis and management.
- Stop potentially contributing medications ± fluids (⚠ 5% dextrose).
- Correct ↓K^+ (📖 p. 534) and ↓Mg^{2+} (📖 p. 546) if present.

Managing hyponatremia without encephalopathy
- Unless patient is encephalopathic, manage conservatively as follows:
    - If volume overloaded, *fluid restrict* <1 L/day (≈ 5 cups/day)
    - If euvolemic, *fluid restrict* as above. An alternative is to give po NaCl tablets ± furosemide 20–40 mg/daily.
    - If volume depleted, *resuscitate* with NS.
- Specific points for managing asymptomatic SIADH:
    - *CAUTION*: Demeclocycline 150–300 mg bid induces nephrogenic diabetes insipidus, reversing ADH effects. Use only if above measures of water restriction and ↑NaCl intake or NaCl tablets fail. Watch carefully if chronic hyponatremia occurs, as diuresis may be brisk. Avoid demeclocycline in renal or liver failure.
    - Newer aquaretics act by inhibiting the ADH V2 receptor; conivaptan IV (hospital available) and tolvaptan, stravaptan (oral forms, but not yet available) have proven efficacy in SIADH.

✱ The brain and ↓Na^+

The skull limits the brain's capacity to increase in size: with ↓Na^+, a falling osmolality → ↑ intracellular water and symptomatic brain swelling. In response, the cerebral ECF is rapidly reduced (to allow more room), as intracellular organic solutes are exported (lessening the osmolar gradient that causes water influx) over days. If too rapid correction of chronic ↓Na^+ occurs, *osmotic demyelination syndrome (central pontine myelinosis)* may occur. Because the brain cannot restore the solute contribution to intracellular tonicity quickly, when the ECF osmolality is rapidly normalized, water leaves cells, causing cerebral dehydration and demyelination (affecting the whole brain, not just the pons as in the original description).

Managing hyponatremia with encephalopathy

1. Manage in ICU or step-down unit.
2. ↑ Na^+ by as little as 3–7 mEq/L will usually treat symptoms.
3. Repeat Na^+ every 2 hours initially, and then 4 hourly.
- If *acute* (<48 hours duration) (often postoperative):
  - Aim for ↑Na^+ by 2 mEq/L/h or until asymptomatic.
  - **Do not correct by >10 mEq/L/24 h.**
- If *chronic* (>48 hours duration):
  - **Always be cognizant of possible osmotic demyelination.**
  - Aim for ↑Na^+ by 0.5 mEq/L/h or until asymptomatic. If severe neurologic symptoms, such as seizures, may initially correct at faster rate.
  - **Do not correct by >10 mEq/L/24 h.**
  - Calculate Na^+ deficit and select appropriate mode of administration.
- Na^+ deficit = TBW × [desired Na^+ − actual Na^+]
  - TBW = 60% body weight in ♂ and 50% body weight in ♀
  - If age is >65, use 50% BW in ♂ and 45% BW in ♀.
  - For example, aiming for a safe Na^+ of 125 mEq/L in a 53-year-old 70 kg ♂ with Na^+ 115, deficit = 0.6 × 70 × 10 = 420 mEq Na^+.
- Generally, use 3% (hypertonic) saline, containing 513 mEq NaCl, respectively, per 1 L (use of NS may worsen hyponatremia if UOsm of patient is over 300 mOsm/kg). Deliver via a central line.
- Estimate effect of infusion by calculating change in Na^+:
  - Change in Na^+ = $\dfrac{\text{infusion fluid } Na^+ - Na^+}{TBW + 1}$ for 1000 mL infusion
  - For example, in the above patient, using 3% hypertonic saline 1 L over 24 hours, change in Na^+ = $\dfrac{513 - 115}{42 + 1}$ = 9.25 mEq/L

  If a rapid increase was required (i.e., if patient is seizing), and a target of >120 mEq/L was desired, over 3 hours (see below) aim to infuse [5/9.25 × 1 L] = 540 mL of 3% saline at 180 mL/h.
- D5W has been used in cases to prevent osmotic demyelination syndrome when there has been overcorrection of Na^+.
5. Other measures:
- Add in furosemide if volume overloaded. The diuresis caused will be hypotonic (i.e., water in excess of salt), adding to sodium correction.
- *Do not correct by* >10 mEq/L/24 h.

Hypernatremia

Serum Na$^+$ >146 mEq/L is usually due to a water deficit and is associated with significant mortality (± 50%). With ↑Na$^+$, ECF osmolality ↑, increasing osmotic drag on the intracellular compartment. This leads to cellular dehydration, most importantly in the brain: loss of volume creates vascular shear stress, resulting in bleeding and thrombosis. As in hyponatremia (📖 p. 522), cerebral compensation begins, but with cellular retention of salts and organic solutes in the brain, increasing cellular tonicity and lessening water losses to the hyperosmolar ECF (occurring over days). Overzealous correction leads to too-rapid intracranial expansion of the brain, with potential cerebral herniation. This is usually accompanied by lack of thirst or access to free water. Causes include the following.

- Excess hypertonic fluids
  - IV infusions (▶ antibiotics), TPN or enteral feeds
  - Rarely, salt ingestion or sea-water drowning
- Excess water loss
  - Nephrogenic or central diabetes insipidus (see Box 9.1) with/without altered thirst
- Excess water loss > Na$^+$ loss
  - Renal
  —Diuretics
  —Osmotic diuresis (glucose in DKA, urea in recovering ATN)
  - GI
  —Diarrhea (most diarrheas and lactulose)
  —Vomiting, NG losses or fistulas
  - Skin
  —Sweating, burns
- Decreased thirst: in the ill and elderly, this occurs especially if they are on psychotropic drugs. Usually associated with a condition above.

Symptoms and signs

Symptoms reflect cerebral dehydration. Thirst, apathy, weakness, and confusion → ↓ consciousness, seizures, and coma. The cause is often apparent clinically. Investigations include urinalysis with specific gravity, plasma osmolality, glucose, UNa, and UOsm. With osmotic diuresis, UOsm is always >300 mOsm/kg.

Treatment

▶ Treat the underlying cause.
- Calculate water deficit (and include ongoing losses in calculations):

$$\text{Change in Na}^+ = \frac{\text{infusion fluid Na}^+ - \text{Na}^+}{\text{TBW} + 1} \text{ for 1000 mL infusion}$$

TBW = 60% body weight in ♂ and 50% body weight in ♀.
If age > 65, use 50% weight in ♂ and 45% weight in ♀.

For example, in a 53-year-old 70 kg ♂ with Na$^+$ 170 mEq/L, TBW = 42 L. Using 5% dextrose (no Na$^+$), [0–170]/43 = –3.95 mEq/L. So 1 L 5% dextrose will reduce Na$^+$ to 166 mEq/L. Aiming to correct only 0.5 mEq/L/h will require 1 L/8 h, or 125 mL/h *if there are no ongoing fluid losses*. As a rule of thumb, allow for 0.5 L insensible loss per day.
- *Reassess patient repeatedly.*
- If ↑Na$^+$ is acute (<24 hours), this can be reversed quickly. Usually this occurs with infusion of hypertonic solutions, but also with rapid loss of hypotonic fluid (sweating, burns).
  - Correct at 1 mEq/L/h.
  - Measure Na$^+$ q2h initially, then q4h.
- If chronic (>24 hours), correct more slowly to prevent rehydration injury to the brain:
  - Document neurological status.
  - Correct at not >0.5 mEq/L/h, or <10–12 mEq/L/day.
  - General rule: correct 50% of the water deficit in the first 12–24 hours. Correct remaining water deficit over the next 24–48 hours.
  - Measure Na$^+$ every 2 hours initially, then every 4 hours.

Choice of fluid
- Water orally if orientated, or per NG if able.
- Use 5% dextrose or consider 0.45% (half-normal) saline IV (if volume depleted as well) if you cannot use the GI tract. If the patient is both water and volume depleted, consider using one IV of 5% dextrose and one IV of 0.9% saline. Patient may require insulin to control hyperglycemia if using 5% dextrose.

Box 9.1 Diabetes insipidus (DI)

ADH (also called arginine vasopressin) binds the V2 receptor on collecting duct cells, leading to surface expression of water channels, aquaporin-2, through which water is rapidly reabsorbed from the urine. DI can be central (i.e., impaired release of ADH):
- Trauma
- Tumors or infiltrative processes (neurosarcoidosis, TB)
- Infections (meningitis, encephalitis)
- Cerebral vasculitis (SLE, Wegener's)

More commonly, DI is nephrogenic (resistance to ADH). Causes include:
- Congenital
- Drug induced (lithium, amphotericin B, foscarnet, demeclocycline)
- Hypokalemia or hypercalcemia
- Tubulointerstitial disease (medullary cystic disease, 📖 p. 421)

Diagnosis rests on finding ↑UO (>3 L/day) with dilute urine (<300 mOsm/kg) in complete DI (vs. 300–700 mOsm/kg in partial DI). Exclude osmotic diuretics, ↓K^+ or ↑Ca^{2+}. A fluid deprivation test ± DDAVP (synthetic analogue of ADH) is diagnostic (▶ seek nephrology advice). See response with DDAVP in central DI. ADH measurements may be required in equivocal cases (<1.5 pg/mL in partial CDI, >2 pg/mL in partial nephrogenic DI).

Treatment depends on the cause. Central DI is treated with intranasal DDAVP 10–20 µg bid. Nephrogenic DI is treated with thiazide diuretics (hypovolemia → ↑ Na^+ reabsorption proximally, ∴ reduced water delivery to the collecting duct, and interferes with distal tubule diluting capacity) and NSAIDs (such as indomethacin, antagonizing effect of ADH). Decreasing solute intake may decrease obligate urine volume as well.

⚠ Simultaneous use of DDAVP and 5% dextrose should be used with extreme caution.

Edema and its treatment

Edema occurs with interstitial expansion of the ECF, becoming clinically apparent if there is >2–3 L of excess fluid in this compartment. It is most obvious in the dependent areas (ankles), but if may affect the face and eyelids, especially in the morning. *Anasarca* refers to severe edema progressing from the lower extremities to the trunk. Edema may occur with other extravascular signs of salt and water retention (pleural effusions, ascites). Causes include the following:
- Congestive heart failure
- Cirrhosis
- Nephrotic syndrome ((p. 384)
- ARF or CKD (↓GFR → ↓ salt excretion)
- Drug induced (NSAIDs, calcium channel blockers)
- Premenstrual or pregnant ♀ (estrogen effect)
- Venous insufficiency (localized edema).

Development of edema

For edema to develop, salt and water retention must occur (to expand the ECF), and/or capillary permeability must increase (to allow fluid shifts into the interstitium). Na^+ retention is the primary factor in the development of edema: any state that leads to ↓EABV (p. 520) → secondary hyperaldosteronism, sympathetic overactivity, and nonosmotic ADH release. This then causes salt and water retention, an increase in ECF volume, and edema. Edema due to nephrotic syndrome is explained in Box 9.2.

Box 9.2 Edema and hypoalbuminemia in the nephrotic syndrome

Edema associated with ↓ albumin (NR 3.6–5 g/dL) in nephrotic syndrome has been attributed to a fall in plasma oncotic pressure (provided largely by albumin) with unchanged hydrostatic pressure resulting in fluid movement into the extravascular space. This then leads to secondary fluid retention.

Experimental evidence suggests this is incorrect with ↓ serum albumin: the transcapillary oncotic gradient is maintained with hypoalbuminemia, as interstitial colloid osmotic pressure (COP) is reduced in tandem with falls in the plasma COP (the interstitial fluid not only maintains a COP-countering plasma COP, but can be varied). Rather, inflammatory cytokines impair capillary permeability, ↑ urinary albumin modifies Na^+ handling directly in the nephron, and renal resistance to ANP develops. The net effect is one of salt retention, with equilibration of the expanded ECF into the interstitium. The exception, with true underfilling and falling EABV with salt retention, may be seen in minimal change disease when albumin <2 g/dL.

Diuretics

All diuretics inhibit the renal reabsorption of Na^+ and, thus, Cl^- and water. Diuretics circulate and are highly protein-bound, and are thus not well filtered by the glomerulus. The diuretic albumin complex is taken up from the peritubular capillaries by proximal tubular-cell ion transporters, and the free diuretic is released into the tubule to block Na^+ uptake by transport proteins in the urinary space (except for spironolactone and other mineralocorticoid receptor antagonists that act from the capillary side). For use in hypertension, 📖 p. 332.

Commonly used diuretics

Loop diuretics
- Site of action: blocks Na^+ uptake at the $Na^+K^+2Cl^-$ (NKCC) cotransporter in the thick ascending limb of the loop of Henle
- Specific side effects: ↑u-Ca^{2+}, ototoxicity
- Examples: furosemide, bumetanide, torsemide.

Thiazide diuretics
- Site of action: blocks Na^+ uptake at the Na^+Cl^- cotransporter in the distal tubule
- Specific side effects: ↓UCa^{2+} (may cause hypercalcemia—look for primary hyperparathyroidism)
- Examples: hydrochlorothiazide, metolazone, indapamide.

Amiloride/triamterene
- Site of action: blocks Na^+ uptake at the apical (side facing urinary lumen) Na^+ channel (ENaC) in the principal cells of the collecting duct.
- Specific side effects: ↑K^+, metabolic acidosis.

Mineralocorticoid receptor antagonists
- Site of action: blocks Na^+ uptake by down-regulating apical Na^+ channel (ENaC) expression in the collecting duct. It enters cells from the circulation rather than the urinary space, and binds the intracellular mineralocorticoid receptor (MR).
- Specific side effects: ↑K^+, metabolic acidosis, antiandrogenic effects (not eplerenone)
- Examples: spironolactone, eplerenone

General side effects of all diuretics include ↓K^+ (*not* with spironolactone), ↓Na^+ (especially thiazide diuretics), ↓Mg^{2+}, metabolic alkalosis (*not* with spironolactone), ↑uric acid, skin rashes, interstitial nephritis, dyslipidemia, ❖ insulin resistance, and impotence.

Using diuretics in edematous states

⚠ Always institute appropriate salt restriction when using diuretics, and consider fluid restriction to <1000 mL/day.
- Assess volume status daily.
- Measure weight daily to assess response.
- Strict input/output charts may be helpful.
- Measure serum electrolytes regularly.
- Monitoring UNa may help in diuretic resistance (if >100 mEq/day and no weight loss, patient is not Na^+ restricting).

Nephrotic syndrome

This often requires high doses of loop diuretics (furosemide 160–600 mg daily po or IV divided in 2–3 doses—beware of ototoxicity), as ↑ urinary albumin binds free diuretic. Consider adding thiazide diuretics (metolazone 2.5–5 mg/day po), but beware of rapid-onset ↓Na^+ and titrate dose against daily weight loss.

♦* Furosemide and albumin infusions have been used in an attempt to improve drug delivery, probably without real benefit because free diuretic may bind back to increased leaked urinary albumin in the tubule, limiting effectiveness. They *may* be of use if albumin <2 g/dL. Administer 6.25–12.5 g salt-poor albumin with 40–160 mg furosemide IV over 2–4 hours.

Renal failure

Use a loop diuretic if GFR <50 mL/min. The patient may require 240–720 mg IV daily, in 2–3 divided doses. The best response is with IV loop diuretic (furosemide 200 mg) or as continuous infusion, which results in increased Na^+ excretion vs. bolus (furosemide 10–40 mg/h to a maximum of 1000 mg/day to prevent ototoxicity). If the patient did not respond at all to the bolus, the continuous drip will not provide any increased benefit. Bumetanide is better absorbed po (not IV) and should be considered in diuretic resistance if on or converting to oral medications (up to 8 mg/day). If response is poor, consider adding on thiazide as above.

Congestive cardiac failure

Loop diuretics are better than thiazides, (furosemide 40 mg qd). Evidence from RALES and EPHESUS trials has confirmed a role for mineralocorticoid receptor blockade, so this class is often used as first-line therapy. Hyperkalemia is a real concern, as these patients are often on an ACEI or β-blockers (📖 p. 336) as well.

If there is pulmonary edema and ARF, the patient may require IV diuretics with gut edema impairing oral absorption and poor delivery of diuretic to kidney with CHF.

Cirrhosis

Spironolactone (50–200 mg qd) prevents secondary hyperaldosteronism with adding thiazide or a loop diuretic (watch for too much diuresis, which may precipitate ARF) if required. Resistant ascites is best treated with paracentesis with albumin infusion.

Potassium

K^+ is the second most abundant cation in the body (~3.5 mol). Dietary K^+ amounts to 80–150 mEq/day. Once absorbed, K^+ is rapidly buffered by removal from the ECF into the intracellular compartment: insulin and β-adrenergic catecholamines stimulate membrane Na^+/K^+-ATPase to pump K^+ into cells. This electrochemical gradient (the cell membrane potential) is critical to nerve conduction, muscle contraction, and normal cell function. Total body K^+ balance is regulated by renal excretion: K^+ is freely filtered at the glomerulus. It is reabsorbed by the PCT (75%), the loop of Henle (15%), and the α-intercalated cells of the collecting duct. As Na^+ enters principal cells from the urine, K^+ exits principal cells into the urinary space. Increased Na^+ delivery to open Na^+ channels (ENaC) increases K^+ secretion. K^+ secretion is tightly controlled by aldosterone primarily by principal cells of the collecting duct. Aldosterone increases Na^+/K^+-ATPase activity and number and opens ENaC channels. Aldosterone is increased directly by hyperkalemia and suppressed by hypokalemia, controlling K^+ in the normal range (3.5–5.0 mEq/L).

Hyperkalemia (see 📖 p. 164 for full discussion)

▶ ↑K^+ is often spurious: *always recheck result*. Traumatic venopuncture → cellular K^+ leakage and pseudohyperkalemia (more common with ↑WBC or ↑ platelet count).

True hyperkalemia is due to either increased shift or release from cells or decreased excretion by the kidney. Since the release of important trials using spironolactone or eplerenone (in addition to ACE inhibitors) in the treatment of heart failure, dangerous hyperkalemia has become more common in those with heart failure.

Common causes
- ARF or CKD
- Drug induced (especially combinations of the following)
  - ACE inhibitors/ARB
  - β-blockers
  - NSAIDs
  - Heparin and LMW heparins (inhibit normal aldosterone release)
  - Cyclosporine and tacrolimus
  - K^+-sparing diuretics (spironolactone, eplerenone, amiloride, triamterene)
  - High-dose trimethroprim, pentamadine (block ENaC)
  - Digoxin *toxicity* (but not therapeutic levels of digoxin)
- Hypoaldosteronism (including type 4 RTA, 📖 p. 557).
- Addison's
- Increased K^+ load with impaired excretion
  - High K^+ diet
  - Salt substitutes
  - Herbal medications (Noni juice)

- Increased release/shift from cells
  - Acidosis (mineral acids)
  - Insulin deficiency (DKA)
  - Hyperglycemia
  - Rhabdomyolysis, hemolysis or tumor lysis.

Rare causes of hyperkalemia
- *Hyperkalemic periodic paralysis:* Mutations in skeletal Na^+ channel lead to episodic paralysis, ↑K^+, and ↓Na^+ in response to varied triggers, as Na^+ and water are pumped into cells in exchange for K^+.
- *Type 1 pseudohypoaldosteronsim* presents in infancy as salt-wasting, ↓Na^+, and collapse. It is due to either resistance to the actions of aldosterone (defect in type 1 mineralocorticoid receptor, with ↑K^+) or defects in ENaC (📖 p. 626).
- *Gordon's syndrome* (type 2 pseudohypoaldosteronism): The clinical inverse of Gitelman's syndrome (📖 p. 538). It presents as ↑BP, ↓ renin and aldosterone, ↑K^+ and acidosis. Mutations in genes encoding WNK-1 and WNK-4 (negative regulators of NCCT, 📖 p. 624) are responsible.

Hyperkalemia since RALES and EPHESUS

These two trials demonstrated a 15%–30% reduction in mortality of CHF patients treated with agents that block the action of aldosterone (spironolactone, eplerenone). Widespread use (occasionally inappropriate) has followed. Since ACEIs/ARBs are also indicated to treat CHF, serious hyperkalemia may occur. If using such combination therapy, use the following precautions:
- Calculate GFR (📖 p. 30)—caution if abnormal.
- Stop NSAIDs.
- Advise patient about dietary K^+ restriction (📖 p. 199).
- If ↓GFR <60 mL/min, add in loop/thiazide diuretic to excrete K^+.
- If patient is acidotic (serum HCO_3^- <20 mEq/L), add $NaHCO_3$ 650 mg bid.
- Caution use of spironolactone above 25mg/day if also on ACEI.
- *Check K^+ regularly. If K^+ >5.5 mEq/L, discontinue either ACEI/ARB or spironolactone/eplerenone.*

⚠ Hyperkalemia arises when volume depletion, concurrent illness, or deteriorating renal or cardiac function is superimposed on patients on combination therapy. *Always check K^+*. Those with K^+ >5.0 mEq/L are at risk.

Hypokalemia

This is one of the most common electrolyte abnormalities, especially with diuretics. Although K^+ of 3–3.5 mEq/L is generally well tolerated except in those with cardiac disease, hypokalemia of <2.5 mEq/L can be life threatening.

Symptoms and signs
See list of causes for specific associations—these are usually picked up on serum electrolyte tests. Fatigue, constipation, weakness, and ↓ muscle tone (progressing to ascending paralysis, respiratory arrest as K^+ ↓) can occur. Cardiac arrhythmias are also found, especially if there is underlying heart disease.

Investigations
Check electrolytes, BUN, Cr, Mg^{2+}, and CK (may have spontaneous rhabdomyolysis). Check digoxin level if patient is on drug. If hypokalemia is not drug related or obviously associated with an underlying illness, consider UpH and urine electrolytes (if urine K^+ <20–30 mEq/day, K^+ losses are extrarenal), renin, and aldosterone tests. Patient may need urine laxative and diuretic screen if you suspect respective abuse. Alkalosis suggests long-standing hypokalemia.

ECG shows small T waves, U wave (after T), PR interval ↑, and ST segments.

Treatment
❶ Is the patient on digoxin? Hypokalemia will potentiate digoxin's arrhythmogenicity. Note that diuretic-induced hypokalemia is exacerbated if dietary Na^+ intake is high. Always aim to treat the underlying cause over time.

Mild (>2.5 mEq/L)
- Give oral slow-release potassium chloride 50–150 mEq/day in divided doses (treatment is limited by GI intolerability).
- Check K^+ regularly.
- ↑ dietary K^+ and ?switch to or add in K^+-sparing diuretic.
- Common options include K-Dur® (20 mEq/tab) or Slow-K® (8 mEq/tab). If patient is acidotic, you may use $KHCO_3$ or K citrate.

⚠ *Severe or symptomatic* hypokalemia (K <2.5 mEq/L, arrhythmias, liver failure or extreme weakness):
- Use cardiac monitor.
- Check Mg^{2+} and correct if needed (📖 p. 546).
- Avoid glucose-containing solutions or sodium bicarbonate.
- Give NS 1 L with 20–40 mEq KCl at no more than 10–20 mEq KCl/h through peripheral vein.
- ▶ *Danger of rapid-onset hyperkalemia*. Recheck K^+.

In volume-restricted patients or those with profound and ongoing hypokalemia, KCl can be given into a central vein as 20–40 mEq/100 mL NS at not >40 mEq/h using a volumetric pump. The patient must be in a monitored setting. If there is chronic hypokalemia, serum K^+ of 2 mEq/L may have an overall deficit of 400–800 mEq that has to be replaced.

Causes

- Inadequate intake <25 mEq/day (either dietary or IV) in conjuction with K^+ loss
- Increased GI losses
  - Diarrhea or laxative abuse, VIPoma, Zollinger–Ellison syndrome, ileostomy or enteric fistula, colonic villous adenoma
- Redistribution into cells
  - β-agonism (any cause of ↑ sympathetic drive, such as delirium tremens)
  - β-agonist drugs (bronchodilators, decongestants, tocolytics)
  - Insulin, theophylline, or caffeine (activate Na^+/K^+-ATPase pump)
  - Alkalosis
- Primary hyperaldosteronism
- Secondary hyperaldosteronism (📖 p. 312)
  - Liver failure, heart failure, nephrotic syndrome
- Renal losses
  - Diuretics (especially thiazides, loops) including abuse of diuretics
  - Vomiting (actually, renal K^+ loss in vomiting → secondary hyperaldosteronism, → delivery of $NaHCO_3$ → renal losses)
  - Acquired renal tubular disease (📖 p. 566) or RTAs (📖 p. 556)
  - Bartter's, Liddle's, and Gitelman's syndromes (📖 p. 538)
- Other drugs
  - Amphotericin and aminoglycosides (tubular toxicity)
  - Glucocorticoids (especially at high dose) or mineralocorticoids
  - Carbenoloxone and licorice (mineralocorticoid effect, prevents breakdown of cortisol, to inactive cortisol. Cortisol binds to mineralocorticoid receptor)
- Familial hypokalemic periodic paralysis
- Thyrotoxicosis
- Correction of vitamin B_{12} deficiency, GMCSF as new cells take up K^+.

Bartter's, Gitelman's, and Liddle's syndromes

Bartter's syndrome

This autosomal recessive disease is caused by impaired NaCl reabsorption in the ascending limb of the loop of Henle. Mutations in a number of channels (including NKCC2 and ROMK) are responsible for salt wasting and mild volume depletion. It is in effect what is seen with *loop diuretic use*. Subsequent secondary hyperaldosteronism (and juxtaglomerular apparatus hyperplasia) leads to a hypokalemic metabolic alkalosis. ↑ luminal Na^+ impairs Ca^{2+} absorption, leading to ↑UCa^{2+}.

Diagnose it in children (or adolescents) with failure to thrive, polydipsia, polyuria, and cramps. Patients have normal BP, ↓K^+, mild metabolic alkalosis, ↑UNa^+, ↑UK^+, ↑UCa^{2+}, ↑Uprostaglandin E2 (not understood reasons), ↑renin, and ↑aldosterone. (One variant has additionally sensorineural deafness and renal failure.)

Treatment

Aim to normalize K^+. Start with amiloride 5–40 mg/day (large doses may be needed) or spironolactone (up to 300 mg/day). Add on oral potassium supplementation as potassium chloride 25–100 mEq/day (for drugs, 📖 p. 536). ⚠ *Recheck* K^+ after 5–7 days to ensure that the dosing is appropriate. NSAIDs (indomethacin) used to inhibit the increased urinary prostaglandins in Bartter's. ACEI may help normalize K^+. This disease is often difficult to treat, and demanding of patient (children) compliance.

Gitelman's syndrome

Marked by autosomal recessive inheritance, this syndrome is caused by loss of function mutations of the thiazide-sensitive NaCl co-transporter (NCCT) in the DCT, resulting in impaired Na^+ reabsorption. ↑Na^+ loss leads to secondary hyperaldosteronism and a hypokalemic metabolic alkalosis. It is in effect what is seen with *thiazide diuretic use*. Increased calcium reabsorption leads to increased urinary Mg^{2+} loss, with significant hypomagnesemia.

Diagnose it in young adults with usually symptomatic ↓K^+ (2.0–3.0 mEq/L). Patients have ↓Mg^{2+}, mild metabolic alkalosis, ↑ renin, and ↑ aldosterone. Urinary Ca^{2+} is low (unlike in Barrter's; see Table 9.1). Genetic testing is available, though not widely so.

Treatment

Generally patients have a good prognosis. Use amiloride or spironolactone, K^+ supplementation (see above).

Liddle's syndrome

This autosomal dominant inherited disorder is caused by gain of function mutations in ENaC (epithelial sodium channel expressed on the apical surface of collecting duct cells), resulting in increased sodium retention. ↑Na⁺ reabsorption leads to ↓BP ± edema, and a hypokalemic metabolic alkalosis, with appropriately suppressed aldosterone.

Diagnose in young, hypertensive patients (often having a positive family history) with ↓K⁺ (may be mild) and mild metabolic alkalosis. There is also ↓renin and ↓aldosterone.

Treatment

Treat with a low-salt diet ± amiloride 5–10 mg qd (or triamterene), which directly inhibits ENaC.

Table 9.1 Differentiating inherited channelopathies

	Bartter's	Gitelman's	Liddle's
BP	N	N	↑
K	↓	↓	↓
Mg	N or ↓	↓	N
UPG E2	↑	N	N
Aldosterone	↑	↑	↓
UCa	↑ or N	↓	N
Age	Infancy	Early adulthood	Childhood

Calcium, magnesium, and phosphorus

Calcium

Nintey-nine percent of total body Ca^{2+} (~1 kg) is stored in bone. Extracellular Ca^{2+} accounts for a small fraction; of this, ~50% is bound to albumin, with 40% available as physiologically active, free (or ionized) Ca^{2+}. Ca^{2+} is important in skeletal health, membrane function, cell signaling, neuromuscular integrity, and coagulation.

The serum normal range is 8.5–10 mg/dL (4–5.2 mg/dL or 1.1–1.3 mmol/L ionized), with Ca^{2+} available from both GI and bone stores. GI Ca^{2+} absorption is controlled by calcitriol (active form of vitamin D). The ionized fraction is freely filtered, and mainly reabsorbed in the PCT and loop of Henle. Falling Ca^{2+} activates parathyroid calcium-sensing receptors, leading to parathyroid hormone (PTH) release. PTH increases renal tubular Ca^{2+} reabsorption and hydroxylation of 25-(OH) vitamin D_3 to the active metabolite, $1.25(OH)_2$ Vitamin D_3, increasing intestinal uptake. PTH also enhances bone osteoclastic activity.

Magnesium

Magnesium (Mg^{2+}) is the fourth most common cation in the body and is found largely in the intracellular compartment, or stored in bone. It is a key component of ATP-requiring reactions and is necessary for the synthesis of protein and maintaining membrane function, nerve conduction, and muscle contraction.

The kidney dominates the control of Mg^{2+} homeostasis. The normal range is 1.8–2.3 mg/dL in plasma. Mg^{2+} is absorbed from the gut and renally excreted. Filtered Mg^{2+} is reabsorbed in the loop of Henle and DCT, and modifying uptake allows Mg^{2+} levels to be maintained in the normal range. Because Mg^{2+} passively follows Na^+ uptake in loop of Henle and DCT, inhibiting Na^+ absorption will result in Mg^{2+} wasting.

Phosphorus

Phosphorus occurs largely as the inorganic fraction, phosphate, in the circulation. Organic phosphorus exists as protein-bound phospholipids and is not measured in clinical practice. Phosphate is essential to almost all biochemical systems. Absorbed from the intestine by passive and vitamin D_3-dependent transport, 80% is found in bone. The normal range for plasma phosphate is 2.5–4.6 mg/dL (higher in children). Freely filtered in the kidney, it is largely reabsorbed in the PCT, depending on oral intake (PTH inhibits tubular reabsorption).

Hypocalcemia

Total serum Ca^{2+} is low with ↓ albumin, though the free fraction may be normal. Always correct for albumin:

Calcium falls 0.8 mg/dL for every drop of 1 g/dL in albumin.

Symptoms and signs

Symptoms include depression and anxiety, (perioral) paraesthesias, carpopedal spasm, tetany, respiratory depression, convulsions, and arrhythmias. Examine for Chvostek's sign (tap over the parotid for facial muscle twitching as cranial nerve VII is excited) and Trousseau's sign (occlude brachial artery with BP cuff inflated >SBP, observe wrist and finger flexion). If it is chronic, cataracts, dental changes, bone pain, and muscle weakness ± skeletal deformities will be seen.

Investigations

▶ ECG shows prolonged QT interval. Check BUN, Cr, electrolytes, Ca^{2+}, phosphate, Mg^{2+}, alkaline phosphatase. If appropriate, also check amylase, CK. Consider PTH, 25-(OH) vitamin D_3, and 1, 25-(OH) vitamin D_3. Consider getting X-ray of long bones and hands.

Treatment

▶ Only treat if patient is symptomatic ± acute illness.

If *mild* (>8): Increase dietary Ca^{2+}. Add in oral Ca^{2+} (e.g., calcium carbonate) 0.5–1.5 g/day 2 hours after meals. If patient is vitamin D deficient, give oral ergocalciferol (25-(OH) vitamin D_3) or calcitriol (1, 25-(OH) vitamin D_3) 0.25–0.5 µg qd or with calcium supplements. If there is ↓Mg^{2+}, supplement as on 📖 p. 547.

⚠ If *acute or symptomatic*, infuse Ca^{2+} at 2 mg/kg/h: start IV 10% calcium gluconate 60 mL in 500 mL 5% dextrose or 0.9% saline (1 mg/mL elemental Ca^{2+}) at 0.5–2.5 mg/kg/h. Recheck Ca^{2+} at +4 hours and adjust infusion rate accordingly.

⚠ If there is *tetany*, give 10 mL 10% calcium gluconate 10 mL (100–200 mg elemental calcium) IV over 10–20 min (⚠ extravasation). Repeat if necessary, ± infusion as above.

Causes of hypocalcemia
- Vitamin D deficiency
  - Malnutrition
  - Malabsorption (gastrectomy, short bowel, celiac disease)
  - CKD
  - Vitamin D–dependent rickets
- Hypoparathyroidism
  - Post-parathyroidectomy—"hungry bone syndrome," 📖 p. 190
    ⚠ Inadvertent after thyroidectomy, radical neck surgery
  - Inherited, autoimmune, pseudohypoparathyroidism
- Hyperphosphatemia (↑ phosphate increases bone Ca^{2+} deposition)
  - Tumor lysis (📖 p. 144)
  - Rhabdomyolysis (📖 p. 138)
- Acute pancreatitis
- ↓Mg^{2+}
- Bisphosphonates
- Cinacalcet
- Cisplatin
- Complexing with EDTA, Foscarnet, citrate, lactate
- Plasmapheresis
- Pseudohypocalcemia after gadolinium, measurement artifact.

Hypercalcemia

This may be the result of increased absorption from gut, bone resorption, or both. It may be due to increased PTH or analogues, or osteolytic metastases. Mild ↑Ca^{2+} (>10.5–11.6 mg/dL) is usually asymptomatic, but rapidly evolving ↑Ca^{2+} >14 may be fatal.

Symptoms and signs

"Bones, stones, groans, and moans" characterize this condition. Nausea, abdominal pain, anorexia, constipation, depression, confusion, polydipsia, and polyuria may be present. Dehydration (?postural drop), renal calculi, and nephrocalcinosis can also occur. There can be signs from associated malignancy. Get a full medication history.

Causes

- Primary hyperparathyroidism (10%–20%)—less commonly tertiary with CKD. Secondary if ESRD with excess Ca^{2+}-based phosphate binders, high Ca^{2+} dialysate, 1, 25-(OH) vitamin D_3, or analog therapy
- Malignancy
  - Local osteolytic bone lesions
  - Tumor-derived PTH related protein, PTHrP, has similar actions to PTH.
  - Common cancers include breast, lung, myeloma, esophagus, renal, prostate, and head and neck primaries. Lymphoma with 1-hydroxylase enzyme not decreased by hypercalcemia results in excess 1, 25-(OH) vitamin D_3.
- Granulomatous diseases (sarcoidosis, TB) with 1-hydroxylase, which causes excess 1, 25-(OH) vitamin D_3)
- Drugs (vitamin D, vitamin A, thiazide diuretics, lithium)
- Immobilization
- Thyrotoxicosis
- Pheochromocytoma
- Milk-alkali syndrome (antacids, calcium carbonate therapy)
- Rhabdomyolysis (later stages after initial hypocalcemia)
- Familial hypercalcemic hypocalciuria.

Investigations

- BUN, Cr, electrolytes, Ca^{2+}, phosphate, alkaline phosphatase, albumin
- PTH ± PTHrP, 25 (OH)- and 1, 25 $(OH)_2$ vitamin D_3. If indicated, serum ACE level, SPEP, PSA. Chest X-ray. Plain KUB
- ▶ ECG shows short QT interval.

Treatment

- Treat the underlying cause.
- Stop thiazide diuretics.
- Primary hyperparathyroidism: Previously, surgery was performed if Ca^{2+} >11 or if there is end-organ damage. Cinacalcet (a calcimimetic activating the calcium-sensing receptor, providing negative feedback on PTH synthesis) may become an alternative.

- Patients with secondary hyperparathyroidism treated with calcium-containing phosphate binders or active vitamin D who become relatively hypercalcemic can be treated with cinacalcet.
- Malignancy: surgical resection, radiotherapy, bisphosphonates
- Corticosteroids (prednisone 30 mg qd) are effective when $\uparrow Ca^{2+}$ is driven by increased extrarenal 1,25-$(OH)_2$ vitamin D_3 synthesis (granulomatous diseases, myeloma, or lymphoma).

Mild hypercalcemia (<12): increase salt intake (promotes urine Ca^{2+} loss). Aim to maintain volume repletion, and treat underlying cause.

⚠ Severe $\uparrow Ca^{2+}$ (>12):
- Vigorous volume replacement with NS, initially at 200–300 mL/h, aiming for + 1–2 L positive balance.
  ▶ Assess fluid balance regularly.
- Furosemide (increases renal $\uparrow Ca^{2+}$ wasting) 10–20 mg 4 hourly, or as IV infusion (5 mg hourly). *Do not cause volume depletion.* Some now skip using this and go right to measures below.
- If urgent control is required (and volume resuscitated), give calcitonin 4 IU/kg SC/IM (inhibits osteoclast activity). Repeat 6–12 hours at 4–8 IU/kg SC. You must add on bisphosphonate therapy, as tachyphylaxis develops with calcitonin.
- Bisphosphonates are powerful and prolonged inhibitors of osteoclasts. Options include zoledronic acid (4–8 mg over 30 min, duration of effect 30 days) or pamidronate (60–90 mg over 4 hours; effect lasts ~7 days). Monitor Cr.
- Treat $\downarrow K^+$ or $\downarrow Mg^{2+}$ with IV supplements.

▶ Hypercalcemia in ESRD may need treatment with hemodialysis on 0 or low Ca^{2+} dialysate. If 0 Ca^{2+} dialysate is used, the patient needs a cardiac monitor during dialysis. This will rapidly lower Ca^{2+} and should be considered if ionized Ca^{2+} >3.5 or there is a depressed level of consciousness.

	Primary HPT	Humoral $\uparrow Ca^{2+}$ of malignancy	Metastases to bone
Phosphate	↓	↔ or ↑	↔ or ↑
PTH	↑	↓	↓
PTH-rP	↓	↑	↓

Hypomagnesemia

This occurs in up to 12% of hospitalized patients. It is often exacerbated by malnutrition, chronic diarrhea, diuretics, and nephrotoxins. Causes include the following.

Renal causes
- Diuretic use (loop or thiazide) or prolonged natriuresis
- Nephrotoxins (aminoglycosides, cisplatin, cyclosporin, amphotericin, foscarnet, pentamidine)
- Hypercalcemia or phosphate depletion
- Gitelman's syndrome (📖 p. 538) or familial hypomagnesemia-hypercalciuria
- Alcohol.

GI causes
- GI losses due to diarrhea, prolonged NG suction, or malabsorptive states
- Pancreatitis (saponification in necrotic fat)
- Alcohol (both GI with diarrhea, pancreatitis, poor intake, and renal loss).

Symptoms and signs

$\downarrow Mg^{2+}$ occurs in conjunction with $\downarrow K^+$ (50% of cases), $\downarrow Ca^{2+}$, and a metabolic alkalosis. Weakness, cramps, carpopedal spasm, positive Chvostek's and Trousseau's signs (📖 p. 542), tetany, and convulsions may occur.

Investigations

Check $\downarrow Mg^{2+}$, $\downarrow K^+$ (<3.0 mEq/L). Hypokalemia is often resistant to K^+ supplementation until Mg^{2+} is normalized. Look for $\downarrow Ca^{2+}$ (if Mg^{2+} <1.2 mg/dL), with inappropriately low/normal PTH.

⚠ ECG changes include ↑QRS width, ↑PR interval, and flattened T waves. Fatal ventricular arrhythmias can occur in the context of underlying heart disease (especially acute coronary syndromes and CHF).

A 24-hour urinary Mg^{2+} (NR <10–30 mg/day) or fractional excretion of Mg^{2+} (renal response should be <2% with hypomagnesemia) will distinguish renal losses from other causes of $\downarrow Mg^{2+}$, but is not usually required for diagnosis.

Treatment

Asymptomatic with modest ↓ Mg^{2+} (>1 mg/dL): oral slow-release Mg^{2+} (slow Mag or Mag-Tab SR have 5–7 mEq; 2.5–3.5 mmol, 60–84 mg per tablet) 5–21 mmol/day in divided doses. Take 2–4 tablets a day if mild.

Symptomatic with hypocalcemia (tetany) or hypokalemia (arrhthymia): 50 mEq or 25 mmol $MgSO_4$ IV in 100 mL 0.9% saline IV over 8–24 hours. Repeat as required.

▶Give oral supplementation once Mg^{2+} >1 mg/dL with 15–21 mmol Mg^{2+}/day in divided doses. Diarrhea may limit use of oral Mg^{2+}. Take 6–8 tablets a day if severe deficienct.

▶▶*With arrhythmias* (e.g., Torsade de pointes): IV $MgSO_4$ 4–8 mmol stat, then 20 mmol/12 hourly against plasma Mg^{2+}. Aim for >1 mg/dL.

Half of administered Mg^{2+} will be lost in the urine, so prolonged therapy may be needed. The total body deficit in symptomatic ↓Mg^{2+} may be 0.5–1 mmol/kg body weight, so up to 300 mEq or 150 mmol may be required over 5 days (with urine losses). In diuretic-induced chronic Mg^{2+} wasting states, adding amiloride 5 mg qd may limit Mg^{2+} losses.

Hypermagnesemia

Urine losses of Mg^{2+} can compensate for rising plasma Mg^{2+}, so ↑Mg^{2+} is unusual. This occurs usually if excess Mg^{2+} is administered IV (as in treating preeclampsia), or in patients with impaired renal function given exogenous Mg^{2+}. Mg^{2+}-containing preparations include antacids (Mg^{2+} hydroxide or carbonate) and $MgSO_4$ enemas.

Clinically

Paraesthesias, hyporeflexia, weakness, and respiratory depression (Mg^{2+} >4.8 mg/dL) occur. Bradycardia and ↓BP with severe toxicity (>8.5 mg/dL) are also seen. ECG shows ↑PR and QT interval.

Treatment

If there is good UO and normal renal function, stop Mg^{2+}-containing preparation and monitor. Excess Mg^{2+} will be rapidly excreted.

▶ If Mg^{2+} >12 mg/dL with bradycardia, consider IV calcium gluconate 10% 10 mL as slow IV bolus. Patient may require repeated doses.

In patients with impaired renal function, hemodialysis provides rapid and effective normalization of Mg^{2+}.

Hypophosphatemia

Important hypophosphatemia occurs in ±1% of hospitalized patients, particularly chronic abusers of *alcohol* and in *diabetics* and those on *TPN*.

▶ It becomes clinically meaningful at <1.2 mg/dL.
Causes include the following:
- Redistribution
  - Refeeding in malnourished (alcoholic) patients[1]
  - Respiratory alkalosis (↑ pH intracellularly stimulates glycolysis)[1]
  - Exogenous insulin administration (DKA, critical care)[1]
  - Hungry bone syndrome (massive Ca^{2+} and PO_4^- deposition)
- ↑Renal losses
  - Primary hyperparathyroidism
  - Impaired vitamin D metabolism
  - Renal tubular disorders (Fanconi's), ATN, or resolving obstructive uropathy
- GI uptake
  - Malnutrition or vitamin D deficiency
  - Chronic diarrhea or malabsorption
  - Antacid (calcium, aluminum, magnesium) abuse.

Symptoms and signs

Proximal muscle weakness → spontaneous rhabdomyolysis, ± diaphragmatic weakness and hypoventilation), ileus, myocardial depression (even heart failure), hemolysis, altered mental state, and seizures. If prolonged, osteomalacia can occur.

Investigations

These include UpH, electrolytes, bicarbonate, Ca^{2+}, phosphate, BUN, and Cr. If indicated, check PTH, FE-phosphate (<5% = nonrenal cause), and calcitriol.

Treatment

If phosphate >1.2 mg/dL, ↑ dietary phosphate (milk and dairy products). Oral phosphate (e.g., K Phos Neutral® or Neutra-Phos® 1 g tid (3 g = ~100 mmol) can be used. Treat vitamin D deficiency if present.

▶ If patient has levels <1 mg/dL or is critically ill, give IV phosphate 2.5 (0.08 mmol)/kg body weight over 6–12 hours in 500 mL 5% dextrose.

---

[1] Glycolysis = intracellular shift of phosphorylated glucose metabolites.

Hyperphosphatemia

This almost always occurs in patients with renal impairment. Calcium and phosphate are at the limits of solubility in plasma, so ↑ calcium:phosphate product leads to precipitation and ectopic calcification. Over time, this leads to vascular calcification (and ↑ mortality in CKD?). Secondary hyperparathyroidism will attempt to ↑ renal losses as compensation.

Usually asymptomatic, causes include:
- CKD
- Tumor lysis (📖 p. 144) and rhabdomyolysis (📖 p. 138)
- Hypoparathyroidism
- Vitamin D toxicity
- Phosphate-containing enemas (usually with renal impairment)
- Lactic and ketoacidosis

No treatment is usually required in the acute setting, though if with ↓Ca^{2+} (tumor lysis, rhabdomyolysis), can be life threatening.

▶ If so, give insulin to redistribute PO_4^- into cells. Promote diuresis through volume resuscitation (NS).

If chronic, aim to restrict dietary phosphate, use oral phosphate binders to limit uptake, and, in those with ESRD or acute renal failure, use hemodialysis or continuous renal replacement therapy if warranted.

Acid–base

Understanding normal physiology

pH is tightly controlled within and without cells, in various tissues, and in fluid compartments of the body. pH is simply the negative log of the concentration of hydrogen ions, or [H^+], in any fluid. In the ECF, pH is maintained at a normal range of 7.38–7.42, where [H^+] at pH 7.40 is 40 nmol/L; at pH 7.0 (the intracellular pH), [H^+] = 100 nmol/L. Remember the pH of water is 6.8—this emphasizes the role of buffers in biological fluids.

Intake and generation

This amounts to 1 mEq/kg acid/day in adults, largely derived from ingested protein breakdown (sulfur-containing amino acids → H_2SO_4) and a byproduct of cellular metabolism.

Buffering

To prevent rapid changes in pH with ↑ dietary intake or excess production of [H^+], a system of local (tissue) and systemic buffers has evolved. These buffers include:
- Bicarbonate (HCO_3^-)
- Bone salts (calcium carbonate and calcium phosphate)
- Blood proteins (hemoglobin).

In the short term, bicarbonate is by far the most important, though bone buffers play a more significant role in chronic acidosis.

Acid math

$$H^+ + HCO_3^- \rightarrow H_2CO_3 \rightarrow CO_2 + H_2O$$

Adding H^+ (acidosis) consumes bicarbonate and generates CO_2 as the reaction is driven rightward. Removing CO_2 (hyperventilation) returns the pH toward normal according to the Henderson–Hasselbach equation:

$$pH = pK \frac{\log [HCO_3^-]}{[H_2CO_3]0.03}$$ where pK = 6.1, the dissociation co-efficient of carbonic acid

This does *not* generate more bicarbonate, so the kidney has to ↑H^+ excretion to balance the system.

Excretion: the kidney in acid–base

Preventing bicarbonate loss

Some 80%–90% of filtered HCO_3^- is actively reclaimed (reabsorbed) in the proximal tubule:
- Proximal tubular cell Na^+ is pumped at the basolateral membrane by the Na^+/K^+-ATPase into the interstitium, creating an inward gradient → Na^+ movement from the lumen.
- Na^+/H^+ antiporter allows Na^+ entry from the lumen, exchanged for H^+.
- In the lumen, $H^+ + HCO_3^- = H_2CO_3$ (carbonic acid).

- Luminal carbonic anhydrase then converts $H_2CO_3 \rightarrow CO_2$ and H_2O, which is taken up into cells.
- Intracellular carbonic anhydrase then $\rightarrow H^+ + HCO_3^-$.
- Intracellular HCO_3^- then passes into the peritubular capillaries.
- The remaining H^+ is available for recycling.

Excreting protons
- Almost all H^+ in the proximal tubule is reabsorbed with HCO_3^-.
- Acid excretion occurs in the collecting duct.
- Na^+ absorbed under the influence of aldosterone (in the principal cells, 📖 p. 626) causes the urinary tubular lumen to become increasingly electronegative.
- K^+ is secreted from principal cells, *and* H^+ is pumped from α-intercalated cells into the lumen to maintain electriconeutrality.
- Aldosterone acts directly to stimulate the H^+-ATPase.

Buffering urinary protons
The luminal pH falls to ~4.0–4.5, which limits the gradient for α-intercalated cell H^+-ATPase. To continue net acid excretion, urinary H^+ is buffered by
- Titratable acids (H^+ incorporated into phosphoric acid, H_3PO_4 or sulfuric acid H_2SO_4)
- Ammonium (NH_4^+).

In normal conditions, titratable acids and ammonium carry ±50% of the dietary H^+ load, but with metabolic acidosis more ammonium is utilized for acid excretion.

Ammonium

Proximal tubular cells deaminate glutamine to form ammonium (NH_4^+) and NH_4^+ may be excreted in the urinary lumen of the proximal tubule.
- NH_4^+ is absorbed into the medullary interstitium from the ascending limb of the loop of Henle into the interstitium, where it dissociates to form NH_3 and H^+.
- NH_3 can now move down a concentration gradient into the lumen of the collecting duct, available to buffer H^+, and is then excreted as NH_4Cl in the urine.
- Ammonia synthesis is enhanced by acidosis, and $\downarrow K^+$.

The urine anion gap = urine $[Na^+ + K^+]$ − urine $[Cl^-]$ is used to determine whether the etiology of a normal anion gap metabolic acidosis is diarrhea or type 1 or 4 RTA. The urine anion gap indirectly measures urinary NH_4^+. If the kidney can respond normally to acidosis (diarrhea), it will $\uparrow NH_4^+$ excretion for H^+ removal. The UAG will then be *negative* (as $\uparrow Cl^-$ will accompany the $Na^+ + K^+$ and $\uparrow NH_4^+$). If the renal response is inappropriate (e.g., distal RTA, 📖 p. 556), the UAG will be 0 or *positive*.

Metabolic acidosis

Acidosis occurs if the systemic pH falls <7.35, and is considered metabolic in origin if ↓[HCO_3^-]. Acidosis is due to excessive acid production, retention, or by ↑ bicarbonate losses. With pure metabolic acidosis, compensation occurs through increasing ventilation and blowing off CO_2 (∴↓pCO_2). For each 1 mEq/L decrease in serum HCO_3^- below normal, the pCO_2 will decrease by 1.2 mmHg to buffer the acidosis.

In assessing metabolic acidosis, it is useful to estimate the anion gap (AG). In health, the difference between cations and anions is made up of organic (negatively charged) acids. An ↑AG occurs if acids other than carbonic acid (→ phosphate, lactate, or sulfate) or ↑ exogenous acids are in plasma.

Calculating the serum anion gap
- AG = [Na^+ + K^+] − [Cl^- + HCO_3^-] = 8–16 in health.
- Albumin is negatively charged: ↓ albumin → *underestimate of* AG.
- To correct for hypoalbuminemia, add 2.5 mEq/L to the AG for every decrease 1 g/dL in albumin from normal.

Normal-AG acidosis
This is due to retained H^+ or HCO_3^- losses—as Cl^- is increased with H^+, such acidoses are also called "hyperchloremic":
- Nonrenal losses of bicarbonate (▶ *negative UAG*)
  - Diarrhea, ileostomy, or ureterosigmoidostomy
- Renal bicarbonate losses
  - Proximal RTA (📖 p. 556) or Fanconi-like syndromes (📖 p. 557)
- Failure of renal acid excretion (UAG > 0)
  - RTA (distal type 1).
  - Type 4: hypoaldosteronism or mineralocorticoid receptor blockers
- Increased acid production or load
  - Toluene poisoning, lysine-HCl or NH_4Cl administration.

Increased AG acidosis ("hypo-" or "normochloremic" acidosis)
This is due to ↑ organic acids in plasma.
- Renal failure
- Lactic acidosis
- Ketoacidosis (acetoacetate or β-hydroxybutyrate)
  - Diabetic, alcoholic or starvation
- Rhabdomyolysis
- Toxins
  - Salicylate, ethylene glycol or methanol poisoning.

Clinically
Systemic effects of severe metabolic acidosis (pH <7.1) are listed below.
- Air hunger (Kussmaul's breathing) and hyperventilation
- ↓ myocardial contractility (↓Ca^{2+} release from sarcoplasmic reticulum), arteriodilatation, and venoconstriction (central blood pooling)
- Resistant arrhythmias (especially VF).

The diagnosis is usually apparent. Investigations might include BUN, Cr, electrolytes, venous pH (in a blood gas syringe) or ABG, and glucose. Check urinalysis (microscopy for crystals), urine electrolytes, and ketones. A toxicology screen is useful.

Treatment
▶ *This involves treating the underlying cause.*
Refer to "Renal tubular acidosis" (next section) for specific conditions—in cases of renal failure, treating acidosis has important benefits, including preventing the following:
- Bone demineralization (bone buffers any chronic acidosis)
- Muscle wasting
- Anorexia and malnutrition
- Progression of renal failure (♦).

Using bicarbonate
If symptoms are mild and prolonged, consider oral $NaHCO_3$ 1.5–4.5 g/day in three divided doses if there is normal AG acidosis.

Treating with IV $NaHCO_3$ is rarely indicated
- It corrects the intravascular pH, not the "treatable body water" (∴ treats the numbers, not patient).
- It generates CO_2 that must be blown off (⚠ fixed or ↓ respiratory rate).
- It *may* worsen intracellular pH, as CO_2 rapidly enters cells → acidosis.
- Na^+ load is substantial (150 mmol in 500 mL 1.26% $NaHCO_3$, and 1 mmol Na^+/mL of 8.4% $NaHCO_3$) and poorly tolerated in volume-overloaded patients.

Managing severe and life-threatening acidosis
Consider $NaHCO_3$ if pH <7.0 in patients with impaired cardiac performance. If correcting this, aim for pH >7.1–7.2 or $[HCO_3^-]$ >10–12, at which pH life-threatening complications of acidosis would be unusual.

$$HCO_3^- \text{ deficit} = (\text{target} - \text{measured } [HCO_3^-]) \times \text{bicarbonate space}^1$$
$$\text{Bicarbonate space} = (0.4 + 2.6/[HCO_3^-]) \times \text{weight (kg)}$$

For example, in a 70 kg ♂ with pH 6.9 and $[HCO_3^-]$ = 4 mEq/L and cardiac instability: deficit = $(10 - 4) \times ([0.4 + 2.6/4] \times 70)$ = 420 mEq HCO_3^-. The target bicarbonate is 10–12 mEq/L, NOT normal (24 mEq/L). Can be given as 150 mEq/L $NaHCO_3$ or D5% water with 3 Amps of $NaHCO_3$.

Respiratory acidosis
This occurs if pH <7.35 and ↑pCO_2; there may be metabolic compensation if chronic (↑$[HCO_3^-]$). Causes include advanced pulmonary disease, respiratory muscle fatigue, or impaired central ventilatory control (drugs or stroke) or it may be a result of mechanical ventilation. Treatment (if warranted) usually involves mechanical ventilation.

---

[1] The intra- and extracellular volume contributing to buffering.

Renal tubular acidosis (RTA)

This refers to a group of disorders characterized by impaired renal handling of acid, usually with normal renal function. The basis for the often confusing terminology used for RTA revolves around physiology: almost all filtered bicarbonate (HCO_3^-) is reclaimed or reabsorbed in the proximal tubule, with little net acid excretion (see Table 9.2). The majority of net acid excretion occurs in the distal nephron (📖 p. 624).

Distal RTA (type 1)

Disordered excretion of acid (H^+) from the α-intercalated cell in the collecting duct leads to acidosis. This presents as a hyperchloremic, hypokalemic metabolic acidosis with renal stones, or diffuse nephrocalcinosis. It is (rarely) inherited, or more commonly acquired secondary to the following:
- Sjogren's syndrome, RA, SLE, and other autoimmune diseases
- Nephrocalcinosis (dRTA is confusingly *both* a cause and result of nephrocalcinosis of any cause)
- Drugs (ifosfamide, amphotericin B, lithium, topiramate)
- Chronic tubulointerstitial disease (of any cause, 📖 p. 408)
- Dysproteinemias (hypergammaglobulinemia, amyloidosis)
- Amiloride, triamterene, trimethoprim, pentamadine, obstructive uropathy block ENaC, causing ↑K^+.

Investigations

↑ urine pH (>5.3 in the face of acidosis), increased, normal, or decreased serum K^+, ↓HCO_3^- <12 mEq/L, normal AG (↑Cl^-), positive urinary AG (📖 p. 553), ↑UCa (chronic acidosis ↑ bone turnover), ↓ urine citrate (absorbed to buffer acidosis). Plain KUB or US. ANA, anti-Ro/La, rheumatoid factor. (If partial distal RTA is suspected where there is decreased acid secretion but normal serum HCO_3^-, you *may do acid loading test*. Give 0.1 g/kg NH_4Cl po and check UpH hourly, HCO_3^- at + 3 hours. If HCO_3^- <21, and UpH >5.3, diagnose distal RTA.)

Treatment

Give potassium citrate 30–90 mEq/day in three divided doses (citrate generates two bicarbonate molecules) or sodium bicarbonate 4–12 g/day or bicitra in four divided doses, aiming for HCO_3^- >20 mEq/L. If treating nephrolithiasis, potassium citrate is better to increase urine citrate because Na^+ load may increase UCa^{2+}. Obviously you will use sodium bicarbonate with hyperkalemic type 1.

Proximal RTA (type 2)

Impaired reabsorption of HCO_3^- in the proximal tubule leads to bicarbonate wasting and a systemic acidosis. This presents as a hyperchloremic metabolic acidosis, usually with other features of proximal tubular dysfunction (so-called Fanconi syndrome, see Box 9.3). Common causes include the following:
- Myeloma and amyloidosis
- Cystinosis, Wilson's disease, or heavy-metal toxicity
- Drugs (acetazolamide, antiretroviral drugs, aminoglycosides).

Investigations

↓ urine pH <5.3 (▶ if IV NaHCO$_3$ 1 mEq/kg/h is given, distal reabsorption is overwhelmed and urine pH ↑ >7), ↓K$^+$, ↓ HCO$_3^-$ (12–20 mEq/L), normal AG (↑Cl$^-$), negative urine AG at steady state as distal acidification is intact (📖 p. 553). Look for findings of Fanconi syndrome (Box 9.3).

Treatment

⚠ High-dose bicarbonate merely ↑ HCO$_3^-$ wasting and increases Na$^+$ delivery to the distal nephron (and so worsens ↓K$^+$). Aim to allow mild acidosis: potassium bicarbonate 1.5–3 g/day in three divided doses (K HCO$_3^-$ is less calciuric and replenishes K$^+$ and Na$^+$ load).

Distal RTA (type 4)

This type is much more common than pRTA or dRTA and is due to hypoaldosteronism or aldosterone resistance, usually hyporeninemic hypoaldosteronism. Aldosterone promotes urinary K$^+$ loss, so its absence → hyperkalemia. ↑K$^+$ impairs NH$_4^+$ secretion, limiting net acid excretion → acidosis. Causes include the following:
- Diabetes mellitus (often with mild renal impairment)
- Drugs (NSAIDs, cyclosporin, tacrolimus, ACEI, ARB, heparin)
- Chronic tubulointerstitial disease of any cause (📖 p. 406) ± CKD
- Addison's or selective aldosterone deficiency.

Investigations

↑K$^+$, ↓ HCO$_3^-$ (rarely <16 mEq/L), normal AG (↑Cl$^-$), positive urine AG (📖 p. 553), (see above). Urine pH is usually <5.3.

Treatment

If RTA is due to hypoaldosteronsim; mineralocorticoid replacement (fludrocortisone 100–300 µg/day) will rapidly reverse the problem.

⚠ Type 4 is often revealed in patients taking ACEI and spironolactone for treatment of heart failure. Advise low-K$^+$ diet (📖 p. 199). Mineralocorticoids are rarely useful because of significant Na$^+$ retention in at-risk patients (CKD, CHF). Give trial of furosemide 40–120 mg qd. Review drugs.

Box 9.3 Fanconi syndrome

A descriptive term for generalized proximal tubular dysfunction, this syndrome is marked by failure of proximal reabsorption of many filtered substances, and classically by phosphate wasting.
- It may present with bone pain ± osteomalacia. Causes are as for proximal RTA.
- Investigations include metabolic acidosis, ↓ s-phosphate, ↓ s-uric acid. Check for glycosuria and proteinuria (amino acids), ↑ urine phosphate, and ↑ urine citrate.

Table 9.2 RTA by numbers

	Distal RTA	Proximal RTA	Hyperkalemic distal RTA
Defect	Impaired net acid excretion	Impaired HCO_3 uptake	↓ aldosterone
Serum K^+	↓ or ↑	↓	↑
Serum HCO_3^-	<10	12–20	>16
UpH	>5.3	<5.3, ↑ with bicarbonate	Variable (<5.3)
Urine AG	Positive	Negative	Positive
Nephrocalcinosis	Yes	No	No

Lactic acidosis

L-lactate is an end-product of anaerobic glucose metabolism: glucose is metabolized to pyruvate. In hypoxic tissue, oxidative regeneration of NAD^+ cannot occur, so pyruvate is used with NADH and H^+ by lactate dehydrogenase to produce NAD^+ (crucial earlier for glycolysis) and lactate. In health, lactate is usually rapidly oxidized by the liver for a plasma concentration of 0.5–1.5 mEq/L. Causes include the following:

- Shock and impaired oxygen delivery
  - Cardiogenic
  - Septic
  - Hypovolemic
- Localized tissue or organ ischemia (infarcted gut, muscle)
- ↑energy-dependent work (usually in skeletal muscle)
  - Seizures
  - Extreme exercise
  - Malignant hyperthermia
- Respiratory failure and hypoxemia
- Metabolic derangements involving oxidation
  - DKA
  - Carbon monoxide poisoning
  - Ethanol poisoning
- Liver impairment
- Drugs (see Box 9.4).

Significant lactic acidosis is present if lactate >4 mEq/L, with an increased anion gap metabolic acidosis. Conventionally, lactic acidosis due to tissue hypoxia is called type A lactic acidosis, and abnormal lactate metabolism, the underproduction or overutilization of ATP or other causes of defective gluconeogenesis (drugs!) cause type B lactic acidosis.

D-lactic acidosis is a rare cause of an increased anion gap metabolic acidosis in which bacterial overgrowth in intestinal blind loops leads to increased lactate absorption—the proliferating organisms (and not humans) are capable of producing the D-isomer.

There is little role for systemic $NaHCO_3$ without fixing the cause. Treatment of type A lactic acidosis involves improving oxygenation: resuscitate shock, restore blood flow, and/or improve gas exchange.

Box 9.4 Drugs and lactic acidosis

Metformin has long been thought to cause a type-B lactic acidosis, particularly in diabetics with renal impairment. There is some doubt about this association, but it is prudent to stop metformin if Cr >1.5 mg/dL.

Recently, reverse transcriptase inhibitors have also been found to cause an often severe lactic acidosis as a result of mitochondrial injury.

Metabolic alkalosis

Metabolic alkalosis is common (as might be expected from its causes), and if severe (pH >7.55), carries a mortality as high as 45%. Either retention of base or loss of acid in the ECF leads to generation of an increasing serum bicarbonate and pH. To buffer such changes, patients can hypoventilate to ↑pCO_2 to as much as 50–55 mmHg). For each 1 mEq/L rise in serum HCO_3^- above normal, the pCO_2 will rise by 0.75 mmHg to buffer the alkalosis (e.g., to buffer a serum HCO_3^- of 34 mEq/L, the pCO_2 will need to rise by 7.5 mmHg). Maintenance of metabolic alkalosis is due to either volume depletion, ↓K^+, chloride depletion, or elevated aldosterone levels. Causes of a metabolic alkalosis include the following:

- Contraction alkalosis
- GI H^+ loss
  - Vomiting, NG suction, self-induced vomiting
  - Chloride-secreting villous adenoma (rare)
- Renal H^+ loss
  - Primary hyperaldosteronism (and less commonly, secondary)
  - Drugs (carbenoloxone, licorice, laxative *abuse*)
  - Diuretics (thiazide, loop diuretics)
  - Bartter's, Liddle's and Gitelman's syndromes (📖 p. 538)
  - Post-hypercapnic
- Alkali load
  - Milk-alkali syndrome (or hypercalcemia of other causes)
  - Overzealous bicarbonate therapy.

Mechanisms for common causes

- Chloride depletion and alkalosis
  - With vomiting of NG losses, the stomach loses gastric HCl. The initial secretion of HCl returns HCO_3^- to the ECF.
  - Diuretics block NaCl uptake, with ECF depletion (secondary hyperaldosteronism), and ↑ salt delivery to the DCT (∴ ↓ exchange of Na^+ for K^+ and H^+). Diuretic-induced ↓K^+ exacerbates alkalosis further.
  - Urinary chloride is exchanged for cell HCO_3^- in intercalated type B cells. If tubular chloride is low as in chloride depletion, normal HCO_3^- excretion is impaired.
- Hypokalemia and alkalosis
  - Hyperaldosteronism leads to ↑Na^+ retention at the expense of K^+ and H^+. Aldosterone also directly increases net acid excretion by stimulating the H^+ ATPase in apical membrane of intercalated A cells.
  - ↓K^+ may increase net acid excretion by the H^+/K^+ ATPase (excretes H^+ in lumen for K^+ reabsorption), which is also on the apical membrane of intercalated A cells and is activated by hypokalemia.

Symptoms and signs
Metabolic alkalosis is often due to associated hypovolemia or hypokalemia. With severe alkalosis there is ↓ cerebral and myocardial blood flow: headaches, confusion, seizures, angina, and arrhythmias may result. Compensatory hypoventilation and hypercapnea may be important in critically ill patients (failure to wean off ventilator).

Investigations
Consider ABG if evaluating respiratory contribution to a mixed acid–base disorder. Check BUN, Cr, electrolytes (↓ K^+, ↓ Cl^-). ? ↑ Ca^{2+}.
- Urine K^+, Na^+, Cl^-
- Urine Cl^- <20 mEq/L if gastric losses (▶ surreptitious vomiting), remote diuretic use, post-hypercapneic
- Urine Cl^- >20 mEq/L if there is current diuretic therapy (abuse), Bartter's, Gitelman's, or hyperaldosteronism.

Diagnosis is usually obvious: get urinary diuretic/laxative screen, and check renin and aldosterone if indicated.

Treatment
This depends on the cause:
- Treat ↓Cl^- alkalosis with *chloride*.
  - If volume depleted: NS IV until volume is repleted
- Treat ↓K^+ alkalosis with KCl (📖 p. 534).
- Reverse the underlying cause:
  - Stop alkali therapy.
  - Stop diuretics if possible, or add K^+-sparing agent, especially if hyperaldosteronism is present (spironolactone).
  - Antiemetics (e.g., metaclopramide 10 mg IMI/IVI) for vomiting
  - If NG drainage is needed, give H_2 receptor antagonist or proton-pump inhibitor.
  - If patient is volume overloaded, acetazolamide 250–500 mg daily will cause Na HCO_3^- wasting.

⚠ Urgent reversal of severe metabolic alkalosis (in ICU)

Indications
- Bicarbonate >45 mmol/L (or pH >7.55) *and*
- Hepatic encephalopathy *or*
- Arrhythmias (including digoxin toxicity) *or*
- Confusion, seizures

Correct K+
Give IV hydrochloric acid (HCl) via *central line*: body weight (in kg) × 0.5 (bicarbonate space = 50% body weight) × required ↓HCO_3^- (mEq/L) = mEq HCl infused at 0.2 mEq/kg/h.

Example: In a 70 kg male, to ↓HCO_3^- by 10 mEq/L, 0.1 M HCl solution (10 × 70 × 0.5 = 350 mEq) at 35 mEq/h for 10 hours to reduce plasma bicarbonate by 10 mEq/L. Alternatives include NH_4Cl or arginine HCl. HD or CVVHD also provide rapid correction of severe alkalosis.

Respiratory alkalosis

This is always a result of overventilation, due to mechanical ventilation, increased central respiratory drive (anxiety, pregnancy, stroke or CNS infection), or hypoxemia (mild asthma, pulmonary edema, or emboli). Treatment can be difficult if alkalosis is severe.

Mixed acidosis and alkalosis

As a rule of thumb, pH will rise or fall by 0.1 if
- [HCO_3^-] changes by 6 mEq/L. For example, a fall in [HCO_3^-] from 24 to 12 = pH from 7.4 to 7.2.

Normal ranges
- pH   7.38–7.42
- pO_2 80–100 mmHg
- pCO_2 36–44 mmHg (mixed venous pCO_2 usually 7.6 mmHg higher)
- HCO_3^- 22–26 mEq/L.

Mixed acid–base disturbances are not uncommon in hospitalized patients: the key to diagnosis is recognizing when compensation is inappropriate. Using Table 9.3, the following should be expected:
- Metabolic acidosis: pCO_2 falls by 1.2 mmHg for every 1 mEq decrease in HCO_3^-.
- Metabolic alkalosis: pCO_2 rises by 0.75 mmHg for every 1 mEq increase in HCO_3^-.
- Acute respiratory alkalosis: [HCO_3^-] falls by 2 mEq/L for every 10 mmHg decrease in pCO_2.
- Chronic respiratory alkalosis: [HCO_3^-] falls by 4 mEq/L for every 10 mmHg decrease in pCO_2.
- Acute respiratory acidosis: [HCO_3^-] rises by 1 mEq/L for every 10 mmHg increase in pCO_2.
- Chronic respiratory acidosis: [HCO_3^-] rises by 3.5 mEq/L for every 10 mmHg increase in pCO_2.

If compensation does not fall roughly within these limits, there is likely to be a mixed component to the disturbance:
1. What is the pH (acidotic or alkalotic)?
2. Is the predominant cause—metabolic or respiratory?
3. Is compensation appropriate?
4. If not, a mixed acid–base disturbance is present.

Table 9.3 Characteristics of pure acid–base disturbances

	pH	pCO_2	[HCO_3^-]
Metabolic acidosis	↓	Ⓓ	↓↓
Metabolic alkalosis	↑	Ⓤ	↑↑
Respiratory acidosis	↓	↑↑	Ⓤ
Respiratory alkalosis	↑	↓↓	Ⓓ

The circled arrows = compensatory mechanism.

5. The correlation between the change in the serum anion gap (ΔAG) from the normal anion gap and the change in the serum bicarbonate concentration (ΔHCO_3^-) from normal value of 24 mEq/L in patients with high anion gap acidosis ($\Delta AG:\Delta HCO_3^-$) has been used to help detect mixed metabolic acid–base disorders. If the $\Delta AG:\Delta HCO_3^-$ <1 a normal anion gap metabolic acidosis and high anion gap acidosis may both be present. If the $\Delta AG:\Delta HCO_3^-$ >1–1.6, a metabolic alkalosis and high anion gap acidosis may both be present. (There is variability in the $\Delta AG:\Delta HCO_3^-$ value.)

Tubular rarities

Cystinuria
Defective uptake of filtered cystine and other dibasic amino acids from the urine leads to cystine stone formation. Autosomal recessive inheritance of genes encoding tubular amino acid transporter proteins presents in childhood or adolescence with flank pain ± haematuria (calculi).

Urine microscopy shows characteristic hexagonal crystals, and there is ↑24-hour urinary cystine excretion (>400 mg/day, NR <40). Radio-opaque calculi appear on plain KUB or US. Aim to increase oral fluids for UO of >3–4 L/day. If urine cystine remains >250–300 mg/L (cystine is insoluble much above this), add in D-penicillamine 1–2 g/day in four divided doses. Alternatives include tiopronin up to 400 mg daily or captopril. All work by increasing cystine solubility. For managing stones 📖 p. 430.

Cystinosis
⚠ *This is not the same disease as cystinuria.*
Cystinosis presents in childhood with growth failure, Fanconi's syndrome, and progressive renal impairment. Eye involvement, hepatomegaly, hypothyroidism, and diabetes develop as cystine deposits impair organ function. An adolescent variant with normal stature and tubular function but renal impairment offers a better renal prognosis. An autosomal recessively inherited defect in cystine export from intracellular lysosomes leads to accumulation and local injury. Oral cysteamine forms a complex with cystine that can leave lysosomes, ameliorating disease.

Primary hyperoxaluria
There are two types, autosomal recessive conditions, presenting in childhood marked by ↑ urine oxalate excretion, calcium oxalate calculi, and nephrocalcinosis. Defective synthesis or targeting of the enzyme AGT, which converts glyoxalate to glycine, leads to compensatory shuttling of glyoxalate to oxalate. Heavy systemic oxalate deposition after onset of moderate CKD results in oxalate deposits in the heart, blood vessels, and joints, causing significant morbidity. The treatment of choice is combined liver–kidney transplantation, although high-dose pyridoxine may offer interim benefit.

Dent's disease
This disease is the result of an X-linked inherited defect in the gene encoding CLC-5, a chloride channel responsible for endosomal acidification in the proximal tubule and elsewhere. This leads to impaired endocytosis and uptake of urinary proteins. It presents predominantly in ♂ (♀ may have urinary abnormalities) as Fanconi's syndrome (📖 p. 557), hypercalciuria, nephrocalcinosis, and CKD. Rickets and osteomalacia are common. Renal transplantation is the treatment of choice for ESRD, and patients generally do well.

Chapter 10

Pregnancy and the kidney

Renal physiology in pregnancy 568
UTI in pregnancy 570
Acute renal failure in pregnancy 572
Hypertension in pregnancy 574
Gestational hypertension 575
Preeclampsia and eclampsia 576
Managing preeclampsia and eclampsia 578
Chronic hypertension in pregnancy 580
Preexisting renal disease 582
Disorders of the renal tract in pregnancy 585
Pregnancy while on dialysis 586
Renal transplantation and pregnancy 588

Renal physiology in pregnancy

Systemic hemodynamics change early in pregnancy, with changes in renal hemodynamics, tubular function, and salt and water homeostasis:
- ↓ systemic vascular resistance and ↑ peripheral vasodilatation
- ↑ cardiac output (by up to 30%–40%)
- ↑ plasma volume (by up to 30%–40%)
- ↓BP and widened pulse pressure (due to vasodilatation).

As early as the sixth week renal plasma flow and GFR increase, under the influence of nitric oxide, vasodilatory prostaglandins, and relaxin. Transglomerular capillary pressure remains the same, with matching dilatation of both afferent and efferent arterioles.

Tubular function

- ↑ fractional reabsorption to compensate for ↑GFR.
- Glycosuria occurs, and does not indicate impaired glucose tolerance. Urinalysis should be repeated, and a blood glucose level measured if glycosuria is heavy or persistent.
- Proteinuria also occurs (not significant unless >300 mg/day). Unlike in nonpregnant women, positive proteinuria on dipstick testing may be normal. Confirm by 24-hour collection; albumin/creatinine ratios on spot urines are less accurate in pregnancy (though a spot urine value of >30 mg albumin/gram creatinine is highly suggestive).
- Tubular handling of bicarbonate and acid is unchanged, but hyperventilation in pregnancy leads to ↓pCO_2, a mild respiratory alkalosis (↑pH from 7.4 to 7.43). HCO_3^- falls to 18–22 meq/L in compensation.

Salt and water homeostasis

Women gain 9–14 kg on average during pregnancy, with up to 8 L as ↑ total body water (TBW). The threshold for arginine vasopressin (AVP) release is lowered: this results in sustained AVP release in the face of plasma dilution, and in a true fall in plasma osmolality of ~10 mOsm/kg.
- Serum sodium falls to 132–140 meq/L (Na^+ >140 meq/L may indicate hypernatremia in pregnancy).
- Rarely, transient diabetes insipidus of pregnancy may develop in the third trimester with marked polyuria, either as pregnancy reveals an incomplete cranial DI in susceptible women, or as a result of increased degradation of AVP. It responds promptly to synthetic DDAVP, an analogue resistant to breakdown.

Anatomical changes

- ↑ kidney volume, weight, and size. ↑ renal length by 1 cm
- Collecting system dilatation may begin at 8 weeks, and is apparent in 90% of women by 20 weeks gestation. It is more obvious on the right (uterine veins, enlarging uterus, and iliac artery compress right ureter → "iliac sign" on intravenous pyelogram (IVP), with abrupt ureteric cutoff at the pelvic brim).
- Collecting system dilatation resolves within 48 hours postpartum in 50% of cases, but may still be present at up to 12 weeks postpartum.

▶ Assessments made during pregnancy should be interpreted with caution when comparing them to findings pre-pregnancy or postpartum.

Normal values for pregnant women

Creatinine falls from a mean of 0.8 mg/dL in nonpregnant ♀ to:
- 0.7 mgl/dL in the first trimester
- 0.6 mg/dL in the second trimester
- 0.5 mg/dL in the third trimester

▶ Cr >0.9 mg/dL in pregnant ♀ may indicate renal impairment and should be evaluated further.

If in doubt, the best measure of renal function is 24-hour urinary creatinine clearance: normal range of 125–150 mL/min, or 30% above the range for nonpregnant subjects, is normal. Formulas that calculate GFR should not be used in pregnancy, as they overestimate actual GFR in pregnancy.

Urate falls in pregnancy: as a rough guide, the intrapartum urate should be 0 (gestational age in weeks), i.e., at 26 weeks, urate should be 0.26 mmol/L.

UTI in pregnancy

Anatomical, functional, and hormonal changes to the urinary tract make UTI more common in pregnancy. Pyelonephritis is the most common renal complication of pregnancy, occurring in 1%–2% of all pregnancies. Preterm labor or low-birth-weight infants may be associated with asymptomatic bacteriuria or UTI (coexisting ascending infection causes amnionitis, with ↑ inflammatory cytokine synthesis provoking uterine contraction). Untreated UTI may be associated with subsequent developmental delay in the child, or even an increased risk of fetal death.

Bacteriology

In 80%–90% of cases, *E. coli*. *Proteus* spp., *Klebsiella* spp., or gram-positive organisms may be implicated. Resistance to first-generation cephalosporins among *E. coli* is ±15% (<1% for cefuroxime). Group B *Streptococcus* (GBS) infection near delivery may lead to vaginal colonization and serious neonatal sepsis. Penicillin prophylaxis should be given during labor if the patient is infected with GBS.

Risk factors

Asymptomatic bacteriuria (>10^5 cfu/mL urine) occurs in 2%–7% of women, and in pregnancy is associated with pyelonephritis in 40% of cases if untreated.

Further risk factors for bacteriuria or UTI prior to delivery include the following:
- UTI before becoming pregnant
- UTI in previous pregnancies
- Diabetes mellitus, HIV positivity, or sickle cell disease
- An abnormal urinary tract

Postpartum UTI is often associated with prolonged labor or delivery by caesarean section, or labor complicated by preeclampsia or placental abruption (and almost always with in-dwelling urinary catheters).

Diagnosis

- Dysuria, frequency, urgency, or offensive urine suggests UTI. Flank pain, backache, vomiting, and fevers are often found with acute pyelonephritis.
- On examination, suprapubic or renal angle tenderness may be found.
- Dipstick testing for leukocytes or nitrites may suggest a frank UTI, but will often miss asymptomatic bacteriuria.
- Get UA, urine for C&S.
- If pyelonephritis is suspected get blood cultures, CBC, and renal function profile, as well as urine culture. Consider US of the renal tract. Fetal well-being should be assessed.

Acute pyelonephritis

Pyelonephritis is more common in the second half of pregnancy and is a significant cause of fetal mortality and maternal morbidity. The increasing size of the uterus may cause ureteral obstruction and impaired urinary flow (particularly on the right), encouraging urinary tract sepsis.

Recurrent UTIs in pregnancy

▶ After more than one UTI (or a single episode in ♀ with an abnormal urinary tract), women should be given prophylactic antibiotics for the duration of the pregnancy.

Postcoital cephalexin 500 mg po or cephalexin 500 mg at bedtime for 1 month alternating with nitrofurantoin 100 mg at bedtime have both proved safe and effective. Ideally the choice should reflect sensitivity of the organism cultured. Postpartum investigation for recurrent UTI is recommended (p. 424).

Treatment of UTI in pregnancy

Asymptomatic bacteriuria or cystitis

As an outpatient:
- Nitrofurantoin 100 mg po bid × 3–7 days or cephalexin 500 mg po qid × 3–7 days
- Midstream urine collection (MSU) for C+S monthly to confirm eradication of bacteria.
- Ampicillin 500 mg po qid × 7–10 days for group B *Streptococcus* infections

Pyelonephritis

As an inpatient:
- IV access and rehydration with 0.9% NaCl as required.
- Ceftriaxone 1 g IV daily, or [gentamicin 1 mg/kg q8h + ampicillin 1–2 g q6h], or ticarcillin-clavulanate 3.2 g q8h

Cephalosporins are not known to be harmful to the fetus, and have not been found to cause any physical or mental damage in children with follow-up beyond 18 months. Trimethroprim may be used after the first trimester as an alternative.

⚠ Fluoroquinolones such as ciprofloxacin should be avoided unless resistant organisms are cultured, and cotrimoxazole needs to be used with caution (sulfonamides should not be used in the third trimester).

Acute renal failure in pregnancy

▶ Preeclampsia is the most common cause of ARF in pregnancy.

Oliguria is most commonly caused by volume depletion and responds to rehydration—renal function is usually transiently and mildly impaired. In the developed world, ARF is now rare during pregnancy and the puerperium, but it is still a significant problem accounting for up to 20% of all ARF in the developing world.

In septic abortion, sudden onset (over hours) of fever (≥40°C), rigors, myalgia, vomiting, and diarrhea (may be bloody) can occur after any attempted abortion. Abdominal pain is common, but vaginal discharge is often absent. Progression to established septic shock with hypotension, tachycardia, peripheral vasodilatation and oliguria is rapid. Organisms include *E. coli* or *Clostridia*.

Investigations
Order blood cultures, CBC (hemolysis), PT, PTT, D-dimers or FDPs (↓Plt and DIC), renal function profile, and LFT. Perform vaginal swabs for C+S. Get plain abdominal X-ray for intrauterine or intra-abdominal gas. Consider US to exclude pyometrium.

Management
Catheterize and monitor UO. Get IV access and administer resuscitation with colloid and blood products.

▶ Ampicillin 2 g IV q6h, PLUS clindamycin 600 mg IV q8h, PLUS gentamicin 1 mg/kg IV q8h (must adjust if patient is in renal failure), PLUS doxycycline 100 mg po bid.

Acute fatty liver of pregnancy

This condition occurs late in pregnancy or immediately postpartum and is part of a spectrum of pregnancy-related diseases characterized by endothelial dysfunction and end-organ damage (such as preeclampsia). Patients present with nausea, vomiting, and an acute hepatitis with jaundice, encephalopathy, and DIC. ARF due to ATN is common (usually successfully managed conservatively).

Investigations
Order CBC, PT, PTT, D-dimers, renal function profile, LFT, glucose. Check ↑ urate. Management is largely supportive, and delivery should be expedited if possible.

Cortical necrosis

Once common, this necrosis is seen especially after placental abruption. It occurs as a result of sudden and profound renal vasospasm (often with marked hypotension), causing patchy infarction of the renal cortex. Severe oligoanuric renal failure (persistent anuria often being the first clue) often progresses to end-stage renal failure.

MAG-3 isotope scanning, contrast-enhanced CT scanning, or MRI angiography will demonstrate perfusion defects.

Hemolytic uremic syndrome (📖 p. 401)

This syndrome used to be known as idiopathic postpartum renal failure—it is very rare, and presents with acute oliguric renal failure progressing rapidly to requiring dialysis in the early puerperium (up until 6 weeks postpartum) after an otherwise unremarkable pregnancy. Again, endothelial dysfunction with a microangiopathic hemolytic anemia and coagulopathy is apparent, usually with severe and uncontrolled hypertension.

Hypertension in pregnancy

Hypertension complicates 6%–10% of all pregnancies and is responsible for 15% of all maternal deaths.

Classification
- Gestational hypertension
- Preeclampsia-eclampsia
- Chronic hypertension
- Preeclampsia superimposed on chronic hypertension.

Measuring BP and proteinuria in pregnant women

A variety of classifications exist for diagnosing raised BP in pregnancy: the International Society for the Study of Hypertension (ISSHP) definitions shown in Box 10.1 seem the most simple. Systolic BP correlates less well with prognosis in pregnancy and hypertension—but ↑SBP should still be matched with more regular review of the patient.

Risks to mother and fetus

Mild-to-moderate hypertension (BP 140/90–159/109 mmHg) carries little risk, though it may progress to more severe ↑BP (>160/110 mmHg), associated with maternal stroke or preeclampsia.

◆* Treatment targets for hypertensive women without preeclampsia remain controversial.

Although there is benefit to the mother in treating high BP, this may come at some cost to the fetus (increased intrauterine growth restriction [IUGR] in particular).

Measuring blood pressure in pregnant women[1]

- Use the bell for auscultation.
- Use a well-maintained sphygmomanometer.
- Use correct cuff: it should encompass 80% of arm circumference.
- Measure with patient sitting after a period of rest with the arm supported at *heart level*.
- Record systolic BP when sounds are first heard *(Korotkoff 1)* and diastolic at the point of disappearance of sounds *(Korotkoff 5)*.

Box 10.1 Defining hypertension in pregnancy

Hypertension
A diastolic BP ≥110 mmHg on any one occasion or
A diastolic BP ≥90 mmHg on two consecutive occasions >4 hours apart

Severe hypertension
A diastolic BP ≥129 mmHg on any one occasion or
A diastolic BP ≥110 mmHg on two consecutive occasions >4 hours apart.

---

[1] International Society for the Study of Hypertension in Pregnancy

Gestational hypertension

Definition
- SBP ≥140 mmHg and/or DBP ≥90 mmHg in the absence of proteinuria in a previously normotensive pregnant woman
- Occurs at or after 20 weeks of pregnancy
- BP readings documented on two occasions 6 hours apart.

Natural history
- 15%–25% will progress to preeclampsia.
- Risk of progression inversely correlates with gestational age.
- BP returns to normal by 12th week postpartum.
- BP remaining elevated after 12th postpartum week = chronic hypertension.
- Mild gestational hypertension (HTN) is associated with favorable maternal and fetal outcome.
- Severe gestational HTN is associated with increased risk of maternal and perinatal morbidity.

Evaluation
- Urine dipstick
- Confirm + dipstick for urine protein with UAB:UCr or 24-hour urine for protein.
- Clinical appraisal for signs of end-organ damage (headache, visual changes, nausea and vomiting, etc.)
- Measure CBC, renal function profile, AST/ALT, LDH.

General principles of management

Bed rest is of no value in mild, non-proteinuric HTN. Although delivery is definitive treatment, non-proteinuric HTN is not an indication for delivery in itself. Drug treatment is not required for non-proteinuric HTN unless
- DBP >105 mmHg or SBP >160 mmHg on repeated measure.

Drug treatment for gestational hypertension
- Labetalol 50 mg po bid, titrate to 100 mg bid or more
  or
- Methyldopa as 250 mg po bid, and titrate up to 750 mg qid (side effects are more common than with β-blockade)
- Blood pressure goal: no end-organ damage, SBP 140–150 mmHg and DBP 80–100 mmHg

Preeclampsia and eclampsia

Preeclampsia (from the Greek *eclampsus*, or lightning) is a rapidly progressive, life-threatening, pregnancy-specific disease characterized by hypertension, proteinuria, and peripheral edema—it is defined as progressing to eclampsia when seizures occur.

This distinction should be thought of as an arbitrary one, as maternal cerebral hemorrhage may complicate preeclampsia prior to seizures. Equally, modest hypertension in the context of preeclamptic proteinuria and edema may progress rapidly to full-blown eclampsia.

Preeclampsia remains a leading cause of maternal and fetal morbidity and mortality, complicating about 3%–5% of all pregnancies (eclampsia occurs in about 0.05%–0.1%). Preeclampsia occurs in the presence of a placenta, and its resolution begins with the removal of the placenta. This has informed the obstetric dogma that preeclampsia is treated by delivery and delivery alone, for more than 50 years.

Pathogenesis

Gestational HTN, preeclampsia, the HELLP syndrome, acute fatty liver of pregnancy, and HUS in pregnancy are all thought to be diseases manifesting endothelial dysfunction. Preeclampsia occurs in a setting of decreased organ perfusion as a result of intense vasoconstriction, affecting almost every organ—the vasculature is highly sensitive to circulating vasopressors (such as AII), reflecting the underlying endothelial abnormality. Decreased intravascular volume as a result of leaky capillaries, and activation of platelets and the coagulation cascade accompany vasoconstriction, exacerbating organ hypoperfusion and leading to formation of microthrombi in small vessels.

In normal pregnancy, endovascular trophoblastic invasion transforms maternal uterine spiral arterioles into dilated low-resistance vessels with little vascular smooth muscle or tone, thus providing a blood supply to the fetus. In preeclampsia, this response is defective. Endovascular invasion occurs incompletely, without remodeling of spiral arterioles, resulting in abnormal flow in the intervillous space of the placenta. Reduced placental perfusion leads to release of a soluble VEGF receptor (sFlt1) that neutralizes circulating VEGF, thus impairing normal vessel function throughout the body.[1] In tandem, increased oxidative stress adds to widespread endothelial damage and intolerance to vasopressors.

Diagnosis

Preeclampsia refers to new hypertension and proteinuria occuring after 20 weeks gestation in a previously normotensive woman. It may evolve from gestational HTN or present abruptly. The development of generalized tonic-clonic seizures in this setting is *eclampsia*.

---

1 Maynard SE, et al. (2003). *J Clin Invest* 111: 649–58.

Criteria for diagnosis
- In ♀ >20 weeks pregnant (who were normotensive <20 weeks)
- Proteinuria >300 mg/day
- ↑BP as one of the following:
  - ↑DBP >15 mmHg or ↑SBP > 30 mmHg on early pregnancy
  - ↑DBP >90 mmHg on two occasions 4 hours apart
  - ↑DBP >110 mmHg on a single occasion.

⚠ New dipstick-positive proteinuria + ↑BP in *any* pregnant ♀ requires exclusion of preeclampsia.

Edema is present in 60% of normal pregnancies, and is not a sign of preeclampsia.

Risk factors for preeclampsia
- Nulliparity
- Maternal age >40 years (or ≤18 years)
- Previous preeclampsia
- Family history of preeclampsia
- Twin pregnancy or fetal hydrops
- Obesity, diabetes mellitus, ↑ insulin resistance or ↑ testosterone
- Chronic hypertension or underlying renal disease
- Anti-phospholipid syndrome, ↑ homocysteine or vascular disease.

Affected organs include
- *Circulation* plasma volume, usually increased to 40% above normal in pregnancy, falls as capillary "leaks" develop. Vasoconstriction and hypoperfusion accompany these changes.
- *Kidney* glomerular endothelial swelling ("endotheliosis") occurs with a fall in renal blood flow (and therefore impaired tubular function with a decreased urate clearance), before proteinuria appears. GFR falls with RBF.
- *Liver* vasoconstriction and hypoperfusion of the hepatic vascular bed may contribute to the evolution of HELLP syndrome.
- *Brain* vasoconstriction leads to abnormal electrical activity that may trigger eclamptic seizures. There may be associated ischemia and edema (often in the parietal and occipital lobes).
- *Coagulation* platelet activation occurs early in the disease and may become associated with thrombocytopenia. Many clotting factors are elevated beyond the already raised levels seen in normal pregnancy.

Managing preeclampsia and eclampsia

⚠ Women with fulminant preeclampsia are at high risk.

- If eclamptic, place patient on left side with a secure *airway*. Protect airway if there is a depressed level of consciousness.
- O_2 by facemask at 4–8 L/min: monitor O_2 sats
- *Observations* as TPR ¼-hourly (more frequently if seizing). Strict intake/output charting
- Insert an in-dwelling *urinary catheter* for hourly UO measurement.
- Get *cardiotocograph trace* (CTG) for continuous fetal heart rate (FHR) monitoring. Request fetal ultrasound to confirm gestational age if need be, and umbilical Doppler US to assess placental capacity.
- *Investigations*: CBC (↓Plt), smear (? hemolysis), clotting, renal function profile, urate, LDH, LFTs
- *IVI access* and give 250–500 mL fluid challenge with colloid prior to giving antihypertensives. After this, administer 0.9% saline at 85 mL/h or as urine output in preceding hour + 30 mL.

Delivery

If the pregnancy is near term, delivery should be expedited. If it is not, and particularly if the fetus is <34 weeks gestational age, the dilemma is one of balancing maternal health against neonatal outcome. If it is clear that a patient has progressive preeclampsia, a decision needs to made on whether or not it is safe for a trial of medical therapy for 24–48 hours after administering corticosteroids to hasten fetal lung maturity. There is rarely a benefit to delaying delivery if placental perfusion is no longer meeting fetal needs, but because the consequences of prematurity are often dire, conservative management of a stable mother is frequently preferred. Maternal complications such as eclampsia, renal, liver, or coagulopathy should be managed by delivery regardless of fetal maturity.

Parameters suggesting a need for delivery

- Gestational age >38 weeks
- Declining renal function (Scr >2 mg/dL, oliguria)
- Platelets <100,000/mL
- Any rise in transaminases
- Severe headaches or visual changes
- Abruptio placentae
- Persistent, severe epigastric pain, nausea and vomiting.

Treating hypertension

Avoid sudden ↓BP that may compromise the fetus.

⚠ The patient is underfilled (reduced plasma volume) and hypertensive!
- If BP >160/110 mmHg, MAP >125 mmHg, or patient is having seizures, consider transfer to the ICU. Consider placing an arterial line—treatment is urgent to reduce risk of *intracranial hemorrhage*. Aim for target of 140–150/90–100 mmHg.
- Give *labetalol* 20 mg IV as a slow bolus (over 1 min). Double dose every 10 min (40 mg then 80 mg IV) to a cumulative maximum dose of 300 mg. Labetalol 5 mg/mL can be infused at 20 mg/h, doubling hourly to a maximum of 160 mg/h. Avoid in asthmatics.
  or
- Give *hydralazine* 5 mg IV as a slow bolus (3–5 min), and repeat every 20 min to cumulative maximum of 20 mg. It can be run as an infusion: 100 mg in 100 mL 0.9% saline at 2 mg/h, doubling hourly to a maximum of 20 mg/h (2–20 mL/h).
- Monitor FHR throughout as hypotension may cause *fetal distress*.

Prophylaxis for and treatment of seizures

At-risk mothers should be treated prophylactically and the underlying pathology reversed—i.e., delivery. Imminent eclampsia is heralded by
- Apprehension and facial itching
- Headache and visual disturbances ("flashing lights" or blurred vision)
- Epigastric pain
- Hyperreflexia
- Worsening proteinuria.

- Give 6 g *magnesium sulphate* IV over 15 min.
- Maintenance dose: 2–3 g/h (give only if patellar reflex is present, respiratory rate >12 + UO >100 mL/h).
- Treatment should continue until 24 hours after delivery.
- Recurrent seizures may be treated with a further bolus of 2 g $MgSO_4$. If seizures persist, consider lorazepam 0.02–0.03 mg/kg IV. You can repeat additional doses up to maximum of 0.1 mg/kg.

Chronic hypertension in pregnancy

Chronic hypertension in pregnancy is ↑BP diagnosed before pregnancy, or before 20 weeks gestation. This group, particularly if newly diagnosed, will have persistently raised BP beyond 12 weeks postpartum.

Most ♀ with mild essential hypertension (DBP <105 mmHg) have uncomplicated pregnancies, but ~10% will develop superimposed preeclampsia that is often early in onset and aggressive in nature.

▶ In ♀ with ↑BP <20th week, consider hydatidiform mole.

Prenatal counseling in hypertensive ♀ seeking to conceive

Most importantly, an antihypertensive regime that has the least potential teratogenicity needs to be planned and implemented. ♀ with poorly controlled BP should be advised about contraception (ideally, with an IUCD or condoms, but progesterone-only pills may be an alternative) and the need to achieve ideal control before attempting to fall pregnant.

Antenatal care

Such care is as per "surveillance," p. 574.

⚠ Evolving superimposed preeclampsia may be severe in this group, associated with placental abruption, multiple organ failure, and maternal and fetal death.

Unplanned conception on antihypertensives

Many women worry about potential harm from routine BP medication when discovering themselves unexpectedly pregnant. ACEIs, associated with fetal renal impairment, IUGR, and fetal death in later trimesters, appear not to be associated with fetal disorders in the first trimester. Nevertheless, they should be stopped as soon as possible.

Optimizing antihypertensives before conception

No drug can be thought of as safe. There are few data about the long-term effects of antihypertensives on child development. This should always be discussed with pregnant hypertensive women—just as importantly, the greater risk to both her and the pregnancy of untreated hypertension should be emphasized. A treatment algorithm might be as follows:
- *Methyldopa* 250 mg po bid, increased to up 1 g po tid
  or
- *Nifedipine SR* 30 mg qd, increased to 60 mg bid (sufficient data suggest that nifedipine is safe in pregnancy—amlodipine is likely to be safe as well, but longer experience with nifedipine makes its use preferable)
  then
- *Labetalol* 50 mg po bid, increased to up to 400 mg po tid (atenolol 25 mg od, increasing to 100 mg qd is an alternative).

Other alternatives
- *Prazosin* 0.5 mg po bid increased to 2–4 mg po tid (doxazosin 1 mg po bd increased to 8 mg po bid is effective, though experience with it is not as extensive as with prazosin)
  or
- *Hydralazine* 50 mg po bid, increased to up to 100 mg po tid

⚠ The following drugs are either contraindicated in pregnancy, or too little experience with them makes their use undesirable: *ACE inhibitors and angiotensin II receptor antagonists and minoxidil, newer α- and β-blockers.*

Preexisting renal disease

The ability to conceive falls with ↓GFR, and the danger a pregnancy carries to both mother and fetus rises substantially. Fetal loss, IUGR, and preterm labor are not uncommon, and irreversible loss of maternal renal function as a result of any pregnancy is a major risk.

↑BP is the single most important predictor of the risk a pregnancy poses to mother and fetus.

Primary glomerular disease with normal renal function
- The type of glomerular lesion has little impact on fetal outcomes—the presence of *proteinuria* is of far greater importance.
- Nephrotic-range proteinuria (>3 g/day, 📖 p. 18) ↑ perinatal loss (up to 23%) and preterm delivery (35%)—this is double expected if there is no proteinuria (12%–15% perinatal loss and 9%–21% preterm labor).
- The rate of spontaneous abortion is not ↑ against the normal population.
- Worsening maternal hypertension occurs in 10%–20% of cases and predicts a worse outcome.
- Relapse of the primary glomerular lesion is rare (▶ ?preeclampsia).
- A permanent deterioration in renal function is unlikely in the absence of renal impairment.

Diabetic nephropathy

Maternal diabetes is usually type 1, but may also be type 2 in young adulthood. Pregnancies may be complicated by prolonged or preterm labor with babies who are large for gestational age (40%). Pregnancy does not accelerate the onset of or progression to diabetic nephropathy, but women with overt diabetic nephropathy fare substantially worse.

Nonglomerular disease and normal renal function

Reflux nephropathy
- There is good outcome if renal function is normal—fetal loss is only about 12%. More frequent and regular UA and C+S should be performed, and bacteriuria treated promptly.
- Acute pyelonephritis is more common.
- Children should be screened in infancy (📖 p. 428).

Adult polycystic kidney disease (APKD) has nearly normal outcomes:
- ↑ risk of preeclampsia
- If Cr is normal but there is ↑BP, up to 45% will develop preeclampsia.
- Cyst complications such as cyst hemorrhage or cyst infection in pregnancy may masquerade as obstetric complications.

Women with APKD and a family history of intracranial aneurysms should be screened prior to conception.

Lupus nephritis (see Table 10.1)

- Lupus affects ♀ of child-bearing age—40% will develop renal disease.
- Fertility is normal if GFR is normal—cyclophosphamide causes premature ovarian failure in up to 60%, especially if total dose >10 g.
- Use progesterone-only pills for contraception if there is active disease or anti-phospholipid antibodies.
- Wait until off cytotoxic agents and on the lowest possible dose of prednisolone before trying to conceive (ideally >6 months after full remission is achieved).
- If active disease is present at conception, disease flares during pregnancy are more likely.
- ♀ with anti-phospholipid antibodies are at increased risk of spontaneous abortion. Consider aspirin and LMW heparins from conception—20 weeks if there is a positive history of venous thrombo-embolism or fetal loss.
- Fetal outcomes depend on disease control, renal function, and the presence of hypertension.
- Active lupus → with increased fetal loss, prematurity, and IUGR.

Table 10.1 Preeclampsia or active lupus nephritis?

	Preeclampsia	Lupus nephritis
BP	↑↑	↑↑
Proteinuria	+++	+++
Hematuria	±	+++
Red cell casts	–	++
ALT	↑	Normal
Complement	Normal	↓
dsDNA titers	Normal	↑
Symptoms of lupus	–	++
Response to steroids	–	+

Antenatal care

Aim to see the mother roughly monthly until the 32nd week, thereafter weekly. Manage as per "surveillance" 📖 p. 574.
- Confirm the underlying diagnosis if possible—if unknown, exclude reflux nephropathy or chronic pyelonephritis.
- Check renal function profile, urate.
- Check Cr clearance and 24-hour proteinuria or albumin/creatinine ratio.
- Assess disease activity in systemic diseases such as lupus or in glomerulonephritis (patient should avoid pregnancy while on cytotoxic agents and until full remission is achieved for at least 6 months).
- Plan antihypertensives and achieve ideal BP prior to conception—test for pregnancy early, aiming to stop ACEIs/ARB.
- Patient should stop smoking, and drinking alcohol and caffeine.

Outcomes in pregnant ♀ with preexisting renal disease

Creatinine <1.4 mg/dL
Good maternal renal prognosis, with usually successful pregnancies.

Creatinine 1.4–2.5 mg/dL
Some risk to pregnancy and fetus—real risk to maternal renal function.

Creatinine >2.5 mg/dL
Poor fetal outcomes, with high risk of maternal end-stage renal failure.

Pregnancy in ♀ with CKD (creatinine >1.4 mg/dL)

Fetal risks
- 60% of neonates will be preterm ± many being small for gestational age.
- Fetal mortality is 7% with good neonatal intensive care facilities.
- If maternal Cr >2.5 mg/dL, fetal IUGR present in 57% of cases.

Maternal risks
Significant risk of loss of renal function:
- Cr <1.4 mg/dL: 16% will experience a transient rise in creatinine.
- Cr 1.4–2.0 mg/dL: 40% will have ↑Cr—50% will not recover lost function.
- Cr >2.0 mg/dL: 65% will have ↑Cr—few regain lost function, and 35% of these patients will be dialysis dependent within 1 year.
- Superimposed preeclampsia occurs in 65%.
- Renal recovery may not be seen until 6 weeks postpartum, if at all.

Diabetics with impaired renal function appear to be at higher risk—pregnancy should be discouraged if significant renal impairment is present.

Disorders of the renal tract in pregnancy

Changes in the anatomy of the renal tract during pregnancy, in particular dilatation of the collecting system (📖 p. 567), need to be borne in mind when assessing women with urinary tract symptoms and signs.

Hematuria

In the absence of proteinuria, hematuria is usually due to anatomical changes, with bleeding from small venules in dilated collecting systems. On microscopy 2–3 RBC/hpf is normal in pregnancy (unlike 1–2 in the nonpregnant population). If Cr is normal and no proteinuria is present, wait until 12 weeks after delivery for further assessment (📖 p. 48).

Obstruction

Obstruction may result from mechanical pressure exerted by the uterus (usually on the right ureter, often where the ureter crosses the iliac artery) or pelvic or ureteric stone impaction. Renal stones occur rarely in pregnancy and usually in women known to have nephrolithiasis prior to pregnancy. Collecting system dilatation with stasis, and 2- to 3-fold increase in urinary calcium excretion may precipitate new stone formation in pregnancy.

Suspect if flank pain, dysuria, and hematuria

- Urine dipstick for hematuria and proteinuria
- Microscopy: red cells (+morphology), casts, WBC, and organisms
- Urine culture ± stone analysis
- CBC, renal function profile, ± PTH (if stones are suspected)

Imaging may include
- Ultrasound
- IVP if obstruction suspected, especially if with coexisting infection
- (Spiral CT—avoid if possible)

In cases where an IVP is requested
- The radiation exposure is low (0.4–1.5 rads).
- Shielding the pelvis further reduces exposure to the fetus.
- Limited films should be taken.

Obstruction can be treated by stenting (📖 p. 500). Limited experience with external shock wave lithotripsy suggests it to be safe, though best avoided if possible. Consider prophylactic antibiotics through pregnancy.

Pregnancy while on dialysis

♀ with ESRD rarely fall pregnant on dialysis: only 0.3%–2.2% will conceive. Nevertheless, offer contraception to women who menstruate while on dialysis (up to 40%). If pregnancy occurs, and progresses beyond the first trimester, fetal outcomes are often poor, and maternal morbidity is significant.

What should women know about pregnancy while on dialysis?

- Between 20% and 70% of pregnancies will result in a live infant.
- 13%–45% of pregnancies result in spontaneous miscarriage <20 weeks gestation.
- Stillbirth, neonatal death, and severe developmental delay are much more common.
- Most pregnancies (up to 85%) will end in preterm labor and delivery, with a mean gestational age of 32 weeks.
- Intrauterine growth retardation and low birth weight are common.
- There is no increase in rate of congenital abnormalities over that of the normal population.
- Difficult to control maternal hypertension complicates up to 80% of pregnancies.

Targets for dialysis

There is no reason for modality switch: HD delivers a higher dialysis dose, but CAPD (especially APD) offers less rapid metabolic changes and allows steady fluid removal. Residual renal function improves pregnancy outcomes.

Hemodialysis

Aim for dialysis for ≥20 hours/week. Titrate dialysate K^+, Ca^{2+}, and HCO_3^- against serum levels (this may require reduction in dialysate HCO_3^- to prevent maternal alkalemia). Heparin requirements may increase. Avoid hypotension if at all possible—expect 0.5 kg/week weight gains from mid-pregnancy onward.

Peritoneal dialysis

As pregnancy progresses and intra-abdominal PD fluid volume is less well-tolerated, automated PD becomes necessary with daytime exchanges and CCPD. Peritonitis should be treated vigorously, bearing in mind the potential teratogenicity of some antibiotics.

Diet, calcium and vitamin D

↑ protein intake to 1.2–1.4 g/kg pre-pregnant weight + 10 g/day. For CAPD, take dialysate protein losses into account and replace. Give daily multivitamin preparation with water-soluble vitamins. ↑ folate to 1.6 mg/day. The placenta produces calcitriol: ↓ vitamin D analogue dose. Supplemental K^+ may be required.

Anemia

Erythropoietin is not teratogenic. Dose requirements in pregnancy will increase by 50%–100%. Supplement oral iron. Use low-dose IV iron if necessary.

Labor and delivery

Most units will deliver pregnant dialysis patients early, usually as a result of worsening hypertension, IUGR, or both: few pregnancies are permitted to progress beyond 38 weeks.
- Monitoring uterine activity should begin as early as the 26th week, as dialysis may induce contractions.
- Caesarian section is performed for standard obstetric indications.
- PD patients should be drained for delivery—dialysis can resume 24 hours after delivery with small volume exchanges. Hemodialysis can be used in cases of leakage.
- Assess fluid status carefully: avoid volume overload.
- Infection should be borne in mind and avoided if possible. Sterile techniques should be used where feasible.
- Neonates should be cared for in specialist units with regular electrolyte assessment.

Renal transplantation and pregnancy

A functioning renal transplant rapidly restores fertility and libido in women with ESRD. About 1 in 50 women of child-bearing age in this group will become pregnant, and over 14,000 such pregnancies have been reported.

Pre-pregnancy counseling

Many women will not want to become pregnant: after successful transplantation, barrier contraception with condoms is the safest but not the most effective method (▶ progesterone-only pill). Oral contraceptives may interfere with immunosuppressants or aggravate hypertension. Pelvic infections may complicate IUD use.

- Review all drugs prior to conception to minimize teratogenicity, with particular attention to antihypertensives.
- Inform blood group Rh− women with Rh+ kidneys (they may develop anti-Rh+ antibodies → neonatal hemolysis).
- Live vaccines (such as rubella) are contraindicated: rubella antibodies should be tested for (ideally, vaccinate before transplantation).
- ±30% of pregnancies will not progress beyond 12 weeks, through miscarriage or termination (similar in general population).
- Beyond this, 95% of pregnancies will succeed. There is ↑ risk of preterm labor and delivery (40%–60%) and IUGR (40%).
- There is no ↑ in congenital abnormalities above that occurring in the general population. Incidence of longer-term developmental delay is probably low.
- Successful live births are related to good graft function, the absence of proteinuria, and length of time after transplantation.
- Maternal hypertension will develop or worsen in 30%.
- Transplant function may worsen transiently or even permanently (up to 10% graft loss in the 2 years after delivery), especially if Cr >2.3 mg/L.
- ±15% of women will experience a decline in GFR with pregnancy.

Ideally

- Patient is 2 years post-transplant with stable renal function (Cr < 2 mg/dL, but <1.6 mg/dL may be a more preferable target).
- Blood pressure control should be good (<135/85 mmHg).
- Proteinuria should be <500 mg/day.
- No recent transplant rejection episodes have occurred.

Potentially teratogenic drugs should have been eliminated.

Drugs in transplantation and pregnancy

Cyclosporin: No ↑ risk of teratogenicity at therapeutic levels, especially if dose ≤5 mg/kg/day. Monitor levels closely, and adjust dose accordingly. Maternal ↑BP and IUGR may be problems.

Tacrolimus: Less evidence is available. Transient neonatal hyperkalemia and renal dysfunction have been reported. Dose adjustment to achieve therapeutic levels is often required. Gestational diabetes and preterm labor may be problems.

Azathioprine: Widespread experience has not borne out experimental concerns: therapy can be safely continued at low dose (<2 mg/kg/day).
Corticosteroids: Safe in pregnancy at maintenance doses (<15 mg/day). Poor wound healing may complicate delivery (especially if by caesarean section). Neonates should be monitored to exclude adrenal suppression.

⚠ Breast-feeding is not advocated on maintenance immunosuppression.

The following drugs commonly prescribed in renal transplantation are contraindicated: MMF, sirolimus, anti-infectives such as ganciclovir, and cotrimoxazole.

Antenatal care
- Check cyclosporin or tacrolimus levels frequently (weekly).
- Check renal function profile, Ca, LFT every 2 weeks or more.
- Measure CBC every 6 weeks.
- Check baseline toxoplasmosis, cytomegalovirus, and HSV status.
- Screen for gestational impaired glucose tolerance every trimester.

Labor
- Vaginal delivery is safe, though short labors are preferable.
- Additional hydrocortisone 100 mg IV should be administered during labor.

Chapter 11

Drugs and the kidney

Prescribing in renal impairment 592
The septic ESRD patient: drug issues 594
Cardiac drugs in renal failure 596
NSAIDs and the kidney 598
Analgesia in renal failure 600
Opioids in renal failure 602
Poisoning and dialysis 604
Lithium and salicylate poisoning 606
Ethylene glycol poisoning 608

Prescribing in renal impairment

⚠ Always check the recommended dose when prescribing a drug to apatient with renal impairment.

Principles
- Most drugs are ultimately excreted by the kidney, though many are broken down in the liver or elsewhere first. Thus renal impairment is likely to affect pharmacokinetics
- In practice, special care is required when using those drugs
  - with a narrow therapeutic index (i.e., the toxic and therapeutic ranges overlap or are close to each other) (▶ digoxin, acyclovir);
  - for which dose reduction and monitoring of plasma levels may be indicated;
  - for which renal toxicity is a possible effect of the drug; in this case a vicious cycle ensues of worsening renal function, decreased drug clearance, and rising drug levels (▶ gentamicin, cyclosporin).
- For many drugs, plasma levels are altered by ~30% with significant renal impairment (▶ many antibiotics). Dose reduction may be required, but the wide therapeutic window may make it possible to use the drug safely with simple guidelines for dose reduction (e.g., "halve the standard dose").

Pharmacokinetics
Renal failure may not just affect the renal clearance of a drug. Other pharmacokinetic changes may also occur.

Absorption
Drugs taken orally are absorbed via the gut. Absorption may be affected by the following:
- Interactions with other substances in the GI tract (▶ cyclosporin absorption is affected by grapefruit juice)
- Interactions with other drugs in the GI tract (▶ phosphate binders)
- Gastric pH may also be important—in renal failure, gastric ammonia production may alter gastric pH, decreasing absorption of some drugs (▶ ferrous sulphate, folic acid).

Protein binding
Changes in albumin concentration affect free drug concentrations of highly protein-bound drugs. In the nephrotic syndrome, hypoalbuminimia → ↓ drug binding to albumin and ↑ free drug. Accumulation of uremic metabolites in renal failure and binding of these compounds to albumin may also affect protein binding by drugs, thus increasing the active fraction of the drug. ▶ Phenytoin is less protein bound in renal failure, and signs of toxicity may occur at "therapeutic" levels.

Volume of distribution
This measures the (theoretical) volume occupied by the drug, assuming uniform concentration in all compartments. Volume of distribution may be affected by renal disease (▶ digoxin, for which a reduced loading dose may be required).

Clearance

Hepatic clearance means breakdown of the drug to inactive metabolites. It usually occurs either by conjugation (to glucuronide or sulphate) to make a lipid-soluble drug more polar (thus increasing renal clearance) or by oxidation or reduction.

Renal clearance

Smaller molecules (MW <60,000) are filtered by the glomerulus to a greater or lesser extent. Polar molecules are more freely filtered than lipid-soluble molecules.

- Tubular reabsorption may be significant, especially of lipid-soluble drugs, as may tubular secretion (acidic drugs tend to be secreted into an alkaline urine and vice versa, e.g., salicylic acid is better excreted via an alkaline urine). ⚠ In general, as GFR falls, drug elimination by all these mechanisms decreases.
- Most drugs approximate to first-order kinetics (the rate of excretion is proportional to the concentration of the drug), and the elimination half life ($t_{1/2}$) is constant (Fig. 11.1). Steady-state concentration in these circumstances depends on $t_{1/2}$, which in turn depends on GFR for drugs excreted by the kidney. Thus, in renal failure, drug levels of renal-excreted drugs accumulate unless a dose reduction occurs.

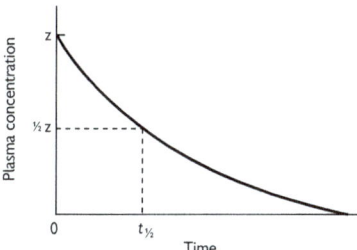

Fig. 11.1 First-order kinetics: if the drug is excreted by the kidneys, renal failure will lead to an increase in $t_{1/2}$. Reproduced with permission from Warrell D, Cox T, Firth J, and Benz EJ (eds) (2004). *Oxford Textbook of Medicine*, 4th ed., p. 469. Oxford: Oxford University Press.

The septic ESRD patient: drug issues

▶▶ Renal failure is an immunocompromised state. Always consider sepsis in the differential diagnosis of any sick patient. The presentation may be atypical and nonspecific. Blood cultures (and any other relevant cultures, e.g., urine, sputum, wound site) should always be collected before the first dose of antibiotics is given in any sick patient.

Choice of antibiotic

- History and examination may reveal the most likely source of sepsis. This should guide the initial choice of antibiotics, but in the sick patient antibiotics should be sufficiently broad range to cover all the most likely and pathogenic organisms. Local antibiotic policies, drawn up in association with the microbiology department, should be adhered to in all but exceptional circumstances.
- Hemodialysis patients: Always consider line sepsis or PTFE sepsis if one of these is present (📖 p. 224).

Empirical therapy in overtly septic HD patients

- Vancomycin 500 mg in 100 mL 0.9% NaCl IV over 30 min *or* if > 75 kg, 1 g in 250 mL 0.9% NaCl IVI over 60 min
- + gentamicin 2 mg/kg IV
- Given during the last hour of dialysis or after dialysis.

Levels are likely to remain therapeutic for at *least* 48 hours, and often much longer for vancomycin. Ototoxicity is unusual.

⚠ The effect on residual renal function (an important long-term prognostic feature in ESRD) remains unknown, but consensus remains that the risks of sepsis far outweigh any decline in UO.

▶ *Always* consider removal of any foreign body (line!)
- Peritoneal dialysis patients: Always consider peritonitis. Do an exchange and send for culture. Remember that peritonitis in APD patients may be less easily diagnosed (📖 p. 228).
- Transplant patients: Consider UTI, chest, atypical infections (especially CMV, pneumocystis). In the sick patient, give broad-spectrum treatment initially until culture results are known (📖 p. 274).

Specific antibiotics

⚠ Consult a local or national formulary and/or get expert advice when prescribing any drug for a renal patient.

Penicillins are safe and effective in the nonallergic patient. The highest doses should be avoided in severe renal failure as clearance is reduced, e.g., penicillin G (give 50% standard dose), piperacillin (4 g every 8 hours IVI maximum), amoxicillin (500 mg po tid maximum).

▶ Neurotoxicity may still occur—watch for confusion and drowsiness.

Cephalosporins are usually safe in renal failure as the therapeutic window is wide, but clearance is reduced. Moderate dose reduction is recommended, e.g., cefuroxime 750 mg IVI bid, cefotaxime 1 g bid IVI, ceftazidime 1–2 g every 48 hours.

▶ Neurotoxicity may still occur—watch for confusion and drowsiness.

Quinolones: dose reduction is required, e.g., ciprofloxacin 200 mg bid IV or 250 mg bid po. If severe sepsis, consider 24–48 hours of full dose prior to dose reduction

Metronidazole: dose should be reduced in severe renal failure, e.g., 3.25 mg/kg every 6 hours IV.

Aminoglycosides in renal failure

⚠ These drugs are renal excreted, have a narrow therapeutic window, and are nephrotoxic.

A vicious cycle of rising drug levels and worsening renal function can develop. Therefore, extreme care is required when prescribing to any patient with renal impairment. Avoid use in acute renal failure, as ischemia is synergistic in causing renal injury.

- Aminoglycosides are freely filtered by the glomerulus (so dosage needs to be adjusted according to GFR) and then partially taken up by tubular cells. They can cause tubular cell injury progressing to frank ATN.
- Standard normograms for calculating dosage regimes must be modified to take GFR into account.
- Peak and trough levels (and renal function) should be measured regularly (after one dose in severe renal impairment). Repeat doses may only be required every few days in severe renal impairment.
- For dialysis patients with no significant residual renal function, gentamicin 80 mg IV may be given at the end of every dialysis session (check trough levels).
- Resolution of renal dysfunction usually occurs over a few days when the drug is withdrawn unless toxicity is severe. Hyperbilirubinemia and other nephrotoxins (NSAIDs) prolong recovery time.
- Amikacin, netilmicin, and tobramycin have similar pharmacokinetics to those of gentamicin—manage in a similar way.

▶ *Avoid* the recommended 5 mg/kg/day dosing schedule unless eGFR is known to be (near) normal.

Cardiac drugs in renal failure

⚠ Most big cardiology trials specifically excluded patients with renal impairment.
► The indications for using drugs shown to be of real benefit in CHF and IHD (in people with normal renal function) in patients with CKD are therefore unknown and may even be *harmful*.
►Ideal dosages in renal impairment are *unknown*.

β-blockers

Some β-blockers require significant dose reduction, i.e, atenolol (30%–50% dose reduction), while others do not (metoprolol, carvedilol, labetolol).

Calcium channel blockers No dose reduction is required.

Aspirin may exacerbate the bleeding diathesis of uremia, but no dose reduction is usually recommended.

Clopidogrel Indications and dose in renal failure are unknown. Most clinicians use it as for nonrenal patients, but caution is required, as the risk of bleeding is (probably) increased, and the benefits unproven.

Thrombolytics No dose reduction is recommended.

Heparin

Unfractionated heparin is usually commenced in standard dosage, titrated against APTT. Low molecular-weight heparin has a significantly increased half-life with ↓GFR. Monitoring of activated factor Xa levels is usually recommended but often impractical (it may take too long to get the result for it to be useful). In practice:
- Give 1 mg/kg every 24 hours.
- Watch for signs of bleeding.
- Monitor activated factor Xa whenever possible.
- If the risk of bleeding is significant, use unfractionated heparin and measure APTT.

Diuretics

As renal failure advances, resistance to diuretics progresses:
- Thiazides used alone are ineffective in advanced renal failure.
- Loop diuretics may require high doses (furosemide 250–500 mg/day, bumetanide 5 mg daily).
- Addition of a small dose of thiazide to a loop diuretic may be effective, but beware of precipitating overdiuresis (metolazone 2.5–5 mg daily).
- ⚠ Avoid combinations containing potassium in renal impairment unless monitoring is regular.

ACE inhibitors (ACEIs)

These are recommended for many patients with chronic kidney disease (📖 p. 58). A drop in GFR can be expected (up to 20% ↑ in serum Cr) when commencing an ACEI, as can a rise in serum K^+. Always check renal function profile 1–2 weeks after commencing an ACEI in any patient with renal impairment. Further falls in eGFR or rises in K^+ may necessitate dose reduction, stopping the drug, ± investigation for RAS (📖 p. 293).

Spironolactone/eplerenone

Effectiveness in advanced renal failure is unknown (the big trials excluded patients with a low GFR).

⚠ Risk of hyperkalemia is significant as GFR falls and needs careful monitoring, especially if used in combination with an ACEI (📖 p. 164).

Digoxin

There is decreased volume of distribution in renal failure, and thus the loading dose should be halved in the dialysis patient. Elimination also depends on GFR, so use a decreased maintenance dose (10%–25% of usual dose every 48 hours) in renal failure. Monitor by therapeutic effect (e.g., ventricular rate in atricular fibrillation) and by plasma levels.

NSAIDs and the kidney

Mechanism

Nonsteroidal anti-inflammatory drugs (NSAIDs) inhibit the enzyme cyclo-oxygenase (COX), part of the major pathway in prostaglandin synthesis. At least 2 COX isoforms have been identified—most NSAIDs inhibit both, while selective COX-2 inhibitors inhibit only COX-2 (purportedly providing fewer GI side effects ♦※).

Their potent anti-inflammatory and analgesic properties make these drugs among the most prescribed in the world. Adverse effects are comparatively rare, but include the following:
- Renal toxicity (see below)
- Gastrointestinal side effects, including peptic ulceration and dyspepsia and small and large bowel toxicity
- Cardiovascular adverse effects, with increased risk of cardiovascular disease and hypertension (?COX-2 > nonselective ♦※)
- Liver toxicity: abnormal LFTs, though liver failure is rare
- Bronchospasm
- Anti-platelet effects (decreased production of thromboxane-A2). This is beneficial when aspirin is given for ischemic heart disease, but potentially an adverse effect in those at risk of bleeding.

Renal effects

⚠ NSAIDS should be avoided in anybody with ARF or at risk of ARF.
- When kidney function is normal, NSAIDs have insignificant effects on renal hemodynamics. When renal blood flow is compromised (renal failure, heart failure, nephrotic syndrome, hypovolemia, concomitant ACEI use), then compensatory afferent arteriolar vasodilation by prostaglandins (prostacyclin and prostaglandin E2) plays a key role in maintaining glomerular perfusion.
- Prostaglandins also affect water handling by the kidney, antagonizing the action of antidiuretic hormone (ADH). With NSAIDs this diuretic effect is lost. Water retention with hyponatremia may result.
- COX-2 inhibitors are equally nephrotoxic (though evidence is limited).
- NSAIDs can also cause direct renal toxicity in the form of an acute interstitial nephritis (📖 p. 404), or may cause a drug-related nephrotic syndrome— (📖 p. 392)
- Chronic analgesic nephropathy → CKD may result from prolonged ingestion (usually in combination with other non-NSAID analgesics), although this occurs rarely, and the causative role of NSAIDs remains unproven.

Analgesia in renal failure

Effective analgesia can be difficult to deliver because certain drugs are difficult to use or contraindicated because of the risk of side effects and toxicity.
▶ Get expert help at an early stage.

Principles in pain control

- Pain should always be treated promptly and appropriately; no patient in the hospital should have uncontrolled pain.
- Always give by mouth if possible
- Give regular analgesic medication, and prescribe prn "top-ups" for breakthrough pain
- Avoid systemic analgesia if possible to minimize toxicity. Ideally, use regional pain relief (use of epidurals, nerve blocks, local anesthetic).
- Use a modified WHO pain control ladder:
  - Start with regular acetaminophen 500 mg–1 g 4–6 hourly po.
  - Avoid compound analgesics.
  - Consider add-on adjuvant treatments where possible (see below).
  - NSAIDs are contraindicated in renal impairment, *but* ▶ NSAIDs may be useful in anuric (functionally anephric) dialysis patients for whom further renal injury is unimportant.
  - Add in weak opioid if required, e.g., tramadol 50 mg 12 hourly po. You *must* monitor dialysis patients for side effects (📖 p. 602).
  - Then add a stronger opiate if needed, e.g., hydromorphone 1–2 mg po 4 hourly, or oxycodone 5 mg every 6 hours titrating up gradually.
  - If the patient has severe pain, consider parenteral morphine (or other opiate) starting at a low dose (1.25–2.5 mg SC, IM, or IV). Be careful to review the patient and drug chart regularly.
  - Fentanyl patches are usually well tolerated by patients with severe chronic pain. Avoid if they are opioid naïve (📖 p. 602).
  - Avoid meperidine, as active metabolites are excreted by kidneys.

Adjuvant therapy

Anticonvulsants

These agents are useful particularly for neuropathic pain. Gabapentin is the best studied, but trials have excluded patients with renal failure. Dose reduction is required depending on GFR with careful monitoring for signs of toxicity. In stage 5 CKD the usual dose is 200–300 mg on alternate days (given after dialysis as partly dialysed out). Toxic effects include fatigue, dizziness, and ataxia. Carbamazepine may be beneficial for trigeminal neuralgia or diabetic neuropathic pain. No dose reduction is usually required in renal failure. Lamotrigine has not been studied in renal failure.

Antidepressants

Tricyclics have analgesic effects at low doses, acting synergistically with opioids. They are metabolized in the liver, and accumulation of metabolites in renal failure may lead to side effects (dry mouth, drowsiness, hypotension). Start with the lowest available dose (e.g., amitryptiline 10 mg qhs, increasing to 50 mg as required) and titrate up slowly. Avoid higher doses, as this produces more side effects with little additional benefit.

Steroids

Steroids may be useful for inflammatory pain and/or spinal cord compression. Side effects limit their long-term use.

Bisphosphonates

These drugs may have a role in chronic bone pain (especially myeloma).

Patient-controlled analgesia (PCA)

A pump provides a continuous IV infusion of opioid, with the patient able to self-administer a controlled extra bolus dose.

- Although many of the drugs (e.g., fentanyl) are thought to be metabolized and inactivated by the liver, in practice, opiate narcosis remains a real problem.
- With severe renal failure or dialysis dependence, omit the basal infusion and allow the patient to give controlled bolus doses.
- Observations should be frequent and directed to excluding opiate narcosis.

PCA can also be given by the epidural route, when a combination of fentanyl and a local anesthetic may be useful. As with IV PCA, avoid basal infusions.

Opioids in renal failure

Opioids act on the endogenous endorphin receptors in the CNS, leading to their narcotic and analgesic effects. As GFR falls, opioid clearance falls, and the dose of opioid should be reduced. Titration is necessary against patient symptoms and side effects. In general, as with all patients, start with a low dose and titrate upward.

Choice of opioid in renal impairment

Tramadol acts both centrally and peripherally. $t_{1/2}$ is ~ doubled (from 5 hours to 10) in severe renal failure. The maximum recommended dose in these patients is 50 mg bid—watch for side effects.

Codeine should be used with caution—it may cause prolonged CNS depression.

Fentanyl is well-tolerated (it can be given as a transdermal patch, but not orally). It is not well dialysed (protein bound, large volume of distribution), so toxicity may be difficult to reverse rapidly. Avoid starting an opioid-naïve patient on a patch as there is risk of toxicity.

Hydromorphone appears to be relatively safe and well-tolerated.

Methadone also appears to be relatively safe, but should be prescribed by someone with experience of using the drug. With all of these drugs watch for slow accumulation of metabolites and associated toxicity.

Morphine and oxycodone may be associated with more side effects (accumulation of metabolites). For morphine start with 25% of the usual dose and titrate upward. Oxycodone should be started at 5 mg orally every 6 hours.

Opiate narcosis in the renal patient

Accumulating opiates and opioid metabolites offer a significant risk to patients with CKD and particularly ARF or ESRD. Patients are often unwell and may even be septic—as such, the side effects of opiates may lead to clinical deterioration. This is a particularly common problem in patients stepped down off the ICU with recovering (but not recovered) ARF, or ESRD.

Signs
- Disorientation and confusion → coma
- Nausea and vomiting
- Constipation
- ▶ Pin-point pupils
- Impaired swallow with risk of aspiration
- Respiratory depression → hypoventilation ± arrest
- Hypotension (and worsening of tissue perfusion)

Be particularly wary of opiate use in the elderly, as they are susceptible to opioid side effects and are likely to have unrecognized ↓GFR.

Treatment
- Sit up and administer face mask O_2.
- If patient has a depressed level of consciousness, secure airway.
- Use IV naloxone 400–800 μg as a bolus. If there is a response (usually the patient "wakes up"), consider infusion as 10 mg in 50 mL 0.9% NaCl starting at 0.5 mL/min, titrating up or down against response.
- ⚠ Many opiates have a long $t_{1/2}$: expect narcotized patients to deteriorate again until drug is removed.
- This may (and often does) require HD.

Poisoning and dialysis

While poisoning (either deliberate or accidental) is common, the need to use dialysis to clear poorly excreted poisons is rare (<1% of all poisonings). Poisonings that lend themselves to extracorporeal therapies are those in which
- toxic effects are severe ± dangerous or potentially irreversible if not treated;
- elimination is quicker via dialysis, or only possible by dialysis (for example if renal or liver failure is present);
- the poison ± its metabolites can be removed by dialysis.

Characteristics of a drug amenable to removal by dialysis are as follows:
- Low molecular weight
- Relatively small degree of protein binding
- Low volume of distribution
- Polar molecule (water soluble).

Dialysis techniques
- The goal is to remove as much of the drug or toxin as possible. Therefore, a dialyser with a large surface area, high pump speeds, and a long dialysis session (4–6 hours or more) are usually recommended. If renal failure is also present, dialysis disequilibrium (📖 p. 128) is a danger and a shorter or gentler dialysis should be prescribed.
- Hemoperfusion may be helpful for some substances not removed efficiently by dialysis (▶ severe cases of phenytoin or digoxin overdose, or paraquat poisoning: blood is passed over a charcoal or polystyrene resin adsorbent and then returned to the circulation). The offending drug is adsorbed onto the charcoal or resin. This technique is not available except in specialist centers.
- Peritoneal dialysis provides much slower clearance and is not recommended in acute poisoning.

Drugs/toxins for which hemodialysis may provide benefit

Lithium (📖 p. 606)
Salicylate (📖 p. 606)
Ethylene glycol (📖 p. 608)
Methanol (📖 p. 609)
Theophyllines
Barbiturates (rare, for severe coma)

Lithium and salicylate poisoning

Lithium
Lithium is an effective treatment for affective disorders. It has a narrow therapeutic window. Blood levels should be measured regularly.
- Toxic effects
  - Nephrogenic diabetes insipidus (📖 p. 523) presenting as polyuria and dysnatremias—lithium may down-regulate aquaporin production.
  - Goiter—check TSH, though usually this remains normal.
  - Acute toxicity causes neuromuscular irritability (tremor, twitching), confusion, and drowsiness.
- Lithium excretion mirrors that of Na^+. Freely filtered, lithium is predominantly reabsorbed in the proximal convoluted tubule (PCT); ~20% is excreted in the urine.
- Lithium accumulation may occur whenever the GFR drops (hypovolemia, NSAID use, diuretics or ACEI therapy).
- Long-term lithium use may be associated with chronic renal impairment, though evidence of causation is limited.
- With progressive renal impairment, it *may* be necessary to stop the lithium. If GFR is declining slowly, it may be more in a patient's interest to continue the drug if well-controlled.

Treatment of lithium intoxication
- Assess severity—signs of neuromuscular toxicity, measure lithium level. Measure renal function.
- Fluid resuscitation—correct hypovolemia. Use 0.9% NaCl ± 0.45% NaCl (if hypernatraemic) to increase UO and maximize renal excretion.
- Hemodialysis removes lithium effectively. Use high pump speed and large membrane for 4–6 hours. Indications for hemodialysis:
  - Lithium level >4 mEq/L
  - Lithium level >2.5 mEq/L with severe symptoms ± ↓ GFR
- Rebound in lithium levels may occur as lithium moves from the intracellular to extracellular space. Recheck lithium levels 6 hours later and give further dialysis if necessary.

Salicylates
Aspirin (acetylsalicylic acid) is rapidly converted to salicylic acid after absorption. It is normally highly protein bound (>90%) and broken down by the liver. Only a small fraction is excreted unchanged by the kidney.

In overdose
- 10–20 g of aspirin may be fatal in an adult.
- If gastric emptying is delayed, peak levels occur hours after ingestion.
- Direct stimulation of the respiratory center → overventilation and *initial* respiratory alkalosis.
- Cellular injury → ↑ anion gap metabolic acidosis.

Symptoms and signs
Symptoms correlate poorly with levels (especially in the elderly), but may include the following:
- Nausea, vomiting, and diarrhea
- Tinnitus, vertigo, and blurred vision
- Sweating and hyperthermia
- Pulmonary edema (increased vascular permeability)
- Confusion and cerebral edema, especially with severe acidosis (salicylate crosses the blood–brain barrier more easily if nonionized).

Once liver conjugation pathways are saturated, most of the clearance is by the kidney. As salicylates are highly protein-bound (and not filterable), secretion occurs via the PCT anion secretory pathway.

Treatment of salicylate intoxication

Exclude other drug ingestions. Urgent salicylate level:
- Therapeutic levels: <300 mg/L (2.2 mmol/L)
- Moderate toxicity: 500–750 mg/L (3.6–5.4 mmol/L)
- Severe overdose: >750 mg/L (5.4 mmol/L)

Obtain renal function profile (↑ or ↓K^+, ↓ HCO_3^-) and blood gas (early respiratory alkalosis, then ↑AG metabolic acidosis), lactate, glucose, LFT, CBC, ↑INR, ECG (?heart block), and chest X-ray (?noncardiogenic pulmonary edema).

 Monitor in ICU setting. Administer O_2 if necessary (avoid intubation if possible)—if needed (hypoxia), hyperventilate to generate alkalosis.
- Level >500 mg/L should prompt aggressive management.
- Gastric lavage up to 12 h after ingestion (delayed gastric emptying)
- Activated charcoal (50 g 4 hourly repeated x 2) may be effective.
- Optimize fluid status. Aim for urine output >100 mL/h (fluids below).
- Alkalinize urine (salicylate is more soluble at ↑pH). Give $NaHCO_3$ IV until urine pH > 7.5. Maintain u-pH using IV or oral $NaHCO_3$.
- Give IV glucose if there is CNS involvement, even if blood levels are normal (salicylates cause neuroglycopenia).
- Correct hypokalemia (allows effective urinary alkalinization).
- Repeat blood gases and salicylate levels every 2 hours until stable.
- Dialysis effectively removes salicylate. Use high pump speeds and large dialyser for 4–6 hours. Indications are:
  - Blood level >700 mg/L (5.1 mmol/L)
  - Renal impairment with toxic salicylate level (If GFR >50 mL/min, trial of aggressive medical therapy may be appropriate if symptoms are not severe. If levels don't fall, resort to dialysis without delay.)
  - Pulmonary edema (prevents use of bicarbonate)
  - Worsening neurological signs or cerebral edema
  - Worsening signs of toxicity despite aggressive medical management

Recheck blood level 2 hours after dialysis. Repeat dialysis may be required if levels rebound (due to delayed absorption).

Ethylene glycol poisoning

Antifreeze contains ethylene glycol (EG).
⚠ Ingestion of as little as 50 mL can be fatal.

EG is freely absorbed, and broken down in the liver by alcohol dehydrogenase in an energy-dependent manner to glycolic acid and then on to oxalic acid. Only a fraction of glycolic acid is metabolized to oxalic acid. It is tissue deposition of metabolites that causes renal failure and (long-term) neurological damage.

Symptoms and signs

▶ Patients may or may not confess to ingestion.
Acute symptoms and signs may include the following:
- Drowsiness, confusion, ataxia (⚠ as with alcohol intoxication)
- Seizures
- Unexplained ↑AG metabolic acidosis (caused by glycolic acid)
- Pulmonary edema and respiratory distress in severe cases
- Symptoms may present late (after several days) with unexplained renal failure and unexplained neurological signs (cranial nerve palsies, visual symptoms, generalized weakness).

Investigations

Blood gas: ↑AG metabolic acidosis with respiratory compensation (mainly glycolic acid, but lactate accumulation may also contribute to the acidosis).

▶ The degree of acidosis correlates with tissue injury and outcome.
Ethylene glycol level (may be normal if ingestion >12 hours before): severe toxicity occurs if >500 mg/L or 8 mmol/L. Check ethanol level if there is co-ingestion.

Get renal function profile, salicylate and acetaminophen levels (in case of co-ingestion), and urine microscopy for oxalate crystals. Check ↓Ca^{2+} (oxalic acid binds calcium to form crystals), LFT, CBC (↑↑WBC).

▶ ↑ Osmolar gap >10 mOsm/kg: measured serum osmolality (raised)—calculated osmolality (often normal, as [2 × Na^+] + urea + glucose)
Renal biopsy will show widespread oxalate crystal deposition.

Management

- Gastric lavage if <1 hour since ingestion
- If within 12 hours of ingestion, give *fomepizole*. It competes with EG for alcohol dehydrogenase receptor, preventing rapid accumulation of toxic metabolites, with $t_{1/2}$ of 14 hours. It has 8000x greater affinity for enzyme than ethanol. Current recommendations are as follows:
  - Load at 15 mg/kg IV.
  - Give maintenance dose 10 mg/kg every 12 hours × 4 doses, then ↑ to 15 mg/kg 12 hourly until EG <200 mg/L (3.2 mmol/L).
  - Fomepizole is dialyzable and dosing frequency should be increased to every 4 hours during HD.
  - ⚠ Many advocate substantially lower doses (perhaps only 25% of the above schedule).

ETHYLENE GLYCOL POISONING

- Ethanol infusion is an alternative (it has much greater affinity for alcohol dehydrogenase than EG), but less preferred due to intoxication and depressed level of consciousness. Monitor blood ethanol concentration every few hours. Aim for ethanol level of 10–15 mmol/L.
- Hemodialysis effectively removes EG and metabolites. It is indicated if there is
  - Suspected ethylene glycol ingestion
  - Presence of unexplained osmolal gap
  - Severe acidosis or neurological signs
  - ▶ *Always err on the side of early and prolonged HD.*
- Adjunct therapies include the following:
  - $NaHCO_3$ 1–2 meq/kg bolus for pH <7.3. Maintenance infusion: 133 meq of sodium bicarbonate in 1 L D5W and infuse at 150–200mL/h. Titrate infusion based on pH.
  - Maintain high urine flow rate with IV fluids to minimize risk of oxalate crystal deposition (care is needed if renal impairment is present).
  - Thiamine and pyridoxine may be beneficial: prevent conversion of metabolites into oxalate.

▶ Late presentations (no EG detected in blood) do not benefit from the above treatment. Management is supportive. Mortality is high, especially in those who present late.

Methanol poisoning

Methanol is contained in de-icing solutions and some varnishes.
⚠ 50 mL may be lethal.
Early signs of toxicity include:
- Confusion
- Headache
- Decreased vision
- May lead to coma

The eye is particularly susceptible. Edema of the retina may lead to permanent blindness, as hypoxia of the optic nerve results in demyelination. Demyelination of white matter in the brain may also occur. As with ethylene glycol, ↑AG metabolic acidosis with ↑ osmolar gap. Diagnosis is confirmed by the history and by measuring blood levels (in early stages). Management is similar to that of ethylene glycol poisoning, with similar indications for fomepizole or ethanol ± hemodialysis. In addition, IV folic acid may be of benefit.

Chapter 12

Appendices

The glomerulus *612*
Regulation of GFR *614*
Tubular function *616*
The proximal convoluted tubule *618*
The loop of Henle *620*
Solute transport in the loop *622*
The distal convoluted tubule *624*
The collecting duct *626*
Insertion of hemodialysis catheters *628*
Renal biopsy *634*
Preparing chronic kidney disease patients for surgery *638*
Plasma exchange *640*
Clinical practice guidelines *644*
Useful Web sites *648*

The glomerulus

Structure

Bowman's capsule is a pocket of epithelial cells that are in continuity with the epithelial cells of the PCT. Within Bowman's capsule are the following elements (see Figs 12.1A, 12.1B).

Capillaries: a knot of capillaries lined by endothelial cells. Blood flows in via the afferent arteriole and out via the efferent arteriole (for a capillary bed to have arterioles on both ends is unique in the circulation). Changes in afferent and efferent arteriolar tone are powerful ways of regulating blood flow and pressure within the glomerulus (📖 p. 614).

The glomerular basement membrane (GBM) consists of a matrix of type 4 collagen embedded with other connective tissue proteins. Part of the filtration barrier in the glomerulus (see Box 12.1), the GBM contains all mesangium and endothelium within, and all podocytes without.

Epithelial cells or podocytes attach to the GBM by specially adapted foot processes (hence the name *podocytes*). Interdigitating podocytes are separated from each other by *slit diaphragms*, the key mechanical and signaling barrier to filtration. Abnormal podocyte function is considered important to proteinuric nephropathies.

The relative contributions of each layer to the filtration barrier for proteins are unclear.

Mesangial cells are important regulating cells in the glomerulus. Most are derived from a smooth muscle lineage (and respond to similar stimuli). They are situated adjacent to the endothelium (within the GBM), and are active in signaling, recruitment of nonresident cells, and maintenance of vascular tone. Some mesangial cells are derived from macrophages and monocytes, and have phagocytic properties. Mesangial cell proliferation and activation occur in response to immune-mediated glomerular injury.

Box 12.1 Filtration within the glomerulus

Substances with a molecular weight <5000 Daltons are freely filtered (unless bound to albumin in the plasma). Larger molecules are partially filtered, the filtration fraction depending not just on size but also charge (negatively charged molecules have a lower filtration fraction than similarly sized cationic molecules). Albumin (MW 61000 D) is scarcely filtered normally by dint of its size and negative charge.

The glomerular filter comprises four levels:
- Endothelium
- The glomerular basement membrane
- The interpodocyte slit diaphragm

The slit diaphragm offers a mesh of interlocking proteins and lipids important in maintaining the barrier: nephrin, podocin, CD2AP, and podocalyxin all contribute. Podocyte dysfunction impairs both the slit diaphragm and foot process adhesion.

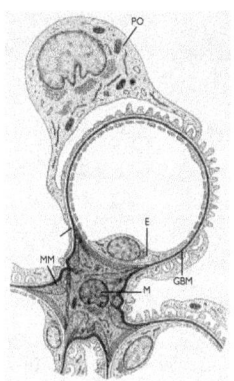

Fig. 12.1A Schematic demonstrating the filtration barrier. The glomerular capillary has a fenestrated endothelium (E). The capillary is surrounded by the glomerular basement membrane (GBM), which deviates to cover the mesangial cells (M). The interdigitating foot processes of the podocyte (PO), separated by slit diaphragms, cover the GBM and form the final barrier to filtration. MM, mesangial matrix Reproduced with permission from Davison AMA, Cameron JS, Grunfeld J-P, et al. (eds)(2005). *Oxford Textbook of Clinical Nephrology*, 3rd ed. Oxford: Oxford University Press.

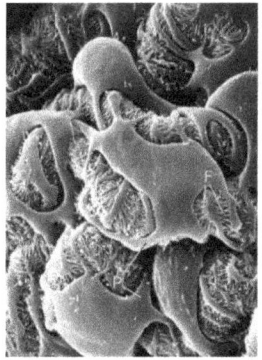

Fig. 12.1B Scanning electron microscopy of rat glomerular capillaries. The capillary is covered by branching podocytes. The primary (P) and secondary (F) processes interdigitate, separated by slit diaphragms, and cover the entire surface of the GBM. Reproduced with permission from Davison AMA, Cameron JS, Grunfeld J-P, et al. (eds)(2005). *Oxford Textbook of Clinical Nephrology*, 3rd ed. Oxford: Oxford University Press.

Regulation of GFR

GFR depends on
- Renal blood flow (RBF)
- Glomerular structure (Fig. 12.2; filtration surface area and permeability)
- Transglomerular capillary pressure (afferent–efferent tone; Box 12.2)
- Plasma oncotic pressure.

> **Box 12.2 Afferent and arteriolar tone**
>
> This controls intraglomerular pressure and flow:
> - Increased afferent arteriolar tone (vasoconstriction) leads to *reduced* flow and *reduced* pressure within the glomerulus.
> - Increased efferent arteriolar tone (vasoconstriction) leads to *reduced* flow and *increased* pressure within the glomerulus.
>
> Angiotensin II (AII) is a potent efferent arteriolar vasoconstrictor (with much weaker vasoconstrictor effects at the afferent arteriole). Thus high local or circulating AII levels raise intraglomerular filtration pressure → maintenance of GFR even if renal blood flow is reduced (hypovolemia, renal artery stenosis, etc.)—this is why ACEIs drop trans-glomerular capillary pressures.

Physiological regulation

Glomerulotubular balance is the process whereby a change (↑ or ↓) in GFR is compensated for by a corresponding change in absorption by the rest of the nephron (mechanism is poorly understood).

Autoregulation preserves glomerular blood flow with variations in systolic BP (local stretch receptors adjust afferent arteriolar tone).

Tubuloglomerular feedback (TGF) allows tubular flow sensing to change GFR: Cl^- delivery to the juxtaglomerular apparatus at the macula densa is sensed. ↑Cl^- delivery distally → afferent arteriolar vasoconstriction, thus ↓GFR (mediators include adenosine, thromboxane, NO, and AII). The importance (and beauty) of this mechanism can be appreciated if large quantities of Cl^- (and thus Na^+) are pathologically delivered to the distal tubule (e.g., nonoliguric ATN). By TGF, ↓ renal blood flow ensures ↓GFR, preventing profound sodium loss and volume depletion.

Systemic factors The sympathetic nervous system (noradrenalin, or norepinephrine) affects vasoconstriction of the afferent arteriole. Thus, in systemic hypotension (↑ sympathetic activity), renal blood flow is reduced (allowing blood to be diverted to the brain and heart). Noradrenalin also stimulates production of renin and AII. AII, with its vasoconstrictive effects at the efferent arteriole, serves to maintain GFR as much as possible in these circumstances. Vasodilatory prostaglandins are also important in these circumstances in maintaining GFR (⚠ hence avoid NSAIDs when renal blood flow is compromised).

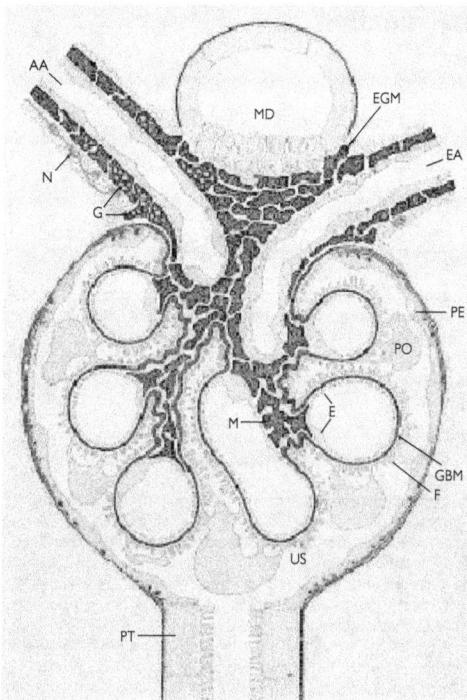

Fig. 12.2 Diagram of a longitudinal section through a glomerulus. Blood enters via the afferent arteriole (AA) and leaves via the efferent arteriole (EA). The capillaries have a fenestrated endothelium (E). The visceral epithelium of Bowman's capsule consists of podocytes (PO), the foot processes (F) of which (with the GBM) cover the capillaries and the mesangium (M). At the vascular pole the visceral epithelium reflects into the parietal epithelium (PE), which itself becomes the proximal tubule (PT) at the urinary pole. US, urinary space. At the vascular pole the juxtaglomerular apparatus is made up of the following:

- Extraglomerular mesangial matrix (EGM) and mesangial cells
- The terminal portion of the AA containing granular cells (G), containing sympathetic nerve terminals (N)
- The efferent arteriole
- The macula densa (MD).

Reproduced with permission from Davison AMA, Cameron JS, Grunfeld J-P, et al. (eds) (2005). *Oxford Textbook of Clinical Nephrology*, 3rd ed. Oxford: Oxford University Press.

Tubular function

The tubules
- Reabsorb most of the filtrate (mainly the proximal convoluted tubule [PCT]).
- Regulate salt and water balance (loop, distal tubule [DT], and collecting ducts [CD])
- Regulate acid–base balance in the body (DT and CD)

The tubule is divided into discrete sections.

Proximal convoluted tubule
- This reabsorbs the bulk of sodium, chloride, bicarbonate, glucose, amino acids, urate, and water (see Table 12.1).
- The "average" PCT is ~14 mm long and offers a large surface area (due to the villous-like arrangement at the apical surface of epithelial cells). The normal kidney contains around 1,000,000 glomeruli, equating to a potential surface area for reabsorption of >50 m^2. The PCT is able to reabsorb up to 60% of the 24,000 mmol of Na^+ and 160 L of water filtered per day.

The loop of Henle
- The loop dives deep into the renal medulla and then back out into the cortex.
- Capillaries serving the loop accompany the loop, enabling a counter-current exchange of urea and electrolytes to exist (p. 622). This helps perpetuate the hypertonic extracellular medium in the medulla, crucial for water homeostasis.
- The loop is divided into thin and thick limbs. The thick (ascending) limb contains cells rich in mitochondria, reflecting the active transport of electrolytes that occurs in these cells.
- The osmotic gradient is maintained by the thick ascending limb, which is impermeable to water but reabsorbs sodium and allows urea to diffuse into the interstitium.
- Filtrate is concentrated in the descending limb by egress of water into the extracellular space and capillaries down an osmotic gradient.

Distal convoluted tubule (DCT) and collecting duct (CD)
- The DCT is responsible for 5% of sodium reabsorption, and is important for urinary dilution and regulation of calcium excretion (PTH).
- The CD is the main regulating site for sodium, potassium, and hydrogen excretion (p. 624).
- Changes in permeability of the CD allow the formation of a concentrated urine (controlled by ADH).

Table 12.1 Sites of reabsorption of the major ions in the nephron (%)

	Na$^+$	K$^+$	HCO$_3^-$	Ca^{2+}
PCT	60	65	80	70
Loop	30	30	10–15	20
DT and CD	0–10	0–5	0–5	10

The proximal convoluted tubule

Sodium/potassium ATPase
- This plays a prime role in tubular reabsorption.
- It is situated on the basolateral membrane (i.e., the capillary side) of the tubular epithelial cell.
- Three Na^+ ions are pumped out of the cell into the capillary network by an active (ATP-requiring) process, in exchange for 2 K^+ ions.
- It maintains a low intracellular Na^+ concentration (20–30 mmol/L). The Na^+ concentration gradient between the tubular fluid and the intracellular compartment helps drive reabsorption of Na^+, other solutes, and water from the urinary space.
- Intra- and extracellular K^+ concentrations are maintained by specific K^+ channels that allow potassium to be extruded from the cell (down a concentration gradient) in a regulated fashion.

Sodium and chloride
- In the early part of the PCT, most sodium is reabsorbed via specific transporters (Fig. 12.3). Na^+ reabsorption is coupled with absorption of glucose and organic molecules. A further transporter exchanges Na^+ with H^+ ions (see below). The energy for these processes comes from the sodium gradient into the cell, itself generated by Na/K ATPase.
- The gap junctions between the cells are slightly leaky. Chloride (an excess is generated when sodium is absorbed with other anions or molecules) is reabsorbed by this route, as is water.
- Late in the PCT, most of the Na^+ is reabsorbed along with Cl^- Fig. 12.4). Na^+ and H^+ are exchanged. Cl^- is exchanged for another base, e.g., formate, bicarbonate, oxalate. This base is then reabsorbed along with H^+ and thus forms a shuttle, the net result being reabsorption of NaCl. Cl^- leaves the cell in exchange for K^+ or HCO_3^-, or via specific chloride pumps.

Potassium is mostly reabsorbed in conjunction with water via the paracellular space down a concentration gradient.

Bicarbonate Carbonic anhydrase in the PCT cells and on the luminal cell surface allows one HCO_3^- ion to be reabsorbed for every H^+ ion excreted. ▶ *Thus, H^+ excretion is equivalent to HCO_3^- reabsorption.* In the PCT, H^+ is exchanged for Na^+. HCO_3^- leaves the cell into the interstitium in exchange for Cl^- or in combination with Na^+

Calcium undergoes paracellular reabsorption, down a concentration (and charge gradient).

Phosphate is cotransported into the cell along with Na^+. It is inhibited by PTH.

Glucose, amino acids are cotransported into the cell along with Na^+.

THE PROXIMAL CONVOLUTED TUBULE **619**

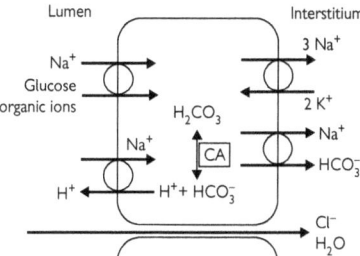

Fig. 12.3 Major pathways of solute reabsorption in the early part of the PCT. Adapted with permission from Greger R (1999). New insights into the molecular mechanism of the action of diuretics. *Nephrol Dial Transplant* **14**: 536–40.

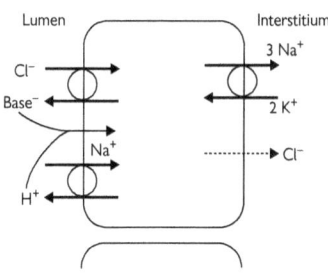

Fig. 12.4 Major pathways of solute reabsorption in the late part of the PCT. Adapted with permission from Greger R (1999). New insights into the molecular mechanism of the action of diuretics. *Nephrol Dial Transplant* **14**: 536–40.

The loop of Henle

The countercurrent exchange mechanism
- The loop dives deep into the medulla and then back up to the cortex.
- The thick ascending limb of the loop is impermeable to water. Na^+ (with K^+ and 2 Cl^-) is actively pumped from the lumen. The result is a decrease in the osmolality of the luminal fluid and an increase in the osmolality of the interstitium (see Fig. 12.5).
- The medullary blood supply functions as a countercurrent—blood flows down into the medulla via the vasa recta and then back up in a hairpin arrangement to the cortex. Countercurrent exchange perpetuates the hypertonicity of the interstitium.
- The descending limb of the loop is permeable to water but not to Na^+. Thus water flows down an osmotic gradient into the concentrated milieu of the interstitium. The effect is a concentration of the luminal fluid, so that at the deepest part of the loop the luminal and interstitial osmolality reaches up to 1200 mOsm/kg.
- Urea also contributes to the osmolality of the medullary interstitium. Diffusion of urea from concentrated urine into the urea-permeable CD helps generate and maintain the hyperosmolality of the inner medulla.

Concentrating and diluting the urine
Tubular fluid leaving the loop and entering the DT is hypotonic, as a result of active transport of NaCl out of the lumen (~200 mOsm/kg, compared with plasma ~285 mOsm/kg). Fluid passes down the collecting duct, through the medulla to the renal pelvis. In the absence of ADH, the CD is impermeable to water. Thus the urine remains hypotonic (dilute). ADH makes the CD permeable to water: with ADH, urine can achieve the same osmolality as that of the inner medulla (~1200 mOsm/kg).

Antidiuretic hormone (ADH)

ADH is released by the posterior pituitary in response to rising plasma osmolality and/or significant hypovolemia. It stimulates thirst, systemic vasoconstriction (V_1 receptors), and in the kidney (via V_2 receptors)
- Conserves water by stimulating water reabsorption in the collecting tubule, thus generating a concentrated urine. The CD becomes permeable to water by the translocation of specific water channels (aquaporin 2) to the apical membrane.
- Increases permeability of inner CD to urea (via the UT-A1 transporter), thus increasing the osmolal gradient in the inner medulla.

High plasma osmolality → ADH release → binds V_2 receptors → aquaporin 2 translocated → ↑ permeability of CD to water → ↑ urine osmolality up to that of the inner renal medulla (~1200 mOsm/kg).

Low plasma osmolality → ADH release suppressed → no aquaporin 2 translocation → CD impermeable to water → ↓ urine osmolality as low as that of tubular fluid entering the cortical CD (~200 mOsm/kg).

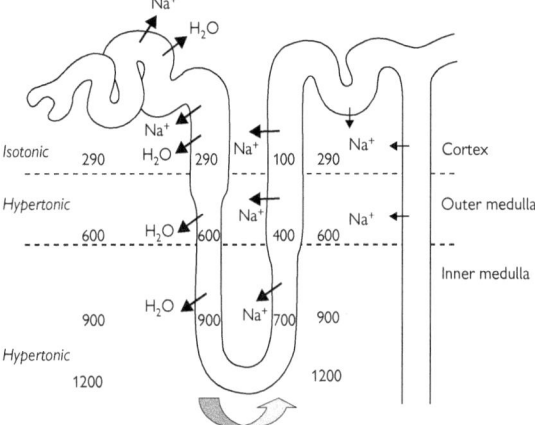

Fig. 12.5 Countercurrent multiplication by the loop of Henle. The thin descending limb is water permeable. The tubular fluid becomes hypertonic (the interstitium is hypertonic). In the ascending limb NaCl is absorbed (via the NaKCC pump) without water, rendering an osmotic gradient of 200 mOsm/kg at any given level. Countercurrent flow in the two limbs of the loop multiplies this gradient longitudinally. The result is a hypertonic interstitium in the inner medulla (urea also contributes to this hypertonicity—see text).

Thus fluid entering the distal tubule is hypotonic. Further Na reabsorption in the distal tubule can make the fluid still more hypotonic. If ADH is not present the CD is impermeable to water and a dilute urine is passed. If ADH is present the CD becomes permeable to water, and the urine becomes hypertonic as it passes through the medulla. All units are mOsm/kg.

Reproduced with permission from Davison AMA, Cameron JS, Grunfeld J-P, et al. (eds) (2005). *Oxford Textbook of Clinical Nephrology*, 3rd ed. Oxford: Oxford University Press.

Solute transport in the loop

The loop
- reabsorbs ~30% of filtrate;
- reabsorbs relatively more NaCl than H_2O, thus generating hypotonic fluid in the lumen, essential for production of a dilute urine;
- helps generate the countercurrent exchange mechanism and hence hypertonicity in the medullary interstitium (p. 621), essential for the production of a concentrated urine.

The loop is divided into
- The descending limb
- The thin ascending limb
- The thick ascending limb

The descending limb is impermeable to sodium. Water moves into the interstitium down the osmotic gradient (p. 621). The result is a high luminal Na^+ and Cl^- concentration.

Solute transport is passive in the thin ascending limb. Na^+ and Cl^- move into the interstitium down a concentration gradient.

In the thick ascending limb, the key transporter is the NKCC cotransporter (see Fig. 12.6):
- NaCl transport without water movement (the thick ascending limb is impermeable to water) allows the loop to generate hypotonic luminal fluid and hypertonic interstitial fluid. This is the fundamental basis of the countercurrent mechanism.
- The energy for this process is derived from the sodium gradient into the cell and, hence, ultimately from Na/K ATPase.
- K^+ is recycled into the lumen via a specific channel (ROMK channel), ensuring its availability and generating a net positive luminal charge.
- This positive charge drives reabsorption of cations across the paracellular junction, including Ca^{2+}, Mg^{2+}, NH_4^+, and (more) Na^+.

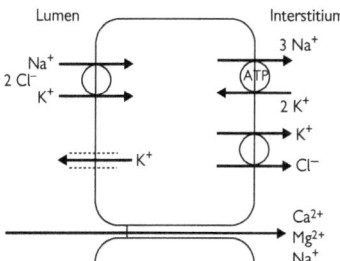

Fig. 12.6 Transport mechanisms in the thick ascending limb of the loop of Henle. The NKCC cotransporter is the key. Potassium can "leak" back into the lumen via the ROMK channel, rendering the lumen positively charged. This charge gradient facilitates passive reabsorption of Ca^{2+}, Mg^{2+}, and more Na^+ via the paracellular junction.

The distal convoluted tubule

The fine-tuning of reabsorption occurs in the distal nephron. The total absorptive capacity of the DCT and CD is not large. Thus mechanisms exist to prevent overdelivery of solute, which would flood the capacity.

The distal tubule is impermeable to passive movement of NaCl (except via specific channels) and water (ADH does not affect water absorption). This allows large-concentration gradients to develop when necessary.

Sodium

Approximately 5% of the filtered Na^+ is reabsorbed in the DCT. The NCCT cotransporter is the major route (Fig. 12.7). Some further Na^+ is absorbed by Na^+/H^+ exchange, and some further Cl^- by Cl^-/HCO_3^- exchange (H^+ and HCO_3^- then combine in the lumen to form CO_2 and H_2O—the CO_2 can be reabsorbed and recycled). The energy for the action of the NCCT cotransporter is derived from Na/K ATPase, and the resulting gradient aids Na^+ reabsorption into the cell.

Calcium

Calcium is absorbed via a specific epithelial Ca^{2+} channel. Reabsorption is partly controlled by PTH and calcitriol.

Thiazide diuretics block the NCCT cotransporter. They also stimulate the pathway for Ca^{2+} absorption (mechanism unknown), thus reducing calcium excretion in the urine.

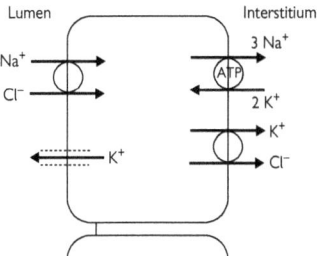

Fig. 12.7 Distal convoluted tubule sodium and chloride reabsorption occurs predominantly via the NCCT cotransporter.

The collecting duct

The vital role of this segment in control of water absorption is discussed elsewhere (📖 p. 620).

From 2% to 3% of the total filtered load is reabsorbed. Two types of cells are important.

Principal cells (~65% of cells)

Sodium

Reabsorption occurs via a specific Na^+ transporter, the epithelial sodium channel (ENaC) (Fig. 12.8). Although only ~3% of filtered Na^+ is reabsorbed by these cells, this is the main site of body Na^+ regulation (aldosterone mediated). Energy is derived from Na/K ATPase. In contrast to mechanisms of Na^+ reabsorption higher in the nephron, it is not the concentration gradient that drives Na^+ from the lumen into the cell (the luminal Na^+ concentration may be as low as 5mEq/L, significantly lower than the intracellular concentration). The system relies instead on a charge gradient: Na/K ATPase, in pumping K^+ out of the cell, generates a net negative charge within the cell. Na^+ flows down this charge gradient into the cell via ENaC. Tubular fluid becomes negatively charged, allowing Cl^- to move across the paracellular junction.

Control of Na^+ excretion

Aldosterone, after binding its mineralocorticoid receptor, increases the number of open ENaC channels, thus regulating Na absorption (and excretion). Increased intracellular Na concentration is another stimulus (with aldosterone) to increased Na/K ATPase activity.

Atrial natriuretic peptide (ANP) also acts on these channels, with ↑ANP → inactivation of ENaC. ENaC activity may also be affected by Na^+ delivery (↓delivery → ↑ENaC activity, reducing Na^+ loss in the urine, thus helping prevent volume depletion). *ADH* may also be important, increasing ENaC activity and numbers. Locally produced *PGE2* also plays a role, decreasing ENaC activity.

Potassium is secreted into the lumen via a specific aldosterone-sensitive K^+ channel, using the favorable charge gradient. High urinary flow rates maintain low intraluminal K^+ concentrations, allowing this channel to operate. Hence hypovolemia can → hyperkalemia.

Amiloride and tramterene block ENaC, thus reducing Na reabsorption and reducing K^+ excretion. Spironolactone inhibits the effect of aldosterone on its receptor, with similar effects on Na^+ and K^+.

Intercalated cells

These cells are important for acid–base homeostasis. Intercalated A cells contain an H^+ ATPase (activity is sensitive to aldosterone) transporting H^+ ions out of the cell into the lumen. Bicarbonate is then returned to the circulation in exchange for Cl^- ions via a cotransporter (see Fig. 12.9). The result is reabsorption of HCO_3^-. Intercalated cells also contain an H^+/K^+ ATPase, as H^+ is secreted into the lumen in exchange for K^+ reabsorption into the cell which is active when patients have hypokalemia.

Intercalated B cells have a Cl⁻/ HCO$_3^-$ exchanger on the apical membrane that excretes HCO$_3^-$ in exchange for Cl⁻ in the lumen. The basolateral side has the H⁺ ATPase.

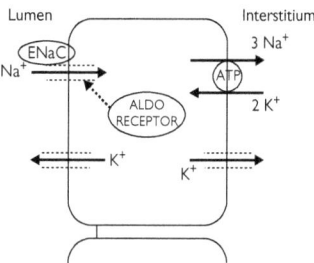

Fig. 12.8 The principal cell in the collecting tubule.

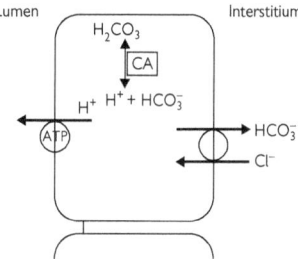

Fig. 12.9 Acid secretion in the intercalated cell in the collecting tubule. Na⁺/K⁺ ATPase is an alternative route for secretion of H⁺ into the lumen (not shown).

Insertion of hemodialysis catheters

Indications
Temporary hemodialysis catheters should be temporary—ideally no line should be in situ for longer than a 7 days. The risk of infection increases significantly if a line remains in place for longer—switch to a tunneled line if continuing access is required.

Routes of insertion
- The right internal jugular vein is the preferred route. It is superficial, easy to cannulate (in a "virgin" neck), and joins the SVC in a straight line. The left internal jugular is an alternative, but the guidewire and the line have to curve in order to reach the SVC. The risk of malposition and malfunction (and perforation of the vein) is greater.
- The femoral veins are suitable for short-term use and may be the safest and quickest option in an emergency.
- The subclavian route should be avoided: there is a high risk of central venous stenoses, potentially rendering the ipsilateral arm unsuitable for permanent access.

Pre-insertion
- Is the line really needed? Check that dialysis is required, that the patient is not suitable for a tunneled line (p. 632).
- Check CBC and PT, PTT.
- Obtain written consent from the patient (verbal and/or family member if in extremis). Consent should be obtained by the operator. Warn patient about potential complications:
  - Failure to cannulate vein
  - Hematoma ± arterial puncture
  - Pneumo/hemothorax (internal jugular [IJ] insertion)
  - Catheter malfunction
  - Infections
- Equipment: You will need the following:
  - An assistant
  - Sterile gown, gloves, drapes, and towels; iodine or chlorhexidine to clean the skin
  - Ultrasound probe to guide line insertion (if available)
  - Dressing pack with a supply of syringes, swabs, and needles
  - Sterile saline for injection
  - Lidocaine (1% or 2%): 10 mL
  - Line pack (if prepacked, this will contain an introducer needle, guidewire, and the line itself). Choose a shorter line (e.g., 16 cm) for the RIJ route, a longer line (e.g., 19 cm) for the left side or the larger patient.
  - Heparin (5000 units/mL) to lock the line once it is in situ
- Wash and dry hands as for a surgical procedure, wear sterile gown, mask, and sterile gloves.
- Position the patient slightly head down (for IJ insertion).
- Clean a wide area of skin around the insertion site. Lay out sterile drapes on all sides.

Tips for problematic line insertions

- Stop if your patient is in *pain*. Seek senior assistance. You might be directing the wire or line into trouble.
- Venous blood looks darker than arterial blood and does not fill a syringe with its own pressure: if in doubt, put a 5 mL syringe on either hub and see if it fills in a pulsatile fashion. If still in doubt, do a blood gas on the blood. ⚠ Don't take the line out yet (see below).
- Arterial puncture with an 18 gauge needle can usually be controlled by pressure for 5–15 min. If the larger introducer needle punctures the artery, it may be safest to abandon the procedure if possible or attempt an alternate location, i.e., femoral. Do not attempt the other side of the neck after significant arterial puncture and hematoma (risk of airway obstruction).
- ⚠ If an artery is accidentally cannulated (i.e., the line is inserted):
  - Check CBC, clotting, and X-match blood.
  - Confirm your concern by aspirating blood (if possible) from both lumens and, if necessary, check PaO_2. If you are unable to aspirate, you are in the *wrong* place.
  - Get a chest X-ray.
  - Monitor closely: BP, pulse, and O_2 sats.
  - Find out where the line is: use either CT or contrast examination to check where the tip is.
  - Once you confirm intra-arterial position, it is best to remove the line under controlled conditions with a vascular or thoracic surgeon available for back-up. Even with a normal quantity of platelets and normal PT/PTT you will need 30–45 min of direct pressure.

Insertion technique

- Establish anatomical landmarks and the planned point of cannulation (see Fig. 12.10).
- Ultrasound-guided insertion is now the technique of choice.
- Use an ultrasound device to compress vein and check for patency.
- Insert local anesthetic under the skin. Always attempt to aspirate before injecting lidocaine to avoid inadvertent IV injection.
- Once the needle is in the vein, use the Seldinger technique. Pass the guidewire through the needle (*there should be no resistance*—if there is do not force it. If the wire is past the needle, remove the wire and needle in tandom to avoid shearing off of wire and embolization). Remove the needle, leaving the guidewire in situ. Use a No. 11 scalpel blade to make a nick in the skin. Pass the dilator over the guidewire until it is in the vein. Remove the dilator, keeping the guidewire in position. Without delay pass the line over the guidewire until it is in position. Remove the guidewire.

Vein localization

Ultrasound-guided cannulation Most probes have a sterile disposable cover. Follow the manufacturer's instructions. After infiltration of local anesthetic, identify the vein with the probe. The introducer needle can be inserted with real-time guidance.

Blind insertion (IJ) The approach can be medial to the SCM muscle, between the two heads, or lateral to the muscle. Local practice and expertise will dictate the optimal route.

- Palpate the carotid artery with one hand (the left for a right-sided insertion).
- Insert the needle just lateral to the carotid pulse, aiming at 45° to the skin in the direction of the ipsilateral nipple. Aspirate gently on the syringe as you go until the vein is reached.
- If unsuccessful, withdraw the needle slowly (continuing with attempted aspiration—you may have gone through the vein). Then reinsert, varying the angle of insertion slightly to the medial side. If still unsuccessful, seek assistance from a more experienced operator.
- Once the vein is identified, pass the introducer needle down the same track in the same manner into the vein, palpating the carotid pulse at the same time.

- Check the flows in both lumens. A 20 mL syringe should fill easily with minimal aspiration. Flush both lumens with saline (which should also be easy), and then lock with heparin (5000 IU/mL). The priming volume will be written on the line (typically 1.3–2.0 mL/lumen). Put caps on the lumens, and suture the line in position.
- Arrange for a chest X-ray and look at it yourself: look for line position (tip should be in SVC for IJ lines) and look carefully to ensure that there is no pneumothorax.

Anatomical landmarks for internal jugular vein cannulation

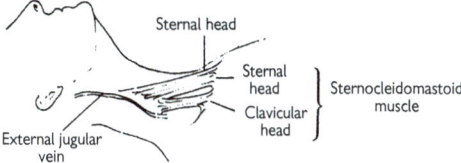

Fig. 12.10A Surface anatomy of external and internal jugular veins.

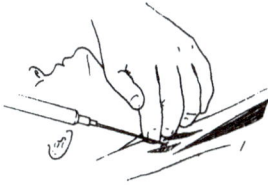

Fig. 12.10B Anterior approach: the chin is in the midline and the skin puncture is over the sternal head of the sternocleidomastoid muscle.

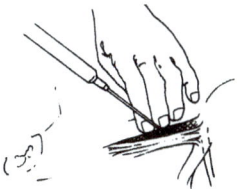

Fig. 12.10C Central approach: the chin is turned away and the skin puncture is between the two heads of sternocleidomastoid. Figure 12.10A–C reproduced with permission from Ramrakha P and Moore K (2004). *Oxford Handbook of Acute Medicine*, 2nd ed. Oxford: Oxford University Press.

Femoral line insertion

Advantages over neck line
- Superficial vein, usually easy to cannulate
- Relatively safe (hematoma can be controlled by pressure, no risk of airway obstruction or pneumothorax)
- No chest X-ray is required post-procedure (saving time in an emergency).

Disadvantages over neck line
- Renders the patient effectively bed-bound
- *There is a high risk of infection*—lines should only be left in for <7 days.

Insertion technique
- The technique is identical to that for neck line insertion. Ultrasound guidance should be used if it is available.
- Position the patient horizontally or with slightly feet down. The hips should be partially abducted. Shave the area if necessary.
- Use gown and gloves, skin preparation, and drapes as above.
- For the right femoral vein, the fingers of the left hand should be used to palpate the femoral pulse. Take care to remain below the inguinal ligament so that any hematoma can be controlled with pressure. The vein runs just medial to this. Infiltrate local anesthetic and try to identify the vein with an 18-gauge needle. Use the track of the 18-gauge needle to insert the introducer needle into the vein. Angle the introducer needle toward the head to facilitate passing of the guidewire.
- The remainder of the procedure is as for the internal jugular line (📖 p. 630).

Tunneled dialysis catheters
- The dual lumen line is inserted into the internal jugular vein (usually), with a subcutaneous tunnel. This acts as a barrier to infection. Tunneled catheters may be used as semi-permanent access while awaiting maturation of a fistula, or permanent access for the patient unsuitable for an AVF or PTFE graft. Long-term complications include poor flows (and thus inadequate dialysis), infection, and/or venous stenosis.
- Tunneled lines should be inserted by a trained operator, ideally with X-ray guidance to ensure the tip of the line lies in the SVC. Complications may arise as for any central-line insertion.

Renal biopsy

Despite improvements in other diagnostic techniques, renal biopsy retains a central role in nephrology.

Indications
- Unexplained acute or chronic kidney disease with normal renal size
- Histology likely to influence treatment
- Histology likely to offer prognostic information
- Information concerning the activity (and reversibility) or chronicity of a known lesion is desirable.

⚠ Renal biopsy is an invasive procedure. An evaluation of the risk/benefit ratio is needed in every case.

Preparation for renal biopsy
- Imaging: confirm two normal-size, unobstructed kidneys with normal parenchyma.
- BP <160/95; lower is better.
- Hb >10 g/dL
- Normal clotting and platelet count
- Antiplatelet agents stopped ~7 days prior to procedure
- Sterile urine
- Informed consent
- If there is renal impairment, the risk of bleeding increases ~2- to 3-fold.

Contraindications
- CKD with small kidneys
- Multiple cysts
- Suspected renal tumor
- Hydronephrosis
- Urinary infection
- Uncontrolled hypertension
- Bleeding tendency
- Uncooperative patient
- Solitary kidney*.

---

* Not an absolute contraindication.

Technique

Renal biopsy is performed percutaneously under local anesthesia, via a posterior approach. Ultrasound is used to locate the kidneys, determine their size, and identify cysts. Either kidney may be biopsied. The lower pole reduces the risk of piercing a major vessel. Real-time imaging can be used with or without a guide device to direct the needle directly to the kidney, though a minority may favor a non-real-time technique once the kidneys have been marked on the surface. CT guidance is a useful alternative when visualization is inadequate with ultrasound, e.g., with obesity. The patient is required to hold their breath when the needle enters the kidney. Disposable TruCut® needles or spring-loaded biopsy devices are generally used. If possible, two cores of tissue are obtained to increase diagnostic yield. Routine processing includes light, immunofluorescence, and electron microscopy. The patient remains on bed rest with a good fluid intake for 12–20 hours (although many radiologic centers now perform biopsies as same-day cases) and is advised not to undertake heavy lifting or exercise for 2–4 weeks.

Open or laparoscopic renal biopsy

This type of biopsy is rarely considered if the percutaneous approach carries an unacceptable risk or has been unsuccessful. It allows direct visualization of the kidney and easier control of bleeding. This type may be of benefit in obese patients and when a coagulopathy prohibits other approaches. More tissue can be obtained. The risk of a GA may exceed that of a percutaneous biopsy.

Transjugular renal biopsy

A technique on loan from hepatology, this biopsy is usually performed by interventional radiologists. The renal capsule is ideally not punctured and the risk of perinephric bleeding may be reduced. High success rates have been demonstrated.

Complications of renal biopsy

- Pain (usually short-lived)
- Bleeding
  - Transient microscopic hematuria occurs in virtually all patients.
  - Macroscopic hematuria occurs in ~2%*, transfusion required, ~1%.
  - Capsular hematoma (pain, ↓ in Hb) occurs in ~2%. A large hematoma may compress the kidney and cause high renin hypertension.
- Arteriovenous fistula
  - ~10% on Doppler US. It is rarely symptomatic; it may cause persistent hematuria and hypertension.
- Incorrect tissue
  - Usually muscle, fat, liver, spleen
  - Colonic perforation
- Nephrectomy (0.1%)
- Death (0.1%)

* Treat with bed rest. Maintain a high urine flow with fluids to prevent obstruction and clot colic. Correct coagulopathy. If severe or persistent, consider arteriography ± embolization and possible surgical intervention.

The role of the renal biopsy

Microscopic hematuria (📖 p. 20)

Proteinuria

Non-nephrotic proteinuria (<3.5 g/24 h)

❧Many clinicians advocate a biopsy at modest levels of proteinuria to ensure potentially treatable lesions such as primary FSGS and membranous GN are not overlooked. Others argue that the benign prognosis of these conditions when proteinuria is below the nephrotic range make biopsy unnecessary. A fixed "cutoff" level of proteinuria is a compromise (e.g., routine biopsy if >1 g/24 h). Renal insufficiency weighs in favor of a biopsy.

Nephrotic-range proteinuria

Biopsy is generally recommended. There are two exceptions:
- Minimal change disease in childhood. Here a trial of steroids may be appropriate before biopsy.
- Diabetic nephropathy (❧ 📖 p. 438).

Acute nephritic syndrome

The desire to confirm the diagnosis and adapt treatment according to the type and severity of the renal lesion leads most clinicians to biopsy, even when the diagnosis is suggested by serological tests (e.g., anti-GBM positive).

Acute renal failure (📖 p. 70)

Chronic kidney disease
The most important determinants of the need for biopsy are as follows:
- Renal size. If <9 cm:
  - Technically more demanding
  - Histology is likely to show chronic irreversible changes (original insult may not be identifiable).
- Clinical context
  - May be sufficient for diagnosis—e.g., renovascular disease or diabetic nephropathy

Preparing chronic kidney disease patients for surgery

Any patient with chronic kidney disease is at higher risk for an operation. Therefore, extreme care should be taken when preparing patients for surgery.

Pre-admission
- Take a full history. Focus on cardiac and respiratory history, dialysis regime (if appropriate), and details about previous anesthesia. Get a drug history.
- Can the procedure be done under regional block (most upper-arm AVFs can and should be done this way)?
- Examination: listen for murmurs and bruits (carotids), examine peripheral pulses, check that lung fields are clear, assess volume status, measure BP (and check BP charts if available). The anesthesiologist will prefer a BP of <150/95.
- Investigations: CBC (? anemia that could be corrected preoperatively), renal function panel (?↑K^+), LFT, Ca^{2+}, ECG if there is any cardiac history (or any patient with ESRD), chest X-ray if patient is breathless or has abnormal signs. Obtain an echocardiogram if there is any new murmur or a suggestion of poor LV function.
- Coordinate surgery with the dialysis unit if the patient is on dialysis. Plan dialysis around the surgery (i.e., usually day before and day after).

On admission
- Repeat full physical examination including BP and volume status assessment.
- Protect access arm. Do not use for BP measurement, IV access, or phlebotomy.
- Send blood tests preoperatively, as well as renal function panel, CBC, PT, PTT, and T&C (if surgery carries risk of bleeding). The anesthesioligst will prefer a K^+ <5.5–6 meq/dL.

Postoperative care
- Avoid nephrotoxic drugs if the patient has residual renal function (e.g., NSAIDs, gentamicin), *especially if on peritoneal dialysis*.
- Ensure that adequate analgesia is given, but be aware of risks of opioid toxicity (p. 602).
- Check volume status and BP. If IV fluids are required, prescribe 1 L and then reassess the patient before prescribing more if there is oliguria.
- Measure electrolytes postoperatively in any patient with significant chronic kidney disease (depolarizing anesthetic agents → muscle K^+ release and may precipitate dangerous hyperkalemia in susceptible patients).
- If an AVF or PTFE graft has been placed, check for a thrill over the fistula and avoid any compression or blood tests in that limb.
- Consider ↓ or no heparin if HD is required.

Plasma exchange

This is a technique in which plasma is separated from the rest of the blood. There are two main methods: one by centrifugation (removing plasma by centrifuging the blood) and the other by filtration. Replacement fluid is usually a combination of albumin solution, saline, and fresh frozen plasma (FFP) (hence "plasma exchange"). See Fig. 12.11.

Indications

Conditions in which there is a pathological buildup of a protein in the plasma should lend themselves to treatment by plasmapheresis. Those for which the evidence is (relatively) strong are as follows:
- Anti-GBM disease (📖 p. 466)
- ANCA-associated vasculitis (certainly if there is associated pulmonary hemorrhage, possibly ♦* if there is severe acute renal failure (Cr >5.7 mg/dL) (📖 p. 458)
- HUS/TTP/TMA (📖 p. 402)
- Cryoglobulinemia
- Hyperviscosity syndrome
- Antibody-mediated rejection in transplant recipient.
- Catastrophic anti-phospholipid syndrome

Other conditions that are sometimes treated by plasmapheresis, though for which the evidence is not strong (♦*), are as follows:
- SLE (only for cerebral lupus or if very severe)
- Recurrent FSGS post-transplant
- Preparation of highly sensitized transplant recipients
- Myeloma with acute renal failure secondary to cast nephropathy
- Crescentic IgA nephropathy
- Nonrenal conditions include Guillain–Barré syndrome, myasthaenic crisis, and familial hypercholesterolemia.

Prescription

One plasma volume exchange will lower plasma levels of macromolecules by ≈60%. Exchanges on 5 consecutive days will achieve ≈90% reduction (some rebound occurs as macromolecules are released back into the circulation).

$$\text{Plasma volume} \approx 0.07 \times \text{Wt in kg} \times (1 - \text{hematocrit})$$

Replacement fluid should consist of a combination of the following:
- *Human albumin solution (5%)*: the predominant plasma protein. At least 50% of the replacement fluid should be albumin. More may be indicated if there is hypoalbuminemia.
- *Normal saline* is cheaper than albumin, but should make up no more than 50% of the replacement solution (usually 20%–40%).
- *Fresh frozen plasma* may be necessary to replace removed clotting factors, especially if there is a high risk of bleeding. Monitor clotting and adjust FFP appropriately. 2 U FFP (more if very high risk) during the last half hour of plasma exchange is an appropriate starting dose. Some conditions (e.g., HUS) require more FFP (📖 p. 401).
- *Anticoagulation*: is usually with heparin (usually 2× dose in HD, as heparin is removed during the process). Citrate is an alternative.

Complications
- Hypotension (usually volume related)
- Hypocalcemia is related to FFP use. Citrate binds calcium, reducing ionized calcium, so is a risk when FFP is used. Hypocalcemia can be prevented or treated by giving IV calcium e.g., 10–20 mL 10% Ca gluconate during the procedure.
- Clotting abnormalities: patients with a high risk of bleeding should receive more FFP and regular monitoring of clotting.
- Infection: risk is increased by IV access and associated immunosuppression but not, it appears, from plasmapheresis itself.

(a) Membrane plasma filtration

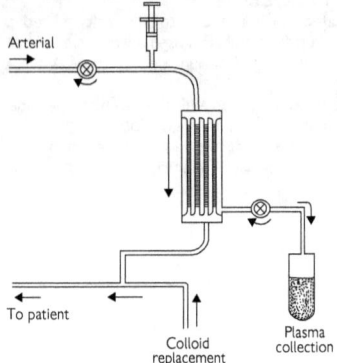

(b) Centrifugal cell separation

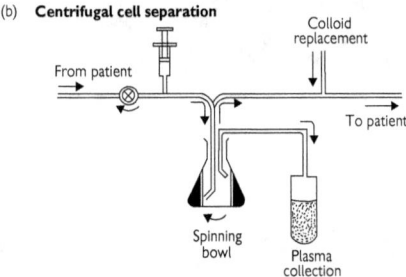

Fig. 12.11 Techniques of plasmapheresis. (a) Membrane plasma filtration: blood flow 100–150 mL/min. With a highly permeable membrane (MW cutoff 2000 kDa), most Igs are removed but some larger immune complexes and cryoglobulins may not be well cleared. Cells are returned to the patient, along with fluid replacement. (b) Centrifugation: plasma is removed by centrifugation using a spinning bowl. Blood is (synchronously or intermittently) returned to the patient, along with replacement fluid. There is no upper limit to the size of protein that can be removed. This can be performed via an antecubital vein. Reproduced with permission from Levy J, Morgan J, and Brown E (2004). *Oxford Handbook of Dialysis*, 2nd ed. Oxford: Oxford University Press.

Clinical practice guidelines

National and international standards (or clinical practice guidelines) outlining the expected level of care for renal patients have been set out by the Renal Association (in the UK), the Kidney Foundation Dialysis Outcomes Quality Initiative (K/DOQI) in the United States, and the European Best Practice Guidelines. See Tables 12.2–12.6.

These guidelines cover the following (among other things):
- Predialysis care
- Dialysis prescription and monitoring
- Vascular access preparation and care
- Anemia management
- Nutrition
- Management of renal bone disease
- Cardiovascular risk factor management
- Management of infection in dialysis patients.

Each of these standards documents makes slightly different recommendations in many of these areas, reflecting the fact that many of the derived standards are the result of expert and consensus opinion rather than good clinical-trial evidence.

These standards have informed the advice contained in this book and, in places, are quoted directly. The full standards documents can be accessed from the following Web sites:

Renal Association: www.renal.org

K/DOQI: www.kidney.org/professionals/doqi

European Best Practice Guidelines: www.ndt-educational.org/guidelines

▶ The Kidney Disease: Improving Global Outcomes (KDIGO) initiative was set up in 2003 with the aim of improving international dissemination and cooperation in the development of guidelines (www.kdigo.org). Many national and international standards documents can be accessed from this Web site.

Table 12.2 Guidelines: anemia management

	UK Renal Association	US K/DOQI
Target Hb (g/dL)	>10	11–12
Frequency of measuring Hb	Monthly for stable HD patients. 3–4 monthly for other stable patients on EPO. More frequently around time of dose adjustments	At least monthly
Assessing iron status	Ferritin >100 ng/mL and TSAT >20% (or <10% hypochromic red cells)	Ferritin >200 ng/mL and TSAT >20%
Frequency of monitoring iron status	At least every 6 months	Monthly if not stable, 3 monthly if stable (3–6 monthly if not on dialysis)
Monitoring of iron status	At least every 6 months	Monthly if not on IV iron, 3 monthly once stable. CKD patients not on EPO: 3–6 monthly

Table 12.3 Guidelines: calcium, phosphate, and PTH management

	UK Renal Association	K/DOQI
Serum phosphate (mg/dL)	<5.7 for nondialysis patients	Stages 3–4: 2.7–4.6 Stage 5 and dialysis: <5.5
Serum calcium (mg/dL)	8.8–10.4	Stages 3–4: within local normal range Stage 5: 8.4–9.5
Serum aluminum (µgl/L)	Every 3 months (HD and/or if on aluminum-containing preparations). DFO test if >60	Yearly, and every 3 months if on aluminum-containing preparations. DFO test if aluminum 60–200
PTH (pg/mL)	<4 × upper limit normal	Stage 3: 35–70 Stage 4: 70–110 Stage 5: 150–300

Table 12.4 Cardiovascular risk factors

	UK Renal Association	K/DOQI
BP	HD: <140/90 predialysis, <130/80 postdialysis PD and transplant recipients: <130/80 CKD patients: <130/80 (<125/75 if proteinuria)	<130/80
HbA1c in diabetics	<7%	<7 %
Lipids–indications for starting statin therapy	10-year risk of coronary disease >30%	Stage 5 CKD: LDL <100 mg/dL; fasting triglycerides <200 mg/dL, non-HDL cholesterol <130 mg/dL
Lipids–targets	Total cholesterol <5 mmol/L or 30% reduction from baseline or fasting LDL <3 mmol/L (whichever is greater)	Non-HDL cholesterol <130 mg/dL

Table 12.5 Nutrition

	UK Renal Association	K/DOQI
Serum albumin (g/dL)	If >3.5 (bromocresol green) or >3.0 (bromocresol purple) then investigate. No standard set	>4.0 g/dL (bromocresol green)
Serum bicarbonate (meq/L)	22–26 (HD), 25–29 (PD)	>22
Screening	BMI, serial weights, albumin, SGA	Serial weights, dietary interviews, nPCR, SGA

Table 12.6 Adequacy, access, and sepsis

	UK Renal Association	K/DOQI
HD		
eKt/V (for thrice-weekly dialysis)	>1.2 (or URR >65%), measured monthly	>1.2 (single pool), measured monthly
Vascular access	>67% patients presenting within 3 months of dialysis start date should commence with a native AVF	>50% of all new HD patients should have native AVF
	80% of prevalent HD patients should have native AVF	40% of prevalent HD patients should have native AVF
PD		
Weekly Kt/V	>1.7 and/or total weekly Cr clearance >50 L/week/1.73 m^2 (may be higher in APD or high transporters)	Weekly Kt/V >1.7
Peritonitis rate	<1 in 18 months	
Negative culture rate	<15%	
Initial cure rate	>80%	

Useful Web sites

Journals

Advances in Renal Replacement Therapy www2.arrtjournal.org
American Journal of Kidney Diseases www.ajkd.org
American Journal of Nephrology www.Karger.ch/journals/ajn/ajn_jh.htm
Journal of the American Society of Nephrology (JASN) www.jasn.org
Kidney International (KI)
www.blackwell-synergy.com/issuelist.asp?journal=kid
Lancet http://www.thelancet.com
Nephrology Dialysis Transplantation www.ndt.oupjournals.org
New England Journal of Medicine http://www.nejm.org
Transplantation www.centerspan.org/pubs/transplantation
Peritoneal Dialysis International www.multi-med.com/pdi

Associations

American Association of Kidney Patients www.aakp.org
American Nephrology Nurse Association www.anna.inurse.com
American Society of Nephrology www.asn-online.com
American Society of Transplantation www.a-s-t.org
Australia and New Zealand Society of Nephrology www.nephrology.edu.au
Australian Kidney Foundation www.kidney.org.au
European Kidney Patients' Federation www.ceapir.org
European Renal Association www.era-edta.org
International Society of Nephrology www.isn-online.org
International Society of Peritoneal Dialysis www.ispd.org
National Kidney Foundation www.kidneyorg
Kidney Research UK www.nkrf.org.uk
UK Renal Association www.renal.org
UK Renal Registry www.renalreg.com
US Renal Data Service (USRDS) www.usrds.org
Vascular Access Society www.vascularaccesssociety.com
World Kidney Fund www.worldkidneyfund.org

Miscellaneous

Atlas of Diseases of the Kidney www.kidneyatlas.org
Cybernephrology www.cybernephrology.org
K/DOQI guidelines www.kidney.org/professionals/doqi
Kidney disease community www.ikidney.com
Kidney school www.kidneyschool.org
Kidney patient guide www.kidneypatientguide.org.uk
Nephron information center www.nephron.com
Nephroworld www.nephroworld.com
Nephronline www.nephronline.com
RenalNet www.renalnet.org
Renal Web www.renalweb.com
Travel Dialysis Site www.dialysisfinder.com

Index

A

ACE polymorphisms 292
Acetazolamide 561
Acid–base 552
  Acidosis 160, 165
Acquired cystic disease 420
Activated clotting time (ACT) 220
Acute coronary syndrome (ACS)
  in CKD 195
Acute hemodialysis 128–9
  complications
    intradialytic hypotension 226–7
Acute interstitial nephritis (AIN) 404
  causes of 404
Acute kidney injury (AKI) 70, 71
Acute nephritic syndrome 636
Acute peritoneal dialysis 133
Acute pyelonephritis 425
Acute renal colic
  investigations 435
  symptoms and signs 435
  treatment 435
Acute renal failure (ARF) 69, 500
  acute hemodialysis 128–9
  acute tubular necrosis 100–1
  AKI classification 70, 71
  assessment
    blood work 84–5
    imaging and histology 90–1
    urinalysis 82
  clinical approach
    recognize problem 78
    reversible cause 79
  contrast-induced nephropathy
    contrast toxic 142
    precautions 142–3
  definition 70
  epidemiology 70–2
  hepatorenal syndrome
    classification 134
    clinical features 135
    diagnostic criteria 135
    hepatic and renal dysfunction combination 134
    management 136–7
    pathophysiology 134, 135
  incidence 71–2
  intrinsic renal ARF 74
    classification 98
    differential diagnosis 98
  ischemic ATN
    pathophysiology 102–3
  isotope study 90
  management
    checklist 104–5
    electrolytes and acidosis 114–15
    hyperkalemia 106–9
    myths 122–4
    nutrition 118–20
    pulmonary edema 112–13
    management of hyperkalemia 110–11
    strategy 116–17
  peritoneal dialysis 132–3
  postrenal ARF 74
  prerenal ARF 74
    causes 94–5
    hypoperfusion 92–3
    volume replacement 96–7
  prevention 76–7
  prognosis 72
  rapidly progressive glomerulonephritis and myeloma 86–8
  renal biopsy 91
  renal replacement therapy 126–7
  rhabdomyolysis
    causes 139
    clinical presentation 138
    investigations 138
    management 140–1
    myoglobin (Mb) 138
  RIFLE classification 70, 71
  in sepsis 146
    causes 146
    clinical findings 147
    kidney 147
    shock 146
  and septic shock
    definitions 148
    general priorities 148
    mean arterial pressure calculation 149
    renal priorities 149
  tumor lysis syndrome 144–5
    clinical findings 144
    investigations 144
    pre- and post-treatment 144
    treatment 124
  urine indices in 82
Acute tubular necrosis (ATN) 100–1
  presentation 100
  prognosis 101
Acyclovir 24, 481
Adefovir 481, 482
Adult dominant polycystic kidney disease (ADPKD) 416–19, 582
  complications of 418–19
    chronic kidney disease 418
    cyst hemorrhage 418
    cyst infection 418
    extrarenal cysts 419
    hypertension 418
    intracranial aneurysms 419
  manifestations 419
  nephrolithiasis 418
  investigations 417
  symptoms and signs 417
Adynamic bone disease (ABD) 176, 180, 193
  factors contributing to 181
Aetaminophen overdose 600
(AA) amyloidosis
  causes of 450
  management of 451
  secondary 450
African American Study of Kidney Disease and Hypertension (AASK) 326, 327
Anion Gap acidosis 554
AL amyloidosis
  management of 451
  primary 450
Albumin/creatinine ratio (ACR) 19
Albuminuria. See Proteinuria
Albustix® 17, 18

INDEX

Aldosterone 294, 626
  extrarenal actions of 294
Allopurinol 264
α-adducin polymorphisms 292
α-blockers 338, 355, 515, 581
  and ALLHAT 339
  and bladder outflow symptoms 339
  mechanism 338
  problems 338
  role 338
α-mercaptopropionylglycine 434
5-α reductase inhibitors 515
Alport syndrome 380
  and transplantation 381
Aluminum toxicity 183
Ambulatory BP monitoring (ABPM) 298–9
  potential indications 299
  reading and interpretation 299
Amenorrhea 4
Amiloride 334, 532, 538, 626
Amino acids 618
Aminoaciduria 65, 66
Aminoglycosides 537
  in renal failure 595
Amlodipine 340
Amorphous phosphates 24
Amyloid fibrils 451
  on renal biopsy 452
Amyloidosis (AA) 450
  secondary 476
Analgesia in renal failure
  pain control principles 600
Analgesic nephropathy 476
  investigations 408
  management 409
  papillary necrosis 409
  symptoms and signs 408
Anasarca 531
ANCA-positive vasculitis 458
  histology 458
  investigations 458
  symptoms and signs 458
  treatment of 460
    induction therapy 460
    maintenance therapy 460
    monitoring response and predicting relapse 461
  WG and MPA 459
    characteristics of 459
Androgen deprivation therapy for prostate cancer 518

Anemia 116, 160, 455
  of CKD 168–9
  dialysis and pregnancy 587
Angiography 45
Angiomyolipoma 508, 510
Angiotensin 293
Angiotensin I/type 1 (AT-1) receptor 292, 293
Angiotensin II/type 2 (AT-2) receptor 293, 295, 581, 614
Angiotensin II receptor blockers (ARBs)
  and ACEIs 345
  examples 344
  mechanism 344
  roles 344
Angiotensin-converting enzyme inhibitors (ACEIs) 355, 581, 596
  and ARBs 345
  examples 342
  mechanism 342
  problems 343
  role 342
Anglo-Scandinavian Cardiac Outcomes Trial (ASCOT) Study 326, 327, 331
  results 330–1
  significance of 331
Antegrade ureteropyelography 45
Anti-CD25 antibodies 265
Antidiuretic hormone (ADH) 521, 522, 530, 620
Anti-GBM (globular basement membrane) disease 61
  antibody for 86
  investigations 466
  pathogenesis 466
  pathology 466
  pulmonary hemorrhage treatment 467
  renal disease treatment of 466–7
  symptoms and signs 466
Antihypertensive and Lipid Lowering Treatment to Prevent Heart Attack Trial (ALLHAT) 326, 327
Anti-neutrophil cytoplasmic antibodies (ANCA) 86, 458, 459
Anti nuclear antibodies (ANA) 86
Anti-phospholipid antibodies 87
  in ESRD 473

Anti-phospholipid syndrome 472
  investigations 472
  symptoms and signs 472
  treatment 472
Anti-streptolysin O titers (ASO) 87
Anti-thymocyte globulin (ATG) 265
Anti-tuberculosis therapy 489
Anuria 63, 496, 500
Aorta coarctation of 317
Arginine vasopressin. See Antidiuretic hormone
Arterial stiffness 294
Arteriovenous fistula (AVF) 222
Atenolol 354, 581, 596
Atherosclerotic renal artery stenosis (ARAS) 410–11
  management of 412–13
    conservative 413
    control BP 412
    intervention 412–13
    prevent renal complications 412
Atrial natriuretic peptide (ANP) 296, 626
Autoimmune diseases
  assays against target antigens in 86
Automated peritoneal dialysis (APD) 230
  special considerations for 238
Autosomal recessive polycystic kidney disease (ARPKD) 420
Azathioprine 264, 265, 369, 370, 389, 470, 589

B

Bacteriuria 22
Balkan endemic nephropathy (BEN) 407
Baltimore longitudinal study 33
Bartter's syndrome
  treatment 538
Basiliximab 265
Benign prostatic hypertrophy (BPH)
  clinical features 514
  differential diagnosis 514
  investigations 514
  management 514–15
β-blockers 355, 581, 596
  examples 337
  mechanism 336
  problems 336
  role 336

β$_2$-microglobulin 32
Birmingham Vasculitis
  Activity Score (BVAS)
  461
Bisphosphonates 545
BK virus nephropathy
  278–9
  clinical assessment 278
  diagnosis 278
  treatment 278
Bladder cancer 512–13
Bladder irritability 64
Bladder outflow obstruction 67–8
  causes of 68
  examination 67
  investigations 67
Bladder outflow symptoms
  339
Bladder stones 431
Bleeding tendency of ARF
  116
Blood pressure. See also
  Hypertension
  in CKD 159
  JNC 7 classification of
    303
  lifestyle interventions for
    reduction 307
  measurement
    ambulatory BP
      monitoring 298–9
    clinic 298
    home 298
  and salt intake 291
Blood Pressure Lowering
  Treatment Trialists
  Collaborative
  (BPLTTC) 325
Brain natriuretic peptide
  (BNP) 296
Bumetanide 334, 533,
  596

C

Calcimimetics 188–9
Calciphylaxis 192–3
  definition 192
  incidence 192
  presentation 192
  risk factors 192
  treatment 192
Calcitonin 545
Calcitriol 542
Calcium channel blockers
  (CCBs) 355, 596
  examples 340
  mechanism 340
  problems 340–1
  putative BP-lowering
    mechanisms 336
  role 340

Calcium homeostasis
  in sarcoidosis 478
Calcium oxalate stones 24,
  430, 433
Calcium phosphate precipitation 144
Calcium phosphate stones
  24, 430, 434
Calcium sensing receptor
  (CaR) 188
  calcimimetic agents 188,
    189
  role 188, 189
Candesartan 344
Captopril 342
Cardiac drugs in renal
  failure 596–7
Cardiovascular disease
  in CKD
    acute coronary
      syndrome 195
    risk factors 194
Cardiovascular risk
  and microalbuminuria 50
Cardiovascular risk factors
  289
  lifestyle measures 307
Carvedilol 336, 596
Cast nephropathy 447
  specific treatment 448
Casts
  broad/waxy 23
  cellular 23
  epithelial cell 23
  fatty 23
  granular 23
  hyaline 23
  noncellular 23
  red cell 23
  white cell 23
Catecholamines 521
Cellulose acetate dialysis
  membrane 216
Central venous pressure
  (CVP) line 97
Cerebral salt-wasting 524
Chapel Hill classification
  of vasculitis 457
Chinese herb nephropathy
  407
Chlorambucil 391
Chlorthalidone 332
Cholesterol crystals 24
Cholesterol emboli
  414–15
Chronic allograft nephropathy (CAN) 272–3
  clinically 272
  histology 272
  prevention and treatment
    272–3
Chronic HD complications
  227

Chronic kidney disease
  (CKD) 58, 80, 418, 454,
  637
  anemia of 168–9
  antihypertensives in 159
  calcimimetics 188–9
  calciphylaxis 192–3
  cardiovascular disease in
    194–5
  complications of advanced
    acidosis 165
    fluid overload 164
    hyperkalemia 164–5
  definition 152
  diagnosis of
    BP importance 157
    identify patients 156
    proteinuria 156, 157
    screening 156
  diet and nutrition in
    198–9
    carbohydrate intake
      199
    fluid restriction 198
    phosphate restriction
      199
    potassium restriction
      199
    protein intake 198
    salt restriction 199
  eGFR for diagnosis and
    management 153
  endocrine problems
    202–3
  erythropoietin
    and kidney 168
    mechanism of
      production 169
    needs 170
    nonhematological
      effects of 170
    nonresponse 171
    preparation 170
  hyperphosphatemia
    184–5
  inflammation in 201
  iron stores and therapy in
    174–5
  malnutrition in 200–1
  NKF-DOQI classification
    152
  palliative treatment of
    advanced 204–6
  parathyroidectomy 190–1
  pathogenesis of
    causes 154
    mechanisms 154–5
  preparing patients for
    surgery
    on admission 638
    posoperative care 638
    pre-admission 638
  pretransplant 196–7

preventing progression
  blood pressure 159
    measurement 160
  progression of 158
renal bone disease
  classification 176
  clinical features 180–1
  definition 176
  high- and low-turnover features 177
  physiology 178–9
  treatment 182–3
uremia 166–7
vitamin D 186
Chronic malarial nephropathy 493
Chronic tubulointerstitial diseases 406–7
  Balkan endemic nephropathy 407
  Chinese herb nephropathy 407
  features 406
  investigations 406
  lead nephropathy 407
  lithium-induced nephropathy 406
Churg–Strauss syndrome 458, 462
  investigations 462
  symptoms and signs 462
  treatment 463
Chvostek's sign 542
Cidofovir 481
Cinacalcet 189, 544
Cirrhosis 533
Classical polyarteritis nodosa 464–5
  investigations 464
  management and history 464
  symptoms and signs 464
  treatment 464
Clinistix® 17
Clonidine 346
Clopidogrel 195, 596
Clot colic 500
Cockcroft–Gault (CG) 30
Collapsing glomerulopathy 395
Collecting duct 616
  principal cells
    intercalated cells 626
    Na$^+$ excretion control 626
  sodium 626
Colloids human albumin solutions 96
Complement-dependent cross-match (CDC) 253
Computerized tomography (CT) 42, 498–9

Congenital adrenal hyperplasia (CAH) 312
Conivaptan IV 526
Continuous ambulatory peritoneal dialysis (CAPD) 230
  technique 231
Continuous positive airways pressure (CPAP) 113
Continuous venovenous hemodiafiltration (CVVHF) 126, 127, 130, 149
Continuous venovenous hemodialysis (CVVHD) 126, 127, 130, 149
Continuous venovenous hemofiltration (CVVH) 126, 127, 130, 149
Contrast-induced nephropathy (CIN)
  contrast toxic 142
  precautions 142–3
Corticosteroids 507, 545, 589
Creatinine 584
  clearance 29
  formulas 30
  GFR measurement 32
  reciprocal 31
  serum creatinine 28
  urea 34
Crescentic GN 476
Cryoglobulinemia 484
Cryoglobulins 87, 485
Crystalloids 96
Cuprophan® 216
Cushing's syndrome 316
Cyclooxygenase (COX) 598
Cyclophosphamide 369, 370, 389, 391, 453, 460, 466, 470
Cyclosporine 369, 370, 392, 470
Cyst 508
  hemorrhage 418
  infection 418
Cystatin C 32
Cystic kidney diseases 420
  acquired cystic disease 420
  autosomal recessive polycystic kidney disease 420
  medullary cystic kidney disease 421
  medullary sponge kidney 421
  nephronophthisis 420
  simple cysts 420
Cystine crystals 24
Cystine stones 430, 434

Cystinosis 566
Cystinuria 566
Cystitis 423
  interstitial 426
Cystoscopy 426, 500, 512
Cysturethroscopy 46
Cytomegalovirus 276–7
  clinical features 276
  prophylaxis 276
  treatment 276
Cytotoxic drugs 4

D

Daclizumab 265
Darbepoetin-α 170
Demeclocycline 526
Dent's disease 566
Deoxyspergualin 461
Dermatomyositis 477
Diabetes 161
Diabetes Control and Complications Trial (DCCT) 438
Diabetes insipidus 530
Diabetes mellitus (DM) 438
Diabetic nephropathy (DN) 438–40, 582
  definition and epidemiology 438
  ESRD management of 444
    peritoneal dialysis versus hemodialysis 444
    renal transparent 444
    survival and cause of death 444
  management of 442–3
  natural history 439
  pathogenesis of 438
  pathology 439
  renal biopsy indication for 439
  renal disease in diabetic patients 440
Dialysate 214
Dialysis and pregnancy
  anemia 587
  diet calcium and vitamin D 586
  hemodialysis 586
  labor and delivery 587
  peritoneal dialysis 586
Dialysis disequilibrium syndrome 129
Diarrhea
  in hemolytic-uremic syndrome 401
Diet and nutrition
  in CKD 198–9
    carbohydrate intake 199

fluid restriction 198
phosphate restriction 199
potassium restriction 199
protein intake 198
salt restriction 199
Dietary Approach to Hypertension Trial (DASH) 306
Dietary protein restriction 161
Digoxin 536, 596, 604
Dihydropyridine CCBs 340
Diltiazem 340
Dipstick tests 16–17
positive for ketones 16
Dipyridamole 225
Distal convoluted tubule and collecting duct 616, 625
calcium 624
sodium 624
Diuretics 355, 596
amiloride/triamterene 532
cirrhosis 533
congestive cardiac failure 533
loop 334, 532
mineralocorticoid receptor antagonists 532
nephrotic syndrome 533
potassium-sparing 334–5
renal failure 533
thiazide and thiazide-like 332–3, 532
using in edematous states 532
D-lactic acidosis 559
Donor-specific antibodies (DSA) 253
Dopamine (DA) 122–3
dosage and effects 122
Doxazosin 327, 338, 339, 354, 581
D-penicillamine 434
Dyslipidemia 160, 386

E

Edema
development 531
and hypoalbuminemia in nephrotic syndrome 531
Effective arterial blood volume (EABV) 520, 521, 522
Effective peritoneal surface area 228

eGFR
creatinine formulas based on 30
Enalapril 342
Encephalopathy
managing hyponatremia with 527
managing hyponatremia without 526
Endocarditis 377
Endocrine problems in CKD
adrenal axis function 202
hyperprolactinemia 202
menopause 202
sexual dysfunction 202
thyroid function 202
Endothelin antagonists 347
Endothelins 295
End-stage renal disease (ESRD) 4, 58
anti-phospholipid syndrome in 473
causes in United States 154
HBV-infected patients with 483
HCV-infected patients with 485
HIV-infected patients with 481
management in diabetes 444
peritoneal dialysis versus hemodialysis 444
renal transplantation 444
survival and cause of death 444
in multiple myeloma 449
in sickle cell nephropathy 454
symptomatic management of 204
Eosinophilia 462
Epithelial sodium channel (ENaC) 626
Eplerenone 311, 532, 596
Eprosartan 344
Ergocalciferol 542
Erythropoietin (EPO) 116
and kidney 168
mechanism of production 169
nonhematological effects of 170
nonresponse 171
preparation 170
prescription 172
Esmolol 355
Ethylene glycol 604
investigations 608
management 608–9
symptoms and signs 608

Extended-duration dialysis (EDD) 129
Extracellular fluid (ECF) 522–3
Extraneal® 234
Extrarenal cysts 419

F

Familial amyloidosis 450
Fanconi's syndrome 65, 557
Fatty casts 23
Felodipine 340
Fenoldopam 355
Ferrlecit® 175
Fibrillary glomerulonephritis (FGN) 453
Fibromuscular dysplasia (FMD) 414
Finasteride 339, 515
Flomax® 339
Flow cytometry 253
Fluconazole 204, 264
Fluid restriction 367, 385
Fluids and electrolytes 519
acid–base 552
buffering 552
excretion kidney in acid–base 552
intake and generation 552
normal physiology understanding 552
Bartter's syndrome treatment 538
diuretics
amiloride/triamterene 532
cirrhosis 533
congestive cardiac failure 533
loop 532
mineralocorticoid receptor antagonists 532
nephrotic syndrome 533
renal failure 533
thiazide 532
using in edematous states 532
edema and treatment development 531
Gitelman's syndrome treatment 538
hypercalcemia
causes 544
investigations 544
symptoms and signs 544
treatment 544–5
hypermagnesemia
clinically 548
treatment 548

hypernatremia 528–30
  symptoms and signs 528
  treatment 528–9
hyperphosphatemia 550
hypocalcemia
  causes 543
  investigations 542
  symptoms and signs 542
  treatment 542
hypokalemia
  causes 537
  investigations 536
  symptoms and signs 536
  treatment 536
hypomagnesemia
  investigations 546
  renal causes 546
  symptoms and signs 546
  treatment 547
hyponatremia
  cerebral salt-wasting 524
  hyperosmolal (dilutional) hyponatremia 522
  hypo-osmolal hyponatremia 522–3
  investigations 524
  iso-osmolal hyponatremia 522
  management of 526–7
  symptoms and signs 523
hypophosphatemia
  investigations 549
  symptoms and signs 549
  treatment 549
lactic acidosis
  and drugs 559
Liddle's syndrome
  treatment 539
magnesium 540
metabolic acidosis
  bicarbonate 555
    increased AG acidosis 554
    $NaHCO_3$ 555
  normal AG acidosis 554
  respiratory acidosis 555
  severe and life-threatening acidosis managing 555
  treatment 555
metabolic alkalosis
  investigations 561
  mechanisms for common causes 560
  respiratory alkalosis 562
  symptoms and signs 561
mixed acidosis and alkalosis
  normal ranges 564
phosphorus 540
renal tubular acidosis
  distal RTA (type 1) 556

distal RTA (type 4) 557
proximal RTA (type 2) 556–7
sodium
  salt and water balance 520–1
tubular disorders (rare)
  cystinosis 566
  cystinuria 566
  Dent's disease 566
  primary hyperoxaluria 566
Focal and segmental glomerulosclerosis (FSGS) 362, 394–5
  histology 395
  investigations 395
  primary 394
  secondary 395
  symptoms and signs 394
  treatment
    disease-modifying treatment 396
Fomepizole 608
Fosinopril 342
Fosrenol® 184
Fresh frozen plasma 402
Fungi 22
Furosemide 334, 354, 533, 545, 596

G

Gabapentin 205, 600
Genitourinary tuberculosis 488
  investigations 488
  symptoms and signs 488
Gestational hypertension
  definition 575
  evaluation 575
  natural history 575
Gitelman's syndrome
  treatment 538
Glomerular bleeding
  hematuria 52
  RBCs in 20
Glomerular damage 154
Glomerular filtration rate (GFR) 26
  measurement 26, 32
  physiological regulation 614–15
Glomerulonephritis
  in adults
    treatment of 483
  diffuse proliferative crescentic 362
  focal and diffuse 364–5
    approaches 366
    principles of management 367

immunosuppressive management 368–71
  drug toxicity pervention 368
  monitor toxicity 368
  side effects 370
  starting immunosuppression 368
  using drugs 368–70
membranoproliferative 378–9
  associations with 379
  complement in 379
  histology 379
  investigations 378
  symptoms and signs 378
postinfectious 376–7
terminology in 363
Glomerulotubular balance 614
Glomerulus
  filtration within 612
  structure 612–14
Glucocorticoid remediable aldosteronism (GRA) 312
Glucocorticoids 537
Glycine 522
Glycosuria 16, 65, 66
Glycyrrhizinic acid 314
Goodpasture's disease. See Anti-GBM disease
Gordon's syndrome 535
Graft dysfunction
  calcineurin inhibitors and early ATN 269
  classification 268
  delayed graft function 268
  early graft dysfunction 269
  late graft dysfunction 269
Granulomatous tubulointerstitial nephritis 479

H

Heart Outcomes Prevention Evaluation Study (HOPE) 326, 327
Heavy-chain deposition disease 453
Hemastix® 17
Hematuria 20, 510, 512, 585
  causes by age and source 53
  glomerular 52
  history 54
  macroscopic 52
  microscopic 52, 56–7
  nonglomerular 52

physical examination 54
transient 52
with urinary dipsticks 21
Hemodiafiltration 213
Hemodialysis (HD) 7, 132, 212, 213, 586
  apparatus 214–15
    alarms and monitors 214
    principle 214
  circuit 215
  prescription
    dialysis adequacy aspects of 218–19
    versus peritoneal dialysis 444
Hemodialysis catheters insertion
  femoral line insertion
    advantages over neck line 632
    disadvantages over neck line 632
    insertion technique 632
  indications 628
  pre-insertion 628
  routes 628
  technique 630–2
  tunneled dialysis catheters 632
Hemofiltration (HF) 132, 212, 213
Hemoglobinuric ARF 141
Hemolytic-uremic syndrome (HUS) 398, 401
  investigations 401
  management of 402
  symptoms and signs 401
Hemoperfusion 604
Henoch–Schönlein purpura (HSP) 373
Heparin 220, 596
Heparin-induced thrombocytopenia (HIT) 220
Hepatitis B (HBV) 482–3
  GN in adults
    treatment 483
  and liver disease
    treatment 483
  and renal disease 482
    with ESRD 483
    investigations 482
    membranoproliferative glomerulonephritis 482
    membranous nephropathy 482
Hepatitis C (HCV) 484–5
  and renal disease
    cryoglobulinemia symptoms and signs with 484

with ESRD 485
investigations 484
management 485
type 1 MPGN ± cryoglobulins 484
Hepatorenal syndrome (HRS)
  classification 134
  clinical features 135
  diagnostic criteria 135
  hepatic and renal dysfunction combination 134
  management 136–7
    establishment 136
    liver transplantation 137
    renal replacement therapy 137
    specific rescue therapies 136
  pathophysiology 134, 135
Hereditary nephropathies 380–1
  Alport syndrome 380
    and transplantation 381
  histology 381
  investigations 380
  symptoms and signs 380
  thin membrane disease 380
  treatment 381
Highly active antiretroviral therapy (HAART) 480
  renal side effects 481
HIV
  patient with ESRD 481
  and renal disease 480
    HIVAN 480
    investigation 480
    renal lesions with 481
    symptoms and signs 480
HIV-associated nephropathy (HIVAN) 480
  management of 480
  and renal disease 480
Hormone replacement therapy (HRT)
  and blood pressure 322
Human leukocyte antigens (HLA) 248
Hyaline casts 23
Hydralazine 346, 355, 579, 581
Hydrochlorothiazide 332
17α hydroxylase (CYP17) deficiency 312
11β hydroxylase (CYP11B1) deficiency 312
11β-hydroxysteroid dehydrogenase 292
11β-hydroxysteroid dehydrogenase 2 (11BHSD2) 314
Hyperaldosteronism

diagnostic algorithm for 313
primary 312
  causes of 310
  congenital adrenal hyperplasia 312
  diagnosis of 310–11
  glucocorticoid remediable aldosteronism 312
  treatment principles of 311
secondary 312
syndromes 314
  mineralocorticoid receptor 314
  pseudoaldosteronism 314
Hypercalcemia
  causes 544
  investigations 544
  symptoms and signs 544
  treatment 544–5
Hypercalciuria 65, 433
Hypercoagulability 385–6
Hyperglycemia 522
Hyperkalemia 106–9, 164–5, 534, 535
  ECG changes 106–7
  insulin and glucose 108
  nebulized albuterol 108
  treatment of severe 108
Hypermagnesemia
  clinically 548
  treatment 548
Hypernatremia 115, 528–30
  symptoms and signs 528
  treatment 528–9
Hyperosmolal (dilutional) hyponatremia 522
Hyperoxaluria 433
Hyperphosphatemia 114, 160, 550
Hypertension 418, 454. See also Blood pressure
  ACE inhibitors 342
    and ARBs 345
    examples 342
    mechanism 342
    problems 343
    role 342
  α-blockers 338
    and ALLHAT 339
    and bladder outflow symptoms 339
    examples 338
    mechanism 338
    problems 338
    role 338
  angiotensin II receptor blockers
    and ACEIs 345
    examples 344

mechanism 344
roles 344
antihypertensive
  centrally acting agents 346
  direct acting vascular smooth muscle relaxants 346
  on horizon 347
ASCOT study
  results 330–1
  significance of 331
β-blockers 336
  examples 337
  mechanism 336
  problems 336
  role 336
calcium channel blockers 340
  examples 340
  mechanism 340
  problems 340–1
  role 340
classification of 288, 302
clinical assessment
  history and examination 300
clinical trials 324
  controversies 324
  designs 324, 326–9
  definition 290
diuretics
  loop 334
  potassium-sparing 334–5
  thiazide and thiazide-like 332–3
emergency 302
  causes of 353
  clinical assessment 352
  definitions 350
  drugs in 355
  investigations 353
  management of 354
  medication 352
  pathophysiology 350–1
  symptoms and signs 352
epidemiology 288
facts and figures 288
hyperaldosteronism
  diagnostic algorithm for 313
  primary 310–11, 312
  secondary 312
  syndromes 314
lifestyle measures 306–7
  alcohol 306
  caffeine 306
  exercise 306
  healthy eating 306
  low-sodium diet 306
  stress management 307
  weight loss 306

orthostatic hypotension 356–7
  causes of 356
  treatment of 357
pathogenesis
  arterial stiffness 294
  genetics 292
  renin–angiotensin system 293–4
  sympathetic nervous system 295
pathophysiology principles in 290
rare single gene causes of 292
in renal disease 60
resistant hypertension 348
  pathophysiology of 348
secondary hypertension
  causes of 316–17
  classification 308–9
treatment thresholds 304
  aim for target 304
urgency 302
  clinical assessment 352
  definitions 350
  investigations 353
  management of 354
  medication 352
  pathophysiology 350–1
  symptoms and signs 352
Hypertension Optimal Treatment Study (HOT) 328, 329
Hypertensive retinopathy 353
Hyperthyroidism 317
Hyperuricosuria 433
Hypervolemia 10
Hypoalbuminemia
  and edema in nephrotic syndrome 531
Hypocalcemia 114–15, 141
  causes 543
  investigations 543
  symptoms and signs 542
  treatment 542
Hypocitraturia 433
Hypokalemia 65, 115
  causes 537
  investigations 536
  symptoms and signs 536
  treatment 536
Hypomagnesemia 115
  investigations 546
  renal causes 546
  symptoms and signs 546
  treatment 547
Hyponatremia 522
  cerebral salt-wasting 524
  (dilutional) hyponatremia 522

hypo-osmolal hyponatremia 522–3
  investigations 524
  iso-osmolal hyponatremia 522
  management of 526–7
  symptoms and signs 523
Hypoperfusion
  causes 92
  physiological response to 92–3
Hypophosphatemia
  investigations 549
  symptoms and signs 549
  treatment 549
Hypothyroidism 317
Hypotonic crystalloids 96
Hypovolemia 10, 94

I

Icodextrin 234
IgA nephropathy 372–4
  histology 373
  investigations 373
  management of 374–5
  pathogenesis 372
  symptoms and signs 372
Ileal loopography 45
Immunoglobulin 87, 447
Immunotactoid glomerulonephritis (ITGN) 453
Indapamide 332
Indinavir 24, 481
Indoramin 338
Infective endocarditis
  kidney in 486–7
  histology 487
  investigations 486
  symptoms and signs 486
  treatment 487
Insulin resistance 296
Intercalated cells 626
Interferon-α 482, 485
Interferon-α$_{2b}$ 483
Interstitial cystitis 426
Intervention as a Goal in Hypertension Treatment (INSIGHT) 328, 329
Intracranial aneurysms (ICAs) 419
Intravenous digital subtraction angiography (IVDSA) 45
Intravenous urography (IVU) 40–1, 499
Irbesartan 344
Ischemic nephropathy 410–11
Islet cell transplantation 285

Isolated systolic hypertension (ISH) 302–3
Isosthenuria 14
Isotope renography 499
Isotopic GFR 32
Isradipine 340
IV iron
 types of 175

J

JNC 7 320
 classifications of BP 303

K

Kayexalate® 110
Ketones
 positive dipstick causes 16
Kidney in systemic disease
 ANCA-positive vasculitis 458
  histology 458
  investigations 458
  symptoms and signs 458
  treatment of 460
  WG and MPA 459
 anti-GBM disease 466–7
  investigations 466
  pathogenesis 466
  pathology 466
  pulmonary hemorrhage treatment 467
  renal disease treatment of 466–7
  symptoms and signs 466
 anti-phospholipid syndrome 472–3
  in ESRD 473
  investigations 472
  symptoms and signs 472
  treatment 472
 Churg–Strauss syndrome 462–3
  investigations 462
  symptoms and signs 462
  treatment 463
 classical polyarteritis nodosa 464–5
  investigations 464
  management and history 464
  symptoms and signs 464
  treatment 464
 diabetic nephropathy 438–40
  definition and epidemiology 438
  ESRD management of 444
  management of 442–3
  natural history 439
  pathogenesis of 438
  pathology 439
  renal biopsy indication for 439
  renal disease in diabetic patient 440
 Hepatitis B–related renal disease 482–3
 Hepatitis C–related renal disease 484–5
 HIV and renal disease 480–1
 infective endocarditis 486
  histology 487
  investigations 486
  symptoms and signs 486
  treatment 487
 lupus nephritis 468
  investigations 469
  ISN/RPS classification of 469
  management of 470–1
  pathogenesis and histology 469
  SLE autoantibodies arise in 468–9
 malaria 492–3
 multiple myeloma 446–7
  diagnosis 446
  ESRD in 449
  histology and pathogenesis 447
  immunoglobulin 447
  investigations 446
  symptoms and signs 446
 non-amyloid dysproteinemias 453
 renal amyloidosis 450–2
  histology 451
  investigations 450–1
  management of 451
  symptoms and signs 450
  types of 450
 renal tuberculosis 488–9
 rheumatoid arthritis 476
 sarcoidosis 478–9
  calcium homeostasis in 478
  investigations 478
  management 479
  symptoms and signs 478
 schistosomiasis 490–1
 scleroderma renal crisis 474–5
  investigations 474
  management 475
  renal histology 475
  symptoms and signs 474
 sickle cell nephropathy 454
  ESRD in 455
  investigations 454
  management of 454–5
  symptoms and signs 454
 vasculitis and renal disease 456
 tubulointerstitial diseases
  acute interstitial nephritis 404
   histology 405
   investigations 404
   symptoms and signs 404
   treatment 405
  urinary tract infections 422–6
   bacteriology 422
   diagnosis of 423–4
   host factors predisposing to 422
   pathogenesis 422
   treatment of 424–6
Kidney in acid–base excretion
 bicarbonate loss preventing 552–3
 protons excreting 553
 urinary protons buffering 553
Kidney stones 430
Klebsiela 431
Kt/V 219
 prescribed versus delivered 221

L

Labetalol 336, 354, 355, 575, 579, 581, 596
Lactic acidosis
 and drugs 559
Lamivudine 483
Lamotrigine 600
Lead nephropathy 407
Leukocyte esterase 16
Leukocytes 22
Leukocytoclastic vasculitis on skin biopsy 458
Levodopa 205
Licorice 314, 537
Liddle's syndrome 292
 treatment 539
Light-chain deposition disease (LCDD) 453
Lisinopril 342
Lithium 604, 606
Lithium-induced nephropathy 406
Liver disease
 HBV treatment of 482
Liver transplantation 137

Living donor (LD) 256
transplantation
 advantages 254
 disadvantages 254
 potential live donor assessment of 254
L-lactate 559
Loin pain 64
Loop diuretics 122, 532, 596
Loop of Henle 616
 countercurrent exchange mechanism 620
 urine concentrating and diluting 620
Losartan 344, 354
Losartan Intervention for Endpoint Reduction in Hypertension (LIFE) 328, 329
Lower urinary tract symptoms (LUTS) 67
Lupus nephritis 468, 583
 investigations 469
 ISN/RPS classification of 469
 management of 470
  experimental therapies 471
  induction therapy 470
  maintenance therapy 470
  monitoring disease activity 471
  prevent CKD 471
  at risk 470
 pathogenesis and histology of 469
 SLE autoantibodies arise in 468–9

M

Macroscopic hematuria 52
 investigation 55
Magnesium ammonium phosphate 24, 431
Magnesium sulphate 579
Magnetic resonance imaging (MRI) 32, 42, 499, 508
Major histocompatibility complex (MHC) 248
Malaria 492–3
 acute malarial nephropathy 492
  investigations 492
  management 492
  symptoms and signs 492
 chronic malarial nephropathy 493
 species causing disease 492

Mannitol 122, 140, 522
Medium-vessel aneurysms in kidneys 465
Medullary cystic kidney disease 421
Medullary sponge kidney 421
Megestrol acetate 200, 204
Membranoproliferative glomerulonephritis (MPGN) 378–9, 482
 associations with 379
 complement in 379
 histology 379
 investigations 378
 symptoms and signs 378
Membranous glomerulonephritis. See Membranous nephropathy
Membranous nephropathy (MN) 390–2
 approaches 34
 histology 391
 investigations 390
 secondary 392, 476
 treatment of 392
 subepithelial deposits 391–0
 symptoms and signs 390
 treatment 391–2
Mesangial cells 612
Mesangial IgA deposits 372, 375
Mesangioproliferative GN 476
Metabolic acidosis 115
 bicarbonate using 555
 clinically 554–5
 increased AG acidosis 554
 $NaHCO_3$ 555
 normal AG acidosis 554
 respiratory acidosis 555
 severe and life-threatening acidosis managing 555
 treatment 555
Metabolic alkalosis
 investigations 561
  respiratory alkalosis 562
 mechanisms for common causes 560
 symptoms and signs 561
Methanol 604, 609
Methyldopa 346, 575, 581
Methylprednisolone 391, 453
Metolazone 596
Metoprolol 336, 596
Microalbuminuria 48
 and cardiovascular risk 50
Microscopic hematuria 52, 56–7
 management of 57

Microscopic polyangiitis (MPA) 458
 characteristics of 459
Midodrine 226
Mineralocorticoid receptor antagonists 314, 335, 532
Mineralocorticoids 537
Minimal change nephropathy 388–9
 histology 388
 investigations 388
 symptoms and signs 388
 treatment 388–9
Minoxidil 346, 581
Mixed acidosis and alkalosis normal ranges 564–5
Monoclonal gammopathy of uncertain significance (MGUS) 448
Multiple endocrine neoplasia type 2A 292
Multiple myeloma (MM) 446–7
 diagnosis 446
 ESRD in 449
 histology and pathogenesis 447
 immunoglobulin 447
 investigations 446
 smoldering 448
 symptoms and signs 446
Multistix Pro® 19
Mupirocin 238, 239
Mycobacterium tuberculosis 488
Mycophenolate mofetil (MMF) 264, 265, 370, 389, 470
Myeloma screen 86–8
Myfortic® 265
Myoglobinuria 477
Myositis 477

N

National Cooperative Dialysis Study (NCDS) 219
Natriuretic peptides 296
Neoral® 265
Nephroblastoma. See Wilm's tumour
Nephrolithiasis 418, 430–1
 bladder stones 431
 calcium oxalate/phosphate stones 430
 cystine stones 430
 staghorn calculi 431
 uric acid stones 430
Nephronophthisis 420

Nephropathy
  analgesic 408–9
  Balkan endemic (BEN) 407
  Chinese herb 407
  lead 407
  lithium-induced 406
Nephrostomy 500
Nephrotic-range proteinuria 636
Nephrotic syndrome 50, 60, 384, 533
  causes of 384
  hypoalbuminemia and edema in 531
  investigations of 384
  principles of management 385–6
    dyslipidemia 386
    hypercoagulability 385–6
    infection 386
    protein restriction and reducing proteinuria 385
    salt and fluid restriction 385
Neurofibromatosis type 1 (NF1) 292
Neurotoxicity 594
Nicardipine 340
Nifedipine 340, 581
Nisoldipine 340
Nitric oxide 295
Nitrofurantoin 571
NKF-DOQI (National Kidney Federation—Kidney Dialysis Outcomes Quality Initiative) classification of CKD 152
Nocturia 454
Non-amyloid dysproteinemias 453
Non-dihydropyridine CCBs 340
Non-glomerular bleeding hematuria 52
  RBCs in 20
Non-heart beating (NHB) 256
Non-nephrotic proteinuria 636
Nonsteroidal anti-inflammatory drugs (NSAIDs) and kidney
  mechanism 598
  renal effects 598
Nordic Diltiazem Study (NORDIL) 328, 329
Normalized protein catabolic rate (nPCR) 219
Nutrineal® 200

Nutrition
  in ARF 118–20

O

Obstructive sleep apnea (OSA) 317
OKT3 265
Oligoanuria 466
Oliguria 63
Olmesartan 344
Oocytoma 510
Open/laparoscopic renal biopsy 635
Opiate narcosis 601, 602
Opioids in renal failure
  choice in renal implantation 602–3
Oral contraceptives and blood pressure 322
Orthostatic hypotension 356–7
  causes of 356
  treatment of 357
Osmoreceptors 521
Osmotic demyelination syndrome 526
Osteomalacia 176
Osteoporosis 176
Oxidative stress 295

P

Pamidronate 545
Papillary necrosis 409, 500
  diseases associated with 409
Paraneoplastic syndrome with RCC 510
Paraproteinemia 448
Paraquat 604
Parathyroidectomy 190–1
  indication 190
  technique 191
Parathyroid hormone (PTH) 178, 181, 540
Pathophysiology
  of ischemic ATN
    repair 103
    tubular cells 102
    vessels and endothelium 102
Patient-controlled analgesia 601
Periaortitis 506
Perindopril 329
Perindopril Protection against Recurrent Stroke Study (PROGRESS) 328, 329

Peritoneal dialysis (PD) 7, 228–9, 586, 604
  adequacy 242–3
  in ARF
    acute PD 133
    catheter placement 132
    demerit 132
    merit 132
  automated peritoneal dialysis (APD) 230, 238
  continuous ambulatory peritoneal dialysis (CAPD) 230, 231
  fluids 232–3
  hypervolemia, diagnosing causes for 245
  patients
    complications 246
    social rehabilitation 246
  prescription 234–5
  types 230–1
  versus hemodialysis (HD) 444
Peritoneal equilibration test (PET) 243
Peritonitis 236–9
  APD special considerations for 239
  clinical features 236–7
    allergy 237
    bacteriology 236
  complications 237
  treatment 237–8
Pharmacokinetics and kidney
  absorption 592
  hepatic clearance 593
  protein binding 592
  renal clearance 593
  volume of distribution 592
Phenoxybenzamine 338
Phentolamine 338, 355
Phenytoin 264, 592, 604
Pheochromocytoma 292, 316
  sensitivity and specificity of screening test 316
Phosphate control 184–5
  adequate dialysis 184
  dietary restriction 184
  phosphate binders 184, 185
Phosphaturia 65, 66
Physical examination
  circulation 10
  elements 8
  hematuria 54
  prerenal ARF 95
  by systems 9
Plain abdominal X-ray 36–7
Plasmacytomas 448

Plasma exchange
  complications 641
  indications 640
  prescription 640
Plasmapheresis (PP) 402
Plasmodium falciparum 492
Plasmodium malariae 492
Plasmodium ovale 492
Plasmodium vivax 492
Podocytes 612
Poisoning
  and dialysis techniques 604
Polyacrylnitrile 216
Polyamide 216
Polyarteritis nodosa (PAN) 482
Polymyositis 477
Polysulfone® 216
Polytetrafluoroethylene (PTFE) graft 222
Polyuria 63, 65, 454
Postinfectious glomerulonephritis 376–7
  acute post-streptococcal
    clinical course 378
    histology 376
    investigations 376
    symptoms and signs 376
    treatment 378
Post-transplant lymphoproliferative disorders (PTLDs) 280–1
Postural tachycardia syndrome (POTS) 357
Potomania 523
Prazosin 338, 581
Prednisone 369, 370, 391, 405, 453, 460, 466, 470, 480
Preeclampsia and eclampsia
  affected organs 577
  diagnosis 576
    criteria 577
  hypertension treating 579
  managing
    delivery 578
    parameters need for delivery 578
    prophylaxis for and treatment of seizures 579
  pathogenesis 576
  risk factors 577
Pregnancy 308
Pregnancy and kidney
  anatomical changes 569
  chronic hypertension
    antenatal care 580
    prenatal counseling 580
    unplanned conception on antihypertensives 580–1
  dialysis and pregnancy
    anemia 587
    diet calcium and vitamin D 586
    hemodialysis 586
    labor and delivery 587
    peritoneal dialysis 586
  gestational hypertension
    definition 575
    evaluation 575
    natural history 575
  hypertension
    BP and proteinuria measuring 574
    classification 574
    risks to mother and fetus 574
  normal values for pregnant women 569
  preeclampsia and eclampsia
    affected organs 577
    diagnosis 576–7
    managing 578–9
    pathogenesis 576
    risk factors 577
  renal disease preexisting
    antenatal care 584
    diabetic nephropathy 582
    lupus nephritis 583
    nonglomerular disease and normal renal function 582
    primary glomerular disease with normal renal function 582
  renal physiology 568
  renal tract disorders
    hematuria 585
    obstruction 585
  renal transplantation
    antenatal care 589
    ideal situation 588–9
    labor 589
    pre-pregnancy counseling 588
  salt and water homeostasis 568
  tubular function 568
  UTI
    acute pyelonephritis 571
    bacteriology 570
    diagnosis 570
    recurrence 571
    risk factors 570
    treatment 571
Pregnancy-associated hypertension 292

Prograf® 265
Prostaglandins 295, 598
Prostate cancer
  clinical features 516
  investigations 516
  management
    early disease 518
    recurrence and late disease 518
  staging and grading 516–17
Prostate-specific antigen (PSA) screening with 517
Prostatic disease 500, 506
Protein electrophoresis 87
Protein restriction 385
Proteinuria 18–19, 48–51, 65, 154, 385, 454
  clinical consequences 50
  detection and quantification of 157
  dipsticks 18
  importance of 48, 156
  levels 49
  nephrotic-range proteinuria 636
  nephrotic syndrome 50
  non-nephrotic proteinuria 636
  pathological proteinuria 48
  persistent 49
  positive dipstick 48
  timed collections 18–19
  transient 49
Proximal convoluted tubule 616
  sodium and chloride 618–19
Proximal tubular cells (PTC) 102
Pseudoaldosteronism 314
Pseudohypoaldosteronsim type 1 535
Pseudohyponatremia 523
Psychogenic polydipsia 523
Pulmonary edema 112–13
  finding 112
  management 112
  ventilatory support 113
Pulmonary renal syndromes 61–2
  causes 61
  clinical features 61
Pulse pressure (PP) 289
Pyelonephritis 423
Pyridoxine 609

Q

Quinapril 342

R

Ramipril 327, 342, 354
Rapamune® 265
Rapamycin 264, 265
Rapidly progressive glomerulonephritis (RPGN) 60, 86
Recurrent stone-formers
  investigation
    imaging in 432
  management of 433
Red blood cells (RBCs)
  dipsticks 20
  urine sediment 20–1
Red cell casts 23
Reflux nephropathy 428–9, 582
  histology 429
  investigations 428
  management 429
  symptoms and signs 428
Renagel® 184
Renal amyloidosis 450
  histology 451
  investigations 450–1
  management of 451
  symptoms and signs 450
  types of 450
Renal biopsy 458
  in ARF 91
  complications of 636
  indications for 439, 634
  preparation for 634
  technique 635
Renal bone disease
  classification 176
  clinical features 180–1
  definition 176
  high- and low-turnover features 177
  physiology 178–9
  spectrum 177
  treatment 182–3
Renal cell carcinoma (RCC)
  clinical features 510
  differential diagnosis 510
  investigations 510
  paraneoplastic syndrome with 510
  preoperative work up 511
Renal damage mechanism in chronic obstruction 503
Renal disease
  primary glomerular disease with normal renal function 582
Renal mass investigation
  cyst 508
  solid renal mass 508

Renal patient clinical assessment 1
Renal replacement therapy (RRT) 137, 207
  acute HD complications
    intradialytic hypotension 226–7
  in ARF 126–7
  treatment 276
  dialysers and membranes biocompatibility 216
  dialysis prescription variables in 220–1
  hemodialysis 212, 213
    apparatus 214–15
    presciption 218–19
  history 208
  pritoneal dialysis (PD) 228–9
    adequacy 242–3
  vascular access 222–3
    complications 224–5
    for hemodialysis 223
    principles 222
Renal tract disorders and pregnancy
  hematuria 585
  obstruction 585
Renal transplantation 455, 467
  in diabetics 444
  and pregnancy
    antenatal care 589
    ideal situation 588–9
    labor 589
    pre-pregnancy counseling 588
Renal tuberculosis 488–9
  genitourinary TB 488
    investigations 488
    symptoms and signs 488
  tuberculous interstitial nephritis 489
    management 489
Renal tubular acidosis (RTA) 65
  distal (type 1) 556
  distal (type 4) 557
  proximal (type 2) 556–7
Renal vein thrombosis (RVT) 414
Renin–angiotensin system (RAS) 169, 293–4, 521, 522
Renin inhibitors 347
Renin-secreting tumors 312
Renovascular disease 410
  atherosclerotic renal artery stenosis 410–11
  cholesterol emboli 414–15
  fibromuscular dysplasia 414

  ischemic nephropathy 410–11
  renal vein thrombosis 414
Resistant hypertension 348
  pathophysiology of 348
Respiratory acidosis 555
Retrograde ureteropyelography 45
Retroperitoneal fibrosis (RPF) 500
  causes 506
  clinical features 506
  investigations 507
  management 507
Rhabdomyolysis
  causes 139
  clinical presentation 138
  investigations 138
  management
    ARF prevention of 140
    compartment syndrome 140–1
    urinary alkalinization and mannitol 140
  myoglobin (Mb) 138
Rheumatoid arthritis (RA)
  renal conditions complicating 476
Rheumatoid vasculitis 476
Risk Injury Failure Loss and End-stage disease (RIFLE) classification 70, 71
Rituximab 280, 370, 392, 461, 471

S

Salicylate 604
  overdose 606
  symptoms and signs 607
Salt intake
  and blood pressure 291
Salt-sensitive hypertension 291
Sarcoidosis 405, 478
  calcium homeostasis in 478
  investigations 478
  management 479
  symptoms and signs 478
Schistosoma haematobium 22, 490
Schistosoma japonicum 490
Schistosoma mansoni 490
Schistosomiasis
  schistosomal glomerulonephritis 490, 491
  treatment 490
  urinary
    diagnosis 490

Scleroderma renal crisis
  investigations 474
  management 475
  renal histology 475
  symptoms and signs 474
Sclerosing encapsulating
  peritonitis (SEP) 241
Secondary hyperparathyroidism (SHPT) 176, 180, 193
  pathogenesis of 179
Secondary hypertension 312
  causes of 316–17
    aorta coarctation of 317
    Cushing's syndrome 316
    obstructive sleep apnea 317
    pheochromocytoma 316
    thyroid disease 317
  classification 308–9
  diagnosis and treatment of 309
Second Australian National Blood Pressure Study (ANBP-2) 326, 327
Sensipar® 189
Sepsis 117, 146
  ARF in
    causes 146
    clinical findings 147
    kidney 147
    shock 146
Serum anion gap calculating 554
Shiga-like toxin 401
Shunt nephritis 377
SIADH diagnosing 524
Sickle cell nephropathy 454
  ESRD in 455
  investigations 454
  management of 454–5
  symptoms and signs 454
Sildenafil 202, 338
Simple cysts 420
Single-pool Kt/V 219
Sirolimus 265
Sjogren syndrome 405, 477
Sodium nitroprusside 354, 355
Sodium/potassium ATPase 618
Solid renal mass 508
Solute transport in the loop 622–3
Spironolactone 311, 532, 533, 538, 596, 626
Staghorn calculi 431
Sterile pyuria 22
Stravaptan 526
Struvite stones 431, 434
Sulfadiazine 24
Suprapubic pain 64

Sustained low-efficiency dialysis (SLED) 129
Swedish Trial in Old Patients with Hypertension-2 (STOP-2) 328, 329
Sympathetic nervous system (SNS) 295
Systemic lupus erythematosus (SLE) 468
  autoantibodies arise in 468–9
  diagnosis 468
Systemic sclerosis (SS). See Scleroderma renal crisis
Systemic vascular resistance (SVR) 290
Systolic blood pressure (SBP) 289
Systolic Hypertension—Europe (SYST-EUR) 328, 329

T

Tacrolimus 264, 265, 269, 369, 370, 589
Tadalafil 338
Tamm–Horsfall mucoprotein 23, 447
Tamsulosin 515
Telmisartan 344
Tenofovir 481
Terazosin 338
Thiazide 532, 596, 624
Thin membrane disease (TMD) 380
Thrombotic microangiopathy (TMA) 269, 398
  causes of 398
  histology 399
  investigations 399
  management of 402
Thrombotic thrombocytopenic purpura (TTP) 398, 400
  investigations 400
  management of 402
  symptoms and signs 400
Tidal APD 230
TNM staging of prostate cancer 516–17
Tolvaptan 526
Total body water (TBW) 521
Trandolapril 342
Transitional cell cancers (TCC) 512
Transjugular renal biopsy 635
Transurethral resection of bladder tumor (TURBT) 513

Transurethral resection of the prostate (TURP) 515
Triamterene 24, 334, 532
Trousseau's sign 542
Tuberculous interstitial nephritis (TIN) 489
  management 489
Tubular function
  collecting duct 616
  distal convoluted tubule 616
  loop of Henle 616
  proximal convoluted tubule 616
Tubular syndromes 65–6
Tubuloglomerular feedback 614
Tubulointerstitial diseases
  acute interstitial nephritis 404
  histology 405
  investigations 404
  symptoms and signs 404
  treatment 405
Tubulointerstitial nephritis and uveitis syndrome (TINU) 405
Tubulointerstitial scarring 155
Tumor lysis syndrome (TLS) 144–5
  clinical findings 144
  investigations 144
  pre- and post-treatment 144
  treatment 124
Tunneled dialysis catheter 222, 632
Tunnel infection 239
Type 1 DM 438, 439
Type 2 DM 438, 439

U

UK Prospective Diabetes Trial (UKPDS) 438
Ultrafiltration (UF) 229
  failure
    causes 244–5
Ultrasound (US) 38–9, 498
Uremia 166–7
Uremic cardiomyopathy 197
Uremic syndrome 58, 59
Ureteric colic 64
Ureteric stenting 502
  retrograde 500
Ureterolysis 507
Ureteropelvic junction and ureterovesicular junction obstruction
  diagnosis 504

management 504–5
symptoms and signs 504
Ureteroscopy 46, 500
Urethral catheters 502
Urethral valves posterior 505
Urethrography 45
Uric acid 24, 144
Uric acid stones 430, 434
Urinalysis 82
Urinary alkalinization 140
Urinary K$^+$ wasting 110
Urinary pH 14
 therapeutic manipulation 15
Urinary schistosomiasis
 diagnosis 490
Urinary tract infections (UTIs) 422–6
 bacteriology 422
 closer attention 424
 diagnosis of 423–4
  investigations 423–4
  persisting or repeated symptoms 423
  positive 423
  symptoms and signs 423
 host factors predisposing to 422
 pathogenesis 422
 in pregnancy
  acute pyelonephritis 571
  bacteriology 570
  diagnosis 570
  recurrence 571
  risk factors 570
  treatment 571
 treatment of 424–6
  catheter-related 425
  complicated lower 424–5
  interstitial cystitis 426
  recurrent 425
  uncomplicated lower 424
Urinary tract obstruction 495
 acute obstruction
  clinical features 500
  investigations 500
  management of 500–1
 approaching
  causes of obstruction 497
  classification 496
  normal physiology 496
 benign prostatic hypertrophy
  clinical features 514
  differential diagnosis 514
  investigations 514

management 514–15
chronic obstruction
 management 502–3
 renal consequences of 502
imaging
 computerised tomography 498–9
 intravenous urography 499
 isotope renography 499
 magnetic resonance imaging 499
 ultrasound 498
prostate cancer
 clinical features 516
 investigations 516
 staging and grading 516–17
prostate cancer management
 early disease 518
 recurrence and late disease 518
renal cell carcinoma (RCC)
 clinical features 510
 differential diagnosis 510
 investigations 510
 preoperative work up 511
renal mass investigation
 cyst 508
 solid renal mass 508
retroperitoneal fibrosis (RPF)
 causes 506
 clinical features 506
 investigations 507
 management 507
ureteropelvic junction and ureterovesicular junction obstruction
 diagnosis 504
 management 504–5
 symptoms and signs 504
urothelial tumors
 bladder cancer 512–13
Urine
 appearance 12–13
 chemical analysis 14–15
 culture 23
 dipstick tests 16–17
 discoloration 13
 indices in ARF 82
 sediment 20–1
 stone risk profile 433
 test strips 17
 volume changes 63
Urobilinogen 16
Urodilatin 296

Uroradiology 45–6
Urothelial tumors
 bladder cancer 512–13
U.S. Renal Data Service (USRDS) 210
UV Flash Compact® 231

V

Valsartan 344
Valsartan Antihypertensive Long-term Use Evaluation (VALUE) 328, 329
Vancomycin 224, 237, 594
Vardenafil 338
Vascular access 222–3
 complications 224–5
 for hemodialysis 223
 principles 222
Vasculitis 456
 Chapel Hill classification of 457
 and renal disease 456
Vasopeptidase inhibitors 347
Vein localization 630
Venofer® 175
Verapamil 340
Vesicoureteric reflux (VUR) 45, 429
Vitamin C 24
Vitamin D 178, 179, 186
Voiding cysturethrography (VCUG) 45
Von Hippel–Lindau (VHL) disease 292

W

Warfarin 225
Water depletion 521
Water-loading 521
Wegener's granulomatosis (WG) 458
 characteristics of 459
White cell casts 23
"White coat" hypertension 299
Wilms' tumor 511
World Health Organization (WHO) 288

X

Xanthogranulomatous pyelonephritis 426
X-ray 36, 180, 274, 498

Z

Zoledronic acid 545

About the Oxford American Handbooks in Medicine

The Oxford American Handbooks are flexi-covered pocket clinical books, providing practical guidance in quick reference, note form. Titles cover major medical specialties or cross-specialty topics and are aimed at students, residents, internists, family physicians, and practicing physicians within specific disciplines.

Their reputation is built on including the best clinical information, complemented by hints, tips, and advice from the authors. Each one is carefully reviewed by senior subject experts, residents, and students to ensure that content reflects the reality of day-to-day medical practice.

Key series features

- Written in short chunks, each topic is covered in a two-page spread to enable readers to find information quickly. They are also perfect for test preparation and gaining a quick overview of a subject without scanning through unnecessary pages.
- Content is evidence based and complemented by the expertise and judgment of experienced authors.
- The Handbooks provide a humanistic approach to medicine—it's more than just treatment by numbers.
- A "friend in your pocket," the Handbooks offer honest, reliable guidance about the difficulties of practicing medicine and provide coverage of both the practice and art of medicine.
- For quick reference, useful "everyday" information is included on the inside covers.
- Made with hard-wearing plastic covers, tough paper, and built-in ribbon bookmarks, the Handbooks stand up to heavy usage.

	Conventional unit	Conversion factor	SI unit
Calcium	mg/dL	0.25	mmol/L
Cholesterol	mg/dL	0.0259	mmol/L
Creatinine	mg/dL	88.4	µmol/L
Lactate	mg/dL	0.111	mmol/L
Magnesium	mg/dL	0.411	mmol/L
PTH	pg/mL (ng/L)	0.105	pmol/L
Phosphorus	mg/dL	0.323	mmol/L
Urea	mg/dL	0.357	mmol/L

Frequently Used Formulas

1. Fractional Excretion of Sodium

$$FeNa^+ = \frac{U}{P}Na^+ \div \frac{U}{P}Creatinine$$

Prenatal < 1%
ATN > 2%

2. Fractional Excretion of Urea

$$Fe\ Urea = \frac{U}{P}Urea \div \frac{U}{P}Creatinine$$

Prenatal < 35%
ATN > 50%

3. Transtubular Potassium Gradient

$$TTKG = \frac{U}{P}K^+ \div \frac{U}{P}OSM$$

With Hypokalemia:
GI K^+ loss < 2
Renal K^+ loss, excess aldosterone > 4

With Hyperkalemia:
Decreased aldosterone < 6

4. Urine Anion Gap

$$UAG = UNa^+ + UK^+ - UCl^-$$

− = GI HCO_3^- loss
+ = Distal (type I) or Distal (type IV) RTA

5. Osmolar Gap

$$Calculated\ serum\ OSM = 2NA^+ + BUN + \frac{Glucose}{18}$$

OSM Gap = Measured OSM − Calculated OSM
Normal = <10 mOsm/kg

6. Free H_2O deficit

$$= (BW)(wt\ Kg) \times \left(\left[\frac{plasma\ NA^+\ actual}{plasma\ NA^+\ desired}\right] - 1\right)$$

BW males = 0.6
BW Females = 0.5

7. Dialysis Access Recirculation

$$= \frac{P - A}{P - V} \times 100$$

P = Peripheral BUN
A = BUN → Arterial Line
V = BUN → Venus Line
(Abnormal > 10%)